SECOND EDITION

CLINICAL ULTRASOUND
a comprehensive text

Abdominal
and
General
Ultrasound

VOLUME 1

This volume is part of a self-contained two volume work entitled *Abdominal and General Ultrasound*. Additionally, it forms an integral part of *Clinical Ultrasound: a comprehensive text* together with its companion title, *Ultrasound in Obstetrics and Gynaecology*, which may be purchased separately.

Commissioning Editor Michael J Houston
Project Development Manager Paul Fam
Project Manager Rolla Couchman
Production Manager Helen Sofio
Designer Sarah Russell
Illustration Manager Mick Ruddy
Illustrator Jenni Miller

SECOND EDITION

CLINICAL ULTRASOUND
a comprehensive text

Abdominal and General Ultrasound

VOLUME 1

Edited by

Hylton B Meire FRCR
Consultant Radiologist, King's College Hospital, London, United Kingdom

David O Cosgrove MA MSc FRCR FRCP
Professor of Clinical Ultrasound, Department of Imaging, Hammersmith Hospital, London, United Kingdom

Keith C Dewbury BSc MBBS FRCR
Consultant Radiologist, Southampton General Hospital, Southampton, United Kingdom

Pat Farrant DCRR DMU
Superintendent Research Sonographer, King's College Hospital, London, United Kingdom

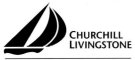
CHURCHILL
LIVINGSTONE

LONDON   EDINBURGH   NEW YORK   PHILADELPHIA   ST LOUIS   SYDNEY   TORONTO   2001

CHURCHILL LIVINGSTONE
An imprint of Elsevier Science Limited

© Harcourt Publishers Limited 2001
© Elsevier Science Limited 2002. All rights reserved.
Growth charts and tables in Appendix, copyright© Lyn Chitty and
Douglas Altman 2001

🌊 is a registered trademark of Elsevier Science Limited

The right of Hylton Meire, Keith Dewbury, David Cosgrove and Pat
Farrant to be identified as authors of this work has been asserted by
them in accordance with the Copyright, Designs and Patents Act 1988

First edition published 1993
Second edition published 2001
          Reprinted 2002

ISBN 0 443 06152 1 (volumes 1 & 2)
ISBN 0 443 06154 8 (volume 3)
ISBN 0 443 06350 8 (3 volume set)

British Library Cataloguing in Publication Data
A catalogue record for this book is available from the British Library

Library of Congress Cataloging in Publication Data
A catalog record for this book is available from the Library of Congress

Note
Medical knowledge is constantly changing. As new information
becomes available, changes in treatment, procedures, equipment and
the use of drugs become necessary. The editors, contributors and the
publishers have taken care to ensure that the information given in this
text is accurate and up to date. However, readers are strongly advised
to confirm that the information, especially with regard to drug usage,
complies with the latest legislation and standards of practice.

The
publisher's
policy is to use
**paper manufactured
from sustainable forests**

Typeset by Expo Holdings, Malaysia
Printed in China by RDC Group Limited

Preface

In the years since the publication of the first edition of this book, the subject of ultrasound has advanced at a dizzying pace, one that could not have been foreseen when we worked on the original edition. Not only have advances concerned technical aspects – harmonic imaging, 3D, power Doppler, contrast agents – which are in the process of rewriting the methodology of ultrasound, but they have also affected the clinical practice of ultrasound where we have seen marked improvements in techniques, understanding and appreciation of the method. Far from being replaced by alternative tomographic techniques, ultrasound has gone from strength to strength as a diagnostic tool to the point where it is now the fastest growing imaging modality. It has consolidated its role in classic applications remaining paramount in obstetrics and in cardiac imaging. It is the primary method for small parts imaging and for biopsy guidance and is carving out new roles in musculoskeletal and vascular investigations. Some of the impetus behind this has been the downward pressure on medical spending – ultrasound is still the most cost-effective way to investigate many medical and surgical problems.

In preparing this new edition – no mean task! – we have tried to retain the basic material that made the first edition useful as a reference and basic learning text, and have tried to provide a systematic description of the proven applications of ultrasound to act as a guide in day-to-day practice. Keeping this balance between the routine and the provisional is sometimes difficult for enthusiasts in a discipline and we crave the reader's indulgence if occasionally we have allowed exciting innovations too prominent a description.

Our great indebtedness to the numerous contributors is obvious and we would like to extend to these experts our most sincere thanks for their patience and labour. The project could not have been completed without the endless support of the publishing team at Harcourt: Michael Houston, who was responsible for cajoling us into taking up the editorial pen again and oversaw the entire effort, Paul Fam and Rolla Couchman who worked with us and our contributors on a weekly and sometimes daily basis keeping the project to schedule and coping with the inevitable technical difficulties that beset such an endeavour.

Pat Farrant was inadequately noted as an assistant editor in the first edition: here she has rightly been recognised as the full editor that she always was.

We all extend our thanks to our colleagues and families who supported us with encouragement and patience, indulging the many hours of time we stole from other activities. We sincerely hope that the result is as useful as before.

Hylton Meire
David Cosgrove
Keith Dewbury
Pat Farrant
2000

Preface to the first edition

Most textbooks, at least in the field of diagnostic imaging, stem from the wish of the authors or editors to make their special expertise more widely available. The origin of *Clinical Ultrasound* is rather unusual in that it is a response to a proposal by the publishers, Churchill Livingstone, that the time was right for a comprehensive ultrasound textbook with a strong clinical content.

At first approach, we have to confess to having been sceptical of the need for such a textbook and we were most reluctant to embark on such a monumental task but, as we began to review the field, it was possible to envisage it being broken down into more manageable components. It was also clear that there really was no comprehensive textbook on the market, all of the available books concentrated on a particular application or body region.

An initial hurdle was to secure the editorship of Dr Peter Wilde to oversee the cardiology section; initially Peter was as reluctant as the rest of us, having heavy commitments on his hands but, fired by the prospect of a comprehensive and strongly clinical reference work, he was persuaded. The cardiology section has been completely under his editorship, though it adheres to the general format and goals of the entire book.

For the remaining large sections, a decisive influence in our agreeing to proceed was the fact that Pat Farrant was enthusiastic, something she may have come to regret as time went by! Pat agreed to take control of the massive task of handling all of the editing and advising that underlay the organising of the extensive text and innumerable figures together with their orientation diagrams, keeping track of where alterations had to be entered, checking that tables referred to in the text were, in fact, contained in the chapter or appendix and generally managing the entire process of creation and collation which extended to double the 18 months that we had originally anticipated. However, that was not all for, as we got further into the project, Pat was also called upon to contribute large portions of chapters that had somehow fallen by the wayside and her input into almost every section has been absolutely invaluable. It was in the knowledge that she would give this kind of support that we entered the 'battle'. None of us foresaw just how protracted a battle it would become nor how large Pat's contribution would turn out to be – 'siege' would have been a more apposite term!

We would also like to thank our families and friends who have borne with us during the past three stressful years. Special thanks are due to Christine Dewbury and Gill Meire for their continuing support and encouragement, and for hosting so many editorial meetings.

From this explanation, our intentions should be clear. We have aimed to provide an up-to-date textbook on clinical diagnostic ultrasound that would cover the entire gamut of its applications, both imaging and Doppler. Because of its clinical basis, the physics of ultrasound does not feature as a formal topic, though its important practical consequences and implications, especially in newer, less familiar areas such as Doppler, are covered.

Diagnostic ultrasound has become so extensive that, inevitably, this had to be a large book and a small team of specialists could not hope to cover the entire field. Therefore, we commissioned a large number of contributing authors from Europe and the Americas, most well known experts in their own areas. We stand to lose friends however, because we have exercised strong editing rights in the interests of maintaining a uniform style – we hope our loyal contributors will feel that our sometimes heavy alterations have contributed to the overall quality of the book and will not take offence that we have freely altered their prose and even sometimes substituted scans that seemed clearer or that made the intended point better.

With respect to the division of material through the book, the separation of cardiology from the other applications already referred to, made it obvious that this should form a separate volume that is available on its own. Obstetrics and Gynaecology formed a second distinct section and so we have arranged that this also be a separate volume with its own page numbering and index. The other two volumes, which contain the remaining applications (abdominal, small parts, vascular, miscellaneous), are offered together as two sections of a single book: pages are numbered through and they have been indexed together in the expectation that few users will need only one of the pair.

We hope that *Clinical Ultrasound* will become a reference work for all who use ultrasound in their clinical practice and that users will find in it comprehensive answers to their everyday needs. It should provide critical information in a form that is easy to look up, as well as form the basis for specialist training.

Hylton Meire
David Cosgrove
Keith Dewbury
1992

Terminology and scan position indicators

The aim of this book is to serve as a reference text and as an aid to education and teaching. During the editorial process it was clear to us that the terminology used to describe ultrasound appearances is extremely diverse, confusing and occasionally inaccurate. We have therefore unified the terminology in *Clinical Ultrasound*. In doing this we have considered the two main interactions between the ultrasound beam and the tissue; namely reflective and attenuation.

Meaningless terms such as 'sonolucent' and 'echo dense' have been eradicated. We also considered the use of the prefixs 'hyper-' and 'hypo-' a source of confusion and found several instances where the secretaries typing the manuscript had confused the two.

Where backscattered amplitude is being discussed the ultrasound appearances are described as of reduced, normal or increased reflectivity (by inference compared with that which would normally be expected).

The above features of *Clinical Ultrasound* have been incorporated in an attempt to make these volumes more valuable and easier to understand, and it is hoped that the terminology we have used will encourage readers to consider more carefully the terminology they use to describe their own ultrasound findings.

The relatively small field of view of modern ultrasound scanners, and the infinitely variable planes of imaging, sometimes lead to difficulties in interpreting the anatomy and orientation of an ultrasound image. Rather than using extensive free narrative to describe the positions from which images have been obtained we have used a system of body markers on which the position of the scans has been indicated. When referring to these the reader should be aware that the scans indicating a lateral area of contact do not necessarily imply that the patient was moved into an oblique or decubitus position, but simply that the transducer was located on a lateral aspect of the patient.

The orientation of the conventional extracavitory images included in this book has generally been adjusted such that longitudinal scans are viewed as if from the patient's rightside and transverse scans as if from the patient's feet. Unfortunately there is no standardisation for the orientation of intracavitory images and, in general, these have been displayed with the orientation unaltered from that supplied by the individual authors. We have not attempted to verify the position of the transducer or the orientation of the image for intracavitory scans as these should be clear from the accompanying text in each case

Hylton Meire
David Cosgrove
Keith Dewbury
Pat Farrant

Contributors

Paul L Allan BSc MBBS DMRD FRCR FRCPE
Consultant Radiologist
Department of Medical Radiology
Royal Infirmary
Edinburgh
United Kingdom

Clive I Bartram FRCP FRCR
Professor of Gastrointestinal Radiology
Intestinal Imaging Center
St Mark's Hospital
Harrow
United Kingdom

Jane A Bates DMU MPhil
Sonographer
Ultrasound Department
St James' University Hospital
Leeds
United Kingdom

Grant M. Baxter FRCR
Consultant Radiologist
Department of Radiology
Western Infirmary University NHS Trust
Glasgow
United Kingdom

Massimo Bellomi MD
Associate Professor of Radiology
Istituto Europeo di Oncologia
University of Milan
Milan
Italy

Roland J Blackwell BSc MSc CEng
FIEE CPhys FInstP FIPEM
Professor of Medical Physics & Bioengineering
Department of Medical Physics & Bioengineering
The Middlesex Hospital
University College London Hospitals
London
United Kingdom

Luigi Bolondi MD
Associate Professor of Internal Medicine
Department of Internal Medicine and Gastroenterology
University of Bologna
Bologna
Italy

Maria Chiara Bossi MD
Senior Researcher in Radiology
Istituto Europeo di Oncologia
Milan
Italy

Rose de Bruyn MBBCh DMRD FRCR
Consultant Paediatric Radiologist and
 Honorary Senior Lecturer
Department of Radiology
Great Ormond Street Hospital for Children NHS Trust
London
United Kingdom

Teresa Cammarota MD
Consultant Radiologist
Ospedale S. Giovanni Battista
Turin
Italy

David O Cosgrove MA MSc FRCR FRCP
Professor of Clinical Ultrasound
Department of Imaging
Hammersmith Hospital
London
United Kingdom

Luca Cova MD
Resident in Radiology
Department of Radiology
General Hospital
Busto Arsizio
Italy

Colin R Deane PhD
Clinical Scientist
Department of Medical Engineering and Physics
King's College Hospital
London
United Kingdom

Lorenzo E Derchi MD
Professor of Radiology
Institute of Radiology
Ospedale S. Martino
University of Genoa
Genoa
Italy

Keith C Dewbury BSc MBBS FRCR
Consultant Radiologist
Southampton General Hospital
Southampton
United Kingdom

Claire Dicks-Mireaux BA MBBS MRCP FRCR
Formerly Consultant Radiologist
The Hospitals for Sick Children
London
United Kingdom

Paul A Dubbins MBBS BSc FRCR
Consultant Radiologist
Imaging Directorate
Derriford Hospital
Plymouth
United Kingdom

Pat Farrant DCRR DMU
Superintendent Research Sonographer
King's College Hospital
London
United Kingdom

John A Fielding MD FRCR DMRD
Consultant Radiologist
Department of Radiology
Royal Shrewsbury Hospital
Shrewsbury
United Kingdom

Richard Fowler MBBS MRCP DMRD FRCR
Consultant Radiologist
Department of Radiology
Leeds General Infirmary
Leeds
United Kingdom

Stefano Gaiani MD
Assistant Professor
Department of Internal Medicine and Gastroenterology
University of Bologna
Bologna
Italy

Wayne Gibbon FRCS FRCR
Consultant Radiologist
Department of Radiology
Leeds General Infirmary
Leeds
United Kingdom

Anders Glenthøj MD
Chief Pathologist
Centralsygehuset Hillerød
Hillerød
Denmark

Christian Görg MD
Professor of Clinical Ultrasound
Department of Internal Medicine
Klinikum Lahnberge
Philipps-University
Marburg
Germany

David E Goss PhD
Vascular Technologist
Department of Medical Engineering and Physics
King's College Hospital
London
United Kingdom

Gail ter Haar MA(Oxon) MSc PhD
Team Leader in Therapeutic Ultrasound
Joint Department of Physics
Royal Marsden Hospital NHS Trust
Sutton
United Kingdom

Christopher M B Hare MB BCh MRCP FRCR
Consultant Radiologist
Middlesex Hospital
London
United Kingdom

Christopher R Hill BA PhD DSc
FIEE FInstP FRCR (Hon)
Emeritus Professor of Physics as Applied in Medicine
Institute of Cancer Research
Royal Marsden Hospital
London
United Kingdom

Hans Henrik Holm PhD MD
Professor and Head
Department of Ultrasound
Chief Surgeon
Department of Urology
Herlev University Hospital
Herlev
Denmark

Henry C Irving FRCR
Consultant Radiologist
Department of Clinical Radiology
St James' University Hospital
Leeds
United Kingdom

Timothy Jaspan MB ChB BSc FRCP FRCR
Consultant Neuroradiologist
Imaging Centre
Queen's Medical Centre
University Hospital
Nottingham
United Kingdom

Robert A Kane MD
Professor of Radiology
Harvard Medical School
Director of Ultrasound
Radiology Department
Beth Israel Deaconess Medical Center
Boston
Massachusetts
USA

Steen Karstrup MD
Department of Diagnostic Radiology
Herlev Hospital
University of Copenhagen
Denmark

Gillian Long MRCP DCH DRCOG FRCR MEd
Consultant Paediatric Radiologist
Radiology Department
Sheffield Childrens Hospital
Sheffield
United Kingdom

Carlo Martinoli MD
Assistant Radiologist
Institute of Radiology
Ospedale S. Martino
University of Genoa
Genoa
Italy

Gebhard Mathis MD
Professor of Internal Medicine
Head, Department of Internal Medicine
Krankenhaus Hohenems
Hohenems
Austria

Hylton B Meire FRCR
Consultant Radiologist
King's College Hospital
London
United Kingdom

Christian Nolsøe MD
Associate Professor
Department of Ultrasound
Herlev Hospital
University of Copenhagen
Denmark

Jacques A van Oostayen MD PhD
Consultant Radiologist
Department of Radiology
Leiden University Medical Centre
Leiden
The Netherlands

Valeria Osti MD
Resident in Radiology
Department of Radiology
General Hospital
Busto Arsizio
Italy

Robert J Peck BSc FRCR
Consultant Radiologist
X-ray Department
Royal Hallamshire Hospital
Sheffield
United Kingdom

Jan Fog Pedersen MD PhD
Head of Ultrasound Laboratory
Department of Radiology
Glostrup Hospital
University of Copenhagen
Denmark

Fabio Piscaglia MD
Department of Internal Medicine and Gastroenterology
University of Bologna
Bologna
Italy

Julien B C M Puylaert MD PhD
Consultant Radiologist
Department of Radiology
Haagland Medical Centre
Westeinde Hospital
The Hague
The Netherlands

David Rickards FRCR FFRDSA
Consultant Radiologist
Department of Radiology
The Middlesex Hospital
London
United Kingdom

Michel Rioux MD
Clinical Professor of Radiology
Hôpital de Matane
Quebec
Canada

Antonino Sarno MD
Senior Registrar in Radiology
Ospedale S. Giovanni Battista
Turin
Italy

Carla Serra MD
Department of Internal Medicine and Gastroenterology
University of Bologna
Bologna
Italy

Philip J Shorvon MA (Cantab) MBBS MRCP FRCR
Consultant Radiologist
Department of Radiology
Central Middlesex Hospital
North West London Hospitals NHS Trust
London
United Kingdom

Marilyn J Siegel MD
Professor of Radiology and Pediatrics
Edward Mallinckrodt Institute of Radiology
Washington University School of Medicine
St Louis
Missouri
USA

Luigi Solbiati MD
Head, Section of Ultrasound
Department of Radiology
General Hospital
Busto Arsizio
Italy

Luc Steyaert MD
Radiologist
Department of Radiology
St-Jan Hospital
Bruges
Belgium

Søren Tobias Torp-Pedersen MD
Head
Department of Ultrasound
Herlev Hospital
University of Copenhagen
Denmark

Joanna M Wardlaw MB ChB(Hons) FRCR FRCP MD
Reader and Honorary Consultant Neuroradiologist
Department of Clinical Neurosciences
Western General Hospital
Edinburgh
United Kingdom

Judith A W Webb BSc MD FRCP FRCR
Consultant Radiologist
Department of Diagnostic Radiology
St Bartholomew's Hospital
London
United Kingdom

Contents

VOLUME 2

1

History: then and now

Christopher R Hill

'History is bunk' – but we can learn from it

Although Henry Ford's famous dictum may be unpopular with professional historians, it finds some justification in the field of investigative ultrasound, whose history includes a considerable mixture of unrecognised achievements and ill-founded ideas. The story is nonetheless a fascinating one for its own sake and has been recorded by several authors in more detail than present space allows,[1-4] as well as in a useful bibliography of the early literature.[5]

In this chapter we look particularly at the development of ideas in the field. The present 'received wisdom' has arisen, on the one hand from some remarkable pioneering work, often carried out in the teeth of professional scepticism, and sometimes even derision, but also from a number of misjudgements and failures of scientific understanding, some of which may still influence current practice and inhibit its effective advance. To learn useful lessons from history one needs, like Henry Ford, to be on the look-out for 'bunk' dressed up for purposes of self-justification.

Origins of the concepts and technology behind investigative ultrasound

Concepts

The dream of being able to explore the living anatomy of the human body must go back at least to the days of the great anatomists, exemplified by the work of Vesalius in the 16th century. The practical means of achieving this non-invasively were of course lacking until recently but the general concept may have arisen earlier, if only subconsciously, as witness the words of Thomas Hardy (in *The Return of the Native*, published in 1878 and thus contemporary with Rayleigh, the great theoretician of acoustics): 'Compound utterances addressed themselves to their senses, and it was possible to view by ear the features of the neighbourhood. Acoustic pictures were returned from the darkened scenery …'. Although still not seen as having application to anatomy, this appears to have been first focused onto practical application by a British physicist, Richardson, in 1912 for detection of icebergs.[6] Somewhat ironically, however, Richardson's Quaker pacifist principles diverted him from following up this idea, on the grounds of its likely military value.[7] The great step that had made an instant reality of medical imaging was, however, Röntgen's discovery of X-rays in 1895, and the concept that this had brought with it, that of the shadowgraph or 'radiograph', dominated people's thinking for the next 50 years or more. Indeed, the first steps towards making an anatomical image with ultrasound were taken

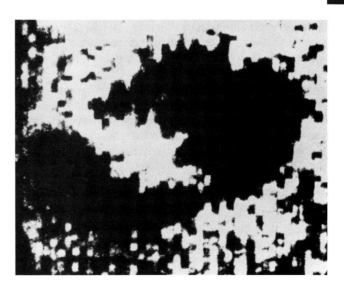

Fig. 1.1 Ultrasound transmission scan ('radiograph') of the human head published by the Dussik brothers[8] in 1942. Hindsight would indicate, however, that the image owes more to artefact than to anatomy (see text).

by the Austrian brothers Dussik in 1937, using essentially that principle.[8] They scanned over a human head, immersed in water, using a transmitter–receiver pair of quartz crystal transducers; the result that they published in 1942 is illustrated in Figure 1.1. However, they gave no grounds for believing that the image portrayed real anatomy and, with the benefit of hindsight, current assessment must be that the data are essentially artefactual.

Technological foundations

The essential technological foundations for modern investigative ultrasound can be described under the following headings: acoustical theory, practical means for electroacoustic conversion ('transduction'), fast electronic pulse technology, and video display and recording. All of these became available in practically usable form in the 75-year period culminating in 1945, with the further important component of contemporary technology – digital processing – following soon afterwards.

Prior to 1870 there seems to have been little coherent intellectual basis for the science of acoustics. Writing in 1873 to the then J. W. Strutt (later, and more generally known as, Lord Rayleigh) Clerk Maxwell remarked 'I am glad you are writing a book on Acoustics. … You speak modestly about a want of sound books in English. In what language are there such, except Helmholtz, who is sound not because he is German but because he is Helmholtz?'. Rayleigh had in fact started work on his book in December 1872, at the outset of a 3-month honeymoon trip on a Nile sailing boat.[9] The result, his *Theory of Sound*[10] immediately became, and has remained, one of the great classic texts in physics and provided the intellectual foundation for the subject of acoustics and, thus, of ultrasonics.

It is a remarkable and double coincidence, first that only 3 years after the publication of *Theory of Sound* came the discovery, quite independently, of the physical phenomenon that makes possible the investigative use of ultrasound, that of the piezoelectric effect[11] and, second, that the two brothers who were its discoverers were those whose surname was shortly to become, for quite other reasons, widely famous in medical science: Jean and Pierre Curie. Their observations were made in single crystals of tourmaline, although the phenomenon was soon recognised as being more general in occurrence and specifically to occur in quartz, which became widely used in practice. It was not until the 1950s that the phenomenon was effectively exploited in the more versatile composite ceramic materials (e.g. lead zirconate titanate – PZT) and, later still, plastics, that are now in almost universal use in medical applications.

In a further manifestation of the apparently small world of turn-of-the-century science it was a graduate student of Pierre Curie, Paul Langevin, who was to go on to develop Richardson's idea and become the practical pioneer of acoustic pulse-echo techniques, in their 1914–1918 wartime application to underwater detection of submarines. This work was secret and unpublished at the time. In a sense it was technologically premature since it predated the thermionic triode valve and thus lacked straightforward means for either generation or amplification of electrical pulses. It, and related work elsewhere, laid the foundations for subsequent developments, first in marine SONAR (Sound Navigation and Ranging) and subsequently in RADAR (Radio Detection and Ranging), non-destructive materials testing and medical imaging.

Interestingly, Langevin's work also was the first to arouse interest in the possible biological consequences, whether harmful or otherwise, of ultrasound exposure, since he noticed damage to the fish in Cherbourg harbour when they strayed into his high-power beam. A remarkable early follow-up of this observation, together with an account of some of the technological problems coped with by Langevin, was reported by Wood & Loomis in 1927.[12]

An important link between Langevin's work in acoustics and its application to medicine was forged by the Russian engineer, S. Y. Sokolov, who pioneered the use of ultrasound echo methods for flaw detection in metals,[13] foresaw the extension of such methods to the gigahertz frequency (and corresponding micron resolution) microscopy applications which have only quite recently been realised, and invented the ultrasonic analogue of the television camera (the Sokolov Camera) which enables direct transformation of ultrasonic image data into electrical signals.[14] During the 1939–1945 war these concepts led naturally into work on ultrasonic non-destructive testing and radar, both of which, in turn, relied on the recently developed cathode ray display tube and the associated technology of television that had been built up by Baird and others during the 1930s.

The 'post-war' period (1948–1960)

With the above background, and following the intensive technological development work stimulated by the needs of the war, particularly that directed towards radar, the essential ingredients had become available for the implementation of investigative ultrasound. In what happened next, although enormous credit is due to the very small number of far-sighted pioneers, the real cause for surprise should not be that the development occurred, but rather how blind was the conventional wisdom to its significance and thus how slowly its potential benefits came to be exploited. Although a relative latecomer, the present author must be numbered among the blind in this context. The reasons behind such blindness can only be speculative. It is nonetheless important to be aware of the influences that can divert otherwise logical and potentially valuable advances.

The Second World War concluded with the nuclear bombing of Hiroshima and Nagasaki, events that led to widespread and deep feelings of awe and guilt. One of the consequences was the creation of the International Atomic Energy Agency, one of whose principal functions was, as some kind of communal reparation, to act as a wealthy patron of a particular phoenix, nuclear medicine. It is ironical that the relatively benign role played by ultrasound in wartime led to its neglect by the post-war, guilt-ridden public imagination.

Also, by this time, diagnostic radiology seemed to have reached a state of relative equilibrium and most radiologists were unreceptive to the prospect of a radically new imaging technology (which nuclear medicine had not become at this stage) that might complement X-ray examination, even for problems in which this was known to be unsatisfactory.

During the war, ultrasonic echo methods had been developed, principally by Firestone in the USA and Sproule in Britain, for detecting cracks in metal structures, and by 1949 three separate groups in the USA had become interested in their medical potential: Ludwig & Struthers at the US Naval establishment at Maryland; Wild, a British-trained surgeon in Minneapolis who recruited help from a local US naval air station; and Howry, a radiologist at Denver. All three groups initially worked with A-scan techniques and while the former, who were interested in locating gallstones and foreign bodies, never apparently progressed beyond that, the two others both developed B-scan imaging methods, but with differences that may have had considerable influence on subsequent development.

Together with his electronic engineering colleague, Reid, Wild, whose interest was in elucidating histopathology, and particularly that of cancer, developed a B-scanner working at 15 MHz and designed to be sensitive even to low-level tissue echoes, at the calculated cost of producing images with a good range of grey scale but of somewhat fuzzy appearance (Fig. 1.2). In retrospect this work can be seen to be the true forerunner of modern imaging procedures, but, perhaps because of failure to solve the technical problem of image display with adequate dynamic range compression, and in spite of an extensive, vigorous and imaginative programme of work,[3] the potential value of the images was not generally perceived in the early days.

Howry's approach was somewhat different, being in essence a prototype of the reconstruction tomography that came into its own with the development of X-ray CT, and had the practical outcome of images that emphasised the location of organ boundaries (Fig. 1.3).[15] In his original 'Somatom' apparatus (although this was shown later not

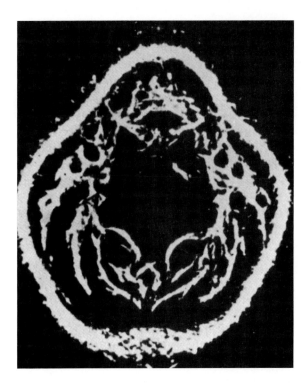

Fig. 1.3 **Cross-sectional image of the neck** obtained by Howry, in about 1954, using a water-immersion compound scanner.[15]

to be essential) the anatomy of interest was immersed in a waterbath and echo data were received from all possible orientations and superimposed in their correct relative locations in order to form the final image. This approach, which became known as 'compound scanning', had the apparent strength, particularly at the height of its development, of providing images reminiscent of anatomical line drawings (Fig. 1.4). It became a standard procedure until the development of high-sensitivity, high-resolution techniques showed both the diagnostic importance of low-level echoes[17] and the serious impact of movement artefact that occurs in compound scanning.[18]

The vogue for compound scanning was in fact lent strength at one stage through developments in display device technology. In the 1950s the only available means, apart from photography, for even temporarily storing complete images was to use display CRTs with 'long persistence' phosphors – an unsatisfactory procedure because their low luminance levels called for scanning in virtually total darkness, and consequent long observer accommodation times. Subsequent developments of 'storage' display tubes initially provided only a bistable (black or white) display, which emphasised the appearances of simple anatomy but provided no half-tones with which to display tissue echoes (Fig. 1.5). However, human conservativeness is such that later developments allowing a return to good half-tone ('grey scale') display were initially greeted by some diagnosticians with appreciable disapproval.

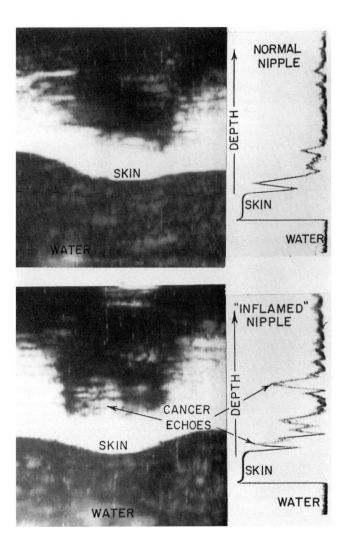

Fig. 1.2 **Early B-scan of the breast**, published by Wild & Reid in 1953 and reported as showing the presence of a tumour in the region of the nipple.[3]

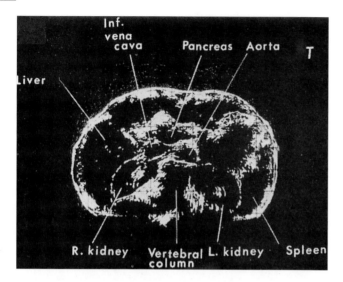

Fig. 1.4 **An outstanding example from the Bistable Image School:** a transverse cross-section of the abdomen, 16 cm above the umbilicus, obtained by Holm[16] in 1970.

A curious aspect of the compound scanning era was the myth (propagated in many standard textbooks and still occasionally resurfacing) that grew up to explain the success of the technique, that the echoes recorded were only those received from 'specularly reflecting' (i.e. essentially flat) interfaces. There seems to be no clear evidence for this model and indeed even simple consideration of the three-dimensional nature of the geometry concerned would indicate that most specular reflectors would not be expected to return echoes in the plane of scan. The more tenable physical explanation of the effect would now seem to lie in the signal-to-noise enhancement that results from multiple sampling of diffusely backscattered echoes, the strongest of which arise from connective tissue around organ boundaries.

A number of other principal items in the technical armoury of present-day diagnostic ultrasound date from this period. For his work on bowel, Wild developed, and used clinically, the first ultrasonic endoscope (Fig. 1.6),[19] while, at about the same time, Edler & Hertz in Sweden opened up applications to cardiology by introduction of M-mode recording.[20] Again at this time it was Wild who took the first steps towards deriving quantitative information about tissue type from features of the ultrasonic echo: in modern parlance, 'tissue characterisation'.[21] What is in a sense a special case of tissue characterisation, although it has come to be seen almost as a technology in its own right – Doppler flow detection and measurement – was developed and published by Satomura[22,23] in Japan in 1956. Finally, these early users of ultrasound were conscious of using an essentially novel form of diagnostic radiation which might have unforeseen consequences for their patients, or even for themselves, and it was once again Wild who seems to have been the first to investigate, in however preliminary a fashion, this possibility,[24] as early as 1951.

Clinically, Wild was interested in cancer, particularly of the breast and large bowel, and time, even with the advent

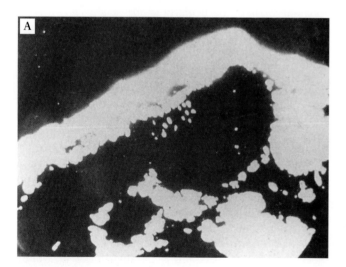

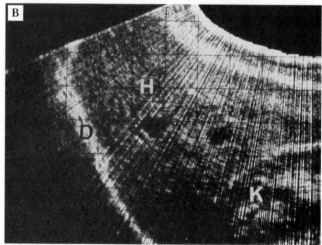

Fig. 1.5 **Two liver scans** published in the same journal issue in 1973 and illustrating the diversity of image appearances at that time. **A:** Scan apparently obtained with an unfocused transducer and recorded through a bistable display device.[33] The author's caption reads: 'Supine transverse scan of a liver showing two transonic nodules bordered by an echogenic band (metastasis of a gastric cancer)'. **B:** Scan obtained on the equipment illustrated in Figure 1.8, with a 3 MHz focused transducer, logarithmic signal compression and 'open shutter' recording directly on to film[18,34] ('scratchy potentiometer artefact' is painfully visible!). The authors' caption reads: 'longitudinal section of liver, 6 cm to right of midline, showing diaphragm (D), normal liver (H), normal right kidney (K) and two small areas of replacement of normal architecture by small discrete areas of Hodgkin's disease.' Copyright © 1973. Reprinted by permission of Wiley–Liss, Inc. A subsidiary of John Wiley & Sons, Inc.

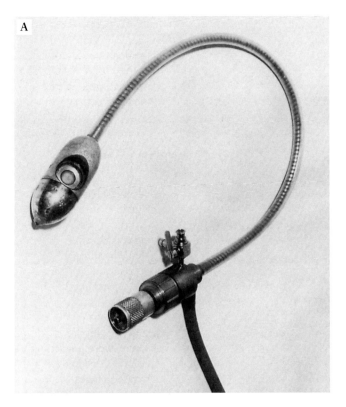

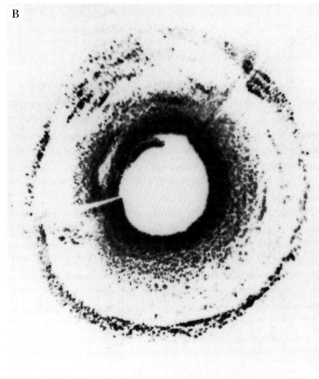

Fig. 1.6 **A: Prototype of an ultrasonic endoscope,** designed and built by Wild[19] in about 1957 (© 1957 IEEE). **B:** Example of a rectal scan obtained with it.

of CT, has vindicated his far-sightedness in these and many other sites of the disease. Equally clearly, however, he was taking on in the breast one of the more difficult areas of diagnostic imaging and it is thus hardly surprising that the clear demonstration of the worth of his results here was slow to come.

Howry's initial interest (as indeed had been the Dussiks', one of whom was a psychiatrist) was, by contrast, in the brain, which was perhaps a natural site for a radiologist to attack at that time, knowing as he did that it presented a substantial set of clinical problems that could not be solved satisfactorily by conventional techniques. Even more than Wild, Howry soon discovered that the adult brain is a very difficult organ to study with ultrasound because of overlying bone, and subsequent authors have confirmed this to present almost insuperable problems.[25] Nonetheless, again in ironic contrast to Wild, Howry's interest in the brain attracted a considerable number of followers, to the extent that a substantial proportion of the 'second generation' of ultrasound pioneers were recruited through an interest in neurology: names such as White in Canada, de Vlieger in Holland, Alvisi in Italy, Mayneord in Britain, and Kikuchi, Tanaka and Wagai in Japan.

As already mentioned, another organ that received relatively early attention was the heart, largely because it was found that useful kinetic information could be derived by relatively simple M-mode techniques. For similar reasons, interest arose at an early stage in studies of the eye, where useful optometric and other information (again with early attempts at 'tissue characterisation') could be derived from straightforward A-scan methods. In this connection it is interesting to note that, as White has pointed out,[5,26] approximately 60% of all papers on echography published prior to the year 1970 were related to applications in either neurology or ophthalmology, a figure that had dropped below 5% by 1982.[27]

The abdomen seems to have proved a difficult region in the early days, probably for the reasons suggested above in relation to cancer investigation, and of the relatively few early published papers in this area the great majority were concerned with location of stones.

Obstetric applications similarly attracted little interest until, from the publication of the early work of Donald and co-workers, commencing in 1958[28] (although with its origins traceable to the work of Mayneord's group[29,30] commencing in 1951), it became apparent that, even with the then somewhat primitive state of the technology, it was quite possible to derive several types of data having vital bearing on obstetric management, for example fetal skull size, placental position and differential diagnosis of hydatidiform mole. Arguably this was the key advance that led to the eventual acceptance of ultrasound as a generally respected clinical imaging tool, as indeed it also led to the production of the first commercial B-scanner – the Diasonograph – designed on Scotland's Clydeside to ship-builders' mechanical specifications and driven by a multitude of wartime electronic valves (Fig. 1.7).

This is to anticipate. Perhaps the event that was to mark the close of the 'classical period' of diagnostic ultrasound was the withdrawal of Wild's US Public Health Service research grant. At $0.5 million this was, at the time of the award in 1962, the largest single medical grant ever given to an individual. The decision to stop payments and confiscate his equipment[31] led to the following entry in the Guinness Book of Records: 'A sum of $16,800,000 was awarded to Dr. John J. Wild, at the Hennepin District Court, Minnesota, USA on 30th November 1972 against the Minnesota Foundation and others for defamation, bad faith, termination of a contract, interference with professional business relationship and $10.8 million in punitive damages'.[4] The award was subsequently much reduced by the Minnesota Supreme Court, but not before its members had resigned *en bloc* over the issue, an event that was itself unique in American legal history.

Modern times

Thus, by about 1963, virtually all the essential concepts underlying modern diagnostic ultrasound had been demonstrated – even something approaching real-time scan acquisition had been achieved by the indomitable Wild.[3] Nonetheless, much remained to be done: the technique was essentially unrecognised outside a very small band of enthusiasts and the only equipment being produced commercially were industrial flaw detectors.

Donald & Brown's Diasonograph went into commercial production in the mid-1960s with an initial run of six units. In this the transducer was mounted so as to move within a rectangular measuring frame (Fig. 1.7), which proved to be good, if somewhat cumbersome engineering design. Some other manufacturers soon followed, however, with what proved to be a more ergonomically satisfactory arrangement of 'compound B-scanner' in which the transducer was mounted on the end of an articulated measuring arm (Fig. 1.8). Thus, by the time of the First World Congress of Ultrasound in Medicine held in Vienna in October 1969,[32] there was already an interesting variety of commercial scanners on offer. However, display devices were still of either the long persistence or the bistable types and this, taken with the remarkable fact that most, if not all, transducers were unfocused and (in abdominal and obstetric scanners) operated at between 1 and 2 MHz, resulted in indifferent image quality (Fig. 1.5).

In relation to the shortcomings in display devices at that time it is noteworthy that the best available technique for recording images of good quality was direct recording

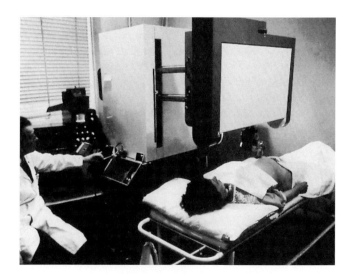

Fig. 1.7 **Professor Ian Donald**, at the Queen Mother's Hospital, Glasgow, working with an early model Diasonograph, manufactured in 1964 by Smiths Industries in Glasgow: the first B-scanner to have been produced commercially. In the background (above Donald's hand) is the Smiths 'Mark 7 supersonic Flaw Detector' that was used by Dr Stuart Campbell in his early work on biparietal cephalometry. Photograph by courtesy of Mr J. E. E. Fleming and with permission of the British Medical Ultrasound Society Historical Collection.

from a non-storage display monitor onto photographic film, with the camera shutter held open during the scanning procedure. It was, to a large extent, careful optimisation of this procedure that enabled Kossoff's group in Sydney to achieve such outstanding results at this time.

Transducer design was, however, being worked on by a number of groups. For example, in 1971 the present author incorporated a 3 MHz, 10 cm focus transducer in an articulated arm abdominal scanner and this, working together with the well-conceived developments in electronics and display that were due to the Sydney group, led to dramatic improvements in image quality[17,35] and corresponding extensions of clinical usefulness.

Perhaps more significant in the long term were developments that had commenced in the late 1960s of transducer arrays – a technology that derived, albeit in miniaturised form, from underwater acoustics. Here Somer[36] and Bom,[37] both working in Holland, pioneered the phased and simple linear array techniques respectively that are in widespread use today. A major practical outcome of array technology was, of course, the facility of real-time imaging, but the alternative of fast automatic mechanical scanning devices – rockers and rollers, or 'whizzers' – was also becoming available,[38] with some substantial advantages for certain applications, once the problems of mechanical reliability had been solved.

The majority of scanners of this period were far from 'user-friendly' – a situation that posed a considerable barrier in terms of training and also of integration into conventional clinical or radiological practice. The

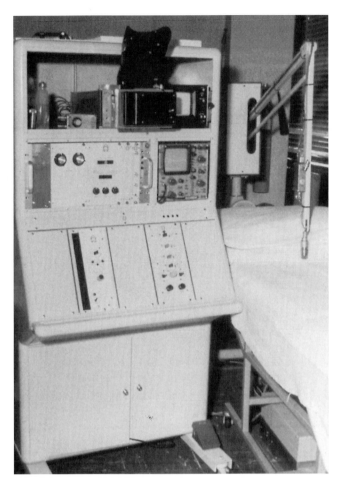

Fig. 1.8 **Early example of an articulated-arm design of compound B-scanner** (scanning arm originally manufactured by Kretz, with electronics developed at the Royal Marsden Hospital[17]).

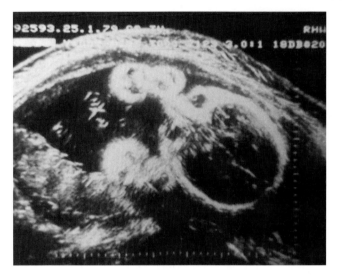

Fig. 1.9 **Image of a pregnant abdomen,** showing a cross-sectional view of a fetal skull, taken at the Royal Hospital for Women, Sydney, in 1979, with the 'CAL Octoson' (courtesy Drs G. Kossoff and W. Garrett).

Australian Octoson, with its derivatives, was a remarkable and imaginative attempt to solve this problem: an automated scanner (not unlike CT, with whose development it was contemporary but conceptually independent) in which the patient lies on a membrane-covered waterbed containing a set of scanning transducers.[39] This device might have seemed ideally suited to the pattern of work of radiology departments and it was certainly capable of producing spectacular and informative images (Fig. 1.9). Eventually, however, it failed to gain general acceptance, and the reason for this failure may have been that it took away from ultrasound the very feature that distinguishes it from the bulk of radiological examinations – its clinical interactiveness.

A strand of thought that has occupied the attention of a number of workers in the field relates to the problems of conveying to the diagnostician, through an essentially two-dimensional image acquisition procedure, information about a three-dimensional object. Developments in this direction are proceeding to this day in spite of a partial solution to the problem offered by effective 'real-time' or 'cine-echographic' procedures but an interesting early approach was that of T. G. Brown, based on the use of a modified articulated arm scanner.[40]

The advances that occurred during the 1980s and 1990s will be familiar to many readers. On the technical side these have often come about through general advances in technology: for example, developments in miniaturisation and in high-frequency transducers have led to much improved equipment for interventional and 'small parts' examination while fast and affordable digital technology has made possible innovations such as colour flow Doppler imaging.

It will have to be for future historians, with the benefit of longer perspectives, to define the factors that have determined the particular patterns of clinical use of ultrasound that we see today. One set of such factors derives of course from the nature of the technology: its successes and failures. Here one can cite, for example, its flexibility and real-time characteristics that contribute to its value for early and rapid extensions of clinical examination, and its apparent safety and patient-friendliness that suit it to both obstetrics and paediatrics. Another factor, however, has been its relationship to complementary imaging methods, particularly CT and MRI, which also underwent a phase of rapid development during this period. The interactions of these different but related developing technologies have been complex, particularly as they have involved the attitudes and activities of both diagnosticians and technologists. To future historians it may well appear that ultrasound in the 1980s and 1990s experienced a period of relatively undeserved neglect, while the attractions, both real and apparent, first of CT and then of MRI, gripped the attention of both radiologists and manufacturers.

The scientific background

Although it could be argued that it has so far had rather limited impact on commercial technology and clinical practice, part of the recent history of medical ultrasound has been in the area of basic physical science, particularly that to do with the propagation and scattering of ultrasound in human tissues. It is difficult to put exact dates to the outset of such work: measurements of tissue absorption coefficient, for example, were being made in the 1950s in connection with experiments on ultrasonic surgery.[41] To the extent, however, that pulse-echo methods rely essentially on the physical process of acoustic backscattering it is indicative that a review of that subject by Chivers in 1973 was only able to find two references to observations of the phenomenon in human or animal tissues (and one of those related to frozen fish).[42,43] While subsequent progress has been impressive,[44] much of the scientific basis for investigative ultrasound is thus quite recently established.

The question of safety

We have already seen that curiosity as to the possible ill-effects of the novel form of biophysical stress represented by pulse-echo ultrasound goes back to Wild's work in the 1950s. Even prior to that, however, there was a considerable body of evidence, albeit often of dubious quality, on the biology underlying attempts to use ultrasound for treatment of conditions ranging from cancer to 'Violinspieler-Krampf'.[45]

In connection with their early work in obstetrics, Donald and colleagues,[46] no doubt correctly concluding with Pope that 'the proper study of mankind is man', carried out what was to be the first (but retrospective, and not rigorously controlled) epidemiological study of the consequences of ultrasound exposure for obstetric examination, with generally negative and thus reassuring findings. Somewhat earlier the present author had been invited to write what was to be the first systematic review of the subject[47] and identified, in addition to epidemiology, the two other and complementary lines of evidence on the subject as being, first, the elucidation of fundamental mechanisms of biological action and, second, the more empirical toxicological type of studies, on both of which there was then an emerging literature.

Subsequently the field has expanded greatly and has survived a number of superficially alarming but subsequently unsustainable claims for evidence of significant hazard. A minor industry has emerged in the writing of reviews on the question of the existence of hazards, with accompanying recommendations for minimising their possible impact.[48,49]

An unfortunate impediment that affected much of the early work on so-called 'ultrasound bioeffects' was the absence of an appropriate experimental and theoretical framework of metrology – the science and practice of measuring and recording – for ultrasonic fields. Until quite recently the conventional wisdom was to report values of acoustic intensity, based on measurements with a radiation force balance. This was not for any clearly defined scientific reason but because the measurement seemed reasonably easy to perform and had become conventional and thus incorporated into a number of national guidelines and regulations. A focus for international collaboration and discussion on this topic was the Medical Ultrasonics Working Group of International Electrotechnical Commission (IEC), whose various members presented the first major symposium on the subject in 1971.[50] From such work has emerged the modern consensus that measurements should be carried out on fundamental acoustic field quantities and that the most appropriate and practical measurement to be carried out is that of acoustic pressure, for which purpose a range of miniature hydrophones have been developed over the past few years.[44]

Is this something of an abstruse technicality that has little to do with the real world of patients and their problems? Indeed not! An important factor in the recent history of diagnostic ultrasound has been the substantial public apprehension, as to both the validity of the evidence on safety and the possible problems that may arise from overdiagnosis.[51]

Conclusion

Arthur Koestler in *The Sleepwalkers* gives a penetrating commentary on the often blind and stumbling manner in which – contrary to the conventional wisdom – many of the major historical advances in scientific perception have actually come about. This theme has resonances in the history of diagnostic ultrasound, where advance, or lack of it, can now, with the benefit of hindsight, be seen often to have been the result of whim, quirks of personality and tides of fashion both in the medico-scientific professions and also in industry.

To derive lessons for the future is always a hazardous task but a good general one would be to avoid the typical attitude of middle-aged conservative professionals that (to paraphrase Keats) 'this is all I know on earth, and all I need to know': many radiologists and others in this category were taken unawares by the advent of diagnostic ultrasound and could be so again.

The current state of the art has come about through empirical and, at times, random processes, with little benefit from systematic insight into the underlying physics of the data-gathering procedure. A lesson from this interim historical review is that one could reasonably anticipate further advances in image quality as and when such insight is eventually achieved. Put another way, if it is indeed true that ultrasound has been relatively neglected as a field of physical science with applications in medical investigation, we should not be surprised if eventually its technical quality, and thus its clinical efficacy, turn out to have potential for advance relatively greater than those of some of the other, complementary imaging methods.

REFERENCES

1 Hill C R. Medical ultrasonics: an historical review. Br J Radiol 1973; 46: 899–905

2 White D N. Ultrasound in medical diagnosis. Kingston, Ontario: Ultramedison, 1976

3 Wild J J. The use of pulse-echo ultrasound for early tumour detection: history and prospects. In: Hill C R, McCready V R, Cosgrove D O, eds. Ultrasound in tumour diagnosis. Tunbridge Wells: Pitman Medical, 1978: 1–16

4 Wells P N T. History. In: de Vlieger M, Holmes J H, Kazner E et al, eds. Handbook of clinical ultrasound. New York: Wiley, 1978: 3–13

5 White D, Clark G, Carson J, White E. Ultrasound in biomedicine: cumulative bibliography of the world literature to 1978. Oxford: Pergamon, 1982

6 Richardson M L F. Apparatus for warning a ship at sea of its nearness to large objects wholly or partly under water. UK patent no. 1125: 1912

7 Ashford O M. Prophet or Professor? The life and work of Lewis Fry Richardson. Bristol/Boston: Adam Hilger, 1985

8 Dussik K T, Dussik F, Wyt L. Auf dem Wege zur Hyperphonographie des Gehirnes. Wien Med Wochenschr 1947; 97: 425–429

9 Rayleigh, 4th Baron (Lord). Life of Lord Rayleigh. London: Edward Arnold, 1924

10 Rayleigh, 3rd Baron (Lord). Theory of sound. London: Macmillan, 1877

11 Curie J, Curie P. Sur l'electricite polaire dans cristaux hemiedres a face inclinees. Compt Rend Seances Acad Sci 1880; 91: 383–389

12 Wood R W, Loomis A L. The physical and biological effects of sound-waves of great intensity. Phil Mag S.7. 1927; 4: 417–436

13 Sokolov S Y. Improvements in and relating to the detection of faults in solid, liquid or gaseous bodies. UK patent no. 477; 139: 1937

14 Hill C R. Ultrasonic imaging: review article. J Phys E 1976; 9: 153–162

15 Howry D H, Bliss W R. Ultrasonic visualization of soft tissue structures of the body. J Lab Clin Med 1952; 40: 579–592

16 Holm H H. Ultrasonic scanning in the diagnosis of space-occupying lesions of the upper abdomen. Br J Radiol 1971; 44: 24–36

17 Hill C R, Carpenter D A. Ultrasonic echo imaging of tissues: instrumentation. Br J Radiol 1976; 49: 238–243

18 Taylor K J W, Hill C R. Scanning techniques in grey scale ultrasonography. Br J Radiol 1975; 48: 918–920

19 Wild J J, Reid J M. Current developments in ultrasonic equipment for medical diagnosis. IRE Trans Ultrasonic Eng 1957; 5: 44–58

20 Edler I, Herz C H. The use of ultrasonic reflectoscope for the continuous recording of movements of heart walls. K Fysiogr Sallsk Lund Forh 1954; 24: 1–19

21 Wild J J, Neal D. Use of high-frequency ultrasonic waves for detecting changes of texture in living tissues. Lancet 1951; i: 655–657

22 Satomura S. A study on examining the heart with ultrasonics: I. Principle; II. Instrument. Jpn Circ J 1956; 20: 227

23 Satomura S. Ultrasonic Doppler method for the inspection of cardiac functions. J Acoust Soc Am 1957; 29: 1181–1185

24 French L A, Wild J J, Neal D. Attempts to determine harmful effects of pulsed ultrasonic vibrations. Cancer 1951; 4: 342–344

25 White D N. The effects of the skull upon the spatial and temporal distribution of a generated and reflected ultrasonic beam. Kingston, Ontario: Ultramedison, 1976

26 White D N. Personal communication, 1989

27 White D N, Carson J, White E. Cumulative bibliography of the world literature 1979–82. Ultrasound Med Biol 1987; 13

28 Donald I, MacVicar J, Brown T G. Investigation of abdominal masses by pulsed ultrasound. Lancet 1958; 1: 1188–1195

29 Mayneord W V. Report for the Physics Department of the Royal Cancer Hospital. In: BECC Annual Report for 1951. London: British Empire Cancer Campaign, 1951

30 Donald I. Sonar – the story of an experiment. Ultrasound Med Biol 1974; 1: 109–117

31 Wild J J. The origin of soft tissue ultrasonic echoing and early instrumental application to clinical medicine. (in press)

32 Bock J, Ossoinig K. Ultrasonographia medica (3 vols) Vienna: Verlag der Wiener Medizinischen Akademie, 1971

33 Melki G. Ultrasonic patterns of tumours of the liver. JCU 1973; 1: 306–314

34 Taylor K J W, Carpenter D A, McCready V R. Grey scale echography in the diagnosis of intrahepatic disease. JCU 1973; 1: 284–287

35 Kossoff G. Improved techniques in ultrasonic cross-sectional echography. Ultrasonics 1972; 10: 221–227

36 Somer J C. Electronic sector scanning for ultrasonic diagnosis. Ultrasonics 1968; 6: 153–159

37 Bom N, Lancee C T, Honkoop J, Hugenholtz P G. Ultrasonic viewer for cross-sectional analyses of moving cardiac structures. Biomed Eng 1971; 6: 500–503, 508

38 McDicken W N, Bruff K, Paton J. An ultrasonic instrument for rapid B-scanning of the heart. Ultrasonics 1974; 12: 269–272

39 Kossoff G, Carpenter D A, Robinson D E, Radovanovich G, Garrett W J. Octoson – a new rapid, general purpose echoscope. In: White D, Barnes R, eds. Ultrasound in medicine 2: New York: Plenum. 333–339

40 Brown T G. Visualization of soft tissues in two and three dimensions – limitations and development. Ultrasonics 1967; 5: 118–124

41 Dunn F, Edmonds P D, Fry W J. Absorption and dispersion of ultrasound in biological media. In: Schwan H P, ed. Biological engineering. New York: McGraw-Hill, 1969

42 Chivers R C. The scattering of ultrasound by human tissues. PhD thesis: University of London, 1973

43 Hill C R, Chivers R C, Huggins R W, Nicholas D. Scattering of ultrasound by human tissue. In: Fry F J, ed. Ultrasound: its applications in medicine and biology. Amsterdam: Elsevier, 1978, 441–493

44 Hill C R, Bamber J C, ter Haar G R. Physical principles of medical ultrasonics, 2nd ed. Chichester: Wiley (in press)

45 Bergmann L. Der Ultraschall. Stuttgart: Hirzel, 1954

46 Hellman L M, Duffus G M, Donald I, Sunden B. Safety of diagnostic ultrasound in obstetrics. Lancet 1970; i: 1133–1135

47 Hill C R. The possibility of hazard in medical and industrial applications of ultrasound (review). Br J Radiol 1968; 41: 561–569

48 Anonymous. Biological effects of ultrasound: mechanisms and clinical implications. NCRP report no. 74. Bethesda: National Council on Radiation Protection and Measurements, 1983

49 Hill C R, ter Haar G R. Ultrasound. In: Suess M J, Benwell-Morison D A, eds. Non-ionizing radiation protection. WHO Regional Publications, European Series, no. 25. Copenhagen: World Health Organization, 1989

50 Hill C R. Ultrasound dosimetry: session summary. In: Reid J M, Sikov M R, eds. Interaction of ultrasound and biological tissues. DHEW publication (FDA) 73-8008. Rockville: US Department of HEW, 1972: 153–158, 159–214 for related papers

51 Anonymous. Future use of new imaging technologies in developing countries. WHO Publication, Technical Report Series no. 723. Copenhagen: World Health Organization, 1985

2

Ultrasound equipment

Roland Blackwell

Introduction

Year by year dramatic claims are made by manufacturers for their latest scanners and many genuine new features have appeared. Machines only 6 years old may well be considered non-diagnostic because diagnostic expectations have risen significantly. Skilled sonographers are in short supply and any design feature that improves ease of interpretation makes the equipment not only more acceptable but also, by reducing user error, safer.

Those who have to spend hundreds of hours scanning know that some machines require little attention to adjustments while others, even among the most modern, seem fussy and time wasting. What is it about images and equipment ergonomics that favours a particular machine?

The related question, 'which is the best machine and probe selection for my purposes?' seems appropriate, but a specific answer is inevitably transient. It is more important for the user to understand the basis of equipment quality and efficiency. This will enable good use to be made of equipment and the most appropriate tool for the job to be selected without being misled by the manufacturers' advertising.

Probe design, digital manipulation of beams and echoes and image processing have been fundamental to the dramatic improvements in image quality that have been achieved recently. Well understood mathematical image processing techniques are not practicable unless the necessary computation can be performed at a speed compatible with the rate at which echoes arrive at the probe. The speed and size of digital components now becoming available are making powerful processing strategies feasible.

In this chapter some aspects of digital manipulation are described and the way they are used in conjunction with probe developments to improve the quality of images is explained in outline.

Features of a diagnostic image

Images that make diagnosis straightforward always have high spatial resolution. Spatial resolution may be loosely taken to mean the ability to see small structures, both along the beam (axial resolution) and across it (lateral resolution). This is important, not only in the centre of the image, but also at the edges. High contrast resolution, the ability to distinguish between different types of tissue, is also crucial. For good contrast resolution, weak echoes must be capable of being displayed at the same time as strong ones without 'noise' and artefacts cluttering the image. Good contrast resolution at depth depends upon the system being sufficiently sensitive for weak echoes to be displayed at all depths of diagnostic importance.

These features depend upon focusing and image forming techniques such as dynamic focusing, aperture control, apodisation, pulse shaping, beam steering, image smoothing and edge enhancement, all of which can best be achieved by digital control. Digitisation, in the context of image processing, will be reviewed before the slightly more complex issue of digital beam control.

Digitisation and storage of echo information

After each ultrasound pulse has been launched into the body, a string of echoes arrive back at the probe where they are turned into a voltage by the transducer (the active element in the probe). The voltage pattern produced by these echoes contains the information required to fill in the grey shaded dots along one line of the image. This voltage pattern could be drawn out as a graph. Just like any other graph, the shape could be recorded as a series of coordinates with the y-axis representing voltage (echo intensity) and the x-axis representing time (equivalent to depth in the body). Given the series of coordinates, the original can be reconstructed. Digitisation is simply the technique of changing the voltage pattern into a series of voltage/time coordinates (Fig. 2.1). For image processing, these values are stored in a computer memory where they are used as the raw data from which the image is modified and later reconstructed for display.

Each computer memory element is essentially a group of electrical switches that can be individually turned on or off under electronic control. The on/off state of each switch is used to represent the binary digits 0 and 1. The computer can write a number into any memory element by setting the switches, or it can read a number from the memory by testing the position of the switches. Thus, a stored binary number can be read as often as desired or it can be changed to a new value.

Measurement of the go-and-return time of the reflected sound pulse requires an extremely accurate timing device. Computers all contain a clock which, like a stopwatch, allows the exact measurement of very small time intervals to be made. It consists of an electronic oscillator that switches a small voltage on and off hundreds of millions of times each second. These voltage pulses are generated with a time accuracy of better than one part in 100 000. The go-and-return interval is represented by the number of clock pulses generated between launch and receipt of the ultrasound pulse. This time, along with the beam direction information, determines the computer address of the pixels to be filled with echo information.

The complete image is stored in computer memory. Each memory element must be filled with a number representing the appropriate echo amplitude. The clock is used to control an analogue-to-digital converter (ADC) which continually reads the echo voltages to be stored. The ADC is an extremely fast voltmeter that reads out each voltage sample as a number. It can obtain an approximate voltage

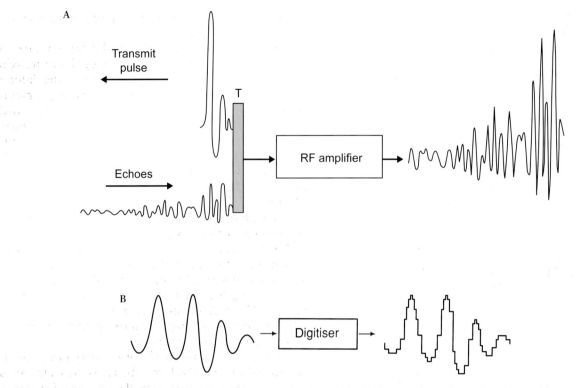

Fig. 2.1 The pulse-echo method. A: The transducer (T) launches a pulse into the body. The returning train of echoes is turned into a voltage pattern corresponding to the sound pressure fluctuations in the echo. The voltage pattern is amplified by a radio frequency amplifier. **B:** The single-echo voltage pattern shown is digitised and appears at the output of the analogue-to-digital converter (digitiser) as a series of voltage steps. The voltage value of each step is stored in digital memory to give a series of coordinates, one being time, the other the voltage, which are later used to reconstruct the image.

reading in about 10 nanoseconds (a rate of 125 million readings per second is used in one machine). This speed enables the radio frequency (rf) voltage signal to be sampled and stored. On the less expensive range of scanners, some smoothing of the signal is first performed to obtain the outline of the echo pulses (Fig. 2.2). This outline is called the 'video' signal, and need only be sampled at a rate of about 4 million readings per second. This less demanding digitisation rate limits processing options but is less expensive to implement.

To turn the stored echo intensity values back into a voltage pattern for display the scan converter uses a device called a digital-to-analogue converter (DAC). This 'reads' each stored number and immediately generates a voltage corresponding to it. By presenting the stored values in

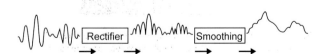

Fig. 2.2 Rectification. The echo voltage signal is sometimes turned into a 'video' signal before digitisation. The negative voltage portions of the waveform are inverted by a rectifier and the envelope of the fluctuations, produced by smoothing, forms the video waveform.

rapid succession to the DAC, a waveform that mimics the original voltage pattern is produced. This can be long after the echoes were recorded.

Accurate digitisation at very high rates, as required by digital beam forming techniques, is difficult. However, a relatively low precision can be tolerated for the process of displaying echo amplitudes. This is because the number of brightness levels that can be displayed on a video screen is many times fewer than the range of echo amplitudes in a typical scan, so echoes with similar amplitudes are all displayed with an identical shade of grey.

The precision to which a voltage reading is recorded is given by the number of significant figures used. Recording, say, 1.3561 V is no more useful than the less precise 1.4 V if the shade of grey is the same at both of these voltages anyway. Computers handle numbers using the binary system. For recording echo voltages, up to 16 binary digits or bits (**BI**nary digi**TS**) are used. For display, eight bits gives 256 shades of grey which is adequate for image interpretation.[1]

The number of bits used to record a voltage is called the word length. The more bits used the more closely the original intensity fluctuations can be followed (Fig. 2.3). Most mid-range scanners record an eight-bit word but

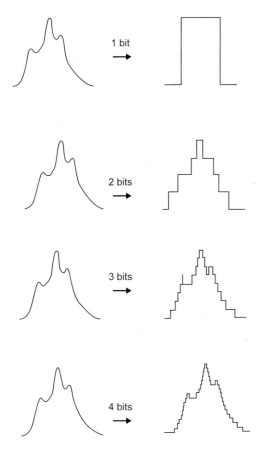

Fig. 2.3 Digitisation. A small portion of video signal is shown alongside the output which is produced after digitisation using different word lengths. When only one bit is used, all voltage samples below a certain value are recorded as 0 (displayed as black) and those above this value are recorded as the digit 1 (displayed as white), producing a bistable image. The shape of the video waveform is recorded more faithfully with intermediate greys as the number of bits used increases.

then use only six bits for display. If complex image processing is to be undertaken the greater word length is required to avoid significant rounding errors when numerical procedures are performed. High-performance machines may use up to a 16-bit word, particularly for beam forming purposes.

Scan conversion

In clinical practice, the obvious choice for image display and storage is in video format. Video monitors, tape recorders, discs and imagers all have remarkably high quality and are inexpensive.

Ultrasound images are built up from a number of vertical or radial lines generated at a rate limited by the speed of sound in the body. The video image, however, is built up from horizontal lines generated at a rate suitable for television transmission. A device is required which will enable an image to be stored in the ultrasound scan format but

displayed in the video format. A digital scan converter performs this conversion.

The scan converter is made up of a large number of computer memory elements which store the entire echo information for the image in digital form. This information is used to produce an image comprising a mosaic of tiny rectangular picture elements, called pixels. Each memory element has an 'address' that relates it to a corresponding pixel in the image. The address where the value of the echo amplitude is to be stored is determined by the direction from which the echo originates and the time taken for the go–return passage of the ultrasound pulse. The stored information enables the appropriate shade of grey to be displayed in each pixel after the stored value is converted back to a voltage.

The scan converter contains enough memory elements to match one to each pixel in the image (Fig. 2.4). There are usually at least 512 pixels across the image and 512 down making 262 144 in all. This arrangement is referred to as a 512×512 memory matrix or memory plane. The addresses may be arranged to identify pixels in columns down and rows across the image.

Consider the formation of a linear array image. As the voltage values from the first pulse arrive they are stored, one to a memory element, in the column of addresses

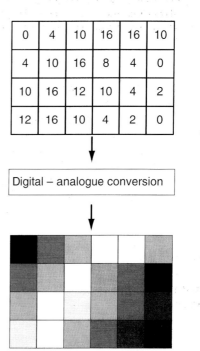

Fig. 2.4 Digital memory. The memory is like a set of addressed 'pigeonholes', each containing the voltage value corresponding to part of the image. A small section of memory elements is shown with the corresponding image pixels, each of which displays a grey level determined by the number in the memory cell. The number in the memory element is translated by the digital-to-analogue converter to a voltage to produce the display.

relating to the first image line. The values from the second ultrasound pulse are stored in the second column of addresses and so on until the memory addresses for the entire image frame are full up. When the memory is full the video system reads out and displays the first video line. This is formed from the values stored in the top row of addresses. The next row is fed out for the next video line and so on until the video image frame is complete.

A real-time ultrasound scanner presents new image frames one after another to produce the real-time effect. Having produced the first frame, the second and subsequent frames can be stored using the same memory elements. As the values for the first column of the second frame are obtained they overwrite the values that are already stored in the memory. The overwriting process continues, line by line, to produce the next frame. It is not essential to wait until the frame is completely overwritten before rows of values for the video display are read out – both read and write processes can proceed together.

Digital processing

Frame freeze

Frame freeze enables a single frame to be examined or a structure measured using the on-screen calipers. The freeze mechanism is simply a mechanical switch that stops new echo values overwriting those already stored. The same stored values are read out time and time again onto the video display. Unfreezing the image restores the overwrite process.

Smoothing the image

The video lines, scan lines and other visible features caused by the scanning process are called 'structured noise', and should be reduced to a minimum by image processing.

A typical linear array is about 10 cm in length and produces, say, 125 ultrasound lines. However, there are likely to be 512 pixels or more in each row across the image to be filled up with echo information. In this case, there is only one echo value available for every 4 pixels across the screen. If the empty pixels are not filled in, an image with obvious gaps between the vertical lines is displayed. The 3 empty pixels between those receiving data can be filled with calculated values. Using the recorded values in the pixels either side of the empty ones, calculated values can be graded to give a smooth transition from one measured value to the next (Fig. 2.5). This process is called 'line interpolation'.

When recording a sector scan a more complex problem is encountered. The directions of the ultrasound vectors cross the grid of pixels at an angle so that some pixels never receive a value, while others have the vector clip the corner of the pixel leaving little time for a voltage value to

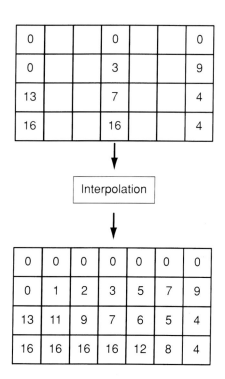

Fig. 2.5 Spatial smoothing. A small section of memory is shown in the upper part of the diagram. The linear array produces only enough echo information to fill every third column. The computer calculates values so that the empty columns are filled with interpolated echo amplitudes.

be obtained. Still others have the ultrasound vector cross the pixel diagonal so that many values of echo voltage are generated for that pixel (Fig. 2.6). A design strategy has to be adopted on how to use the digitised data. The voltage value actually recorded for the pixel may be the largest, smallest or some sort of average of the digitised voltages.

If nothing is done about the empty pixels, a series of black spots appears over the image, as if pepper had been sprinkled on it. These spots are called 'drop-out'. The strategy used to smooth drop-out gives a distinctive appearance to the scan. One solution is to adapt the size of the pixels so that some are square and others are oblong, the shape being chosen to ensure that the ultrasound vector always passes through the middle of the cell. The vertical spacing of the pixels may also be chosen so that they always fall on video lines. This technique makes good use of all available information but, unless further processing is undertaken, produces a slightly 'smeared' appearance to the image in the deep part of the scan where the scan lines are diverging significantly.

There are other strategies that can be used. One is the 'moving nine point average' smoothing technique. In this process a complete frame is stored and then smoothed by replacing the value in each pixel by the average of that value and its eight surrounding neighbours. This smoothing strategy can produce visually pleasing results. Other variants use matrix convolution to produce images with,

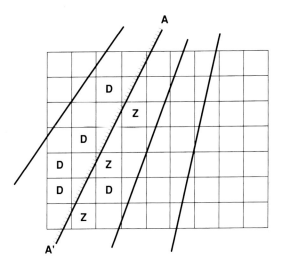

Fig. 2.6 Image smoothing. The diagram illustrates the way in which the axes of several consecutive ultrasound beams cross the corresponding pixels in the image. One vector (line A–A′) has time intervals marked on it indicating the instants at which digitisation takes place. As the vector crosses the corners of the pixels marked Z, it remains within the pixel for too short a time for the voltage to be measured. Similarly, the pixels marked D are not entered at all by the ultrasound vector. Conversely, many pixels have the ultrasound vectors cross them in such a way that there are a substantial number of voltage readings, and a representative reading must be stored for these memory locations.

for instance, sharpened outlines (edge enhancement) to make measurements easier.[2]

Smoothing out coherent radiation speckle (frame averaging)

The limit of axial resolution for a scanner is about half the pulse length and for lateral resolution is equal to the width of the beam across which, after processing, the structure can be detected, i.e. the 'effective' beam width (Fig. 2.7). In practice, the resolution of parenchymal echoes appears to be better than the theoretical limit of resolution. The reason is that parenchymal tissue gives rise to small echoes that are so close together that they interfere with each other and generate a random pattern (Fig. 2.8). There is a loss of the 'one-to-one' correspondence between the tissues and the image. This 'tissue texture' pattern is called 'coherent radiation speckle'. It must be remembered that

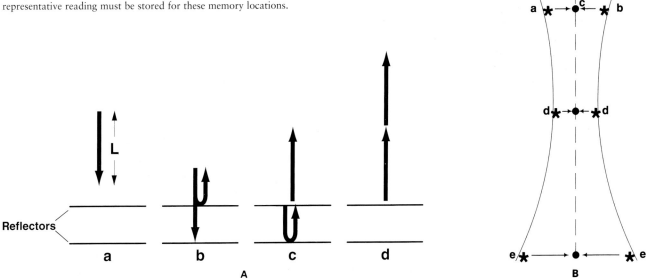

Fig. 2.7 Spatial resolution. A: Axial resolution. Two reflecting surfaces are separated by half of the pulse length. The diagram suggests that this is the limit of axial resolution. The broad arrows represent the physical length of an ultrasound pulse which, in (a), is travelling towards the two reflecting surfaces. In (b) the pulse is crossing the first surface and has just reached the second. An echo, half a pulse length in extent, has already been reflected from the first surface. In (c) an echo of the entire pulse length has been reflected from the first surface and the transmitted energy has now been reflected from the second surface and follows the first echo. In (d) both echoes are travelling back towards the transducer and the head of the second echo just touches the tail of the first echo. This is the condition required for the two surfaces to be resolved. **B:** Lateral (azimuthal) resolution. A reflector detected anywhere within the beam is displayed as if it was on the axis of the beam. Thus, reflectors a and b (*) are displayed as if they were situated at c and only show as a single echo (i.e. they will not be resolved as separate structures). Lateral resolution is equal to the effective (processed) beam width and is best at the focus (d–d) and worst where the beam is widest (e–e). **C:** As a beam is swept in the direction of the arrow across a small reflector (*) a line (L) is displayed instead of the ideal spot (S). Sections 1–5 illustrate the beam at the point where the reflector is situated. In 1 the beam has just reached the reflector, which is displayed on the axis of the beam (a). In 2 the reflector is nearer to the position where it is actually displayed, while in 3 the reflector is on the axis and is displayed in its correct position. As the beam moves still further across the reflector (4 and 5), the error increases in the opposite direction. The result is that a point reflector is displayed as a line (L) which has the same length as the effective beam width.

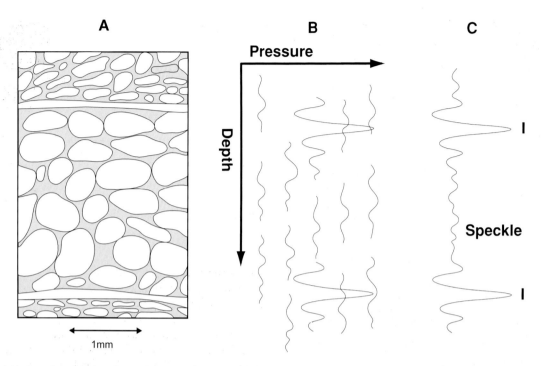

A   **B**   **C**

Pressure

Depth

Speckle

1mm

Fig. 2.8 Production of speckle. A: The small interfaces in this section of tissue each give rise to a scattered echo which arrives at the probe before the previous echo has died away. **B:** These reflected pressure waves are from a single pulse. For clarity they are drawn staggered across the page to show their relationship. (Each wavelet is oscillating around a zero pressure, i.e. the waves to the right are not at higher pressures.) As the pressure waves overlap, interference occurs. At some positions the echoes cancel out and at others they reinforce, and **C:** a random pressure pattern, called coherent speckle, is produced. The large echoes (I) from the boundaries to the central region are correctly identified, but the correspondence between 'an echo' displayed on the image and the presence of a reflecting structure in the tissue is lost in the regions where significant interference occurs.

the texture does not necessarily relate to the physical texture of the tissue.

In some diagnostic situations the ability to determine small changes in the reflectivity of tissues is essential. In these cases the speckle pattern can be obtrusive. The speckle pattern may be smoothed out to leave an impression of the overall reflectivity of the tissue. Smoothing relies on small movements of the speckle pattern as the tissue is moved by cardiac or muscular action or as the probe is moved. Although the speckle pattern moves, the general brightness of the region does not change. Thus, if successive frames are superimposed, the movement averages out the speckle but leaves the average brightness of an area on the display. The way the speckle pattern moves has itself been used as an indication of pathology by 'elastography'.[3]

For this smoothing technique a number of identical computer frame store memories, perhaps nine, have to be provided. The first frame is stored in the first memory in the usual way. The second frame does not overwrite the first, but is stored separately in the second memory, the third in the third and so on until the eighth frame has been stored. The value of the echo in the first pixel in each frame store is now averaged and the result stored in the first pixel of the ninth memory. Similarly, the series of echoes in all the second pixel addresses are averaged and

stored in the second pixel of the ninth memory and so on until all of the elements in the ninth memory are full. This ninth frame store is then read out to give the video information for display. Subsequent frames sequentially overwrite the eight originally stored, the values for the displayed ninth store being recalculated as each new frame is stored. A common variant calculates a weighted average value for each pixel so that the most recent frame has a greater influence on the image.

The initial phase of any clinical ultrasound examination requires a rapid survey of the structures of interest. Frame averaging is only meaningful when the slice to be averaged is identical in each frame. If the probe or tissues are moving rapidly (e.g. when imaging the heart), different sections are averaged together and result in an unhelpful smeared image. If detailed study of small changes in tissue reflectivity is not required, the frame averaging should be turned off.

Volume and three-dimensional scanning

The reduction in the cost of computer memories has made it realistic to use many frame stores. This has made it possible to take sequential images through a large number of anatomical planes and store them all. An image can then be

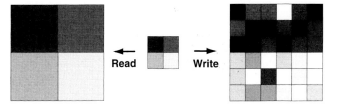

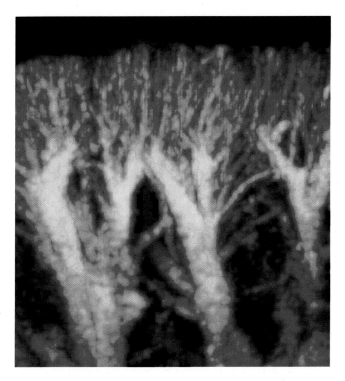

Fig. 2.9 In this image the vessels in the renal cortex are displayed with the impression of depth. A series of parallel scans provide the data to enable display of the vessels from any desired angle. (Picture by kind permission of ATL UK Ltd.)

Fig. 2.10 Zoom. The four pixels in the centre of the diagram represent part of the image which is to be enlarged by the zoom control. 'Zoom on read' is achieved by displaying each pixel larger than it was originally. There is no new information presented. In 'zoom on write' the pixels are the original size but more of them are used to display the section of the original image. There is a consequent increase in displayed information.

reconstructed in any desired plane, even those which were not originally scanned (Fig. 2.9). A related technique is the combination of echoes from many planes selected by application of appropriate rules to produce a three-dimensional representation of anatomical structures such as the prostate, the fetal heart or the intraluminal architecture of blood vessels.[4] A developing area is the automatic estimation of the volume of organs from the three-dimensional data set.[5–8]

Zoom

An area of the scan can be magnified on the display by the use of the zoom control. There are two types of zoom (Fig. 2.10). Read zoom is used to enlarge a frozen image and write zoom is used to enlarge the display magnification while scanning is taking place.

In read zoom, grey level values are read from only a small part of the computer memory and the pixels are displayed larger. The effect is rather like taking a magnifying glass to the image. If the magnification scale factor is too large the image matrix becomes rather obvious and the grainy effect becomes obtrusive.

In write zoom, use is made of the fact that digitised echo samples are usually received fast enough for several samples to occur in each pixel. When this is the case, the image scale may be enlarged up to the point when only one sample occurs in each pixel. The amount of tissue represented by each pixel is decreased but the displayed dimensions of each pixel are unchanged. Thus, there is magnification without loss of definition.

As the scale factors are increased there is a larger space between the scan lines so that further interpolation and smoothing may be required to maintain an acceptable image. It is possible, using sophisticated signal processing, to introduce more real scan lines so that definition is improved (see below, 'Focus on receive').

Recording the image (gamma correction)

When a film record (or other medium) of a scan is viewed, it should look just like the image that was seen on the screen. This situation is difficult to achieve because the eye can respond to a huge range of brightness levels, but film has a far more limited range (Fig. 2.11). Film density swings from black to white over a small range of subject brightness so that a direct photograph of the display screen results in a film with a loss of grey levels. To achieve an acceptable recording, it is necessary to photograph an image in which the change in greys is limited by compression of the contrast so that a rather 'muddy-looking' image is photographed.

The scan converter can perform a process rather like 'painting by numbers', each stored voltage value representing an arbitrary shade of grey. A child who drops the painting-by-numbers box and gets the colours muddled up can still paint a consistent, if somewhat strange, picture. The stored values of voltage can similarly be changed by an electronic 'look up' table before they are fed to the DAC. With look up tables the stored values can be used to generate simultaneously one image for viewing and another for display on the camera tube or laser imager. This process is called gamma correction, the gamma characteristic being the name given to the plot of the film response to different light levels.

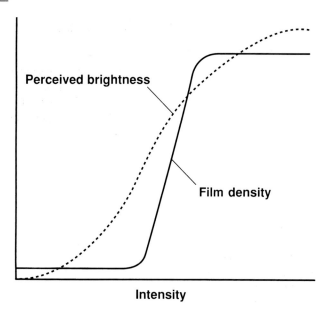

Fig. 2.11 Gamma correction. The eye can perceive a range of brightness of over 100 000 000 to 1 (dashed line). Conversely, exposed film changes from clear to maximum density over a relatively small range of brightness (solid line). The contrast of the image must be reduced to match the film characteristic if the film image is to look like the display seen directly on the screen.

Post-processing

The facility to change the displayed grey shade assigned to each echo amplitude also enables the contrast and brightness of the viewed image to be altered after storage in the memory. This is only useful if the image was originally stored with an adequate word length. Post-processing implies that the image is modified after storing it in the memory.

The range of echo intensities coming from the tissues (the signal dynamic range) may be extremely large, typically 100 dB (i.e. the amplitude of the strongest echo voltage is 100 000 times that of the weakest). Roughly half of this range is attributable to the attenuation of the pulse intensity as it travels into the tissue, and may be compensated for by the time-gain compensation (TGC) function. The other half results from the change in tissue reflectivity which is an important feature mapped in the ultrasound image. Even assuming that the time-gain compensation TGC was set perfectly, the strongest reflection from a soft tissue interface gives a stored voltage about 300 times bigger than the smallest. A video display screen is limited in the range of brightnesses it can display, so the large range of reflectivities to be displayed results in loss of information. In some way the echo information must be compressed before it is displayed. A compression characteristic is chosen, using a front panel control, to emphasise the diagnostic feature of interest.

If linear compression is chosen, the echo amplitude is allowed to increase substantially before a change in grey shade is registered on the display (Fig. 2.12). This is particularly appropriate if outlines, showing the shape and size of organs, are to be measured. If, however, it is the small variations in reflectivity of tissues that are diagnostically important, then these need to produce a detectable change in grey on the display. In this case it is usual to display all large echoes, perhaps half the total range, as white. The remaining echoes are graded so that small variations in reflectivity give noticeable changes in grey. The changes that are important may be among the smallest echoes, in which case a logarithmic characteristic is used. To emphasise mid-range echoes a sigmoid characteristic ('S' curve) is appropriate. Selection of the best characteristic to use has a strong subjective element because individual perception of detail varies from one person to another and there may be no 'correct' setting.

Analogue processing

Pre-processing

Before a series of echoes is stored some signal processing usually takes place. This is termed pre-processing. The exact functions performed before or after storage vary slightly from machine to machine. TGC is usually per-

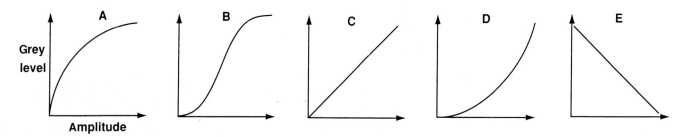

Fig. 2.12 Compression. Compression characteristics show how the grey tone of an echo displayed on the image varies with the echo amplitude. Characteristics are usually a variant of one of five types. **A:** A logarithmic curve which emphasises changes in small echoes. **B:** A sigmoid curve which suppresses the smallest echoes but emphasises changes in mid-range echoes. **C:** A linear characteristic where the input amplitudes are evenly distributed across the available grey tones. **D:** An exponential characteristic which gives heavy emphasis to outlines. **E:** Characteristics with a negative slope reverse black and white on the image (this may be necessary for photographic recording).

formed as a pre-storage function, and radio frequency digitisation is obviously performed before storage.

Automatic time-gain compensation

As a sound pulse progresses though tissues, it loses energy. Some is scattered out of the beam, like a car headlight trying to penetrate fog. Some is turned into heat by absorption and relaxation processes. The whole process is termed attenuation, and is directly proportional to frequency in the diagnostic frequency range.

The TGC compensates for this attenuation in such a way that echoes from identical structures, whether superficial or deep, appear equally reflective. Echoes from deep structures are amplified more strongly than those from superficial structures. This can be controlled by the user who manipulates a series of sliders controlling the gain at each depth until the image looks 'right'. Accurate adjustment of the TGC characteristics has always been a source of difficulty for inexperienced operators. To obtain an automatically compensated scan is very desirable. There are several successful designs of automatic TGC[9] but there are also some that introduce artefacts in the region beyond large fluid spaces, such as *liquor amnii*, the bladder or gallbladder.

In essence, automatic TGC is based upon detection of the fall of echo intensity along each ultrasound line. By smoothing out the rapid fluctuations due to the changes in reflectivity, an approximation to the shape of the attenuation profile is obtained. When inverted, the profile gives the ideal shape for the TGC characteristic (Fig. 2.13). The averaging may take place over just one line, by using one line to correct the next, or by strategies that use the information contained in an entire frame.

Edge enhancement and phase-sensitive processing

To achieve good axial resolution, well-defined echoes must be displayed. Echo definition may be enhanced in some clinically important measurement and visualisation situations. This is achieved by processing the echo voltages so that the sharp upswing of a relatively intense echo from the wall of a structure is artificially enhanced before the echo is stored (differentiate and add techniques). This is called edge enhancement.

The phase of the pressure fluctuations in an echo is altered by the relative densities of the two tissues forming the reflecting surface. By making use of ultrafast processing circuitry this phase condition can be detected. An image in which the phase change is detected is sensitive to the direction of density variation changes and enables structures spaced closely in the lateral direction to be more clearly differentiated.

Digital beam control

Uncertainty in the position of echo origin

The major problem in generating an image is to know the exact origin of each echo. The range of an echo is determined from the time delay from launching a pulse and its subsequent arrival back at the transducer. The round trip distance is derived from the product of the time delay and the speed of sound. There is a variation of some 5% in the speed of sound in soft tissues either side of the weighted average value of $1540\ ms^{-1}$ which is the value used in the design of most scanners.[10] Consequently, there is an

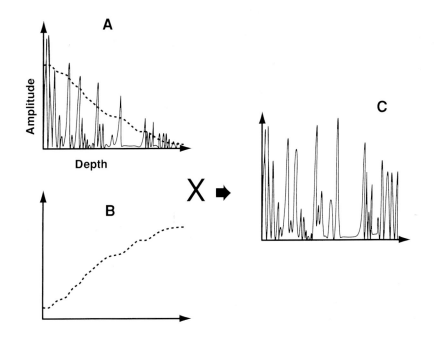

Fig. 2.13 Automatic TGC. A: Attenuation results in deep echoes having progressively less intensity. The average rate of decrease (dotted line) of the voltage produced by the echoes is measured at every instant to define a decay characteristic. B: The decay characteristic is inverted (i.e. the reciprocal of each voltage value is derived) to give the 'ideal' TGC characteristic. C: The original echo amplitudes are multiplied by the TGC values to give automatically corrected amplitudes.

uncertainty in determining the depth from which an echo originated. The resulting image distortion is usually imperceptible and cannot be corrected for unless a sound velocity map is first produced (velocity maps have been used experimentally where 360° anatomical access is possible, such as with breast scanning).[11]

Of greater significance is the uncertainty in the direction from which an echo originates. The direction is conventionally taken to be along the axis of the beam as it leaves the probe, but echoes, in fact, occur from anywhere across the beam which is disturbingly wide over much of its path and also suffers small degrees of refraction. An echo from one side of the beam will be displayed at exactly the same point as a similar echo from the other side (Fig. 2.7). This makes for inherently poor lateral resolution. The fact that the beam is most intense along its axis helps to give reasonable results because axial echoes will be most intense. The beam intensity and the probe sensitivity patterns must be multiplied together to obtain the overall response. This accentuates the high-intensity region and narrows the effective beam width. However, active improvements through focusing are necessary for high-quality images. The beam may be focused electronically, both on send and receive.

Grating lobes

A related problem is caused by grating lobes. These are low-intensity beams generated at an angle to the main beam from all array probes (the acoustic analogue of diffracted beams from an optical diffraction grating). Although of low intensity, strong reflectors situated in a grating lobe give echoes that are easily detected. These are erroneously displayed as if they came from the axis of the main beam, though the true origin may be a substantial distance away. Grating lobe artefacts limit the maximum amplification factor that can be used. The amplification needs to be as high as possible to boost small echoes to a size that can be displayed. If the amplification is too high, the resulting grating lobe artefacts from strong reflectors introduce unacceptable amounts of noise. The artefact can be significantly reduced by a technique called apodisation (see below). If apodisation is used, a much wider range of echo amplitudes can be displayed (Fig. 2.14).

Synthetic aperture techniques

Array probes can be made to behave as though they had a flexible shape, focusing and directing the beam in unexpected ways. Thus, an 'aperture' is synthesised.

Wave interference

Fundamental to the technique is the way in which sound waves interact with each other. Sound is a longitudinal compression wave. Any small volume of tissue in the beam

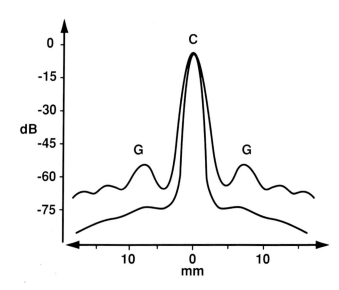

Fig. 2.14 Apodisation. The figure shows how the relative intensity of two beams varies from one side of the beam to the other. The large peak is the main lobe with the central axis at C. The upper trace has prominent grating lobes (G). When apodisation is applied (lower trace) the grating lobes are heavily suppressed.

contains an excess of molecules during the high-pressure phase of the wave and a reduction during the low-pressure phase. Two ultrasound transducers, separated by a small distance but operating at the same frequency and amplitude, give rise to waves that cross each other. A small volume of tissue, situated where the pressure peaks coincide, receives an excess of molecules from one wave and a further excess from the other. Consequently, the amplitude of the pressure wave in this volume is doubled. Conversely, a volume of tissue, situated where a pressure peak and trough coincide, experiences an increase in molecules from one source and a reduction from the other, leaving the net number of molecules in the volume unchanged. Thus, the pressure waves cancel out. All intermediate situations exist.

A row of small sound sources can generate a wavefront (a region where all of the molecules move synchronously), in a direction tangential to the waves from each transducer at the points where reinforcement occurs by wave interference (Fig. 2.15). A beam always propagates in a direction at right angles to the wavefront.

Groups of transducer elements

Highly directional beams of ultrasound are produced by wave interference, but the necessary conditions for interference can only be achieved if the transducer is large compared to the wavelength. An equivalent size transducer can be approximated by grouping a number of narrow transducer elements and triggering them all together. Array transducers are made from a sheet of piezoelectric material that has been cut into small elements. A wire connects

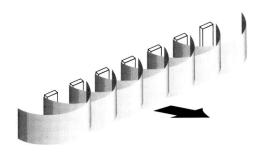

Fig. 2.15 Wavefront from an array. Each element in the array produces a sound wave at the same moment. The wavelet from each element spreads out and crosses the wavelets from the other elements. At the crossing points, constructive interference occurs and reinforces the wave. The waves combine as shown to produce a wavefront which propagates as a beam in the direction of the arrow. In other directions there is cancellation due to destructive interference.

to each element, and the number of elements selected in the group can be changed by electronic switches. The number of elements selected in a group, and the timing and processing of the voltages on each element, is the basis of synthetic aperture techniques.

Channels

For array transducers to achieve their full potential, each element must be accessed by its own electronic circuit. In one arrangement, a wire connects the transducer element to a voltage generator which energises it after the voltage passes through an attenuator and a delay. Another wire connects to an amplifier and a delay to form the receiving side. The whole system connecting to each element is called a channel (Fig. 2.16). Every component in a channel may be adjusted independently and instantaneously by

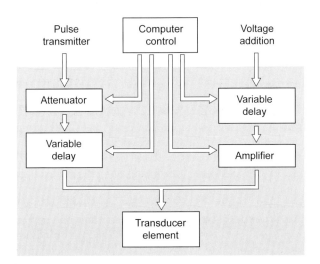

Fig. 2.16 Array channel. An arrangement of computer-controlled electronic components of a channel is shown in the shaded area of the diagram. For dynamic focusing and apodisation, and for beam steering, each transducer element in the group is connected to a channel.

computer control. To economise, many scanners use fewer channels than there are elements by switching groups of elements into the channels as required.

On the pulse generation side, the pulser generates the trigger voltage that makes each element vibrate. Older machines used shock excitation in which a voltage spike of about 500 V was applied to the element for perhaps one-tenth of a microsecond and the transducer 'rang' at its natural frequency. In recent designs, the transducer may be driven with an exact waveform. The attenuator can reduce the voltage that reaches the transducer element and controls the output power. Delays are devices, in principle, which pass a voltage pattern, unchanged in shape, from the input to the output, but with a small, but controllable, time delay between the signal entering and emerging.

On the echo reception side the amplifier is a radio-frequency amplifier whose amplification factor can be varied. The delay performs the same function as on the send side.

Apodisation

Grating lobes can be suppressed by apodisation. In this technique, elements at the outer edges of a transducer group in the array are energised less strongly than the central elements. Similarly, if the echo voltage is amplified less by the amplifiers connected to the outer elements then the echoes received from the residual grating lobes are reduced further. Apodisation enables the dynamic range displayed to be increased, facilitating the ability to display small changes in tissue reflectivity. The consequent improvement in contrast resolution has considerable diagnostic advantage.

Phased array scanners

Phased array scanners produce a sector scan by steering the beam electronically. This has the advantage over mechanical sector scanners that there are no moving parts to wear out and, more significantly, that the beam can be switched instantly to any direction without passing through the intermediate scan line directions. This facility makes it possible to produce Doppler displays, or time-position traces, simultaneously with an image. The pulses producing the Doppler spectral display or time-position can be interleaved with image lines sufficiently fast for the two to be displayed together.

A phased array probe contains a large number (commonly 128) of narrow transducer elements. There is a small time delay between the application of the trigger pulse to each element (Fig. 2.17). The wavefront from each element is circular because the elements are small compared to the wavelength. The wave from the first element to be triggered has time to propagate further than the wave from the adjacent element, which is triggered

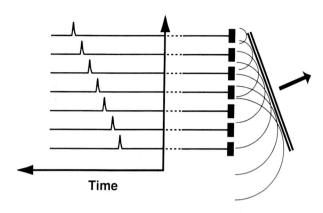

Fig. 2.17 Electronic beam steering. A few transducer elements from a phased array probe are portrayed along with a timing diagram showing the time delays between the trigger pulses applied to each element. The waves propagating from the lower elements have time to travel further than those from the upper elements. The interference between the waves causes the wavefront to be at an angle to the probe face. The pulse travels in a direction determined by the delays.

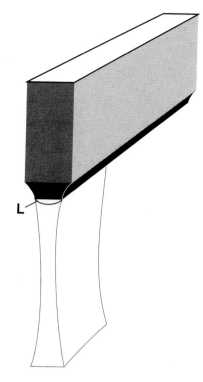

Fig. 2.18 Orthogonal focusing. A cylindrical lens along the face of a linear array focuses the beam in a direction at right angles to the scan plane. The consequent reduction in the beam width reduces the slice thickness, thus improving the 'partial volume' artefact.

fractionally later. The wave from the second element, in turn, propagates further than its neighbour and so on.

Because the composite wavefront is tangential to the wavelets, the result is that the ultrasound pulse propagates at an angle to the probe face. The angle of propagation is dependent only upon the time delay between trigger pulses. This time delay is altered for each new ultrasound pulse so that the beam angle changes to give the required 'windscreen wiper' sector scanning action.

When the beam is steered to angles greater than about 30° to the probe axis, the first cycle of the pressure wave from one of the last elements to be triggered may interfere with the second cycle from one of the elements triggered first. This particular interference results in a relatively intense grating lobe, the direction of which is at a large angle to the primary beam and so may cause significant artefacts.

Focusing

Weakly focused lenses on single element transducers in mechanical sector scanners are used to narrow the beam over the central part of the image at the focal depth. However, mechanical lenses are fixed focus, improving the image in the focal region but degrading it further away.

It is not obvious how the beams from linear and phased array probes could be focused. In this case cylindrical lenses can be used to focus the beam, but only at right angles to the scanning plane (Fig. 2.18). This reduces the slice thickness of the scan in the focal region, which is desirable because images improve in both contrast and spatial resolution with reduced slice thickness.

Electronic focus 'on send'

An electronic focusing technique is required to bring the beams from array scanners to a focus in the image plane, again using the wave interference principle. The beam is produced by an electronically selected group of elements in the array, the channels being used so that the trigger pulses to the inner elements are delayed with respect to the pulses applied to those further out. The circular wavefronts from the outer elements have time to propagate further than the waves from the inner elements. By constructive interference, the resulting wavefront will be curved (Fig. 2.19).

The beam propagates at right angles to the curved wavefront which brings the beam to a focus. Adjustment of the values of the delays applied to the trigger pulses changes the curvature of the wavefront and alters the focal depth. As the selection of the group of elements producing the pulse move along the probe, the delays are changed accordingly. The focal depth can be selected by the user.

It is often desirable to focus at more than one depth in each image. This can be achieved by building up the scan in strips, or zones, with the focus centred on each strip in turn. The delays are adjusted under computer control so that the focus is first set close to the probe. All echoes occurring beyond the focal zone are rejected by an electronic 'range gate' and are not stored in memory. Having

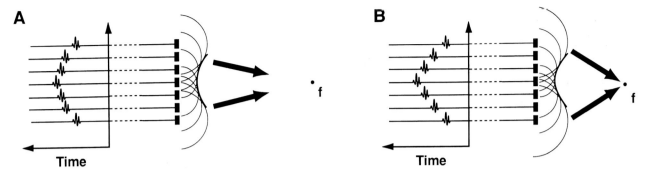

Fig. 2.19 Electronic focusing. A small group of transducer elements is shown with a timing diagram of the trigger pulses applied to each element. The outer elements are triggered first so that the wave has time to propagate further than the waves from the inner elements. Interference effects cause the wavefront to be curved and the pulse propagates toward a focal area, f. In **A**: the time delays between the trigger pulses are smaller than in **B**: so the focus is further from the probe.

collected the echoes for the first strip, the delays are reset to give a deeper focus. The next zone starts at the depth at which the first zone cuts off and ends beyond the new focal point. The process is repeated to collect successively deeper strips until the image is complete.

The disadvantage of this technique is that the image frame rate is slowed down, making it more difficult to follow moving structures. (However, the video display frame rate is maintained so that flicker is eliminated.) It is of some concern that the total sound energy deposited in the scanned tissues is increased but, conversely, the improved resolution may significantly reduce the total scanning time required to reach a diagnosis.

With modern multi-frequency probes, the frame rate can be increased substantially by sending out a second pulse before all the echoes from the previous one have been collected.[12] The image is built up as a patchwork of areas. Thus, say, the first pulse may interrogate the top left part of the image. Almost immediately the second pulse can be launched from the middle of the probe and produce the information for a deeper part of the image. The physical separation of the two pulses means that there is little interference from late echoes from the first pulse interfering with those from the second pulse. Separation of interfering echoes can be enhanced further by generating the second pulse at a different frequency from the first and changing the tuning of the receiver amplifiers to detect the second pulse and reject the remnants of the first. The sequence can be optimised to maximise the frame rate and minimise interference.

Dynamic slice thickness focusing

A simple dynamic focus in the plane at right angles to the image plane is now available for linear and phased arrays. Each transducer element is divided into three or more sections. The trigger pulses to the inner sections are delayed with respect to the outer sections resulting in a relatively coarse, but variable, focus that reduces slice width.[12] Probe

technology is improving rapidly, and it is expected that much better dynamic slice width focusing will soon be available.

Annular arrays

Focusing techniques may also be applied to annular array probes. Annular arrays have the potential for producing excellent spatial resolution because focusing is achieved equally both in the image plane and across it (i.e. in both scanned and orthogonal planes). The shape of the beam is conical rather than the wedge shape produced by linear and phased arrays. These probes are constructed from a series of concentric ring-shaped transducers fitting around a small disc at the core. For annular array transducers to achieve their full potential they need a relatively large diameter and many rings. However, the beam cannot now be steered electronically. The mechanical problems of scanning the beam by oscillating a large array with all its electrical connections are considerable. Some instruments keep the array stationary and reflect the beam into the patient from an oscillating acoustic mirror.

'Focus on receive'

The scanner can be continuously refocused during the passage of the pulse, like refocusing a pair of binoculars to follow a race, to track the position from which echoes are being received. This gives a beam that is well focused at all points from only a single pulse. It is achieved by computer control of the channels as the echoes are received.

All elements on the array receive some of the sound energy from each echo, but at slightly different times. A reflector will produce an echo that is detected first by the nearest element in the array and at slightly later times by elements at a greater distance (Fig. 2.20). If the echo voltages from all of the elements are added together as they arrive, the time differences between them result in interference and loss of intensity.

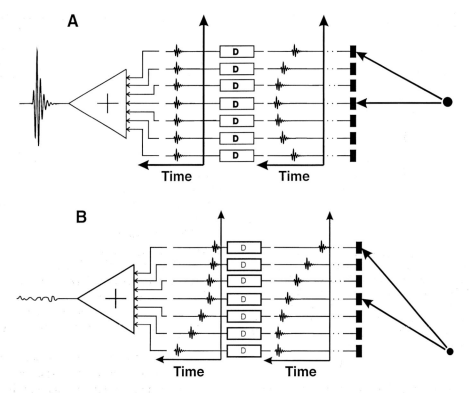

Fig. 2.20 Receive focusing. A: There is a reflector on the axis of the beam. It takes longer for the echo to reach the outer elements than the central element. The timing diagram of the arrival of the echo at each element is shown. The voltages are passed through delays which bring the waves back into phase. When the waves are summed a large echo voltage is produced. **B:** The reflector is off-axis. The relative arrival times at the elements is now different. The same delays are applied as in (A) but this moves the echo voltages further out of phase so that no 'in phase' voltage summation occurs and low-level noise results.

A correction for the time delays can be made assuming that the echoes came from the axis of the beam. The distance from an on-axis reflector to each element in the array can be calculated for reflectors at any depth. Because the speed of sound in tissues is fairly constant, the expected time delays between the reception of the echoes can be estimated. The echo voltages at each of the elements can then be synchronised by a computer that adjusts the delays in each channel. After synchronisation, the voltages are summed and result in a large signal.

If the echo did not originate on the beam axis, the delays, which have been calculated for an on-axis echo, will not synchronise the signals: summing produces only a low intensity randomly fluctuating voltage. Thus, on-axis echoes will be preferentially amplified. This is the same result as achieved by focusing with a fixed lens.

As the ultrasound pulse moves into the body, the delays are constantly recalculated to give a focal point that moves to coincide with the depth where echoes are currently originating. This gives real-time focal tracking. In general, the more channels there are in the array the more accurately the beam can be focused. The complexity and cost of equipment rises with the number of channels, but the additional image quality is impressive.

Dynamic aperture and f number

Photographers are familiar with the fact that a large lens aperture enables a photograph to be strongly focused on a subject in the middle foreground. The same considerations apply to ultrasound scanning. In optics, the focal length divided by the aperture is the familiar unit known as the 'f number'. The same term is used in ultrasound. The width of the beam at the focus determines the lateral resolving power of the system and is calculated (approximately) as the product of the wavelength and the f number.[13]

The resolving power in the focal zone improves as the f number decreases and also as the frequency increases. However, there is a limit. From other physical considerations it is known that it is impossible to obtain a focal spot smaller than a wavelength. A good f number to achieve is f2, where the beam width at the focus is twice the wavelength (e.g. 1 mm at 3 MHz). Systems designed at the limiting value of f1 are available. It follows that an aperture of f2 can be achieved with a small number of elements when echoes originating near to the probe are being focused. To retain a low f number as echoes are received from deeper into the tissues, more and more elements are switched into circuit. This is termed 'dynamic aperture'.

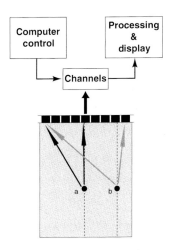

Fig. 2.21 Off-axis focus. Figure 2.20 illustrates how an on-axis reflector is brought into focus electronically by delaying the echoes at the inner elements to bring them into phase with echoes arriving at the outer elements slightly later. By selecting different delays it is equally possible to bring the echoes from an off-axis reflector into phase. Thus, by suitable computer control of the channels the reflector at (b) can be emphasised while the on-axis echo (a) is rejected. The process depends upon a calculation of the distances from the reflector to each element in the array.

To obtain high resolution at 20 cm depth, at f2 the aperture would need to be 10 cm, implying that the entire length of the linear array was used. At first sight it would seem that this would result in the disastrous situation of only a single ultrasound line being available to produce the scan!

A solution is found in the same principle that lay behind 'focus on receive'. If all of the elements in the array are used, the sound field floods the target area. The sent beam is weakly focused and steered in the general direction of the desired line. This maintains the advantage of reducing the effective beam width. Again, the required delays can be estimated, but this time so that echoes from an off-axis point are synchronised. Instead of emphasising echoes from the axis of the beam, a line of echoes parallel to the axis can be focused (Fig. 2.21). The possibility of following the off-axis echoes as the pulse propagates frees the designer from being constrained by where the axis of the ultrasound beams lies – the lines are created on receive rather than send.

The technique is valuable for the zoom function since the spacing between the lines created can be adjusted by appropriate selection of delays to that required by the magnification factor.

One pulse, many lines

If the digitised echoes from each element were split into two receive channels and processed, each with a different set of delays, two focused lines of image information could be achieved with a single transmitted pulse. This is the basis of the 'send one, display two' system.

The idea can be extended further. If the signal from each element was further split into a whole series of different sets of delays and memories, a corresponding series of focused lines could, in principle, be generated simultaneously. To provide a large number of delay circuits and memories is bulky and expensive.

A more elegant device, in outline, consists of a single large memory matrix. In it, the digitised rf echoes from each element in the array, and from a single pulse, are stored (Fig. 2.22). Once stored, the columns of the memory addresses represent the sequence of echo voltages on the corresponding element, while the rows represent the voltages recorded from each element at identical times.

Adding the values in cells with the same row address gives the net voltage value that would have occurred from a single element probe of the same length as the array. However, if values in adjacent columns, but with slightly different row addresses are added, the result is the same as applying delays to those channels. The amount of delay increases as the row addresses get further apart (Fig. 2.23).

Selection and addition of one value from each column, but with different row addresses, produces the required value for a single pixel in the image at the synthesised focal point in exactly the same way as passing the signals through a set of delays. There is total flexibility because selecting values from the same matrix, but with an appropriate set of row addresses, gives the value for any desired new focal point.

Thus, the delay values in each channel necessary to find the voltage that would have occurred if the beam had been focused at each point in the image, can now be achieved simply by selecting appropriate row addresses of the memory before summing the voltage values stored. Each summation of a set of row values generates the 'focused' value for one element in the image.

The 'focus on receive' system now consists of adding the stored values from addresses representing different times from the launch of the pulse. Any image line can be reconstructed from the same stored data by incorporating the desired amount of delay for each element simply by selecting the values stored in the appropriate addresses. The delays selected can be changed at will to reconstruct each line. Thus the delay is performed after storage of the digitised echo rather than before.

If the digitisation rate is high and the word length is large, this technique produces excellent results. All the values are stored before any focal area can be selected, and selection can go on as a parallel process so that many lines can be reconstructed from a single pulse. The 'one pulse, many lines' image, in which the pulse is first stored and focused in the direction of the lines to be generated, has the advantage of speed and offers the possibility of noise reduction by averaging.

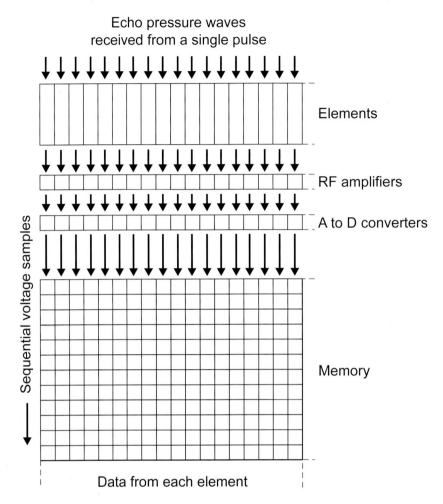

Fig. 2.22 Recording of echo sequence from full array. After a pulse has been sent out, the echoes are received at each element in the array. The voltage from each transducer element is amplified by its channel amplifier and converted by the analogue-to-digital converter to a series of voltage values which are stored sequentially in the memory.

Aperture and sensitivity

The large apertures produced by selecting many elements in the array not only enhance focusing but also improve sensitivity. The transducer is rather like a sail on a ship – extensive canvas experiences significant force even when the breeze is light. Similarly, a large area transducer collects more ultrasound energy and makes the transducer more sensitive. In this way the large apertures used for imaging at depth enhance the sensitivity available for detecting deep echoes which undergo significant attenuation.

Probe construction

The digital techniques described would be of little value without high-quality probes. Probe manufacture has steadily improved but there are inevitable design compromises. Thus, damping produces short pulses which improve resolution but degrade sensitivity. More channels improve performance but, despite some ingenious technical improvements, make the cable relatively stiff and bulky, the plugs difficult to change, and the manufacture of internal connections difficult and expensive to implement. A decision must always be reached on the best balance between options, and the optimum probe design usually has to be found by experience gained in a particular clinical situation.

Resolution and frequency

As was shown in Figure 2.7, lateral resolution improves as the effective beam width decreases. Narrower beams can be produced as the frequency increases. Similarly, the axial resolution is about half of the pulse length. Since there is usually much the same number of cycles in a pulse, regardless of frequency, the pulse length will also decrease and the resolution will be improved as frequency increases. The use of high-frequency probes allows both lateral and axial resolution to be improved.

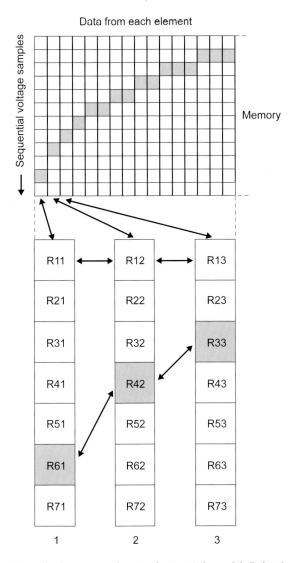

Data from each element

Sequential voltage samples

Memory

R11	↔	R12	↔	R13
R21		R22		R23
R31		R32		R33
R41		R42		R43
R51		R52		R53
R61		R62		R63
R71		R72		R73

1   2   3

Fig. 2.23 Delay by memory element selection. Columns labelled 1, 2 and 3 represent the memory addresses storing sequential voltages from just three channels. The values in row 1, R11, R12, R13 are all stored at the same instant. A delay in one channel with respect to another is achieved by adding voltages that were stored at different times. Thus, adding R42 to R33 is the equivalent of delaying the element in column 2 by 1 clock interval with respect to the element in column 3, and adding R61 to R42 the equivalent of delaying the echo recorded in column 1 by 2 clock pulses compared to column 2. The section of memory shown above has shaded cells which, when added, give the voltage value for 1 pixel, the same value that would have been recorded for a highly focused beam. The values for every other pixel in the image are similarly calculated by summing the appropriate memory elements.

However, a compromise must be made between resolution and sensitivity. Attenuation of sound at diagnostic frequencies is approximately proportional to frequency. Consequently, higher frequencies are absorbed more strongly by the tissues so that deeper tissues cannot be imaged without using unacceptably high power levels. This consideration usually restricts the diagnostic frequency

range to between 1 and 20 MHz (up to 100 MHz for imaging skin and the anterior chamber of the eye[14,15] with the most used frequencies being between 2 and 12 MHz.

Pulse frequency spectrum

The frequency of a wave can be estimated by measuring the time between similar parts on successive cycles of the waveform, and taking the reciprocal. For instance, if the time measured is 0.5 millionths of a second the frequency is 2 MHz, and so on. If this process is performed on a pulse, different results are achieved according to where on the waveform the timing points are measured. This is because a pulse does not have a single frequency but a spectrum of frequencies. The Fourier Transform is a mathematical process of defining the spectrum. The frequency quoted for a probe is actually that at which the spectral power is maximum (Fig. 2.24).

Damping

To achieve high axial resolution the ultrasound pulse must contain as few cycles as possible. Efficient damping is required to stop the transducer ringing. This is achieved by moulding a 'backing block' made of a material possessing optimum mechanical and acoustic properties, onto the back of the transducer. Sometimes, an electronic resonant circuit applied across the transducer is used to give further damping. Pulses as short as 2 cycles are achieved. Regrettably, efficient damping also makes the transducer insensitive. The shorter the pulse, the wider the spectrum of frequencies comprising the pulse. Broad band probes are those which produce short pulses of sound.

Sensitivity and pulse shaping

The effective depth of penetration of a pulse depends on the sensitivity of the probe which, in turn, depends upon many factors including frequency, damping, quarter wave matching, transducer material and aperture.

Because the attenuation of a sound wave is proportional to its frequency, the higher frequencies in the echo spectrum are preferentially removed as they originate from deeper in the patient causing the centre frequency of echoes to drop. Some scanners use a radio frequency amplifier which is progressively retuned to lower frequencies as echoes return from increasing depth to keep track of the expected centre frequency. Retuning allows a higher amplification factor to be used and makes the equipment more sensitive.

One form of tissue characterisation that has been offered on commercial scanners is based on the change in frequency content of echoes from different tissues. The results are dependent upon the equipment used but the

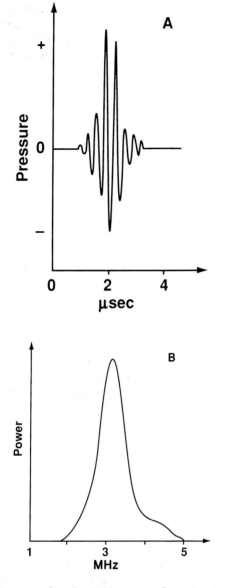

Fig. 2.24 Spectrum of a pulse. A: The pressure fluctuations in a pulse from a commercial probe, marked 3 MHz by the manufacturer, are displayed. **B:** A Fourier power spectrum of the pulse in (A) shows that a wide range of frequencies is present in the pulse. The plot shows that maximum power (i.e. the predominant frequency) is at 3 MHz but there is a significant amount of power at other frequencies.

technique has been developed to the point where there is some clinical promise.[16]

The natural frequency of a transducer is determined by the thickness of its piezoelectric sheet. This frequency is produced by a 'shock' of an extremely brief high voltage applied across the piezoelectric element. To alter the shock excited frequency the entire probe is changed. Multi-element mechanical sector probes are available where each element produces a different frequency. However, if the probe is heavily damped, it is possible to drive a trans-

ducer at a different frequency to its resonant frequency with a shaped voltage pulse rather than a 'shock'.

The move of the pulse spectrum to lower frequencies by differential attenuation is equivalent to a lengthening of the pulse with a consequent degradation of the axial resolution. A heavily damped transducer can be made to change dimensions in close correspondence to the applied voltage pattern. In the unique case when the Fourier spectrum of the applied voltage has a bell-shaped 'Gaussian' profile, and if the attenuation is directly proportional to frequency, it turns out that the shifted spectrum still has a Gaussian profile of the same band width, so the pulse length is not increased. Thus the axial resolution is maintained throughout the depth of the image. This feature is available on some machines.[12]

Probe efficiency and reverberation

Reverberation is an annoying artefact in which a cloud of false echoes is displayed extending deep from the proximal edge of an area known actually to be echo-free. It is mainly caused by the poor absorption of echo energy by the transducer material. The echo energy that is not absorbed (typically 80% in an uncorrected probe) is reflected back into the tissues, producing a 'ghost' image. To minimise reverberation, the sound energy in the echo must be transmitted into the transducer more efficiently.

The technique that is commonly used to improve sensitivity is 'quarter wave plate' matching. The transducer is coated with a layer of a material with an impedance that is the geometric mean of the acoustic impedance of the tissues and the transducer material. The thickness is made equal to one-quarter of the wavelength used. For long pulses the energy in the pulse is transferred to the transducer with very high efficiency but, since the short pulses used in imaging encompass a range of wavelengths, matching is, in practice, imperfect.

A further problem is the production of a material with the correct impedance. It is simpler to manufacture a series of materials of graded acoustic impedance, which produces identical results and achieves high efficiencies. These are described as multiple matching layer transducers, and give good results reducing reverberation and allowing higher frequencies to be used with improved resolution.

Another technique, which has been used for high-frequency probes, involves the use of a transducer material with a specific acoustic impedance much closer to that of soft tissue than the traditional ceramic materials. Transducers have been made from specially treated plastics such as polyvinylidene difluoride (PVDF), which is more widely used for wrapping chocolate boxes! These have the additional advantage of being acoustically rather 'dead' so that there is no need for backing material. Although these transducers are good at receiving ultrasound, they are inefficient at producing it. Their major use is as hydrophone transducers for measuring beam profiles.

Composite probes

The efficiency of ceramic materials and the low mismatch impedance of epoxy materials has led to the development of probes that make use of both.[12] Typically the ceramic material is set as tiny rods into a base of the plastic, so that it has a chequered appearance. The net efficiency of this structure is better than the ceramic material alone. The improved sensitivity implies that more of the sound energy in an echo is absorbed in the probe, so there is less reflected to produce reverberation artefacts. Thus, an additional benefit is the reduction of image noise.

Some refinements for noise reduction

Modern equipment designs have made effective use of some less obvious features of the ultrasound process which previously were ignored.

Split-band non-linear amplification

Broad-band probes (used for short pulse, high-resolution imaging) require broad-band amplifiers that amplify a wide range of frequencies by the same factor. All electronic circuits generate a small amount of random 'noise' as a tiny fluctuating voltage. This noise voltage occurs at random at all frequencies. Similarly, ultrasonic speckle occurs independently in different parts of the spectrum. A wide-band amplifier picks up the power of these noise components and displays the unwanted echoes on the display.

The incoming signal can be split between a number of rf amplifiers, each having a narrower band width, but with their pass bands overlapping. The noise in each occurs at random times. The amplifiers are made non-linear in some way, perhaps logarithmically, so that intense echoes are amplified less than low-level echoes. If the outputs of the amplifiers are added together, the result is equivalent to multiplying the outputs, and the noise tends to cancel out. However, the wanted signal occurs simultaneously in each amplifier, and the outputs combine to give a coherent reconstruction for wanted echoes. Thus noise can be reduced and a higher amplification factor used.[12]

Non-linear effects

The speed of an ultrasound pulse actually depends slightly upon the excess acoustic pressure. For small-amplitude waves the change in speed for each part of the wave is negligible and the change is imperceptible. However, diagnostic pulses have amplitudes many times in excess of atmospheric pressure. Under these circumstances, the

high-pressure parts of the wave steadily catch up with the low-pressure parts, and distort the wave shape until a shock wave is formed. This is called non-linear propagation. The effect becomes more evident as the sound pressure amplitude increases.

The Fourier spectrum of the pulse changes as it travels through the tissues because the non-linear propagation pushes energy into higher frequencies. The deeper the pulse goes, the more the Fourier harmonics of the fundamental frequency increase in amplitude. This is opposite to the changes in the spectrum due to attenuation.

Tissue harmonic imaging

If the amplifiers attached to the array elements are tuned to twice the frequency of the probe, then the displayed echo pattern will come from echoes that are frequency shifted by non-linear propagation. These harmonics are more intense for deeper echoes where the shock wave has had time to build up and, in a focused beam, where the intensity is increasing.

Much of the noise in the image is in the frequency range of the transmitted pulse. In particular, conventional imaging of obese patients is made difficult by reverberation of the pulse in the superficial fat/muscle layers. This produces a dense haze of echoes obscuring the deeper parts of the image. In the harmonic technique, these strong reverberant echoes tend to remain at the fundamental frequency because the intensity of the pressure wave is relatively low near to the probe. As the intensity increases towards the focal area, the harmonics are generated more strongly. Consequently, by imaging the harmonics the reverberant echoes are eliminated giving a much cleaner image.

Measurement

The design of 'on-screen' measurement user controls often makes a substantial difference to the acceptability of a particular scanner. The design should enable the system to be rapid and convenient to use. If the measurement process is cumbersome, requiring a number of key strokes, a single measurement may easily take a few seconds longer. In many investigations perhaps 10 measurements are made. A poor system can easily require an additional minute of measurement time per patient. Over a day this amounts to sufficient time to see another patient.

Systems for linear dimensions that require the operator to depress a control and wait while a caliper moves slowly across the screen are time wasters, as are systems that move the caliper spots back to the middle of the screen and destroy the previous reading as soon as the frame freeze is released. Calipers that remain on screen and are controlled by a tracker ball or joystick are generally quicker to use.

Freehand area measurement requires a steady hand. The fact that the caliper spots tend to deviate from the required position randomly on either side of the outline produces positive and negative errors that tend to cancel. Since many area measurements are of oval shapes, systems that produce an ellipse on the screen which can be superimposed on the image can give results quickly, often without significant loss of accuracy over the manual system.

Probe ergonomics

The majority of what has been explained is profoundly important to image quality, but is not immediately obvious to users unless they read the manufactures' literature. Of more direct interest is the selection of probes. The range of available probes is huge. In general, probes should have a very flexible cable and be lightweight, robust, convenient to hold and easy to change.

General considerations

Mechanical probes have the advantage that they are simple to produce. However, a typical scanner produces about 3 million frames per year. Clearly even a well-engineered mechanical probe will wear out after a couple of years of use.

The lenses used on phased and linear array scanners are often made of silicone rubber to form a convex shape. Silicone rubber is hygroscopic and lenses can be damaged if left in coupling gel for long periods of time. Similarly, cleaning spirits can cause damage.

Transducer ageing

Well over a billion pulses are produced by a typical probe in its lifetime. The transducer material may ultimately start to lose its piezoelectric properties as the crystal structure becomes more disordered. The probe becomes less sensitive. Probes must be regarded, rather like X-ray tubes, as consumable items with a typical lifespan of about 5 years of intensive use.

Footprint

For many applications, the access area of the patient through which a satisfactory scan can be obtained is small. In such cases the region of the probe in contact with the patient, the 'footprint', must be appropriate. An obvious example is cardiac scanning where a sector scanner is essential because of the small footprint that will fit into the window afforded by the intercostal spaces.

If good visualisation of superficial tissues is important, a larger footprint gives a better view. A linear or curvilinear array is required. Sometimes angling of a probe into an anatomical area involves pressing one end of a linear array hard against the skin, causing discomfort. A curvi-

linear array may be preferable and produces good results. An instance is a longitudinal scan into the pelvis. Linear array probes are available, from which the beam can be steered into the pelvis by phasing the last group of elements in the array.

Intracorporeal probes

It is desirable to place the transducer close to the target organ; this may often be achieved by intracorporeal scanning. There are a number of reasons for this. The near-complete reflection of sound at gas or air/tissue interfaces make an external approach to some organs effectively impossible. Similarly, the scattering and absorption of sound by tissues make the use of high frequencies, with their potential for markedly improved resolution, unusable for structures at depth if an external approach is used. Finally, although the speed of sound changes only slightly in soft tissues, angulated fat/muscle interfaces refract the sound beam by several degrees and may produce significant artefacts. Avoidance of superficial musculature is then helpful.

There is a wide range of intracorporeal probes operating in most of the traditional modes of scanning, including linear and curvilinear arrays, mechanical sectors and radial (plan position indication) probes. These are used as endoscopic, trans-oesophageal, trans-rectal, trans-vaginal, trans-urethral and intra-vascular probes.

In all cases, taking the probe inside a patient makes additional demands on the design. The electrical integrity of the probe and cable must be significantly better than that acceptable for external scanning. The contours of the entire device must be smooth and able to be satisfactorily disinfected, or be 'single use'. The size and shape must be acceptable to the patient.

Because of the often restricted nature of access to the probe contact area, needle guides may be useful to constrain the passage of the needle to the plane of the scan and along a marked vector on the image.

Intra-operative probes

Intra-operative probes, like other intracorporeal probes, are capable of high resolution. There is a wide range of application because there are few parts of the anatomy that cannot be effectively scanned. Once the skull or abdomen is opened, ultrasound access without interference from bone or gas is usually assured. These probes are particularly useful for guiding a surgical team to a particular structure or foreign body.

The features of intra-operative probes are a small footprint and a probe casing and cable that do not get in the way of the operative field. In addition, the microbiological integrity of the device must be of a higher order than for any other probes.

'Panoramic' extended field of view displays

It is possible to move an array probe in the direction of the image plane and extend the image as far as desired beyond the edge of the original frame (Fig. 2.25). As the probe is moved, the advanced software identifies major features in the previous frame and calculates the new position of the probe, both in translation and angle, by aligning the common features in the new frame. The new frame is moved and rotated so that the echoes not on the original image frame are added into the display. Thus, the image can be extended indefinitely, the current position being in real time, but the rest displayed as a static image.[4] The system does not work well if moving features such as cardiac structures are in the scan because the system is confused when trying to lock onto principal features in the previous frame that have moved anatomically rather than by movement of the probe.

Ultrasonic safety

Improvements in resolution and sensitivity, particularly in some Doppler and colour flow mapping techniques, and the use of annular array transducers have led manufacturers to raise the acoustic output power of equipment. Machines are available that produce beams 1000 times more intense than some of those used a decade ago.[17] Spatial peak pulse average intensities of 10 W cm^{-2} and peak negative pressure of -4 MPa (-40 atmospheres) have been measured from commercially available scanners. At these levels there is no question that mechanisms for cellular modification exist. It is important that all users make a risk–benefit judgement and know the output of their equipment.

Duplex scanners ensure that pulsed Doppler signals are obtained from the desired vessel. If the same elements are

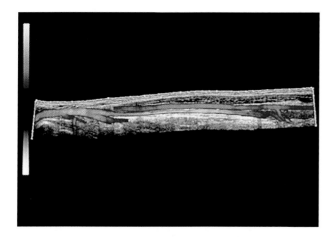

Fig. 2.25 Extended field of view image: This image shows a 38 cm view of the femoral artery, vein and the main branches, produced by a single sweep of a linear array probe. SieScape image by kind permission of Siemens Medical Imaging.

used to generate the image and to derive the Doppler signal it is certain that the image and the Doppler vector are co-planar. This ensures that the Doppler signal comes from the desired vessel. These systems are set up to optimize the image processing chain, rather than the Doppler signal. The consequent low sensitivity of the system and the broad band width of the pulse make it very difficult to detect the minute echoes from blood corpuscles. The solution is to use high-intensity pulses with the attendant uncertainties about hazard. This is of particular concern with trans-vaginal probes.

The alternative of using separate imaging and Doppler paths has attractions. The Doppler and the imaging processors can be optimised independently so that substantially less power is required in the Doppler interrogating pulse. However, the system is now seldom used.

Safety indices

It is good practice to give the operator an 'on-screen' indication of the potential of the equipment to produce biological changes at the settings selected. There are two basic indicators, the thermal and mechanical indices.[18] These should be displayed if either value is more than 1.[19]

The thermal index (TI) is equivalent to the temperature rise that can be produced by the beam, usually at the focus. (NB. The transduction process is inefficient and the probe itself may become hot, quite apart from the heating effect of the beam.) The thermal index is subdivided into effects on soft tissue, and at a bone/tissue interface, the condition being indicated by additional letters: TIS for soft tissue, TIB for bone and TIC for the cranium. It is left to the user to decide if the temperature rise is acceptable. A temperature rise of 1.5°C is generally regarded as tolerable but a temperature rise of more than 4°C for more than 5 minutes would require very clear justification.

The mechanical index (MI) is less intuitive, but indicates the likelihood of cavitation occurring. Cavitation becomes less likely as frequency is increased, but more likely as the peak negative pressure in the wave is increased. The MI is equal to the peak rarefaction pressure in the pulse divided by the square root of its fundamental frequency. The mechanical index is of particular importance if a gaseous contrast medium is being used, or if a gas/tissue interface is insonated. There does not seem to be general consensus on an appropriate threshold for the mechanical index, but peak values are about 1.3.[20]

REFERENCES

1 Geiger M L, Ohara K, Doi K. Investigation of basic imaging properties in digital radiography. 9. Effect of displayed grey levels on signal detection. Med Phys 1986; 13: 312–318
2 Sonka M, Hlavac V, Boyle R. Image processing, analysis and machine vision. London: Chapman Hall Computing, 1995; 68–82

3   Cespedes I, Ophir J, Ponnekanti H, Maklad N. Elastography: elasticity imaging using ultrasound with application to muscle and breast in vivo. Ultrason Imaging 1993; 15(2): 73–88

4   Whittingham T A. Modern developments in diagnostic ultrasound – 2. Radiography 1996; 2: 311–325

5   Evans J L, Ng K H, Wiet S et al. Accurate three-dimensional reconstruction of intravascular ultrasound data. Spatially correct three-dimensional reconstructions. Circulation 1996; 93(3): 567–576

6   Kyei-Mensah A, Zaidi J, Pittrof R, Shaker A, Campbell S, Tan S L. Transvaginal three-dimensional ultrasound: accuracy of follicular volume measurements. Fertil Steril 1996; 65(2): 371–376

7   Marks L S, Dorey F J, Macairan M L, Park C, deKernion J B. Three-dimensional ultrasound device for rapid determination of bladder volume. Urology 1997; 50(3): 341–348

8   Moritz W E, Pearlman A S, McCabe D H, Medema D K, Ainsworth M E, Boles M S. An ultrasonic technique for imaging the ventricle in three dimensions and calculating its volume. IEEE Trans Biomed Eng 1983; 30(8): 482–492

9   Hughes D I, Duck F A. Automatic attenuation compensation for ultrasonic imaging. Ultrasound Med Biol 1997; 23(5) 651–664

10 Duck F A. Physical properties of tissue. London: Academic Press, 1990; 76–84

11 Jago J R, Whittingham T A. The use of measured acoustic speed in reflection ultrasound CT. Phys Med Biol 1992; 37: 2139–2142

12 Whittingham T A. Modern developments in diagnostic ultrasound – 1. Radiography 1995; 1: 61–73

13 Wells PNT. Biomedical ultrasonics. London: Academic Press, 1977; 39

14 Aslanides I M, Reinstein D Z, Silverman R H et al. High-frequency ultrasound spectral parameter imaging of anterior corneal scars. CLAO J 1995; 21(4): 268–272

15 Semple J L, Gupta A K, From L et al. Does high-frequency (40–60 MHz) ultrasound imaging play a role in the clinical management of cutaneous melanoma? Ann Plast Surg 1995; 34(6): 599–605

16 Stetson P, Sommer G. Ultrasonic characterization of tissues via backscatter frequency dependence. Ultrasound Med Biology 1997; 23(7): 989–996

17 Henderson J, Willson K, Jago J, Whittingham T A. A survey of the acoustic outputs of diagnostic ultrasound scanners in current clinical use. Ultrasound Med Biol 1995; 21(5): 699–705

18 Duck F A. The meaning of thermal index (TI) and mechanical index (MI) values. British Medical Ultrasound Society Bulletin 1997; 5(4) 36–40

19 American Institute of Ultrasound in Medicine/National Electrical Manufacturers Association. Standard for real-time display of thermal and mechanical acoustic output indices on diagnostic ultrasound equipment. Rockville, Maryland: AIUM, 1992.

20 Patton C A, Harris G R, Phillips R A. Output levels and bioeffects indices from diagnostic ultrasound exposure data reported to the FDA. IEEE Transactions in Ultrasonics, Ferroelectrics and Frequency Control 1994; 4: 353–359

FURTHER READING

Bamber J, Tristam, M. Diagnostic ultrasound. In: Webb S, ed. The physics of medical imaging. Bristol: IoP Publishing, 1995: 319–386

Fish P. Physics and instrumentation of diagnostic medical ultrasound. Chichester: Wiley, 1997

McDicken N. Diagnostic ultrasonics, 3rd edn. Chichester: Wiley, 1990

Safety of diagnostic ultrasound

Gail ter Haar

Introduction

The increasingly widespread use of diagnostic ultrasound techniques means that safety considerations have become more important. The main applications for which safety is of paramount importance are those in obstetrics and neonatology. It seems probable that the most sensitive targets that are exposed to ultrasound are those in the embryo or fetus, and thus the potential for inducing adverse effects will be greatest here.

Although the bioeffects literature is apparently very extensive, the overwhelming majority of studies reported concern the interaction of therapeutic ultrasound with biological systems and very few deal with 'diagnostic' exposures, let alone diagnostic machines used in clinical practice.

Therapeutic ultrasound uses either continuous or tone burst exposures whereas diagnostic ultrasound employs short pulses. It can be seen from Table 3.1, in which a number of important exposure parameters are compared, that there is some overlap in the amount of acoustic power emitted during a pulse, even though the time-averaged intensities are generally lower for therapy devices. It is clear that therapy devices can induce changes in biological systems (albeit beneficial), so it is important to ascertain whether or not diagnostic devices can also induce changes, which, in this case, would be unwanted.

It is now generally accepted that the two main mechanisms that may produce biological change are heat and cavitation. These two mechanisms are discussed, and methods of minimising their potential effects suggested.

Biological effects

Heating

As an ultrasonic wave travels through tissue, the energy it carries with it reduces. Some of the energy is scattered out of the path of the beam (and may be used to form images), and some is absorbed within the tissue. It is this energy absorption that leads to tissue heating.

Although it is known that therapeutic ultrasound can raise tissue temperatures significantly, very few measure-ments of the temperature rises induced by diagnostic exposures have been made. ter Haar *et al*[1] have reported biologically insignificant temperature rises measured in liver tissue *in vitro* following pulse-echo exposures (I_{SPPA} 183 W cm^{-2}, I_{SPTA} W cm^{-2}, 3.3 MHz), but rises up to 1.9°C following 1 min of exposure to Doppler ultrasound (I_{SPPA} 190 W cm^{-2}, I_{SPTA} 6.2 W cm^{-2}). However, greater temperatures have been measured at bone surfaces; this is because of the high energy absorption in bone. Bosward *et al*[2] studied the temperature rises induced in fetal guinea pig brains, both in the mid-cerebral region and adjacent to the occipital and parietal bones. They measured the great-est temperature rises next to bone, and these increased with increasing mineralisation (gestational age). Mid-brain temperature rises never exceeded 1°C in live animals when the incident power was 260 mW at 3.2 MHz, but at the bone surface of the oldest fetuses studied, the temper-ature rise was 5.2°C. A similar dependence of temperature rise on gestational age was shown in human fetal femurs by Drewniak *et al*.[3] Duggan *et al*[4] measured the temper-ature rise in fetal sheep brains *in utero* (124 days, where full term is 147 days). The temperature sensor was placed 1 mm deep in the cerebral cortex. 3.5 MHz pulsed Doppler transducers were operated at either 600 mW (I_{SPPA} 8.9 W cm^{-2}, I_{SPTA} 0.3 W cm^{-2}) or 2 W (I_{SPPA} 27.3 W cm^{-2}, I_{SPTA} 1.7 W cm^{-2}). The maximum temper-ature rises recorded were 3°C (600 mW) and 12.5°C (2 W) in the dead fetus, and 1.7°C (600 mW) and 8.8°C (2 W) in the live, perfused fetus. The greatest temperature rise occurs when the Doppler beam meets the bone surface at normal incidence (ter Haar, unpublished data). It can be seen from Table 1 that current machines do not yet have maximum power outputs as high as 600 mW.[5] Current FDA regulations limit the *in situ* I_{SPTA} to 720 mW cm^{-2} for machines that have an output display, and to 94 mW cm^{-2} for those that do not. It is therefore unlikely that low-output devices will lead to significant heating in human fetal brains, but these results demonstrate the potential of Doppler ultrasound to heat tissue at the top end of their available outputs, and give emphasis to the importance of users being aware of the heating potential of Doppler beams. It should be remembered that uncalcified fetal bone is unlikely to show these temperature rises.

Table 3.1 Ultrasound exposure parameters for therapy, imaging and pulsed Doppler

	Therapy	Imaging	Pulsed Doppler
Pulse length	1–10 ms	11 µs	110 µs
Frequencies	0.75–3.0 MHz	3–7 MHz	3–7 MHz
Pulse repetition frequencies	100–300 Hz	11 kHz	110 kHz
Power	≤ 3 W	0.3–300 mW	10–450 mW
Spatial peak, temporal average intensity (I_{SPTA})	500 mW cm^{-2}	11–430 mW cm^{-2}	175–9000 mW cm^{-2}
Peak negative pressure (p.)	0.5 MPa	0.45–5.5 MPa	0.7–5.3 MPa
Typical beam widths	11 cm	12 mm	12 mm

Tissue heating is likely only to be a significant biological problem in obstetric applications. Here, some data on the effects of supra-normal temperatures on the well-being of the fetus or embryo are available. Although there is very little information about the effect of hyperthermia on humans during pregnancy, all other mammalian species that have been studied appear to be susceptible to heat damage.

The effect of a hyperthermic insult depends on the stage of embryonic or fetal development and on both the temperature rise and the time for which it is imposed. Thermally induced embryonic death is possible at any stage, but is most likely before implantation stage. The uterus and its secretions change significantly at this stage and are vitally linked to the stage of development of the embryo. If embryonic development is delayed, it may be put out of phase with the nutrient uterine secretions. It appears that hyperthermia during this stage either kills the embryo outright or the embryo goes on to develop normally. Death, resorption or abortion may, however, occur at any stage of development.

Abortion is a well-known consequence of elevated temperatures. There may be a number of causes for this, including increased uterine activity or severe cellular damage that is incompatible with the continued development of the fetus or embryo.

Hyperthermia is known to be a teratogen in a number of mammalian species, for example, rats, mice, sheep, pigs and monkeys.[6] Adverse effects may be found if the temperature is elevated during a crucial stage in organogenesis. It appears that the central nervous system is most susceptible to damage. Examples of defects found are neural tube defects, microphthalmia, microcephaly and micrencephaly.

It is the temperature elevation above normal that is important in producing effects rather than the actual temperature reached. Temperature rises above normal that can produce death, resorption, abortion or teratogenesis in the mammalian species that have been studied are in the range of 1.5–2.5°C.

Thus, it is known that death and teratogenic effects are possible outcomes of raised temperatures *in utero*. Early embryos are more likely to show lethal effects than are late embryos or fetuses. Teratogenic effects are most likely during early stages of organogenesis, the central nervous system being most at risk. The most sensitive stages are those when cell proliferation is most intense. It should be noted that adult proliferative tissues may also be at risk (e.g. testis and bone marrow).

Diagnostic ultrasound that heats the embryo or fetus by less than 1°C can be used without reservation for any length of time. At higher temperature rises, the risk of causing adverse effects increases with the length of exposure time. Duggan & Cowan[7] have shown that the median time for a Doppler examination of the carotid artery for singleton pregnancies (18–34 weeks gestation) was 31 s. It is probable that this is representative of the time that a Doppler probe may be held stationary during an investigation. A review of the thermal bioeffects literature[8] has shown that a temperature of 43°C can be maintained without hazard for 60 s, and 44°C may be maintained for 30 s. It should, however, be noted that hyperthermia research has in general heated the whole body of the fetus. The consequences of selective heating, as would be achieved for example from a Doppler beam, have not been studied.

It seems likely that pulse-echo imaging can be used safely from purely thermal considerations, whereas some degree of caution should be exercised where Doppler examinations are to be used, although if examinations are kept as short as possible, it is unlikely that the elevated temperatures produced will lead to significant biological damage.

Biological effects of cavitation

Cavitation is the term used to describe the activity of microscopic gas bodies when they are influenced by an ultrasonic field. The behaviour of a bubble depends on its size and on the characteristics of the acoustic field with which it interacts. For every ultrasonic frequency there is a bubble diameter that is 'resonant'. If the acoustic amplitude is sufficiently high, these bubbles oscillate violently in the ultrasonic field and may undergo a cycle of rapid growth and implosion, resulting in very high local temperatures and shear stresses. For lesser amplitudes and for smaller bubbles, the bubble may be set into forced oscillations, setting up streaming motions around it. These small bubbles may grow to resonant size and undergo collapse. Large bubbles may also oscillate and may disintegrate, thus seeding the population of smaller bubbles. (For more detailed information, see reference 9.)

This bubble activity requires that stabilised microscopic gas bodies exist in tissue, or that the nuclei from which they may be formed (nucleation sites) exist. It has been shown that such bubbles do exist in tissues[10] and that therapeutic ultrasound exposures can cause these to grow to a detectable size. Very little is known about nucleation sites in tissues, but it seems likely that the same tissue type in different individuals, or even in different sites within one individual, may have significantly different gaseous content and therefore different likelihood of cavitation.

It has not been demonstrated that diagnostic pulses of ultrasound can induce cavitation in mammalian tissues, although effects have been seen in Drosophila[11] and in agar gels.[1]

The biological consequences of cavitation activity due to diagnostic ultrasound are not well understood. It is known from work at therapeutic output levels that tissue immediately around the site of a collapse cavitation event is completely disrupted. Cell lysis is seen, but on a very localised scale, a few microns across. Bubbles that are oscillating in a stable fashion, without collapsing, set up streaming patterns around themselves. In fluids, the shear stresses associated with the liquid's movement may be quite considerable, and cells in the vicinity may be lysed. In more structured tissues, such fluid movement may not be possible and the effect of oscillating bubbles will be considerably damped.

The greatest hazard from diagnostic ultrasound lies in the possibility that a cavitation event may occur in amniotic or body fluids close to a developing organism, lysing a cell or group of cells such that irreparable damage may occur. Cavitation may occur in blood plasma, but no reports of thrombus formation have been published.

Experimental evidence indicates that acoustic cavitation associated with the activity of microbubbles is not likely to be an important source of hazard during clinical diagnostic examinations. There is, however, some experimental evidence emerging from work in animals that some damage can occur at relatively low acoustic intensities, when ultrasound is incident on pre-existing stabilised gas bodies in tissue, such as, for example, the alveoli in the lung. Lung haemorrhage (more accurately described as capillary extravasation) has been observed in mouse lungs following exposure to ultrasonic pulses with pressure amplitudes around 1 MPa.[12–14] Similar damage has been reported in the lungs of mini-pigs[15] and monkeys.[16] The physiological significance of these findings is not fully understood. It is clear, however, that such haemorrhage cannot occur in the non-aerated fetal lung. The presence of stabilised gas bodies in intestine has also been implicated in the observation of haemorrhage in mouse intestine.[17,18]

It appears to be very difficult to induce cavitation in whole blood. Brayman *et al*[19] found a threshold of 17 MPa. Other investigators[20–23] have shown that the presence of gas contrast agents can reduce this threshold (a range of 11–24 MPa is quoted), but that it still lies well above the pressure amplitudes available from commercial diagnostic units.

Biological effects from other mechanisms

There are a number of other ways in which ultrasound may interact with tissues, but the biological consequences of these are even more poorly understood than those of cavitation. In particular, for diagnostic ultrasound where there may be significant non-linear propagation effects, nothing is known about the biological effects of non-linearity on tissues.

Epidemiological surveys

There are few published epidemiological studies of the effects of ultrasound exposures in humans. The literature has been extensively reviewed by Ziskin & Petitti.[24] Effects that have been studied include birthweight,[25–30] structural fetal anomalies,[31,33–35] neurological effects,[32,33] incidence of childhood cancer,[36,37] dyslexia,[30,33,38–40] speech development[41,42] and hearing in children.[34]

No association could be found between ultrasonic exposures *in utero* and the incidence of childhood malignancy in either of two well-conducted studies.[36,37] There is one study[33] that showed that a significantly higher number of children exposed to ultrasound *in utero* were dyslexic than in the control group, but this finding was not repeated by two published Norwegian studies.[30,38–40] There was an association with ultrasound exposure for only one of the outcomes studied by the Norwegians.[38,40] This was handedness. A weak association between non-right handedness and ultrasound exposure was found. However, the results are not conclusive, and a prospective randomised trial with this as its prior hypothesis is required to answer this question definitively.

Two surveys have been published in which the subject of speech development has been addressed. In one survey[41] it was reported that the odds of suffering delayed speech were higher for children exposed to ultrasound before birth than for those who were not. A second survey[42] suggested that ultrasonically exposed children were less likely to be referred to a speech therapist. Both these studies have statistical limitations, and so further information is required.

The vast majority of reports on the effect of *in utero* ultrasound on birthweight and subsequent growth have failed to show any effect.[27–30] One study[26] found a nonsignificant 25 g reduction in birthweight following five Doppler examinations in the third trimester. Other groups have reported an increase in mean birthweight following ultrasound exposure.[27,28] No difference in growth during childhood could be found between exposed and unexposed groups of children up to 6 years of age.[27,29,30]

One can summarise from epidemiological evidence to date that there is no association between diagnostic ultrasound exposure *in utero* and childhood malignancies, and associations between such exposure and dyslexia, speech development and handedness have not been confirmed. The data on birthweight are conflicting, with one report suggesting a decrease in birthweight following Doppler examinations, and others suggesting an increase following B-mode imaging.

Minimising the possibility of harm

What has gone before has been somewhat theoretical and hypothetical. We need to know the answer to the question: how can the user minimise the probability of producing biologically significant heating or cavitational effects using the controls provided on the machine?

We know that the amount of heating obtained increases with acoustic output intensity, exposure (or dwell) time and ultrasonic frequency. If the time-averaged intensity is increased, for example by increasing the pulse repetition frequency without altering pulse amplitude, then the amount of heating may be expected to increase. Important quantities for determining whether cavitation may be produced are peak negative pressure, pulse length, pulse repetition frequency and exposure time. Thus, for example, for all modes of operation of diagnostic scanners we can deduce that increasing the exposure time and output power will increase both the amount of heating obtained and the probability of cavitational effects, while increasing the transducer frequency increases the probability for biologically significant thermal effects because of the increased absorption, but decreases the probability of cavitational effects.

Table 3.2 illustrates the way in which thermal and cavitational effects may vary when different machine settings are altered for different operating modes. Where possible, settings that minimise the possibility of producing significant heat or cavitation should be used. It should be noted that this is a broad generalisation as there are probably as many ways of driving transducers as there are machines available, highlighting the need for a good understanding of each individual machine and for good exchange of information between manufacturer and user.

Since it is, in practice, impossible to know the temperature rise induced by a specific application of an ultrasound beam *in vivo*, or to assess the probability of inducing cavitation, two biophysical indices have been introduced.

Table 3.2 Table showing in general terms how variation of machine controls may alter the probability of producing biologically significant thermal or cavitational effects.

	Probability of biologically significant: thermal effects	cavitation effects	Comments
All operating modes			
Exposure time	↑↑	↑	These lead to greater energy absorption
Output power	↑↑	↑	
Transducer frequency	↑	↓	Absorption increases with increasing frequency Cavitation threshold drops with decreasing frequency
Switching to freeze	↓/0	↓/0	
Imaging and m-mode			
Selection of M-mode imaging mode	↑	↑	This gives repeated exposure of the same small tissue volume
Sector format	↑	↑	Line density is increased near the transducer
Choice of narrow sector resolution	↑	↑	Increase in line density
Focal zone depth	↑↑	↑	For some machines, power is increased to account for attenuation losses
Receiver gain	0	0	These are 'receive' variables so have no effect
Grey scale	0	0	
M-mode time base	0	0	
Pulsed Doppler			
Range gate length	↑↑	↑	In some machines power is increased to account for attenuation losses
Range gate depth	↑↑	↑	
Velocity range	↑↑	↑	
Receiver gain	0	0	These are 'receive' variables so have no effect
Doppler audio gain	0	0	
Doppler time base	0	0	

↑ indicates an increase; ↓ indicates a decrease; 0 indicates no change expected.

These are the thermal index (TI) and the mechanical index (MI), and they have been introduced with the intention of giving the user information on which to make safety judgements.[43,44] The thermal index is a number which provides an estimate of the tissue temperature rise in °C which might be possible under 'reasonable worst case conditions'. Three forms of the index are available: TIS, which is intended for soft tissue exposures; TIB, which is used when bone lies near the beam focus; and TIC, which is designed for the heating of bone situated close to the transducer. The mechanical index is designed to give some indication of the probability that cavitation will occur in target tissues, and relies on the fact that there is a frequency-dependent threshold acoustic pressure above which cavitation may occur. The US Output Display Standard[44] requires that at least one of these indices is displayed on the equipment monitor, depending on the mode of operation, clinical application and the maximum value that the indices may achieve. If an index may reach 1.0 for any machine setting, then it must be displayed from 0.4 upwards. In practice, it is MI that is usually displayed in B-mode, and TI that is displayed in Doppler or M-mode.

General guidelines

In conclusion, a few general recommendations may be made to ensure the continued safe use of ultrasound.

1. Machine default output conditions should be set to give low output power and high receiver gain.
2. The time that a transducer is in contact with the skin while transmitting should be kept to a minimum.
3. The acoustic output should be kept to the minimum level consistent with good clinical accuracy and performance.

Appendix

There have been a number of statements issued by national and international bodies concerning the safe use of medical ultrasound. The most recent is a statement issued by the European Federation of Societies for Ultrasound in Medicine and Biology (EFSUMB)[45] in 1999:

Diagnostic ultrasound has been widely used in clinical medicine for many years with no proven deleterious effects. However, as the use of ultrasound increases, with the introduction of new techniques, with a broadening of the medical indications for ultrasound examinations, and with increased exposure continuous vigilance is essential to ensure its continued safe use.

A broad range of ultrasound exposure is used in the different diagnostic modalities currently available. Doppler imaging and measurement techniques may require higher exposure than those used in B- and M-modes, with pulsed Doppler techniques having the potential for the highest levels.

Modern equipment is subject to output regulation. The recommendations contained in this statement assume that the ultrasound equipment being used is designed to international or national safety requirements and that it is used by competent and trained personnel.

B- and M-modes

Based on scientific evidence of ultrasonically induced biological effects to date, there is no reason to withhold B- or M-mode scanning for any clinical application, including the routine clinical scanning of every woman during pregnancy.

Doppler for fetal heart monitoring (CTE)

The power levels used for fetal heart monitoring (CTE) are sufficiently low that the use of this modality is not contraindicated, on safety grounds, even when it is to be used for extended periods.

Doppler mode (colour flow imaging, power Doppler and pulsed Doppler)

Exposures used in Doppler modes are higher than for B- and M-modes. There is considerable overlap between the ranges of exposure which may be used for colour flow imaging and power Doppler, and for pulsed Doppler techniques. The clinical user should be aware that pulsed Doppler at maximum machine outputs and colour flow imaging with small colour boxes have the greatest potential for biological effects.

In general, the informed use of Doppler ultrasound is not contraindicated. However, at maximum machine output settings, significant thermal effects at bone surfaces cannot be excluded. The user is advised to make use of any exposure information provided by the manufacturer (for example in the form of displayed safety indices) to gain awareness of the highest output conditions, and to act prudently to limit exposure of critical structures, including bone and regions including gas. Where on-line display is not available, particular care should be taken to minimise exposure times.

The embryonic period is known to be particularly sensitive to any external influences. Until further scientific information is available, investigations using pulsed or colour Doppler ultrasound should be carried out with careful control of output levels and exposure times.

With increasing mineralisation of the fetal bone as the fetus develops the possibility of heating fetal bone increases. The user should prudently limit exposure of critical structures such as the fetal skull or spine during Doppler studies.

In addition, the World Federation for Ultrasound in Medicine and Biology (WFUMB)[46] surveyed the existing literature in 1994 and issued the following statements:

Thermal issues

The following safety statements were endorsed as policy of the World Federation for Ultrasound in Medicine and Biology following recommendations from the 1991 WFUMB Symposium on Safety of Ultrasound in Medicine on Thermal Issues. The conclusions from the 1996 WFUMB Symposium on Safety in Ultrasound in Medicine are that there is no scientific evidence to alter the existing safety statements on thermal issues. Hence, the WFUMB Safety Statements for Thermal Bio-effects are reiterated to complete the current safety guidelines.

B-mode imaging

Known diagnostic ultrasound equipment, as used today for simple B-mode imaging, operates at acoustic outputs that are not capable of producing harmful temperature rises. Its use in medicine is, therefore, not contraindicated on thermal grounds. This induces endoscopic, trans-vaginal and trans-cutaneous applications.

Doppler

It has been demostrated in experiments with unperfused tissue that some Doppler diagnostic equipment has the potential to produce biologically significant temperature rises, specifically at bone/soft tissue interfaces. The effect of elevated temperatures may be minimised by keeping the time for which the beam passes through any one point in tissue as short as possible. Where output power can be controlled, the lowest available power level consistent with obtaining the desired diagnostic information should be used. Although the data on humans are sparse, it is clear from animal studies that exposures resulting in temperatures less than 38.5°C can be used without reservation on thermal grounds. This includes obstetric applications.

Transducer heating

A substantial source of heating may be the transducer itself. Tissue heating from this source is localised to the volume in contact with the transducer.

REFERENCES

1 ter Haar G R, Duck F A, Starritt H, Daniels S. Biophysical characterization of diagnostic ultrasound equipment – preliminary results. Phys Med Biol 1989; 34: 1533–1542

2 Bosward K, Barnett S B, Wood A F K, Edwards M J, Kossoff G. Heating of guinea pig fetal brain during exposure to pulsed ultrasound. Ultrasound Med Biol 1993; 19: 415–424

3 Drewniak J L, Carnes K I, Dunn F. In vitro ultrasonic heating of fetal bone. J Acoust Soc Am 1989; 86: 1254–1258

4 Duggan P M, Liggans G C, Barnett S B. Ultrasonic heating of the brain of fetal sheep in utero. Ultrasound Med Biol 1995; 21: 553–560

5 Henderson J, Whittingham T A, Dunn T. A review of the acoustic output of modern diagnostic equipment. BMUS Bull 1997; 4: 10–14

6 Edwards M J. Hyperthermia as a teratogen: a review of experimental studies and their clinical significance. Teratogenesis, Carcinog Mutagen 1986; 6: 563–582

7 Duggan P M, Cowan L M E. Reference ranges and ultrasound exposure conditions for pulsed Doppler studies of the femoral carotid artery. J Ultrasound Med 1993; 12: 719–722

8 Miller M W, Ziskin M C. Biological consequences of hyperthermia. Ultrasound Med Biol 1989; 15: 707–722

9 ter Haar G R. Ultrasonic biophysics. In: Physical principles of medical ultrasound, 1986: 379–435

10 Daniels S, ter Haar G. Bubble formation in guinea pigs and agar gels during ultrasonic irradiation. Proc I O A 1986; 8: 147–157

11 Child S Z, Carstensen E L, Smachlo K. Effects of ultrasound on Drosophila III. Exposure of larvae to low temporal average intensity, pulsed irradiation. Ultrasound Med Biol 1981; 7: 167–173

12 Child S Z, Hartman C L, Schery L A, Carstensen E L. Lung damage from exposure to pulsed ultrasound. Ultrasound Med Biol 1990; 16: 817–825

13 Raeman C H, Child S Z, Carstensen E L. Timing of exposures in ultrasonic haemorrhage of murine lung. Ultrasound Med Biol 1993; 19: 507–512

14 Frizzell L A, Chen E, Lee C. Effects of pulsed ultrasound on the mouse neonate: hind limb paralysis and lung haemorrhage. Ultrasound Med Biol 1994; 20: 53–63

15 Zachary J F, O'Brien W D. Lung haemorrhage induced by continuous and pulsed wave (diagnostic) ultrasound in mice, rabbits and pigs. Vet Pathol 1995; 32: 43–54

16 Tarantal A, Canfield D R. Ultrasound induced lung damage in the monkey. Ultrasound Med Biol 1994; 20: 53–63

17 Miller D L, Thomas R M. Thresholds for hemorrhages in mouse skin and intestine induced by lithotripter shockwaves. Ultrasound Med Biol 1995; 21: 249–257

18 Dalecki D, Raeman C H, Child S Z, Carstensen E L. Intestinal haemorrhage from exposure to pulsed ultrasound. Ultrasound Med Biol 1995; 21: 1067–1072

19 Brayman A A, Azadniv M, Cox C, Miller M W. Haemolysis of albunex supplemented, 40% haematocrit human erythrocytes in vitro by 1 MHz pulsed ultrasound: acoustic pressure and pulse length dependence. Ultrasound Med Biol 1996; 22: 927–938

20 Miller D L, Thomas R M. Ultrasound contrast agents nucleate inertial cavitation in vitro. Ultrasound Med Biol 1995; 21: 1059–1065

21 Miller D L, Thomas R M. Contrast agent gas bodies enhance haemolysis induced by lithotripter shock waves and high intensity focused ultrasound in whole blood. Ultrasound Med Biol 1996; 22: 1089–1095

22 Brayman A A, Azadniv M, Makin I R S et al. Effect of stabilised microbubble echo contrast agent on haemolysis of human erythrocytes exposed to high intensity pulsed ultrasound. Echocardiography 1995; 12: 13–21

23 Ivey J A, Gardner E A, Fowlkes J B, Rubin J M, Carson P L. Acoustic generation of intra-arterial contrast boluses. Ultrasound Med Biol 1995; 21: 757–767

24 Ziskin M, Petitti D. Epidemiology of human exposure to ultrasound – a critical review. Ultrasound Med Biol 1988; 14: 91–96

25 Moore R, Diamond E, Cavaliere R. The relationship of birth weight and intrauterine diagnostic ultrasound exposure. Obstet Gynecol 1988; 71: 513–517

26 Newnham J, Evans S, Michael C, Stanley F, Landau L. Effects of frequent ultrasound during pregnancy: a randomised controlled trial. Lancet 1993; 342: 887–891

27 Waldenström U, Axelsson O, Nilsson S et al. Effects on routine one-stage ultrasound screening in pregnancy: a randomised controlled trial. Lancet 1988; ii: 585–588

28 Neilson J P (1993) Routine ultrasound in early pregnancy. In: Enkin M W, Keirse M J N C, Renfrew M J, Neilson J P, eds. Pregnancy and Childbirth module 'Cochrane database of systematic reviews' Review no. 03872 Oxford update software, 'Cochrane update on disc'.

29 Lyons E, Dyke C, Toms M, Cheang M. In utero exposure to diagnostic ultrasound: a 6 year follow-up. Radiology 1988; 166: 687–690

30 Salvesen K, Jacobsen G, Vatten L, Eik-Nes S, Bakketeig L. Routine ultrasonography in utero and subsequent growth during childhood. Ultrasound Obstet Gynecol 1993; 3: 6–10

31 Bakketeig L S, Eik-Nes S H, Jacobsen G et al. A randomized controlled trial of ultrasonographic screening in pregnancy. Lancet 1984; ii: 207–210

32 Scheidt P D, Stanley F, Bryla D A. One year follow-up of infants exposed to ultrasound in utero. Am J Obstet Gynecol 1978; 121: 742–748

33 Stark C R, Orleans M, Haverkamp A D, Murphy J. Short- and long-term risks after exposure to diagnostic ultrasound in utero. Obstet Gynecol 1984; 63: 194–200

34 Hellman L M, Duffus G M, Donald I, Sunden B. Safety of diagnostic ultrasound in obstetrics. Lancet 1970; i: 1133–1135

35 Bernstine R L. Safety studies with ultrasonic Doppler technique: a clinical follow-up of patients and tissue culture study. Obstet Gynecol 1969; 34: 707–709

36 Cartwright R A, McKinney P A, Hopton P A et al. Ultrasound examination in pregnancy and childhood cancer. Lancet 1984; ii: 999–1000

37 Kinnier-Wilson L M, Waterhouse J A. Obstetric ultrasound and childhood malignancies. Lancet 1984; ii: 997–999

38 Salvesen K, Bakketeig L, Eik-Nes S, Undheim J, Okland O. Routine ultrasonography in utero and school performance at age 8–9 years. Lancet 1992; 339: 85–89

39 Salvesen K, Vatten L, Jacobsen G et al. Routine ultrasonography in utero and subsequent vision and hearing at primary school age. Ultrasound Obstet Gynecol 1992; 2: 243–247

40 Salvesen K, Vatten L, Eik-Nes S, Hugdahl K, Bakketeig L. Routine ultrasonography in utero and subsequent handedness and neurological development BMJ 1993; 307: 159–164

41 Campbell J, Elford R, Brant R. Case-control study of prenatal ultrasonography exposure in children with delayed speech. Can Med Assoc J 1993; 149: 1435–1440

42 Salvesen K, Vatten L, Bakketeig L, Eik-Nes S. Routine ultrasonography in utero and speech development. Ultrasound Obstet Gynecol 1994; 4: 101–103

43 European Committee for Ultrasound Radiation Safety. EFSUMB tutorial paper: Thermal and mechanical indices. Eur J Ultrasound 1996; 4: 145–150

44 American Institute of Ultrasound in Medicine/National Electrical Manufacturers Association (AIUM/NEMA) Standard for real-time display of thermal and mechanical acoustic output indices on diagnostic ultrasound equipment. Rockville, Maryland: AIUM, 1992

45 European Committee for Medical Ultrasound Safety. http://www.efsumb.org.

46 World Federation for Ultrasound in Medicine & Biology. 1998 WFUMB Symposium on Safety of Ultrasound in Medicine, Kloster-Banz April 1996: Conclusions and recommendations on thermal and non-thermal mechanisms of ultrasound. Barnett S B (ed) Ultrasound Med Biol 24 Suppl 1.

FURTHER READING

Fowlkes J B, Holland C K. Mechanical Bioeffect from Diagnostic Ultrasound: AWM Consensus Statements. Jounal of Ultrasound in Medicine 2000 19: 68–168.

Artefacts in B-mode scanning

David O Cosgrove

Introduction

Strictly, an artefact is any man-made object; in radiology the term is used in a looser sense to describe unwanted information generated in the process of image formation.[1,2] Most artefacts interfere with interpretation, though there are occasional 'friendly artefacts' which contain diagnostically useful clues (e.g. acoustic shadowing). Ultrasound is particularly prone to artefacts: their recognition and avoidance form a major part of the skill and art of sonography.[3]

Noise

Two types of noise beset all imaging systems: random and structured. All electrical components produce random voltage changes at low level; when these are amplified they appear as a fluctuating, moving pattern of fine grey spots resembling a snowstorm. Since the scanner's electronic components are designed to keep such noise at low levels, it is only seen when high degrees of amplification are applied and so is usually most obvious in the deeper parts of the image where the Time-gain Control (TGC) amplifier adds most to the overall receiver gain (Fig. 4.1). Noise is also produced by tissue where it arises from random vibrations of molecules. Noise sets the limit to the maximum depth that can be reached at a given transducer frequency. Because this type of noise is random in time, its effects can be reduced by temporal smoothing (the scanner controls for this are labelled 'frame averaging' or 'persistence' on some machines). With this technique the information in

two or more images is added together. The 'real' information is reinforced while the random noise tends to cancel out. Another way to reduce the impact of noise is to encode the transmitted pulses so that the corresponding echoes can be picked out from the noise by recognising the encoded signature in the receive circuitry. This approach has been implemented in high-end scanners and allows the use of higher frequency transducers, thus improving the spatial resolution of the images.

Random noise may also be produced by electrical interference but in this case it usually forms patterned signals such as flashes or bars in the image; structured noise such as this is known as clutter (Fig. 4.2). It is caused by pickup of extraneous signals in the radio-frequency band, the transducer acting as an antenna, or by electrical pulses breaking through into the mains or interconnecting cables to attachments such as recorders. The noise they produce is usually obviously artefactual, the interference appearing randomly or intermittently, sometimes coinciding with the switching of a nearby motor or diathermy unit. Transient pulses can also wreak havoc with the digital circuitry of the scanner computer, causing it to lock up or otherwise misbehave. Mains filters or even shielding of the scanning room may be required in severe cases.

Structured noise can also be caused by body or probe movements. In practice these are usually too low in amplitude to produce detectable signals in B-mode but they are important as motion artefacts in Doppler. However, in phase inversion harmonics, used either in the tissue harmonic mode or with microbubbles, motion artefact can be

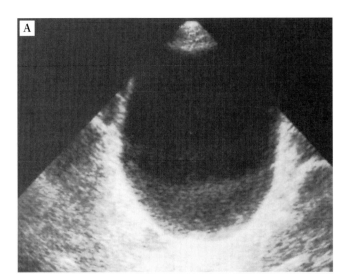 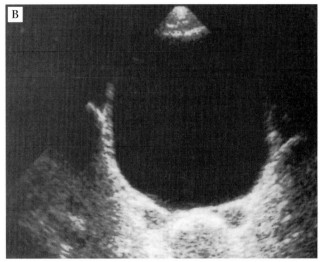

Fig. 4.1 Gain-related noise. A: The combination of high overall gain and the high TGC amplification at depth may produce random noise in the image. Though this is present throughout the deeper parts of the image, because it is masked by the echoes from tissue structure, the noise is most obtrusive in echo-free regions such as within the urinary bladder. **B:** In this case, correction of the excessive gains removed the noise but this cannot always be achieved without also darkening the structure whose display is required.

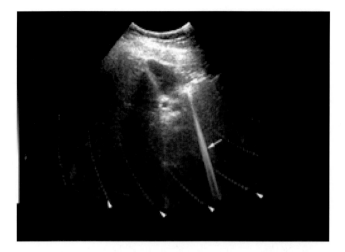

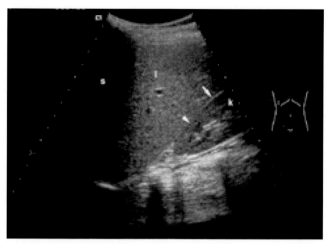

Fig. 4.2 Structured noise. Persistent oblique bars (arrowheads) on these images were found to be due to electrical interference to the scanner by a nearby diathermy apparatus. Similar effects can be produced by radio transmitters and by stray fields from poorly shielded television monitors and video recorders. CB radio transmitters are particularly troublesome offenders. Note also the comet-tail artefact (arrow) (see also Fig. 4.15).

Fig. 4.3 Specular and scattered echoes. Scattered signals account for the low intensity parenchymal echoes from the liver (l) and kidney (k). Their appearance is independent of the direction of the ultrasound beam. Specular echoes arise from the flatter structures of the peritoneal and fascial layers separating the liver from the kidney. These echoes are strongly dependent on the angle between the beam and the surface, being intense when the surface is aligned at 90° (arrow) but weak or even completely absent when the beam runs along the interface (arrowhead). Note also the rib shadow (s).

apparent as flashes of grey highlights when the probe is swept across a structure.[4] This arises because the system is sensitive to differences between sequential pulses (see Ch. 5).

There are numerous other sources of noise such as interference from the scan-head motor and faulty connections and soldered joints which may affect ultrasound scanners, but they are uncommon and generally not diagnostically confusing, though rectification requires specialist service engineers. Structured noise due to multiple reflections and side lobes is discussed on page 54.

Scattering and specular interfaces

Two distinct types of ultrasound echo formation are recognised and each produces important artefacts. Echoes arising from small regions[5] (around the ultrasound wavelength, say 0.1–1 mm) where there is a change in impedance are known as scattered echoes because they are sent out more or less uniformly in all directions.[6] It follows that the amount of ultrasound energy returning to the transducer from each scattering structure is extremely low (e.g. if the scattering is truly omnidirectional, then only some 0.25% is received by the transducer, depending on its diameter and on the depth of the scatterer); generally this signal will be too weak to be detected. However, when a group of such weak scatterers lies in the beam (this is the usual situation when, for example, they are the surfaces related to liver lobules or renal tubules), the echoes

combine to form an interference pattern, cancelling out in some directions but summing in others to produce signals strong enough to be detected (Fig. 4.3). The near-random pattern that results is known as speckle: it is the acoustic equivalent of the speckled texture seen under laser light, for example in a hologram. The ultrasound pattern, though isotropic (i.e. uniform regardless of scanning direction), is only indirectly related to the real tissue structure: the displayed texture is actually a convolution of the real structure by the ultrasound pulse shape. Thus a pixel on the ultrasound image of the parenchyma of, say, the liver, cannot be expected to correspond to a histological interface in the organ. Because the speckle pattern is as much produced by the transducer as by the tissue, the same organ will produce a different texture with different transducers and tissues with different histological structures may have indistinguishable appearances on ultrasound – an example is the near-identical texture of liver and spleen.

When the reflecting surface is flat (relative to the ultrasound wavelength), it behaves like a mirror so that the direction of reflection equals the angle of incidence. Since the focused beam of ultrasound is not dispersed, all of the reflected energy can be picked up by the transducer so that the signals are much stronger than for scatterers. However, they are intensely directional and thus are only detected when the transducer is correctly directed, i.e. when the surface is at right angles to the beam in standard pulse-echo imaging. As the surface is tilted away from the right angle, the signal intensity falls off rapidly; in fact, were it not for the tolerance afforded by the beam width and the fact that real biological surfaces are rarely mirror-smooth, any tilting of the surface from 90° would cause the echo to be lost and this constraint would apply in both the scanned and orthogonal planes. In practice most interfaces are detectable up to angles of more than 60°, albeit with diminished intensity, depending on the particular structures involved (Fig. 4.3). A situation where this may cause confusion is in scanning tendons, whose fibrilar structure gives strong echoes when they lie at right angles to the beam but at oblique angles appear as relatively echo-poor, simulating a tear or tendinosis.[7,8]

However, beyond some limiting angle, flat surfaces are not imaged and this can be confusing (Fig. 4.4). It

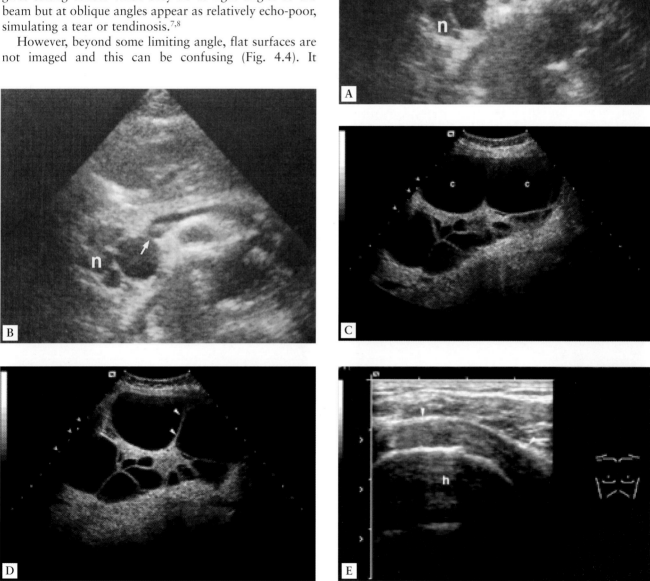

Fig. 4.4 Missing echoes. When flat surfaces that lie along the beam are not depicted, very confusing images are produced. **A:** An example is the wall between a dilated lower common bile duct and the adjacent portal vein in the head of the pancreas. The duct seems to form part of the vein and may be missed altogether. **B:** The interface is readily detected when the transducer is appropriately angled (arrow). (The obstruction was caused by enlarged lymph nodes (n) in the head of the pancreas.) **C:** A similar situation can be seen in this hyperstimulated ovary: when the ultrasound beam runs along the interface between the largest cysts (c) it is hard to make out, but **D:** moving the transducer a little to one side reveals it clearly (arrowheads). **E:** In this scan of a normal rotator cuff in the shoulder, the tendon (arrowheads) appears more reflective where the beam strikes it at right angles anteriorly. As the ligament curves laterally, it seems to be less reflective. This artefact can erroneously suggest tendon damage. h – head of humerus.

accounts for the apparent communication sometimes seen between the inferior vena cava and the aorta when these lie close together, for the failure to image the sides of the globe of the eye and for the invisibility of the superior surface of the urinary bladder in ascites scanned from certain angles. Such 'missing' surfaces can be demonstrated by scanning from other angles: the sonographer needs to be aware of the problem to avoid serious diagnostic errors.

Shadowing and increased sound transmission

The commonest form of shadowing (and its counterpart, increased through transmission of sound) are perhaps not true artefacts and their presence provides important diagnostic information about the attenuation of the tissues responsible for them (Table 4.1).[9,10] Shadowing occurs when a region of the tissue has a higher attenuation coefficient than the majority of the tissue in the scan; since

Table 4.1 Types of shadowing

Type	Source
Attenuation	Attenuation higher than TGC compensation
Reflective	Near-total reflection
Edge	From curved surfaces

the TGC (which corrects for the attenuation with depth) can only be set for an average value, an inadequate correction will be applied to this region so that both it and the tissues deep to it are depicted as less reflective than they actually are (Fig. 4.5). The dark band is referred to as an acoustic or distal shadow. Conversely, if a region of tissue attenuates less than its surroundings, echoes from it and the deeper tissue are overcorrected and appear as a bright band known as 'enhancement' but, in view of the enhancing effects of microbubble contrast agents (see Ch. 5), it is perhaps better termed 'increased through transmission' or 'distal bright-up' (Fig. 4.6). The degree of shadowing and increased sound transmission is determined by the difference in attenuation from the surrounding structures as well as the path length through the anomalous region. Thus these effects provide clues to the attenuation of the tissue regions responsible – they can be thought of as 'friendly artefacts'. Ways to reduce shadowing and increased through transmission have been developed and promise to facilitate correct setting of the TGC.[3]

Since shadowing is simply loss of acoustic signal for a tissue region, it can also be produced by an extremely efficient reflector (Fig. 4.7).[11] Gas bubbles or regions of calcification for example, where 99% and 80% of the incident sound beam is reflected back respectively, cast acoustic shadows because very little of the sound energy penetrates to insonate the deeper tissues (in addition, any echoes from them would probably not cross the reflective layer on the return journey since they would be re-reflected distally).

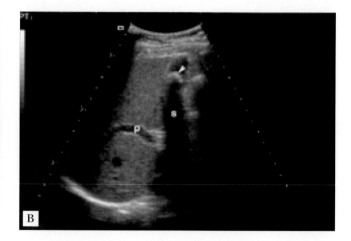

Fig. 4.5 Acoustic shadowing. When a structure absorbs more sound energy than its surroundings, the TGC correction is inadequate for that region and the deeper structures appear darker: this is known as acoustic or distal shadowing. **A:** Produced by fibrosis in a breast surgery scar and **B:** by gallstones in the gallbladder (arrowhead). p – portal vein, s – shadowing.

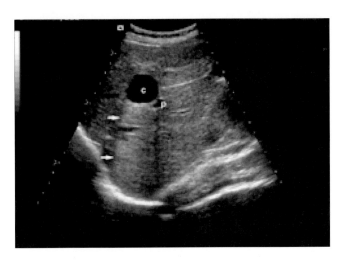

Fig. 4.6 Increased through transmission. The fluid in a cyst absorbs very little of the sound energy passing through it so that the TGC, which has been adjusted to correct for attenuation in the surrounding tissues (here, the liver) is locally excessive. The deeper tissues are depicted as being more reflective giving a lighter band (arrows) known as distal or acoustic enhancement. c – cyst, p – portal vein.

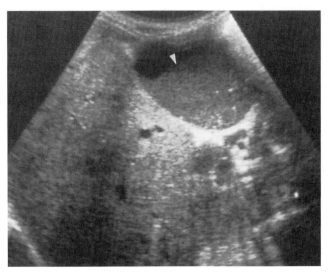

Fig. 4.8 Echogenic fluid. Since in many real situations only a small amount of energy is removed from the beam by reflection, it is quite possible to encounter debris-containing fluids that are accompanied by enhancement. In this example echogenic bile (arrowhead) partly fills the gallbladder.

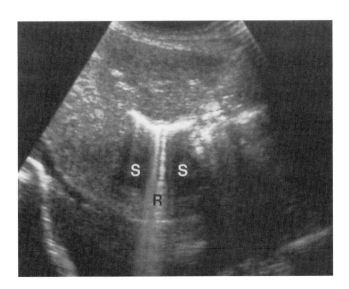

Fig. 4.7 Reflective shadowing. When an interface reflects all or almost all of the incident sound energy, a situation that is typical of gas (here, gas in the common bile duct), so little penetrates that a band of distal shadowing (S) results. Though the effect is the same as with absorptive shadowing (compare with Fig. 4.5), the mechanism is different. The intense flat reflector that the gas forms often leads to reverberation artefacts (R) that partially fill the shadow (compare with Fig. 4.14).

However, it should be noted that, for most soft tissues, only a small proportion of the loss of energy from the beam (i.e. the attenuation) is due to reflection (in fact only between 1% and 20%) so that echogenicity does not correlate closely with attenuation. Echogenic fluids (e.g. crystalline bile or a pyonephrosis) are examples where strong echoes are associated with increased through transmission (Fig. 4.8).

An interesting and sometimes confusing form of shadowing occurs deep to the edges of strongly curved surfaces such as vessels, cyst walls and fetal skull (Fig. 4.9). Fine, dark lines are seen extending distal to such edges; in the case of a cyst, they are striking by contrast with the increased through transmission behind the cyst itself. Two explanations have been offered (Fig. 4.10). In the refractive model, the ultrasound beam is dispersed as it is reflected from the curved edge because the leading edge of the ultrasound beam strikes it at a different angle than the trailing edge. Thus the ultrasound energy is spread through a larger tissue region and so the returning echoes are weaker, resulting in a 'shadow'; at the same time, the velocity differences may focus the beam in the region immediately deep to the structure, increasing the signals here.[12] Simple geometric reflection, as from a flat surface, would not have the same effect, for a mirror image of the tissues it strikes will be superimposed on the band immediately behind the edge; this is the mirror image artefact (see below). The other explanation presumes that the tissue of the wall of the curved structure has a higher attenuation than the surrounding tissue; the ultrasound beam passing along the edge must pass through three to four times as much of this tissue than that crossing at the diameter and therefore will be attenuated more. The effect is familiar to those who have used a hacksaw in plumbing: cutting a pipe is difficult at first, becoming easier towards the centre of the pipe before becoming more difficult again as the full thickness of the other side is cut. In this model the edge shadows are a form of attenuation, but only of the wall material, not of the contents. The two mechanisms could coexist in different situations.

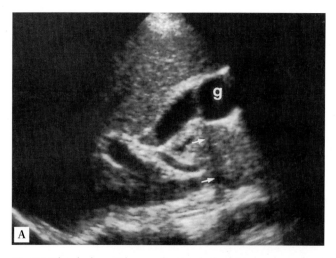 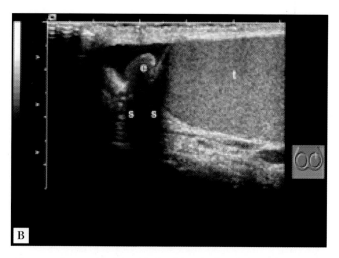

Fig. 4.9 Edge shadows. Edge or refractive shadows (s) are commonly produced by smooth curved surfaces. In **A:** such a shadow (arrows) is seen beyond a fold within the gallbladder (g), while in **B:** the upper pole of a normal testis (t) and the surface of the head of the epididymis (e) have had the same effect.

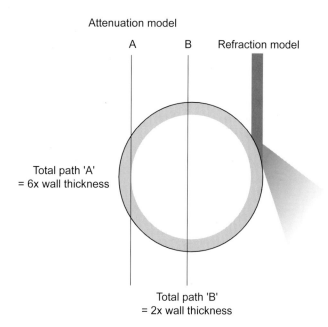

Fig. 4.10 Mechanisms of edge shadows. Edge shadows are fine echo-poor lines extending deep to the edges of strongly curved structures. Two possible mechanisms are illustrated. On the left is the attenuation model which proposes that the wall is more attenuating than the surrounding tissue; since the beam traversing the edge of the wall 'B' must traverse three times the thickness of the wall as the beam 'A' passing through the diameter of the curved structure, it is more heavily attenuated. On the right is the refractive model which proposes that the beam is dispersed as it reflects from the curved edge which is struck at more than the critical angle; the returning echoes from the spreading beam have less energy than echoes from a confined beam, so that, even though they are reflected from the interfaces they encounter, their intensity is reduced. In either case the shadows should not be construed as signifying high attenuation, as would ordinarily be the case.

Edge or refractive shadows do not have the same diagnostic significance as bulk shadowing. Unfortunately, edge shadows commonly occur in situations where shadowing suggests calcification (e.g. in the kidney, arising from vessel walls in the renal sinus) or malignancy (e.g. in the breast, where they arise from Cooper's ligaments); they must be recognised for what they are and dismissed.

Multiple echoes

A basic and critical assumption in pulse-echo ultrasound is that the ultrasound beam returns directly to the transducer after a single reflection.[13] Where the geometry allows multiple reflections to occur, multiple images are formed, and sometimes these are confusing. Repeat echoes are more likely to occur where the reflections are strong and this implies flat surfaces giving specular echoes. Since the path lengths for multiples are longer, the corresponding images are depicted as lying deeper in the body and they are weakened as the ultrasound is attenuated. Therefore, multiple echoes are more likely to be observed when the surfaces are close together and when the intervening tissue is of low attenuation, for example, when it is a fluid.

An example of a single echo is the mirror image artefact where a repeat of a structure is depicted on the 'other side' of a specular reflector and equidistant from it.[14,15] This effect is readily demonstrated for the diaphragm: imaged from below through the liver, echoes commonly appear above the diaphragm and sometimes discrete structures in the normal liver or focal lesions can be recognised there (Fig. 4.11). This is not the appearance of lung (which is seen as an intensely reflective band when imaged intercostally) and is attributable to the beam reflecting back into the liver from the diaphragm.[16] Actually the reflecting

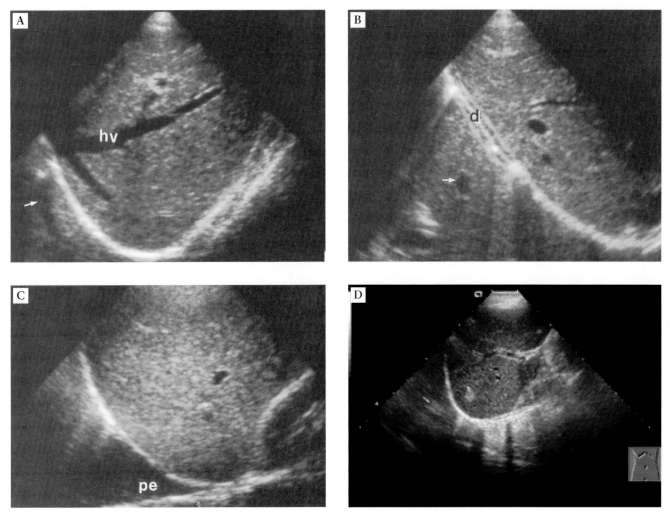

Fig. 4.11 Mirror image artefacts. The apparent tissue normally visualised above the diaphragm in the right lower zone of the chest is actually artefactual, being produced by the air–pleura interface acting as an acoustic mirror. Sometimes recognisable structures feature in the artefact, forming 'ghost images'. **A:** An example is a branch of the right hepatic vein (arrow) while in **B:** a blood vessel (arrow) is cut in cross-section. In this image the diaphragm appears as a triple-layered structure: probably this is a mirror image of thickening of the diaphragmatic peritoneum. **C:** Since the artefact depends on reflection from the air surface, where this is replaced, such as by consolidation or a pleural effusion (pe), the artefact no longer occurs. **D:** Pathological changes may appear as 'ghost lesions'; an example is the haemangioma in the upper part of the right lobe of the liver. It has its mirrored counterpart (arrow), seemingly within the chest. d – diaphragm, hv – hepatic vein, k – kidney.

surface is probably the air–pleura interface since the muscle of the diaphragm itself would be expected to act as a scatterer rather than a specular reflector.

Generally this artefact is not a diagnostic problem and on rare occasions it may actually be useful, for example when it reveals increased sound transmission beyond a peripheral liver cyst where it would otherwise be invisible as it falls onto the diaphragm; since this is already shown as a full white on the screen no further increase in intensity can be depicted. In other situations the mirror artefact is confusing; in the pelvis for example, a repeat echo of the bladder or of structures immediately posterior to it (the rectum or sigmoid) may appear as a deeper line

marking the back of an echo-poor mass (Figs 4.12 and 4.13). In fact the echo-poor region is the mirror image of the bladder. The typical position should arouse suspicion that it is artefactual and the back wall of the 'mass' often lies beyond the position of the sacrum and so is anatomical nonsense. A further clue is the weak superior and inferior walls compared to the strong anterior and posterior walls.

Multiple repeat echoes are known as reverberations. They are produced when two strong reflectors lie parallel to each other. By far the commonest example of this is when a flat surface such as a gas pocket or a stone is parallel to the skin surface where the skin–transducer

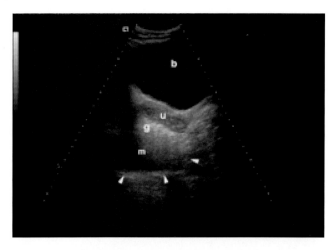

Fig. 4.12 False pelvic mass. Ultrasound reflecting from the gas surfaces in pelvic bowel loops may be re-reflected into the tissues and produce a second-time-around echo depicted at twice the depth of the gas surface (arrow). Here it may simulate a deep interface forming the back wall of a pseudomass which is nothing more than a mirror artefact. The typical geometry, the anatomical impossibility of a mass lying so far posteriorly and the lack of superior and inferior walls are clues to its artefactual nature. b – bladder, g – gas in bowel, m – mass, u – uterus.

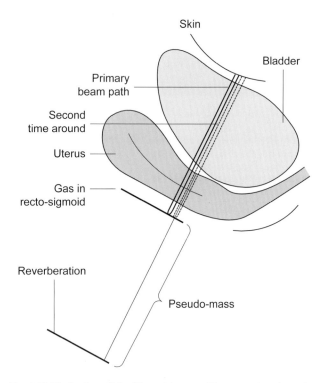

Fig. 4.13 Mechanism of the false pelvic mass. The strong interface of bowel gas immediately posterior to the bladder acts as a mirror, reflecting the sound beam back to the transducer from which a proportion is re-reflected into the tissues to give a repeat or second-time-around image that simulates the back wall of a large pelvic mass.

interface forms the second reflector (Fig. 4.14). Ultrasound reflected from the gas travels back to the transducer in the usual way to generate a correctly placed image, but a proportion of the echo is re-reflected back into the tissue, retracing its path. On its second reflection from the gas surface it produces a second image at twice the depth of the real image. Sequential repeat echoes are depicted deeper behind the first ('real') echo. A striped pattern results, with the deeper multiple echoes becoming weaker because of loss of sound energy due to incomplete reflection at the surfaces and to attenuation by the intervening tissues. Since weaker echoes appear to be narrower than stronger ones, the reverberating bands become shorter as well as less intense with depth. The spacing between the bands depends on the distance between the reflectors; if they are very close together the echoes may merge to form a reflective band in which the individual components cannot be discerned (Fig. 4.15). A bright streak appears on the display, forming a tail distal to the image of the causal structure, itself usually strongly reflective. The whole complex looks rather like a comet with its bright tail.[17,18] This 'comet-tail' artefact is commonly seen deep to calcifications[19] and foreign bodies such as surgical clips, implants (including IUCDs) and catheters. Bullets and shrapnel may also cause the comet-tail effect, as may small fluid cavities such as the Aschoff-Rokitansky sinuses in the wall of the gallbladder in adenomyosis. Presumably here the sound reverberates within each fluid space, echoing repeatedly from its walls. The same phenomenon probably accounts for the comet tail commonly seen distal to frothy or foamy collections of gas bubbles, the sound reflecting repeatedly from the outer surfaces of the gas bubbles in all directions within the intervening fluid so that a continuous stream of sound escapes, some of which returns to the receiving transducer. The effect is often observed from gas within the duodenal cap and is transient as a peristaltic wave moves the gas on.

Velocity errors

An important assumption of the pulse-echo technique used in ultrasound imaging is that the velocity of ultrasound in soft tissues is constant. In fact this is not quite true, fat, for example, conducting ultrasound some 15% more slowly than most other soft tissues (Table 4.2).[20–23] Prosthetic materials show more marked deviations; for example, silicone used for breast augmentation and testicular implants has a sound speed of about half that of soft tissue.

The average velocity of 1540 m/s used to calibrate scanners corresponds to a delay-to-depth conversion constant and the scanner is calibrated so that every 13 µs delay in the echoes after the transmit pulse corresponds to 1 cm depth on the final image. Where a tissue conducts more slowly the echoes from deeper structures are further

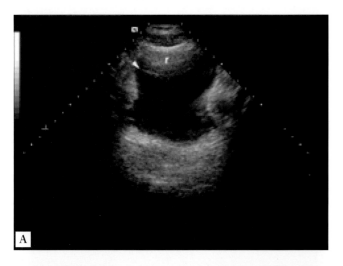

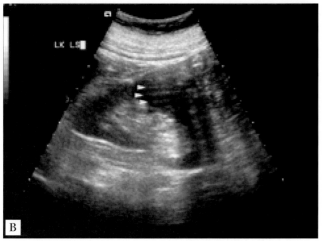

Fig. 4.14 Reverberation artefacts. A: A second-time-around signal occurs when a strong reflector, in this example the anterior surface of the bladder, lies parallel to the skin-transducer surface so that some of the received signal is re-reflected into the tissue to be received as a false surface (arrowhead) at twice the depth of the real surface. The mechanism is the same as for the false pelvic mass (see Fig. 4.13) There are also complex reverberations (r) giving an impression of noise in the anterior part of the bladder. **B:** The same effect occurs in solid tissue, here across a kidney (arrowheads), though here it is often masked by the tissue echoes themselves.

Table 4.2 Velocity of ultrasound in biologically important materials (from Wells 1969, Goss 1978 and Bamber 1986)

Tissue type	Velocity (m/s)
Air	330
Fat	1450
Water (20°C)	1480
Amniotic fluid	1510
Brain	1565
Blood	1570
Kidney	1560
Muscle	1580
Liver	1600
Uterus	1630
Skin	1700
Lens of eye	1650
Fascia	1750
Perspex	2680
Bone	3500
Soft tissue average	**1540**

delayed and are therefore depicted as originating from deeper in the body (Fig. 4.16A).[23,24] This geometric distortion does not affect lateral dimensions of the image since this is set by the scanning action of the transducer rather than by the speed of sound. For the most part, velocity errors are too small to be clinically important, though, especially for silicone implants, the effects may be surprisingly marked. However, in ophthalmic measurements, where great precision is required, the distortion caused by the significantly higher velocity in the lens can be important. The speed of sound in the lens of the eye is 1620 m/s; regions of the retina imaged through it appear closer than the parts imaged through the sclera so that a shelf-like anterior distortion is produced (known as Baum's bumps after the sonologist who first described them; Fig. 4.16B).[25]

Changes in velocity also produce refractive artefacts: the ultrasound beam deviates from its straight line path

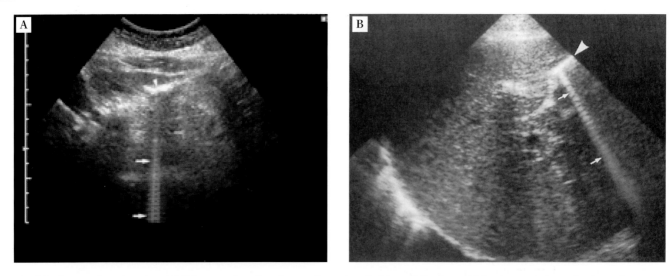

Fig. 4.15 Comet-tail artefact. A and **B:** When a pocket of gas forms a foam, there is the possibility for multiple, almost random reflection paths between the bubbles to produce trains of echoes. They are seen as intensely reflective lines (arrows) extending deep to the gas. This is most commonly seen from the duodenum (arrowheads).

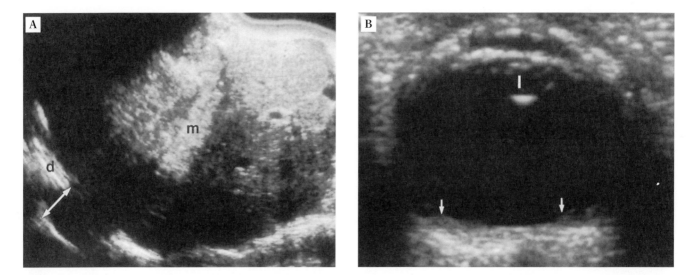

Fig. 4.16 Velocity errors. When traversing a region where it is conducted slowly, the sound beam takes longer to complete the go-and-return pathway, so that echoes from beyond it are depicted deeper in the image than their real positions. **A:** In this example, a fatty metastasis (m) in the liver has slowed the sound beam so that the diaphragm (d) appears to have a shelf (arrow). **B:** The reverse situation, where a high-velocity region is traversed, as is the case for the lens (l) of the eye, moves the portion imaged through it closer. The resulting distortion, known as Baum's bumps (arrows), can cause serious errors in eye diameter measurements.

when it crosses obliquely between two tissues of different velocities (Fig. 4.17). The beam is bent towards the 90° line when entering a 'slower tissue' and vice versa. The scanner, of course, continues to operate on the assumption that the beam follows a straight line so that reflectors distant to the surface are incorrectly plotted to the side of their true position. The degree of displacement depends both on the speed of sound difference and on the distance of the object from the surface. A particular situation where this lateral distortion is important clinically is in trans-abdominal pelvic scans. The beam crossing the wedge-shaped fat space around the rectus muscles is refracted so that deep pelvic structures (e.g. the uterus or prostate) can appear stretched laterally (Figs 4.18 and 4.19).[26,27] A transverse obstetric measurement made under these circumstances may be in serious error. In extreme cases the object, for example a gestational sac, may seem to be duplicated giving rise to the false appearance of twins – this is one reason for the phenomenon of the 'vanishing twin' noted when ultrasound was first used in early pregnancy. The

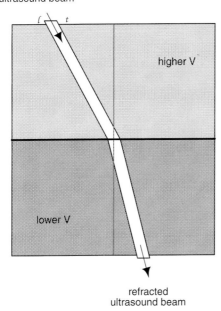

Fig. 4.17 Refraction of ultrasound. When the ultrasound beam crosses obliquely between two tissues of differing velocities, the beam is refracted to emerge in a new direction. The situation is exactly the same as the refraction of a light beam. The diagram illustrates the effect of crossing into a material that conducts the ultrasound more slowly: the sound in the leading edge of the beam (l) is slowed first, while sound towards the trailing edge (t) is affected later. This results in the entire beam being refracted towards the 90° direction. The converse occurs when the deeper medium conducts faster.

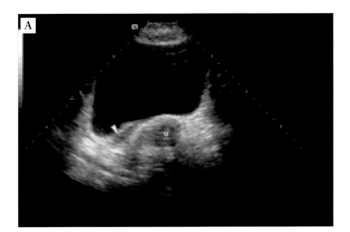

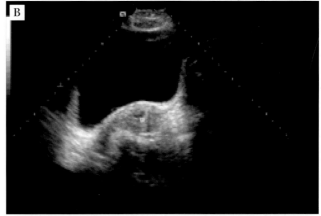

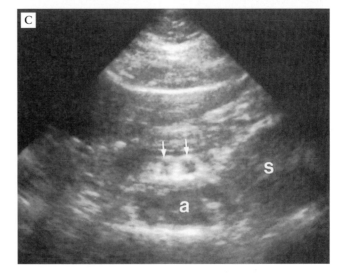

Fig. 4.18 Refractive artefacts. A: Refraction of the ultrasound beam by the fatty tissues in the anterior abdominal wall can produce split or double images such as this apparent double wall at the back of the bladder (arrow). **B:** Its artefactual nature is clear when the duplication disappears on moving the transducer slightly to one side. **C:** The 'split image' artefact is less common in the upper abdomen, perhaps because there is usually less fat and less muscle here, but occasionally apparent duplication of the super mesenteric artery is seen (arrows). The aortic wall also appears to be stretched laterally. a – aorta, s – stomach.

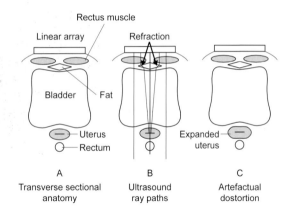

Fig. 4.19 Double images in the pelvis. When the ultrasound beam strikes the slower-conducting layer of fat, it is bent towards the midline so that medial structures are displayed lateral to their true position (B). They therefore appear laterally stretched (C) or even duplicated, leading to confusing or even serious diagnostic errors.

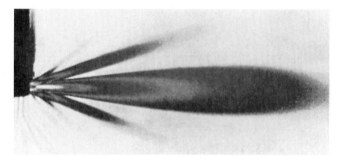

Fig. 4.20 Ultrasound beam shape. In this Schlieren tank photograph of the ultrasound field from an unfocused disc transducer, the main beam is accompanied by several side lobes emitted at angles from the central axis. The width of the main beam limits resolution in the transverse direction. The side lobes cause falsely positioned images. From Bergmann L. Der ultraschall und sein unwendung in wissenschaft und technik. Stuttgart: S. Heizel Verlage, 1954.

distortion disappears when the transducer is moved so as to image the pelvis through the centre of the muscle and this allows the appearance to be recognised as artefactual. It is also less common in longitudinal scans (because the alignment of the fat–muscle interface is changed) and in the epigastrium (presumably because there is less fat here).

The mechanism by which the ultrasound beam is focused depends on the compression and rarefaction waves of which it is composed coinciding in their proper phase at the focal zone and, in the same way, at the transducer surface during receive focusing. If the velocity in the intervening tissue is different from the calibrated value, the focal zone is shifted and, when the intervening tissue has heterogeneous velocities, defocusing will occur because the waves no longer coincide precisely, some arriving early when the propagation path includes tissues of a high velocity, others arriving late when the path includes fat, for example. The beam is thus defocused, degrading the lateral resolution. This effect partly accounts for the marked variation in ultrasound image quality from patient to patient, despite which the quality of images from obese subjects is sometimes surprisingly good. The larger the transducer aperture used, the worse the effect; this is probably why sophisticated systems such as high-resolution linear arrays in which 500 or more elements are used to form each ultrasound line give such exquisite images in 'easy' subjects, but perform badly with 'difficult' subjects, in whom images from smaller, simple transducers may be less degraded.

Beam width

Unfortunately the real ultrasound beam shape falls far short of the desired uniformly narrow laser-like configuration that would be optimal.[28] A typical actual focused beam (Fig. 4.20) consists of a disturbed region immedi-

ately in front of the transducer surface, then a near field that progressively narrows to the focus, after which it spreads rapidly in the far field. In addition to this main beam there are side lobes, low-energy beams directed at angles away from the centre line.

Axial resolution depends on the pulse length which is mainly determined by the wavelength; typically this might be 0.3 mm for a 5 MHz transducer and it does not change greatly with depth. In contrast, the width of the main beam defines the lateral resolution of the ultrasound image because adjacent objects can only be resolved separately if the beam is narrower than the distance between them.[29] If the beam is wider, they are depicted as one larger object on the screen. Because of the complex trumpet shape of the typical practical ultrasound beam, lateral resolution varies with depth, being best at the focal zone and deteriorating rapidly beyond it.

The edges of the beam are not sharply defined; the ultrasound energy is concentrated on the centre line of the beam and falls off progressively from the centre line with a Gaussian distribution. This means that a strong reflector will continue to give detectable echoes further from the central axis than a weak reflector. In clinical terms this means that the resolution of ultrasound is better for weak reflectors. Strong reflectors tend to blur laterally and are therefore seen as cigar-shaped smears or streaks so that their width is exaggerated. This is the 'beam width artefact' (Fig. 4.21), and is most obvious when the smearing overlaps an echo-free structure, often encountered when a gassy or bony structure lies adjacent to a fluid space.[30] However, it also leads to the general tendency to fill in small echo-free regions, such as ducts, and in part for the discrepancy between the ultrasound and X-ray measurements of the calibre of the bile and pancreatic ducts (the remaining discrepancy being attributable to the magnification on X-ray and to duct dilatation caused by contrast agents).

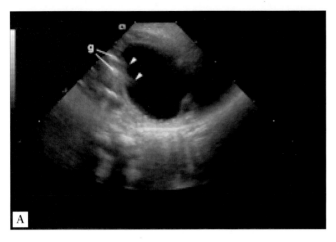
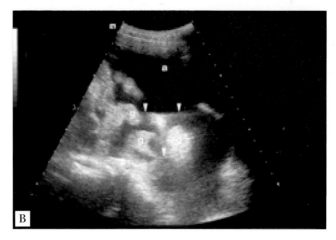

Fig. 4.21 Beam width artefact. Echoes arising from structures at the edge of the ultrasound beam, which has a finite width, are depicted as lying in the centre line of the beam. The more intense the reflection, the further off-axis its echoes will be received. **A:** In this example the strong echoes from a pocket of gas in pelvic gut loops (g) smear across the bladder (arrowheads). **B:** A beam spread artefact misplaces echoes from the reflective gas in gut loops (g) spread across the ascitic fluid (arrowheads). As is often the case with artefacts, they are more obvious when the false signal overlies an echo-free region but, in fact, are present everywhere to a greater or lesser extent, depending on the beam shape (mainly determined by focusing) and the reflectivity of the off-axis interfaces. a – ascites.

Beam width artefacts also occur in the orthogonal plane, i.e. in the slice thickness. With circular transducers (either the simple disc type or annular arrays) the beam is symmetrical in all planes but, for linear and phased arrays, the beam is wider in the orthogonal plane. These artefacts are exactly the same as the slice thickness artefact in CT except that the ultrasound beam is not uniform with depth; low-level information derived from signals in adjacent planes is spuriously depicted in the image plane.[31,32] Typically, bands or lines are noted within echo-free spaces (Fig. 4.22). They may mislead the operator into thinking that the fluid contains debris. Because the 'offending' reflector is not visualized within the image, the orthogonal

beam width artefact is more difficult to recognise than the same artefact occurring within the scanned plane.

Unfortunately, even this rather complex description of the shape of the ultrasound beam is incomplete because the profile is even further complicated by the inevitable presence of side lobes and, for array transducers, of grating lobes also.[33–35] Both these are misdirected, aberrant lines of ultrasound energy transmitted alongside the main beam. They have their exact counterpart in off-axis regions of sensitivity when the transducer is in the receive mode. Side lobes are generated as part of the beam focusing mechanism, whether by applied lenses or by curving of the transducer face, and consist of ill-defined beams, the

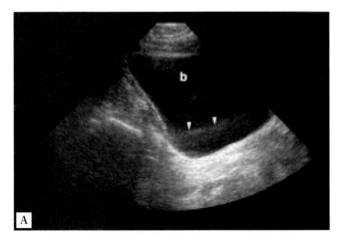
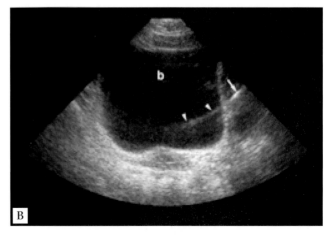

Fig. 4.22 Orthogonal beam width artefact. A: The low-level echoes (arrowheads) within this longitudinal section of the bladder are not due to debris or echogenic urine but are a beam width artefact arising from gas in adjacent bowel loops seen in **B:** the transverse section (arrow); because the artefact arises out of the plane of the tomogram, this variant of the beam width artefact is more difficult to recognise. b – bladder.

first some 20° away from the main beam and much weaker than it (by about 40 dB). For a disc transducer they form a series of rings, while in the case of linear arrays they are asymmetrical, being differently positioned in the two planes.

Grating lobes are similar but are produced by array transducers of all types; however, they tend to be more discrete and powerful. Grating lobes are less marked when the elements are small and numerous because the array then approximates more closely to a continuous transducer. Because they are weaker than the main beam, only strong reflectors cause serious side and grating lobe artefacts in clinical practice but if a gas bubble or bone surface happens to lie at the position of a side lobe then its grating lobe echo will be depicted in the line of the main beam (Fig. 4.23). The result is a convex-shaped streak that has been dubbed the 'Chinese hat artefact' (Fig. 4.24). Because these artefacts may appear consistently on rescanning the same region, they may be rather confusing. Often the cause can be visualised within the image, but side lobes can extend beyond the imaged area and do also occur in the orthogonal plane. Because the same focusing mechanisms are used in Doppler, the same misregistration of signals may occur and be quite difficult to recognise (see Ch. 6).

The introduction of tissue harmonic modes has reduced some of these artefacts and produces cleaner images, especially in 'difficult' subjects.[36] They operate by exploiting the fact that harmonics are only generated at relatively high acoustic powers and so the lower powers that occur in side and grating lobes and in reverberations do not excite harmonics and therefore echoes are not detected

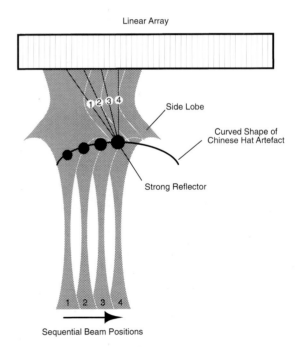

Fig. 4.24 **Mechanism of the Chinese hat artefact.** When a side or grating lobe strikes a strongly reflective target (1), a weak signal will be received and registered as originating slightly deeper than the real target depth because the oblique line of sight takes longer for the beam to traverse than the direct line that results when the beam is correctly centred on the target (4). The result is a cigar-shaped artefact whose ends are depicted as lying deeper than the centre, recalling the shape of a Chinese hat.

(Fig. 4.25). Such harmonic signals are generated because tissue resists compression more than it resists expansion so that an ultrasound pulse that begins as a symmetrical sine wave becomes asymmetrical as it propagates through the tissue. The harmonics are represented by the asymmetry, and are much more strongly formed with higher sound pressures. There are two ways to exploit the phenomenon. In one, the receiver circuitry is tuned to accept echoes at twice the frequency of the transmitted sound. In another approach, the phase inversion mode, each image line is formed from the sum of the echoes from a pair of pulses sent in the same direction, the second of which is inverted with respect to the first. Where the sound is conducted in a linear fashion, the echoes are out of phase and cancel out, but asymmetries caused by non-linear conduction result in differences that do not cancel and these are used to form the image. Both modes give cleaner images with less clutter; the phase inversion mode images have the same spatial resolution as fundamental mode images but at half the frame rate, while dual frequency harmonics have some compromise in spatial resolution because they use narrower band pulses. Both have limited depth penetration because the high powers that are critical to the generation of the harmonics are attenuated at depths greater about 10–15 cm.

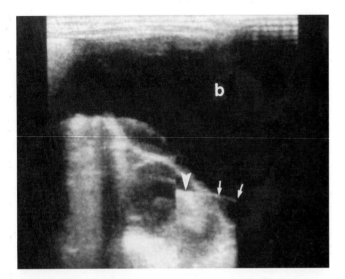

Fig. 4.23 **Grating lobe artefact.** Grating lobe artefacts have essentially the same effects as simple beam spread artefacts but are more severe and only occur with array transducers. They often have a convex shape (arrows). This example arose from a gas-containing pelvic gut loop (arrowhead). b – bladder.

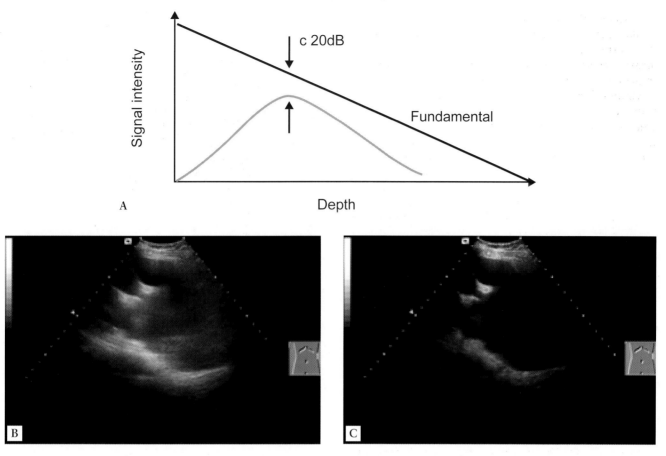

Fig. 4.25 Tissue harmonics. A: Because their generation depends on the amount of acoustic pressure applied to the tissue, harmonics are always weaker than the fundamental echoes and fade off more with depth. They take a few centimetres to develop and so are less obvious in superficial tissues. Their effect is to improve contrast in the tissue because there are fewer reverberant and beam width artefacts since these both require higher energy levels than are seen in the reflections and in the side/grating lobes. **B:** In this example of a hydronephrosis, marked reverberant and beam width artefacts partly fill the pelvis with artefactual echoes; **C:** in the dual frequency harmonic image they have been greatly reduced and the image has been 'cleaned up'.

Time sampling problems

Some interesting and important artefacts arise from the fact that there is an upper limit for the rate at which ultrasound pulses can be repeated. This is set by the speed of sound in tissue and the depth penetration required. If the next pulse is sent before the deepest echoes from the first have faded away, then these late echoes will be received soon after transmission of the second pulse. The scanner has no means of identifying which pulse is responsible and wrongly plots these deep echoes as nearby reflectors from the second pulse (Fig. 4.26). The process is repeated for subsequent pulses. Thus a distant structure is imaged as though it lies close to the transducer. Flickering 'objects' are seen in the near field and their depth can be altered by changing the pulse repetition frequency (PRF).[37] Since the PRF is usually linked to the depth of field, they move with a change in scale. Properly adjusted scanners should not allow this effect to occur, though the constraints affecting

duplex Doppler (both pulsed and colour) may force a compromise in this respect.

The limited frame rate can also obscure the motion of fast-moving structures such as heart valves, because their position is not being sampled sufficiently frequently for a true rendition of their movement to be displayed. Generally this results in a jerky, cartoon-like rendition of the movement, but in some cases the movement can seem to be slowed or even reversed in direction.[33] This phenomenon, known as aliasing, is rare in real-time imaging but is important in Doppler (see Ch. 6).

Artefacts in three-dimensional scanning

Some artefacts are only encountered in three-dimensional ultrasound.[38] They may stem from errors in the data collection process, for example movements of the probe that

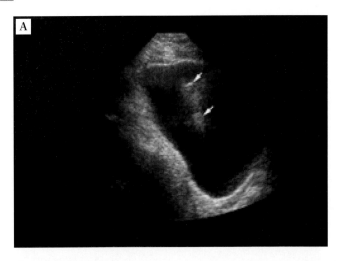

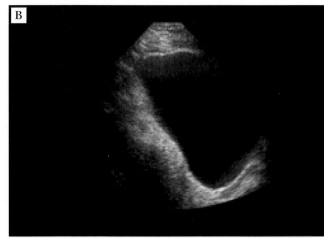

Fig. 4.26 Ranging artefact. If the manufacturer exceeds the limit in the pulse repetition frequency – in an attempt to increase the frame rate – late echoes from pulse 1 overlaps early echoes from pulse 2, etc. and signals are falsely depicted in the near field. **A:** The phenomenon is most obvious when a fluid path is traversed and so is well seen in transabdominal pelvic scanning, as in this example (arrows). **B:** Reducing the PRF eliminates this range overlap or 'wraparound' artefact.

are too rapid result in gaps in the final image that may be depicted as such in registered 3D but when the data are collected freehand (where no correction is made for the *z*-plane movement), they produce errors in the geometry of this axis that are not necessarily apparent in the image: this is why measurements from this type of unregistered three-dimensional scan are unreliable.[39] Obviously errors in the system that generated the spatial coordinates of the raw images distort the final rendered image.

Speckle in the ultrasound data also produces defects in the final image and they are particularly obvious in surface-rendered displays where they show as serpiginous holes.[40] Though unaesthetic, they do not affect the validity of the image; speckle reduction techniques can be used to mitigate the problem.

If the rendering algorithm does not interpolate adequately for missing slices, a 'gappy' rendered image results giving a toothcomb appearance when the three-dimensional set is rotated to align the z-axis.

If the structure being imaged moves during the data collection, the final rendered set will be distorted. This is particularly a problem with an active fetus and produces bizarrely distorted three-dimensional images. It is also a problem with vascular three-dimensional imaging because of vessel pulsations.

REFERENCES

1 Robinson D E, Kossoff G, Garrett W J. Artefacts in ultrasonic echoscopic visualisation. Ultrasonics 1966; 14: 186–194
2 Laing F C. Commonly encountered artifacts in clinical ultrasound. Semin Ultrasound 1983; 4: 1–25
3 Sanders R C. Atlas of ultrasonographic artifacts and variants. In: Year Book of Ultrasound. Chicago: Mosby, 1986
4 Hope-Simpson D, Burns P N. Pulse inversion Doppler: a new method for detecting nonlinear echoes from microbubble contrast agents. IEEE Ultrasound Symposium, 1999
5 Wells P N T, Halliwell M. Speckle in ultrasonographic imaging. Ultrasonics 1981; 19: 225–232
6 Burchard C B. Speckle in ultrasound B-scan. IEEE Trans Son Ultrason 1978; SU-25: 1–6
7 Grechenig W, Clement H G, Fellinger M et al. Value of ultrasound imaging of the Achilles tendon in traumatology. Radiologe 1997; 37: 322–329
8 Bachmann G F, Melzer C, Heinrichs C M et al. Diagnosis of rotator cuff lesions: comparison of US and MRI on 38 joint specimens. Eur Radiol 1997; 7: 192–197
9 Suramo I, Paivanslo M, Vuoria P. Shadowing and reverberation artifacts in abdominal ultrasonography. Eur J Radiol 1985; 5: 147–151
10 Robinson D E, Wilson L S, Kossoff G. Shadowing and enhancement in ultrasonic echograms by reflection and refraction. JCU 1981; 9: 181–188
11 Sommer F G and Taylor K J. Differentiation of acoustic shadowing due to calculi and gas collections. Radiology 1980; 135: 399–403
12 Ziskin M C, LaFollette P S, Blathras K et al. Effect of scan format on refraction artefacts. Ultrasound Med Biol 1990; 16: 183–191
13 Bly S H, Foster F S, Patterson U S et al. Artefactual echoes in B-mode images due to multiple scattering. Ultrasound Med Biol 1985; 11: 99–111
14 Cosgrove D O, Garbutt P, Hill C R. Echoes across the diaphragm. Ultrasound Med Biol 1978; 3: 388–392
15 Gardner F J, Clark R N, Kozlowski R. A model of a hepatic mirror image artefact. Med Ultrasound 1980; 4: 18–21
16 Fried A M, Cosgrove D O, Nassiri D K et al. The diaphragmatic echo complex: an in vitro study. Invest Radiol 1985; 20: 62–67
17 Thickman D I, Ziskin M C, Goldenburg N J et al. Clinical manifestations of the comet tail artifact. J Ultrasound Med 1983; 2: 225–230
18 Lichtenstein D, Meziere G, Biderman P et al. The comet-tail artifact: an ultrasound sign ruling out pneumothorax. Intensive Care Med 1999; 25: 383–388
19 Ahuja A, Chick W, King W et al. Clinical significance of the comet-tail artifact in thyroid ultrasound. JCU 1996; 24: 129–133
20 Wells P. Physical principles of ultrasonic diagnosis. London: Academic Press, 1997
21 Goss S A, Johnstone R A, Dunn F. Comprehensive compilation of principle properties of mammalian tissues. Ultrasound Med Biol 1978; 3: 373–379
22 Bamber J C. Attenuation and absorption. In Hill C R, ed. Physical principles of medical ultrasonics. Chichester: Ellis Horwood, 1986

23 Pierce G, Golding R H, Cooperberg P L. The effects of tissue velocity changes on acoustical interfaces. J Ultrasound Med 1982; 1: 85–187

24 Richman T S, Taylor K J W, Kremkau F W. Propagation speed artefact in a fatty tumour (myelolipoma). J Ultrasound Med 1983; 2: 45–47

25 Baum G. Ultrasonography in clinical ophthalmology. Trans Pa Acad Ophthalmol Otolaryngol 1964; 68: 265–270

26 Müller N, Cooperberg P L, Rowley V A et al. Ultrasonic refraction by the rectus abdominis muscles: the double image artefact. J Ultrasound Med 1984; 3: 515–520

27 Sauerbrei E E. The split image artefact in pelvic ultrasonography: anatomy and physics. J Ultrasound Med 1985; 4: 29–34

28 Goldstein A, Parks J A, Osborne B. Visualization of B-scan transducer transverse cross-sectional beam patterns. J Ultrasound Med 1982; 1: 23–35

29 Jaffe C C, Taylor K J. The clinical impact of ultrasonic beam focusing patterns. Radiology 1979; 131: 469–472

30 Finet G, Cachard C, Delachartre P et al. Artifacts in intravascular ultrasound imaging during coronary artery stent implantation. Ultrasound Med Biol 1998; 24: 793–802

31 Fiske O E, Filly R A. Pseudo-sludge. Radiology 1982; 144: 631–632

32 Goldstein A, Madrazo B L. Slice-thickness artifacts in gray-scale ultrasound. JCU 1981; 9: 365–375

33 Laing F C, Kurtz A B. The importance of ultrasonic side-lobe artifacts. Radiology 1982; 145: 763–768

34 McKeighen R E. The influence of grating lobes on image quality using real-time linear arrays. J Ultrasound Med 1982; 1(S): 83

35 Balthez P Y, Leveille R, Scrivani P V. Side lobes and grating lobes artifacts in ultrasound imaging. Vet Radiol Ultrasound 1997; 38: 387–393

36 Tranquart F, Grenier N, Eder V, Pourcelot L. Clinical use of ultrasound tissue harmonic imaging. Ultrasound Med Biol 1999; 25: 889–894

37 Goldstein R, Downey D B, Pretorius D H. Three dimensional ultrasound. Philadelphia: Lippincott, 1999

38 Eckersley R J, Goldberg B B, Cosgrove D O et al. Vessel beading in normal vessels using three dimensional ultrasound imaging. Radiology 1999; 213: 396

39 Tong S, Cardinal H N, Downey D B et al. Analysis of linear, area and volume distortion in 3D ultrasound imaging. Ultrasound Med Biol 1998; 24: 355–373

40 Rohling R, Gee A, Berman L. Three-dimensional spatial compounding of ultrasound images. Med Image Anal 1997; 1: 177–193

5

Ultrasound contrast agents

David O Cosgrove

Introduction

Contrast agents are widely used in all imaging modalities but until recently have not been available for ultrasound. Now this gap has been bridged with the development of very effective echo-enhancing agents in the form of gas microbubbles smaller than 10 μm in diameter[1,2] (Fig. 5.1). Following intravenous injection these bubbles flood the vascular space and produce a marked boost to the ultrasound signals from blood. Depending on the conditions (the agent itself and its dose), the vascular space and the scanner, the effect can be imaged in grey scale or by Doppler (Fig. 5.2). Microbubbles can also be instilled into other body spaces, e.g. the bladder or the uterus, to delineate them better[3,4] (Fig. 5.3).

The striking reflectivity of microbubbles results from the fact that gases are much more compressible than soft tissues so that the bubbles resonate in the sound field and thus return much stronger echoes than passive reflectors (Fig. 5.4). Because microbubbles behave in more complex ways than the scatterers that make up tissue or blood, they can be driven to produce signatures that allow them to be depicted separately from the tissue echoes; the use of these non-linear modes reduces the interference from tissue motion (clutter) in Doppler and has the important advantage of depicting stationary microbubbles.[5,6] This extends the frontiers of ultrasound by enabling the detection of capillary flow (which moves at only 1 mm/s), and of targeted microbubbles that are retained in tissues such as normal liver.[5,7,8] These interactions represent a new mode for radiological contrast agents in general, because the interrogating beam affects the behaviour of the agent: in X-ray and MRI the contrast agent is a passive component in the process.

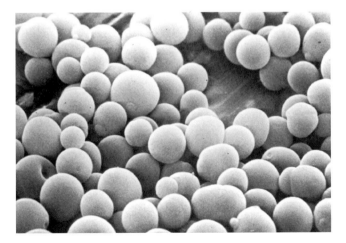

Fig. 5.1 An encapsulated microbubble. In an electron micrograph of the albumin-encapsulated microbubble Quantison the tight distribution of bubble sizes can be appreciated. They are around 4 μm in diameter (scale 10 μm). (Figure courtesy of Richard Johnson, Andaris Ltd, Nottingham.)

An important additional way to use microbubbles is to track the time course of the arrival and departure of a bolus injection through a region of interest[9–12] (Fig. 5.5). By quantifying the changing signal strength time–enhancement curves can be generated and the shape of these contains valuable functional information, analogous to the data in dynamic radioisotope tracer studies or functional CT. These similarities should not be pressed too far because although the small molecules used in these techniques diffuse across the capillary membranes so that they have an interstitial phase, the size of microbubbles (2–8 μm) means that they do not diffuse (although some are phagocytosed by the reticuloendothelial system). They may therefore offer complementary functional information.

Basic principles

Obviously, for intravenous use microbubbles must be smaller than the diameter of capillaries or they would embolise and be ineffective and perhaps dangerous. Because the reflectivity of particles increases with their diameter, structures smaller than 10 μm in diameter would be expected to be poor reflectors – this is why only weak echoes are obtained from red blood cells, so that the cardiac chambers and major blood vessels generally appear as echo-free spaces. However, the gas in microbubbles is highly compressible and, when subjected to the alternating compression and refraction pressures that constitute an ultrasound pulse, they oscillate.[13,14] Like all oscillating systems such as springs or swings, they have a natural frequency at which they resonate most strongly (Fig. 5.6). This is determined chiefly by their size (smaller bubbles resonate at higher frequencies) but is also influenced by the composition of the gas and the microbubble envelope. Serendipitously, clinically useable microbubbles resonate at the frequencies used in diagnostic ultrasound. This fortunate coincidence makes microbubbles such extremely effective reflectors that, even in the low concentrations achieved after they have been dispersed throughout the systemic circulation, they produce 20 dB or more enhancement in echo strength, an increase of some 100-fold.

The techniques for making microbubbles are legion and often cunning, and have been devised both to control their size and to make them sufficiently stable to provide a clinically useful enhancement time of at least a few minutes.[15] Levovist (Schering AG, Berlin), for example, consists of galactose ground into tiny crystals whose irregular surfaces act as nidation sites on which air pockets form when it is suspended in water, much as bubbles form at small irregularities on the surface of a glass of champagne. A trace of palmitic acid is added as a surfactant to stabilise the resultant microbubbles: they are in effect tiny soap bubbles. Optison (Malinkrodt, St Louis) represents another class of

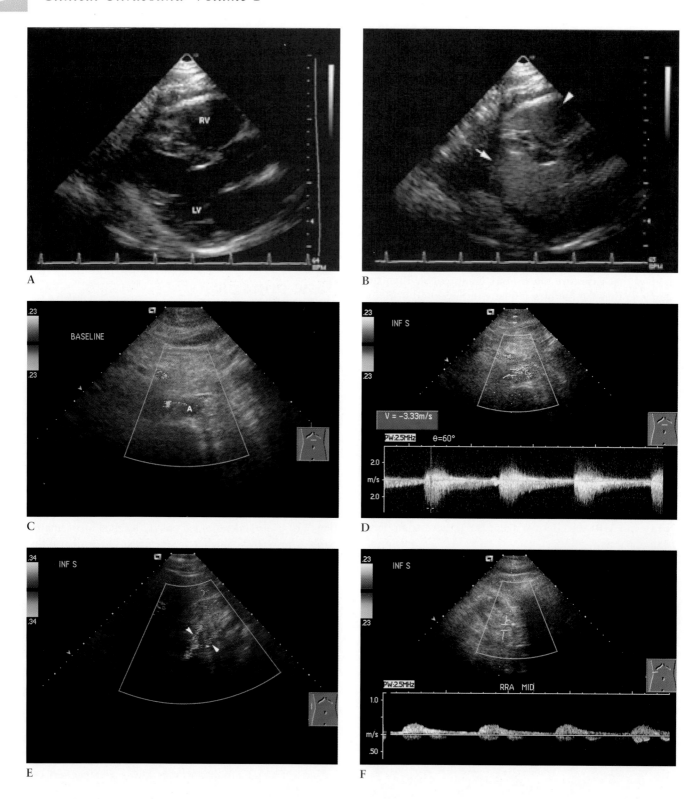

Fig. 5.2 Echo enhancement. A: Baseline. **B:** Contrast-enhanced grey scale echocardiogram showing the right and left ventricles. Following i.v. injection of Optison enhancement can be seen in the right (arrowhead) and left (arrow) ventricles. **C:** Baseline. **D:** Contrast-enhanced Doppler study of the renal artery. No usable signals could be obtained from the origin of the renal artery on the baseline scan; following an infusion of Levovist, signals adequate to make a measurement of the high velocity at the stenosis were obtained (velocity over 3 m/s). **E:** A previously unsuspected double renal artery was also found after enhancement (arrowheads). **F:** Within the kidney, the typical slow rise and fall (parvus and tardus) pattern of a tight stenosis was demonstrated. (**A** and **B** courtesy of Dr Petros Nihoyannopoulos, Hammersmith Hospital, London.) a – aorta.

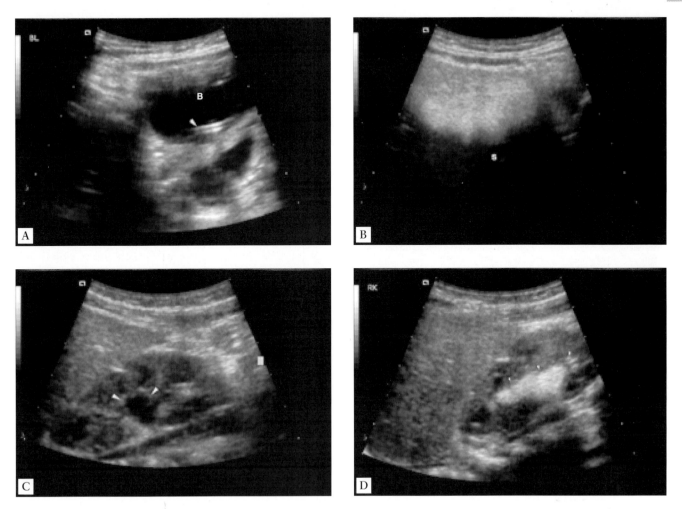

Fig. 5.3 Ultrasound contrast micturating cysto-urethrogram (MCU). A and **B:** Following administration of Levovist into this child's bladder via a urethral catheter (arrowhead) the bladder becomes echogenic, with transient self-shadowing that obscures the deeper parts of the pelvis. **C:** The right kidney before contrast instillation shows moderate dilatation of the collecting system (arrowheads). **D:** Following micturition, echogenic contrast has refluxed into this space, demonstrating at least grade 3 reflux. (Scan courtesy of Dr Ruth Williamson, Hammersmith Hospital.) B – bladder; S – shadowing

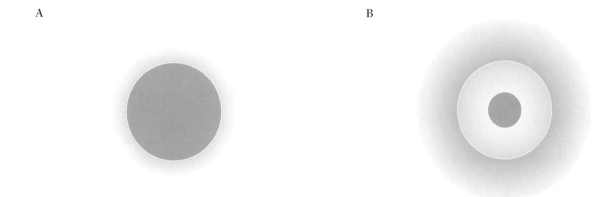

Fig. 5.4 Bubble resonance. A: A scarcely compressible scatterer such as a red blood cell returns echoes in a passive way. **B:** The compressibility of gases means that microbubbles resonate actively in the sound field and therefore return very much stronger signals. The shaded circles indicate the fluctuating diameter of a microbubble in response to the pressure changes in the sound field.

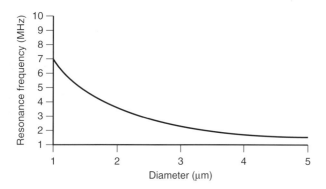

Fig. 5.5 Microbubble resonance frequency. The chance correspondence between the resonance frequency of a 2–3 μm bubble and the ultrasound frequencies used in clinical diagnosis underlies their effectiveness as echo-enhancing agents. This chart depicts the resonance of an air microbubble in water. This is likely to be modified by blood and by the wall and the content of clinically useful agents.

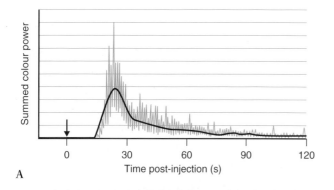

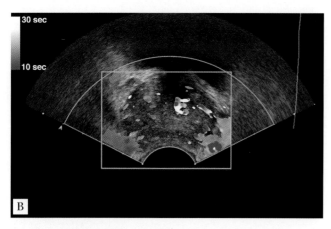

Fig. 5.6 Transit time curve. A: The Doppler signal intensity in the region of interest has been quantified and its change with time plotted to form a wash-in/wash-out curve. The blue curve is the raw data and is irregular because of cardiorespiratory variations; the red curve has been smoothed. **B:** Indices derived from this can be used for differential diagnosis and to form true functional images, this one showing the arrival time of Levovist in seconds after a bolus injection in a carcinoma of the prostate. The heterogeneity of the haemodynamics is highlighted by the irregularity of the tints across the prostate.

microbubble, with a shell formed by sonicating a solution of human serum albumin. The resulting capsules are filled with a perfluorocarbon gas (perfluoropropane) whose high molecular weight slows dissolution and thereby prolongs the enhancement for several minutes. In EchoGen (Abbott, Chicago) a liquid perfluorocarbon (perfluoropentane) is prepared as an emulsion in an aqueous medium; the physical properties of the compound have been carefully chosen so that it becomes a gas when warmed to body temperature. Thus, following injection the minute droplets become gas bubbles of around 3 μm diameter, a so-called phase-change agent. Sonovue (Bracco, Milan) and Definity (DuPont Merck, Billericay) are examples of an important family of microbubbles whose membrane consists of phospholipids. The respective gases are sulphur hexafluoride (SF_6) and perfluoropropane, which diffuse slowly and so prolong the bubbles' life after injection.

Thus, the gas content can be used as a definition of the family to which bubbles belong, the air-containing bubbles being shorter-lived than those containing high molecular weight gases such as perfluoro compounds. The membrane can be classified as surfactants (e.g. Levovist), soft shelled (e.g. Optison and Sonovue) or firm shelled (e.g. Sonavist (Schering AG, Berlin), a polymer-coated agent) (Fritszch 1998, personal communication). A few special-purpose bubbles have no coating, such as Echovist (Schering AG, Berlin), used for ultrasound salpingography.

Although it may seem unwise to inject a gas intravenously, the total amount used is minute (less than 200 μl in the case of Levovist) and the small size of the bubbles makes immobilisation most unlikely.[16] Extensive preclinical and clinical trials have demonstrated an excellent safety profile, the main unwanted effect being a mild and transient local discomfort at the injection site, which results from the high osmolality of Levovist. Although each agent has its own profile of adverse effects, all have so far been trivial. In fact, tolerance of these agents is much higher than that of most X-ray or MRI agents, a reflection perhaps of the higher expectation of safety and convenience for ultrasound (see Ch. 3).

The signal boost referred to allows microbubbles to be visualised on grey scale in larger vascular spaces such as the cardiac chambers using standard scanners. In the periphery, more sensitive techniques such as Doppler or non-linear modes must be used because of the dilution of the microbubbles in the blood pool (see Fig. 5.2).

An important general concept in the practical use of microbubble enhancing agents is their fragility, such that they are readily destroyed by the insonating beam.[17] In some situations strategies to preserve them by limiting their exposure to the ultrasound beam greatly improve their effectiveness. The most important example is in echocardiography, where the entire microbubble population generally passes through the beam. A marked increase in both the amount and the duration of enhancement can be achieved by scanning intermittently (triggered by the ECG) rather than continuously. Such approaches allow grey-scale visualisation of myocardial perfusion; a development whose importance is hard to exaggerate.[18] In radiological applications the destruction is less complete because usually only a small proportion of the bubbles is exposed at each recirculation, but the destructive effect can be exploited in a different way: if the bubbles in a tissue slice are deliberately destroyed, their reappearance is related to the rate of inflow of fresh bubbles, which depends on the tissue flow rate.[19] This 'destruction–reperfusion' method has been used for the myocardium and can be expected to be useful also in the kidney and other abdominal organs.

When microbubbles resonate in the ultrasound beam they behave like a musical instrument and emit harmonic signals at double their resonance frequency[20,21] (Fig. 5.7). If a scanner is modified to detect these harmonic signals and use them to form the image or Doppler trace, the confusing clutter signals from tissue, either stationary or moving, are suppressed and a cleaner image or trace is produced, allowing weak signals from tumours and the myocardium, for example, to be detected. The effect depends on the fact that it is easier to expand a bubble than to compress it so that it responds asymmetrically to a symmetrical driving force, i.e. the ultrasound wave. This is an example of a non-linear mode.

An important non-linear mode relies on the signals given out by bubbles when they are inactivated by strong ultrasound pulses (at the upper range recommended for diagnostic use).[5] Colour Doppler is a correlation technique that works by comparing the echoes from one pulse with

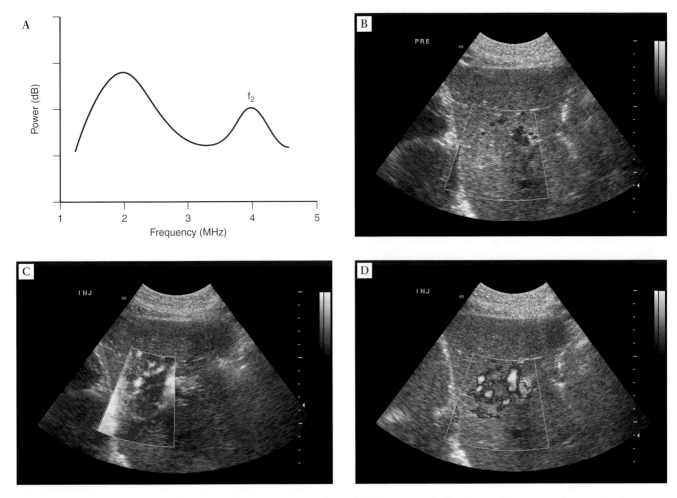

Fig. 5.7 The harmonic mode. A: Diagram of the frequency response of microbubble resonance in the ultrasound beam: note the second peak response (f_2) which is selectively filtered to form the harmonic image. Generally tissue gives only a small harmonic signal (owing to non-linear propagation rather than to non-linear response) and so the ratio between the echogenicity of the microbubble and of the tissue is increased. An important advantage is the suppression of motion artefact. **B:** Fundamental baseline and **C:** Levovist-enhanced scans of a poorly vascularised liver metastasis; the enhancement was not clinically useful because of overwhelming flash from movement of the adjacent heart. **D:** In the harmonic mode the tumour vascularity is better seen.

those from a second (in practice, to obtain accurate motion information, ensembles of up to eight sequential pulses are used). Changes between sequential echo trains are detected and the mean frequency of the Doppler signals represented by a colour overlay on the image. If a microbubble lying in the line of sight is inactivated by the first pulse, a major change in the signal from that location results: the correlation circuitry recognises this as a large Doppler shift. Perhaps 'pseudo-Doppler' would be a better term as there has, of course, been no true movement but simply the disappearance of a microbubble from the scan line, although it is generally referred to as 'stimulated acoustic emission' (SAE). The display shows Doppler shift signals at the extreme colours, so that it looks like severe aliasing (Fig. 5.8). Their detection does not depend on actual motion: stationary or very slow-moving microbubbles are equally well sensed, and this is especially useful for imaging targeted agents which are held within particular tissues, for example those that are phagocytosed by the fixed reticuloendothelial system, such as the liver's Kupffer cells in the case of the firm-shelled agent Sonavist (SHU

563A, Schering, Berlin), or those that pool in the extensive sinusoids of the liver and spleen, as probably occurs with Levovist. Because the bubbles are inactivated in some way, this is a consumptive process and therefore transient, disappearing within a frame or so with Levovist. It has been referred to as 'transient scattering'.

Another way to improve the signal/clutter ratio is to use a pair of pulses to form each B-mode line, the second of each pair being inverted in phase[22] (Fig. 5.9). The line in the final image is formed by summing the two resultant echo trains. Because the echoes from linear reflectors such as tissue are inverted they cancel out but the non-linear response of the microbubbles means that their echoes are not exactly symmetrical in the compression and expansion phases and so they do not cancel out completely. This 'phase inversion' mode has a similar effect in reducing clutter as the harmonic mode but, with the important advantage of retaining the spatial resolution of B-mode, which is compromised in the latter because a narrow-band pulse must be used. Obviously this has some kinship with the SAE colour Doppler approach both being multipurpose techniques. New modes

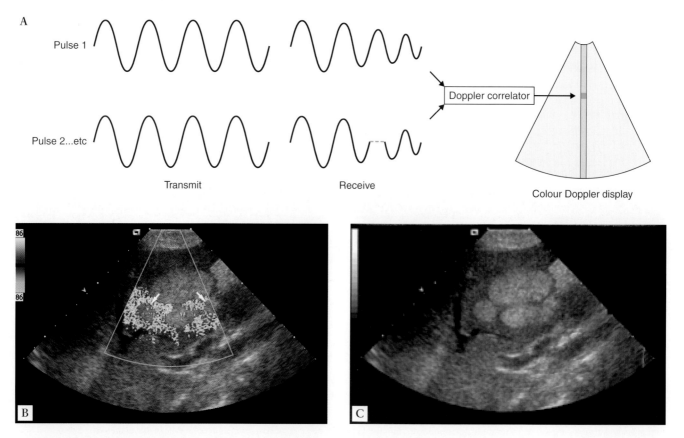

Fig. 5.8 Stimulated acoustic imaging (SAE). A: When the acoustic intensity of the ultrasound pulse is increased above a threshold (usually corresponding to a mechanical index (MI) of 1), the microbubbles are inactivated. Echoes from the next pulse (pulse 2) along the same line have changed (dotted portion) and this is interpreted by the Doppler correlator as a marked signal, which is displayed as a colour pixel in the corresponding position. **B:** In this example using Levovist in the late (post-vascular) phase, the SAE highlights normal liver as a coloured mosaic pattern, demonstrating the fact that SAE is not dependent on microbubble movement. **C:** Small metastases (arrows) are more clearly seen than on the control scan.

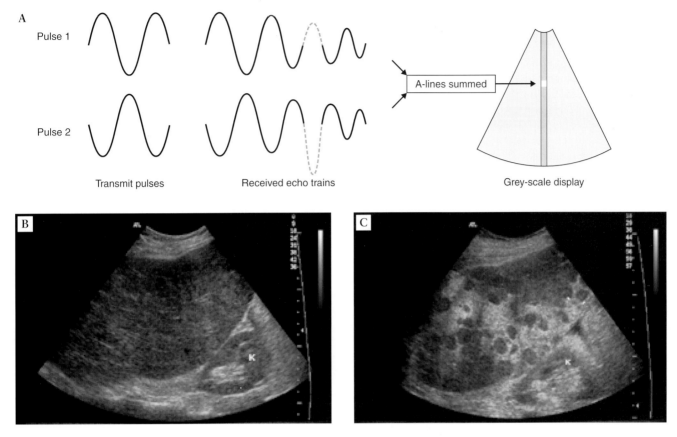

Fig. 5.9 Phase inversion mode. A: In this non-linear mode a conventional ultrasound pulse is followed by a second phase-inverted pulse (pulse 2) along the same line. The final ultrasound image line is made by summing the resulting echoes. Because tissue generally scatters in a linear fashion, its echoes cancel out. However, microbubbles are highly non-linear reflectors, resisting compression more than they resist expansion, and therefore their echoes do not cancel. Thus, the bubble signature is highlighted in the image and, because the pulses are the same as those used for conventional B-mode imaging, the spatial resolution is better than in SAE mode. **B:** In this patient with a bronchial carcinoma, the liver is enlarged and heterogeneous but discrete lesions are not clearly delineated. **C:** in the late phase after Levovist injection, normal liver tissue is highlighted, so that the individual metastases are shown with much more contrast than on the baseline scan. Lesions smaller than 1 cm diameter are clearly revealed (arrowheads). K – kidney.

using series of inverse pulses are under development and can yield bubble-specific Doppler information.[22]

Artefacts

Some microbubble-specific artefacts need to be recognised if interpretative errors are to be avoided.[23]

On the spectral Doppler tracing 'bubble noise' in the form of sharp spikes, corresponding with crackles on the audio output, sometimes occur (Fig. 5.10). This may be caused by microbubble collapse or perhaps represent aggregates of macrobubbles.

Just as occurs when the Doppler gain is set too high, excessive signal intensity can overload the Doppler discriminator circuitry and produce channel breakthrough, so that flow is artefactually displayed in the reverse as well as the correct direction (see Ch. 6).

An important effect that is sometimes observed is an increase in the highest velocities displayed.[24] This is

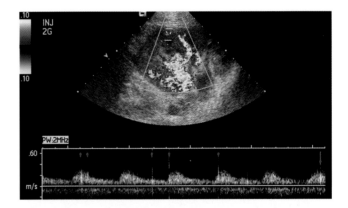

Fig. 5.10 Bubble noise. Late in the vascular phase after microbubble injection spectral Doppler artefacts termed 'bubble noise' may occur. In this example a renal transplant was being studied and the tracing from an arcuate artery shows several transient signals (arrowheads) that are heard as crackling sounds. They may arise from bubbles being inactivated by the sound beam. There is also a lower-frequency transient (arrow), which may arise from a clump of microbubbles flowing through the vessel.

probably the result of signals that were previously too weak to be detected being raised above the system's sensitivity threshold. This effect is a potential clinical problem when absolute (i.e. angle-corrected) values are used as criteria for disease, for example in carotid and renal artery stenosis. Revised values for the upper limits of normal may have to be determined and, awkwardly, they will probably vary with the degree of enhancement produced. The problem is minimised if peak systolic ratios are used to define normal limits (e.g. the internal-to-common carotid (IC/CC ratio), or the renal/aortic ratio (RAR)).

Because in velocity Doppler only the mean frequency shift is displayed, it may be asked why echo-enhancing agents (which do not alter blood flow velocity) produce an increase in signal strength. The enhancement presumably occurs because of the same sensitivity threshold effect that changes the peak signals in spectral Doppler: flow velocities that were too weak to be registered before enhancement are now displayed, leading to a more complete depiction of the vascular bed. This improves the detection of slow flow and of weak signals from small vessels, as well as of poor signals caused by attenuation in overlying tissues or because the beam-to-vessel angle is close to 90°. The increased signal intensity produced by echo-enhancing agents is directly displayed in B-mode and by power Doppler, and so these are the natural 2D modes to use for contrast studies unless flow direction is critical to the diagnosis. Spectral Doppler shows signal intensity as loudness (or brightness of the screen tracing), and is useful as a direct measure of enhancement.

'Blooming' appears in colour Doppler as a spread of the colour pixels beyond the confines of the blood vessel, particularly when the signals are very strong (Fig. 5.11). It is probably attributable to a combination of overloading of the Doppler circuitry by the strong signals and of multiple re-reflections between adjacent microbubbles which is equivalent to the 'comet-tail' artefact on grey scale ultrasound. Although not a serious concern for subjective diagnosis, blooming may corrupt quantitative measurements.

Clinical applications

The earliest and still most important application of microbubbles is in echocardiography to 'opacify' the cardiac chambers.[11,25] This improves delineation of the left ventricular endocardial border and thus allows better estimates of left ventricular function and measurements of the ejection fraction. In many cardiology units microbubble-enhanced echocardiography has replaced isotope studies for left ventricular function: it is cheaper and quicker, and avoids the use of ionising radiation. The development of means to detect microbubbles in the myocardial capillaries is making myocardial perfusion estimates possible, and ultrasound contrast stress echo studies are becoming more widely used. The possibility of studying the coronary arteries directly is also becoming an option.

For the larger peripheral vessels the main clinical application is rescuing a Doppler study that has been a technical failure because of attenuation by overlying tissues, perhaps combined with weak signals because of slow or low-volume flow. Trans-cranial Doppler (TCD) is a situation where the skull attenuates the signal so strongly that routine use is difficult, time-consuming and subject to failure, but most patients can be studied satisfactorily after the administration of a microbubble agent. In neurological centres, enhanced TCD is becoming a routine test, for example to study arterial spasm after stroke or subarachnoid haemorrhage.[26]

Similar considerations apply to Doppler of the extra-cranial circulation and of deep abdominal vessels: ultra-

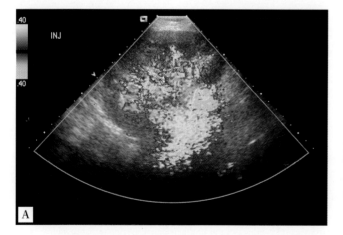 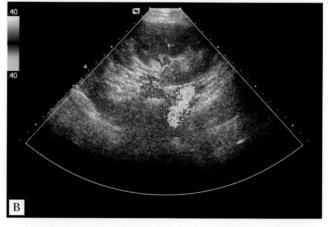

Fig. 5.11 Blooming. A: At the peak of enhancement the intensity of the Doppler signals may overload the scanner's electronics, so that the colour Doppler signals spread on the display. This produces a smearing artefact known as 'blooming', where the Doppler signals extend over a much larger area than the vessels occupy. **B:** In this renal transplant the precontrast study is a truer representation of the vasculature.

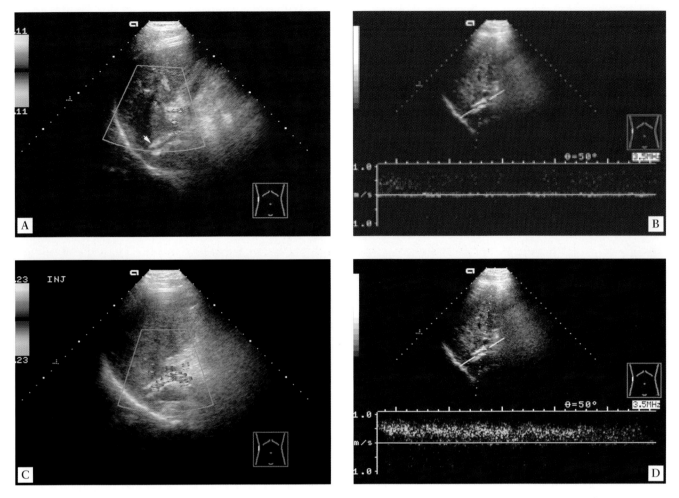

Fig. 5.12 TIPS shunt. A and B: No useful signals could be obtained from this portohepatic shunt on colour (arrow) or spectral Doppler until Levovist was infused. C and D: The enhancement produced adequate colour signals in the shunt and a spectral trace could be obtained. Note that the flow was reversed: the subsequent venogram showed disturbed flow caused by a dilated stenosis.

sound has long been used as a screening test for renal artery stenosis in the evaluation of hypertension and of progressive renal failure in arteriopaths, but is subject to a high failure rate because of technical difficulties. With the use of a microbubble agent successful studies are the rule, so that the study can be completed more quickly and more invasive procedures such as angiography can be avoided[27] (see Fig. 5.2). For the portal circulation, a common use is evaluation of the patency of the portal vein in cirrhosis, where the highly attenuating overlying liver and the slow flow often make the study technically difficult (Fig. 5.12). An enhanced scan is usually much simpler to interpret.[28] Similarly, in patients with TIPS shunts, an enhanced Doppler study usually succeeds where no signals could be obtained previously and many other vascular studies can be improved in a similar way.[29] A particularly important example is the hepatic artery of the transplanted liver: reliable Doppler signals may be difficult to obtain in the early postoperative period because of the small size of the vessel

and because of the barriers posed by the wound, as well as by dressings and drains. Hepatic artery patency is critical for the survival of the transplant, and urgent angiography or re-exploration is required if it is occluded. Microbubble agents, which are not hepatotoxic, rescue such failed Doppler studies and, as they can be performed in the intensive care unit, are very useful in excluding hepatic artery occlusion.

An extension to current Doppler capabilities is the additional information that microbubble enhancement gives on the microvasculature, especially in tumours. Unenhanced Doppler has proved useful in characterising malignant neovasculature for differential diagnosis as well as for predicting aggressiveness and monitoring response to treatment, but only relatively larger vessels can be accessed. After enhancement many more smaller vessels can be depicted, making these evaluations more complete (Fig. 5.13). It also improves the 3D display of the malignant neovasculature, and this seems likely to enhance

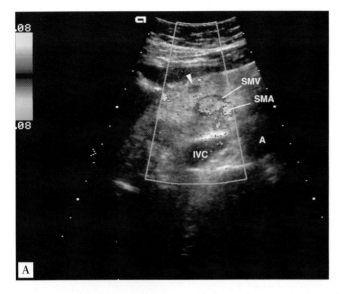
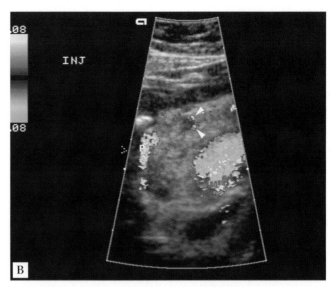

Fig. 5.13 Tumour enhancement. A: A small echo-poor area with no Doppler signals was seen in the neck of the pancreas (arrowhead) in this patient with carcinoid syndrome, but it was difficult to be sure that it was other than a simple cyst. **B:** Following Levovist infusion the supply vessels were demonstrated (arrowheads), indicating that this was a real lesion and that it was solid: at surgery it proved to be the primary carcinoid tumour. A – aorta; IVC – inferior vena cava; SMA – superior mesenteric artery; SMV – superior mesenteric vein.

appreciation of its anatomical complexity. Though as yet unproven as a clinical tool, the potential value of micro-bubbles in oncology is great, particularly at a time when the new class of anticancer drugs that inhibit angiogenesis is being introduced.

Transient response imaging of Levovist in its liver-specific phase (using SAE or phase inversion mode) has been shown to improve the detectability of liver metastases, and very likely reveals hitherto occult lesions.[30-32] It may also improve specificity, because some benign lesions, notably focal nodular hyperplasia and haemangiomas, show marked or modest retention of Levovist. This approach could develop into an important method for staging malignancy.

The non-vascular use of these agents is established for demonstrating the patency of the fallopian tubes by instill-ing the agent (usually Echovist) into the uterine cavity and watching the contrast track along the tubes with real-time transvaginal scanning. Thus it can replace X-ray salpingo-graphy as a screening test for tubal patency in the investigation of infertility (see ultrasound in obstetrics and gynaecology, Ch. 5). Because HyCoSy (hystero contrast salpingography) does not give as detailed an image of the tubal anatomy, conventional salpingography must be used for complex cases, e.g. where tubal microsurgery is planned.

Another non-vascular use of great potential is in ureteric reflux: currently this requires a micturating cystourethrogram, but similar and possibly better inform-ation can be obtained using Levovist instilled into the bladder and watching the ureters and renal pelves with ultrasound (see Fig. 5.3). Because X-rays are not used

continuous or prolonged scanning can be performed, so intermittent reflux is more likely to be detected.[33]

New uses

The development of microbubble contrast agents for ultra-sound has opened up major new uses, some of which have already been mentioned as they are entering clinical use. An exciting area is the ability to track the transit of a bolus of microbubbles through a tissue of interest, such as a tumour or kidney (see Fig. 5.6). Using quantitative methods wash-in/wash-out curves that embody functional information on the local circulation can be generated. Indices derived from these can be expected to yield important information on organ function that are analo-gous to functional nuclear medicine studies.[34,35] Similar approaches using contrast agents with CT and MRI have become routine. Ultrasound offers a simpler, cheaper method with a difference: microbubbles are confined to the vascular bed, unlike CT and MRI contrast agents, which are small enough to diffuse into the interstitial space. Thus functional studies with ultrasound can be expected to provide unique and probably complementary functional information. The indices derived from these transit curves can be used to create functional images by depicting them on a pixel-by-pixel basis as an overlay on the grey scale scan.[12] These registered structural and func-tional images are intriguing and full of promise.

They can also be used in simple and very practical ways to derive functional information about vascular transits – an important example is the arrival time of the agent in the hepatic veins after a peripheral venous bolus injection. Normally there is a delay of around 45 seconds while the microbubbles cross the intervening capillary beds (lung, gut or spleen and liver sinusoids) but, in diseases where there is arteriovenous shunting, as in cirrhosis and liver malignancy, the contrast arrives earlier.[35,36] In preliminary studies this test seems to be a sensitive and reliable way of discriminating between chronic hepatitis and cirrhosis, and between haemangiomas and liver metastases.

The therapeutic potential for microbubbles is a topic of active research. They may be used in two distinct ways: to enhance the effects of high-intensity focused ultrasound (Hifu) by increasing the amount of energy deposited, or by acting as vehicles for therapeutic agents.[7,37] In this mode the loaded microbubbles are ruptured at the desired site by applying sufficiently intense sound to achieve a local high concentration of a gene, a thrombolytic agent or an anticancer drug.[38]

REFERENCES

1 Burns P N. Overview of echo-enhanced vascular ultrasound imaging for clinical diagnosis in neurosonology. J Neuroimag 1997; 7(Suppl 1): S2–14

2 Cosgrove D. Echo enhancers and ultrasound imaging. Eur J Radiol 1997; 26: 64–76

3 Degenhardt F. Contrast sonography in gynaecology. Stuttgart: Thieme, 1996

4 Darge K, Dutting T, Zieger B, Mohring K, Rohrschneider W, Troger J. Diagnosis of vesicoureteral reflux with echo-enhanced micturition urosonography. Radiologe 1998; 38: 405–409

5 Blomley M, Cosgrove D, Albrecht T. Stimulated acoustic emission in the liver. Radiology 1998; 224: 124–134

6 Kono Y, Moriyasu F, Mine Y et al. Gray-scale second harmonic imaging of the liver with galactose-based microbubbles. Invest Radiol 1997; 32: 120–125

7 Unger E C, McCreery T P, Sweitzer R H, Shen D, Wu G. In vitro studies of a new thrombus-specific ultrasound contrast agent. Am J Cardiol 1998; 81: 58G–61G

8 Schwarz K Q, Chen X, Steinmetz S, Phillips D. Harmonic imaging with Levovist. J Am Soc Echocardiog 1997; 10: 1–10

9 Villanueva F S, Kaul S. Assessment of myocardial perfusion in coronary artery disease using myocardial contrast echocardiography. Coronary Artery Dis 1995; 6: 18–28

10 Sehgal C M, Arger P H. Mathematical modeling of the dilution curves for ultrasonographic contrast agents. J Ultrasound Med 1997; 16: 471–479

11 Kaul S. New developments in ultrasound systems for contrast echocardiography. Clin Cardiol 1997; 20: 127–130

12 Eckersley R, Cosgrove D, Blomley M, Hashimoto H. Functional imaging of tissue response to bolus injection of ultrasound contrast agent. Proc IEEE Ultrasonics Symposium 1998; 2: 1779–1782

13 Leighton T. The acoustic bubble. London: Academic Press, 1994

14 de Jong N, Hoff L, Skotland T, Bom N. Absorption and scatter of encapsulated gas-filled microspheres: theoretical considerations and some measurements. Ultrasonics 1992; 30: 95–103

15 Dawson P, Cosgrove D, Grainger R. Contrast agents in radiology. Oxford: Isis Medical Press, 1999

16 Schlief R, Schurmann R, Niendorf H P. Blood-pool echo enhancement after intravenous injection of galactose-based microbubbles: results from European phase III clinical trials in Doppler sonography. Academ Radiol 1996; 3: S466–467

17 Porter T, Xie F, Li S, D'Sa A, Rafter P. Increased ultrasound contrast and decreased microbubble destruction rates with triggered ultrasound imaging. J Am Soc Echocardiogr 1996; 9: 599–605

18 Wei K, Kaul S. Recent advances in myocardial contrast echocardiography. Curr Opin Cardiol 1997; 12: 539–546

19 Wei K, Jayaweera A R, Firoozan S, Linka A, Skyba D M, Kaul S. Quantification of myocardial blood flow with ultrasound-induced destruction of microbubbles administered as a constant venous infusion. Circulation 1998; 97: 473–483

20 Newhouse V, Ullendorf V. Second harmonic characteristics of the ultrasound contrast agents. Ultrasound Med Biol 1997; 23: 453–459

21 Burns P, Powers J, Fritzsch T. Harmonic imaging, a new imaging and Doppler method for contrast enhanced ultrasound. Radiology 1992; 185: 142

22 Hope-Simpson D, Burns P. Pulse inversion Doppler: a new method for detecting nonlinear echoes from microbubble contrast agents. IEEE Ultrasound Symposium 1997

23 Forsberg F, Liu J B, Burns P N, Merton D A, Goldberg B B. Artifacts in ultrasonic contrast agent studies. J Ultrasound Med 1994; 13: 357–365

24 Petrick J, Zomack M, Schlief R. An investigation of the relationship between ultrasound echo enhancement and Doppler frequency shift using a pulsatile arterial flow phantom. Invest Radiol 1997; 32: 225–235

25 Nihoyannopoulos P, Zamorano J. Applications of contrast media in echocardiography. Rev Esp Cardiol 1998; 51: 428–434

26 Bogdahn U, Becker G, Fröhlich T. Contrast enhanced transcranial color coded real time sonography of cerebrovascular disease. Echocardiography 1993; 10: 678

27 Missouris C G, Allen C M, Balen F G, Buckenham T, Lees W R, MacGregor G A. Non-invasive screening for renal artery stenosis with ultrasound contrast enhancement. J Hypertens 1996; 14: 519–524

28 Braunschweig R, Olif S, Oliff J. Echo-enhanced liver and portal system ultrasound imaging with Levovist. Angiology 1996; 7(Suppl): 23–29

29 Goldberg B, Liu J-B, Forsberg F. Ultrasound contrast agents: a review. Ultrasound Med Biol 1994; 20: 219–333

30 Blomley M, Albrecht T, Cosgrove D, Jayaram V, Butler-Barnes J, Eckersley R. Stimulated acoustic emission in liver parenchyma with Levovist. Lancet 1998; 351: 568

31 Harvey C, Blomley M, Eckersley R et al. Improved detection of hepatic malignancies using pulse inversion mode in the late phase of enhancement with the ultrasound contrast agent Levovist (SH U 508A): early experience. Radiology 2000; (in press)

32 Harvey J C, Blomley M J K, Eckersley R J, Heckemann R A, Butler-Barnes J, Cosgrove D O Pulse-inversion mode imaging of liver specific microbubbles: improved detection of subcentimetre metastases. Lancet 2000; 355: 807–808

33 Darge K, Troeger J, Duetting T et al. Reflux in young patients: comparison of voiding US of the bladder and retrovesical space with echo enhancement versus voiding cystourethrography for diagnosis. Radiology, 1999; 210: 201–207

34 Blomley M, Albrecht T, Eckersley R, Butler-Barnes J, Jayaram V, Cosgrove D. Renal arteriovenous transit time measured noninvasively using bolus injections of microbubble contrast. Radiology 1998; 209: 461

35 Blomley M J, Albrecht T, Cosgrove D O et al. Liver vascular transit time analyzed with dynamic hepatic venography with bolus injections of an US contrast agent: early experience in seven patients with metastases. Radiology 1998; 209: 862–866

36 Albrecht T, Blomley M J, Cosgrove D O. Non-invasive diagnosis of hepatic cirrhosis by transit-time analysis of an ultrasound contrast agent. Lancet 1999; 353: 1579–1583

37 Fry F J, Sanghvi N T, Foster R S, Bihrle R, Hennige C. Ultrasound and microbubbles: their generation, detection and potential utilization in tissue and organ therapy. Ultrasound Med Biol 1995; 21: 1227–1237

38 Birnbaum Y, Luo H, Nagai T et al. Noninvasive in vivo clot dissolution without a thrombolytic drug: recanalization of thrombosed iliofemoral arteries by transcutaneous ultrasound combined with intravenous infusion of microbubbles. Circulation 1998; 97: 130–134

Doppler

Hylton B Meire

Introduction

The basic principles of ultrasound pulse–echo imaging have been covered repeatedly in numerous texts and are not therefore included in this book. However, the application of the Doppler principle to detect moving blood has only relatively recently gained clinical acceptance and is a rapidly expanding field.[1–5] Correct interpretation of the information obtained from Doppler ultrasound presupposes a knowledge of the principles of both blood flow and Doppler ultrasonics, and for this reason both are discussed in some detail in this chapter.

The characteristics of blood flow

Blood is a viscous medium and as it moves throughout the vascular tree there is a drag effect between the moving blood and the vessel walls.[6,7] As a result of these two factors the speed of the blood near the vessel wall is generally less than that toward the centre of the vessel. There is thus a 'velocity profile' across the vessel (Fig. 6.1).[8] If the vessel is straight the profile is symmetrical and, in steady venous flow, generally parabolic in shape (Fig. 6.1). In this situation the blood can be considered to be flowing in a number of concentric laminae (streamlines), the velocity within each lamina increasing towards the centre of the vessel. This form of flow is frequently referred to simply as 'laminar flow', but the use of this term does not imply any particular velocity profile or gradient across the vessel.

Normal venous flow

Normal flow in peripheral veins at rest is slow, continuous and unmodulated, with a velocity of typically only 2 or 3 cm per second (Fig. 6.2A and B). As limb perfusion increases as a result of exercise the venous velocities increase dramatically, but flow usually remains unmodu-

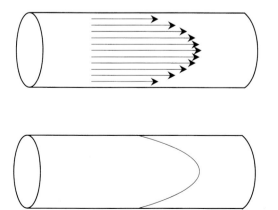

Fig. 6.1 Normal blood flow. The vessel walls exhibit a drag effect upon the adjacent blood, giving rise to a parabolic flow profile across the vessel.

lated. Flow within more central veins – typically the jugular, iliac, intra-abdominal and intrathoracic veins – is normally modulated to a variable extent by the cardiac pulsations. The atrial (a) and ventricular (v) waves are conducted from the right atrium into the superior and inferior venae cavae and cause transitory reductions in flow velocity, or even flow reversal (Fig. 6.2C and D). In addition there is usually also some modulation of venous flow induced by normal breathing movements. The degree to which flow is modulated by both cardiac pulsations and respiration is very variable from patient to patient but in general is greatest in the vessels closest to the heart.

It is generally assumed that the flow profile in major veins is approximately parabolic in shape (see below). This assumption is probably valid for most medium-sized veins. In larger veins the drag has little or no effect on the peripheral streamlines and most of the central blood moves at the same velocity, thereby approximating to plug flow (Fig. 6.3).

On the occasions when volume flow calculations are attempted the vessel is often assumed to be circular in cross-section. Although this is almost always true for arteries, it is seldom true for veins: most are normally somewhat elliptical and those that lie superficially are particularly prone to distortion by pressure from the overlying transducer.

Normal arterial flow

The characteristics of blood flow within arteries are extremely complex. The arterial wall is elastic and dilates significantly as the systolic pressure wave passes.[9–11] This radial expansion causes a transitory increase in cross-sectional area of 20–25% in medium-sized healthy arteries, and during the expansion phase there is necessarily some radial movement of blood to fill the increased lumen size. The pulsatile changes in vessel dimensions and the radial component of flow are almost invariably ignored in current Doppler studies and calculations.

During systole there is rapid acceleration of the moving blood column, with a subsequent rapid deceleration in early diastole. Flow throughout diastole is determined by a wide range of factors, including cardiac dynamics, the state of the local vascular tree and the nature of the circulation supplied by the artery under examination. These factors, commonly referred to as upstream, local and downstream, are discussed in more detail later in the chapter.

The flow velocity in diastole is invariably lower than that in systole (Fig. 6.4A) and, when there is little distal perfusion (for example in the vascular bed of a muscle at rest), diastolic flow is very low; in addition, the elastic recoil of the distal arterial tree may cause transitory reversal of flow during early diastole (Fig. 6.4B). The waveform shown in Figure 6.4A characterises flow in vessels supplying capillary beds with low flow resistance – typically the

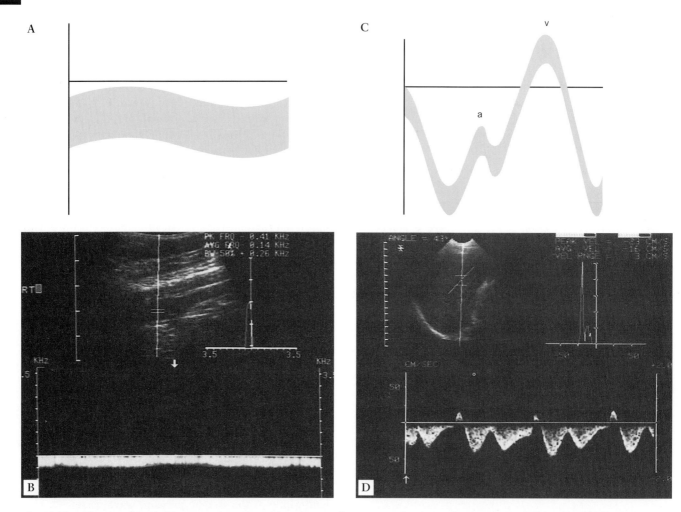

Fig. 6.2 Normal venous flow. A: Diagrammatic representation of venous flow in a peripheral vein showing gentle respiratory modulation.
B: Spontaneous low-velocity flow in a femoral vein, showing minimal respiratory modulation. **C:** Schematic representation of blood flow in a central vein. Forward flow is reduced by the atrial 'a' wave and is temporarily reversed by the ventricular 'v' wave transmitted from the right ventricle.
D: Normal pulsatile flow in a hepatic vein. Note that in all the above examples flow is away from the probe and forward flow is therefore below the baseline.

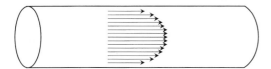

Fig. 6.3 Normal flow in a large vein. In large veins the drag effect does not reach the centre of the vessel, thus giving rise to central flattening of the velocity profile.

brain, liver, kidneys, placenta and pregnant uterus – and is commonly described as a 'low-resistance' waveform. The waveform in Figure 6.4B is termed 'high resistance' and, in addition to normal muscles at rest, may be seen in a range of pathological conditions elsewhere in the body.

Simultaneous with the changes in velocity throughout the cardiac cycle the velocity profile across an artery also changes (Fig. 6.5). As a general rule, flow during diastole approximates to parabolic flow, but in systole the power of the left ventricular ejection forces almost all of the blood to move with the same velocity, giving rise to a profile approximating to plug flow. The temporal changes in velocity profile in arteries supplying a higher vascular resistance bed may be extremely complex, with the different flow laminae showing simultaneous flow in opposite directions during certain phases of the cardiac cycle (Fig. 6.6).

Flow axis

For the purpose of making measurements from Doppler signals it is always assumed that all the flow streamlines within a vessel are moving in a direction parallel to the vessel wall. This is only true in parallel-walled straight vessels: the direction and parallelism of the flow streamlines

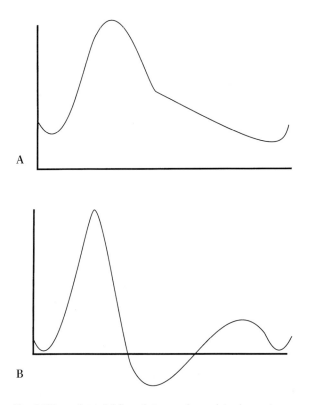

A

B

Fig. 6.4 Normal arterial flow. A: In vessels supplying low-resistance vascular beds there is continuous forward flow throughout the cardiac cycle. B: Arterial flow to high-resistance vascular beds shows varying degrees of diastolic flow reduction, with early diastolic flow reversal if the resistance is high.

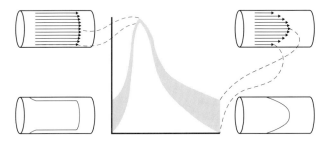

Fig. 6.5 Changes in arterial velocity profile throughout the cardiac cycle. During peak systole most of the blood is moving at one velocity, giving rise to a flat flow profile and a narrow range of frequencies in the Doppler spectrum. During diastole the velocities are lower and the range of velocities wider, giving rise to a parabolic flow profile and a wide range of frequencies in the spectrum.

may be very different in the region of junctions, bends and branches (Fig. 6.7)[12], which may give rise to areas of physiological vortex formation or flow reversal (Fig. 6.8).

Flow in abnormal arteries

Narrowing, for example due to atheromatous plaques, disturbs the normal flow streamlines[13] and the nature and

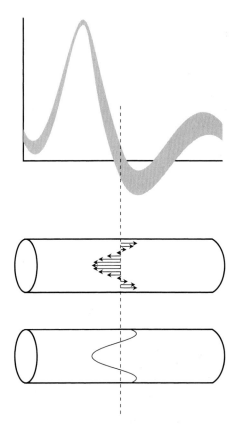

Fig. 6.6 Velocity profile during early diastolic flow reversal. When flow reverses in early diastole the reversal occurs first in the centre of the column of moving blood, whereas the blood nearer the vessel wall is still moving in a forward direction. This gives rise to a biphasic velocity profile and simultaneous forward and reverse flows in the spectral analysis.

degree of this disturbance varies according to the size and characteristics of the plaque.

It is generally assumed that smooth plaques which reduce the lumen by less than 50% do not reduce the volume of blood flowing through a vessel segment. However, if the volume flow is maintained despite a reduction in the vessel cross-sectional area, there must necessarily be an increase in flow velocity at the site of the narrowing (Fig. 6.9). The flow velocity and velocity profile are normal both proximal and distal to the lesion.

If the surface of the plaque is rough or ulcerated, even if the plaque itself is quite small, local flow disturbance occurs over the surface of the plaque, usually with small vortices developing within the craters on the plaque surface (Fig. 6.10). The flow characteristics above and below the lesion remain normal, the vortices usually only propagating for a few millimetres downstream. Stenoses of greater than 50% are associated with a more marked increase in flow velocity through the stenosis, with flow disturbance (Fig. 6.11). The increase in peak velocity is approximately

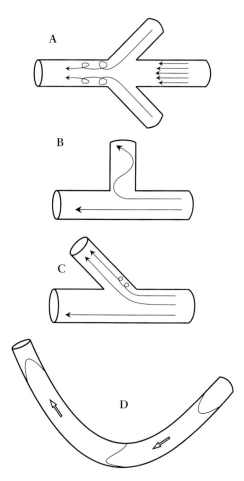

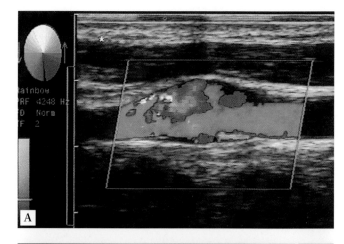

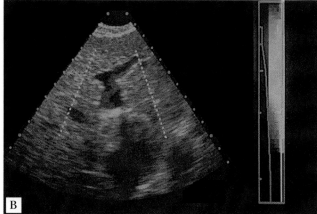

Fig. 6.7 Normal flow at junctions, branches and bends. A: Normal venous laminar flow is disturbed at major junctions, for example between the renal veins and IVC, giving rise to vortex formation at and just beyond the junction. B: A coarse vortex may arise at an acutely angled branch, for example at the bifurcation of the portal vein within the liver (see Fig. 6.8B). C: As blood enters the origin of an obtusely angled branch flow near the wall may become disturbed owing to 'boundary layer separation', and give rise to small localised vortices (see Fig. 6.8A). D: In curved vessels the normal symmetry of the velocity profile is distorted in the region of the curve.

Fig. 6.8 Physiological vortices. A: Longitudinal scan of the carotid bulb. Complex vortices (red) are present owing to boundary layer separation. This is a normal flow characteristic. B: Transverse scan of the left portal vein. The CDI sensitivity has been reduced to show only the highest velocity flow, which can be seen to follow a spiral course through this vessel (compare with Fig. 6.7B).

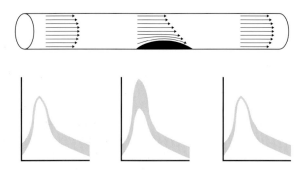

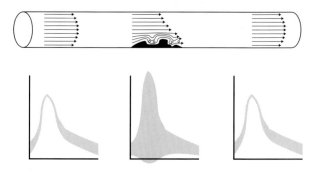

Fig. 6.9 Flow over a low-grade stenosis. Proximal and distal flow remains normal but there is a slight acceleration at the site of the stenosis, resulting in an increased range of velocities in the Doppler spectrum during systole.

Fig. 6.10 Flow over an ulcerated atheromatous plaque. If the stenosis is less than 50% flow above and below the plaque is normal. As the flow streamlines enter the craters in the plaque, small vortices are generated and propagate for short distances downstream. These give rise to widening of the spectral breadth, with true simultaneous forward and reverse flow that is usually only apparent during systole, as they are most likely to be produced when the flow velocity is fast.

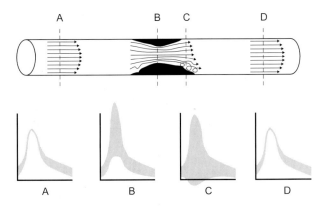

Fig. 6.11 Flow through a 50–90% stenosis. Although the proximal and distal profiles are normal there is an overall velocity reduction roughly in proportion to the severity of the stenosis. At the site of the stenosis there is an increase in peak velocity and gross spectral broadening with true flow reversal. The flow disturbance may be propagated for 2–3 cm downstream.

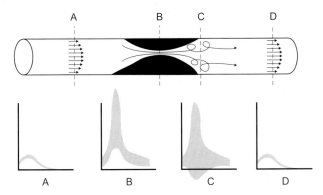

Fig. 6.12 Flow through a high-grade stenosis. Proximal and distal flow is drastically reduced (A and D). The flow velocity through the stenosis is greatly increased (B) and there is severe vortex formation beyond the stenosis (C).

proportional to the severity of the stenosis[14] and the high-velocity jet may propagate for 2–3 cm distal to the lesion. Proximal to the lesion there is a reduction in flow velocity below that which would normally be expected at that anatomical site.

Stenoses of greater than 90% produce a drastic reduction in volume flow, with a high-velocity and extremely disturbed flow through and beyond the stenosis (Fig. 6.12).

The basis of Doppler ultrasound

The detection of blood flow with ultrasound depends on the Doppler principle (Fig. 6.13), which determines that, when ultrasound is reflected from a moving structure, the frequency of the reflected waves is different from that of the incident waves. The degree to which the frequency is altered is determined by both the speed and the direction of movement of the blood cells, movement towards the

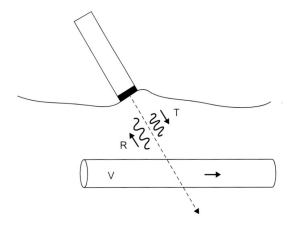

Fig. 6.13 The Doppler principle. The frequency of the transmitted ultrasound pulse (T) is altered when it is reflected from a moving structure, in this case blood flowing within the vessel (V). When the direction of blood flow is away from the transducer the frequency of the returning wave (R) is reduced.

transducer increasing the frequency and *vice versa*. Analysis of the Doppler-shifted frequency permits assessment of the speed and relative direction of the blood flow. The equation which describes the value of the Doppler shift frequency is:

$$f_d = \frac{2V\,(\cos\theta)\,f}{c}$$

where f_d is the Doppler-shifted frequency, V is the speed of the moving blood, θ is the angle between the ultrasound beam and the direction of movement of the blood, f is the transmitted ultrasound frequency, and c is the speed of ultrasound (1540 m/s).

In any Doppler examination the ultrasound frequency and speed are fixed and the Doppler-shifted frequency therefore depends on the speed of the blood and the beam/vessel angle. The beam/vessel angle (θ) is of great importance in clinical Doppler examinations,[15] as when θ is 90° its cosine is 0 (Fig. 6.14) and therefore no Doppler signal is obtained. Conversely, if the ultrasound beam can be aligned along the direction of the long axis of the vessel θ is 0, the cosine of θ is 1 and the maximum possible Doppler shift frequency is obtained. In practice this alignment is seldom achievable and a compromise has to be accepted. In general, however, it is advisable to try to position the ultrasound transducer in such a way that the beam/vessel angle is no greater than 60°.

In clinical examinations there is never a single Doppler shift frequency and the returning ultrasound signal contains a spectrum of frequencies determined by the distributions of different blood velocities across the vessel.

The interpretation of the Doppler signal, and any calculations made from information derived from it, assumes that the whole width of the vessel under interrogation is exposed to a uniform ultrasound field. This is termed

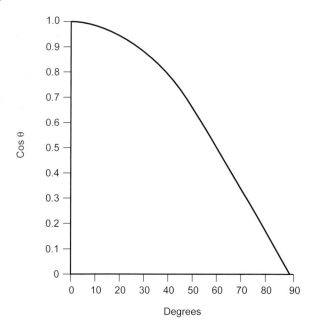

Fig. 6.14 Cosine θ.

'uniform insonation', and the degree to which this is achieved in practice is determined by the size, depth and orientation of the blood vessel, together with the characteristics of the ultrasound beam (Fig. 6.15).[16] If the beam is significantly narrower than the blood vessel little or no signal is obtained from the slow-moving blood at the periphery of the vessel. This may lead to an overestimation

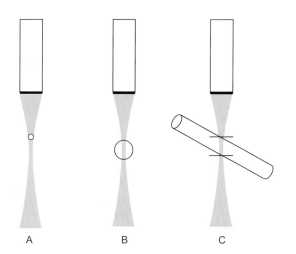

Fig. 6.15 Uniform insonation. A: If the vessel is no larger than the effective width of the ultrasound beam the whole lumen can be assumed to be uniformly insonated. **B:** If the vessel is significantly wider than the beam a high proportion of the slow-moving peripheral blood may not be sampled, giving rise to a falsely high assessment of the overall flow velocity. **C:** The sample volume is also determined by the size of the range gate, which should match the vessel diameter (see Fig. 6.16).

of the mean flow velocity, or to failure to detect areas of flow disturbance near the vessel wall.

The simplest of medical ultrasound Doppler equipment uses two separate transducers, one transmitting a continuous ultrasound tone while the second receives the returning echoes.[2] These devices still have wide clinical application in such areas as fetal heart detection and for the assessment of patency of peripheral arteries. These 'continuous wave' (CW) machines can be small, simple and inexpensive, but suffer from the major disadvantage that there is no information concerning the depth from which any Doppler-shifted signals originate. Any vessel or other moving structure anywhere along the length of the ultrasound beam gives rise to a signal and all such signals are mixed together in the resulting Doppler output.

In clinical situations where it is necessary to identify signals from within individual closely adjacent vessels, or from limited areas within a single vessel, it is necessary to employ pulse–echo ultrasound similar to that used for conventional imaging. In imaging ultrasound, the depth from which each individual echo originates is calculated from a knowledge of the speed of transmission of ultrasound in the tissues and the time taken between transmission of the ultrasound pulse and reception of a specific echo. Provided the duration of the transmitted pulse is sufficient for its frequency to be measured accurately, the frequency of the returning echoes can also be measured, in addition to determining the depth from which they arose. The combination of Doppler with conventional imaging has been responsible for the rapid increase in the clinical applications of Doppler ultrasound. Modern Doppler systems permit the operator to identify the depth from which Doppler signals are to be acquired, while ignoring signals arising from outside the defined sample volume. The depth and dimensions of the sample volume are determined by a combination of the ultrasound beam width and the position of the 'range gate' markers, which are set by the operator (Fig. 6.16).

Colour Doppler/colour flow imaging

In colour flow imaging (CFI) the Doppler-shifted information is used to generate a colour overlay on the conventional 2D grey scale image.[17-19] In order to achieve this, it is necessary to detect the Doppler flow information at a large number of sites within the image in rapid succession. This necessitates the use of a great deal of additional electronic hardware and sophisticated software and significant compromises are generally employed by equipment manufacturers in order to limit both the complexity and the cost of the equipment.

The principle is similar to that of conventional single range gate Doppler but, instead of detecting flow in a single large sample volume, numerous small adjacent sample volumes are created along the lines of site of

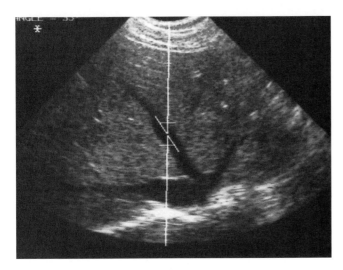

Fig. 6.16 Sample volume and range gate size. The portion of the ultrasound beam from which Doppler signals are received is marked by the operator using 'range gates', which appear in this figure as short lines at right-angles to the ultrasound path. The separation of these range gates determines the sample volume, and this should be adjusted to ensure that the whole vessel cross-section is being sampled.

several consecutive pulses (Fig. 6.17). Calculating the Doppler frequency content for each individual range gate takes a significant time and computational power and there is thus a limit on the number of picture elements that can be interrogated in a given time interval. If the user requires a large number of picture elements to produce finer detail in the colour image a significant time penalty is suffered, with the frame rate falling to as low as 4 per second. Conversely, if a high frame rate is required, for example in cardiological imaging, it is only possible to display a smaller number of relatively large picture elements, giving rise to poor spatial and frequency resolution.

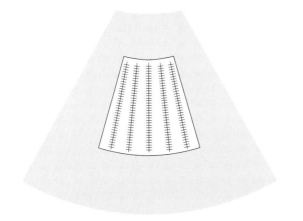

Fig. 6.17 Colour flow imaging. Within the colour flow region of interest there are large numbers of sequential range gates along each line of sight. The number and spacing of the range gates and lines of sight vary with make of equipment and control settings.

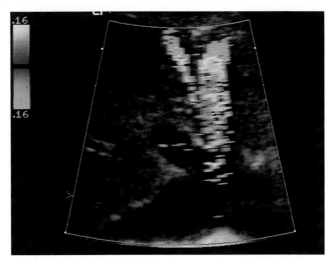

Fig. 6.18 Pixels in the colour image. The pixels within CDI images are much larger than those in grey scale imaging, giving rise to jagged vessel margins and usually leading to an inappropriately wide display of narrow vessels. This image has been magnified to demonstrate this.

These compromises dictate that manufacturers generally optimise their equipment either for cardiac or for abdominal purposes, and machines optimised for one are usually inappropriate for use in the other.

The Doppler information obtained from each range gate is analysed to determine the direction of movement and a relatively crude assessment of the mean velocity. This information is then turned into a colour signal, which is added to the appropriate pixel in the 2D display (Fig. 6.18). Flow towards the transducer is customarily coded red and flow away is blue. However, the user is able to change this or to substitute a wide range of other colour maps to the velocity information.

In the majority of clinical applications it is not necessary to interrogate the entire field of view for Doppler information. When a smaller region of interest is selected all the available colour picture elements can be allocated to this region, thereby reducing pixel size and significantly improving the resolution of the colour image as well as the frame rate.

A great many technological refinements have been developed in modern colour Doppler imaging systems to improve flow detection, suppress confusing signals from moving soft tissues and to improve both spatial and temporal resolution. The effects of some of these are discussed further in the section on artefacts below.

Power Doppler

Introduction

The term power Doppler is becoming accepted to describe a number of alternative forms of colour Doppler display offered by a range of different equipment manufacturers under a variety of other names. These include 'ultrasound angio', 'colour Doppler energy', 'colour power angio' etc. The theme common to all these forms of display is the use of colour to code the amplitude or power content of the Doppler signal, rather than its frequency shift. Because the frequency information is discarded power Doppler display contains no directional information, but the colour hue at any point within the image is determined by the strength of the Doppler signal from the relevant area.[20] This is approximately proportional to the number of moving red cells within the volume element, and thus high signals are obtained from within the lumina of large vessels and weaker signals are obtained when only part of the beam width impinges on moving red cells. In common with conventional spectral and colour Doppler there are frequency and velocity limits below which moving cells will not be detected, and thus weak or absent signals may result from low velocity rather than absence of moving red cells.

Advantages of power Doppler display

There are two major advantages, both of which arise from discarding the frequency information. The first is most apparent in areas where colour Doppler display may be confusing because of the wide range of velocities and directions of blood within a relatively small area. The colour Doppler information may either be self-cancelling or may give rise to a mosaic of colours, which may be difficult or impossible to interpret. The distribution of the power signal from such a situation is shown in Figure 6.19, where it can be seen that the power signals from both the advancing and the receding blood are in a positive direction and therefore summate, giving rise to a relatively uniform colour hue irrespective of red cell velocity or direction. The advantages of this for clinical display are shown in Figure 6.20.

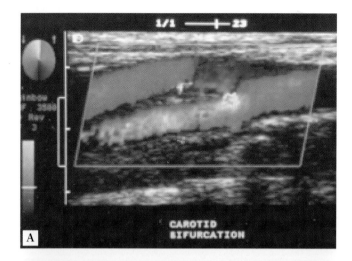

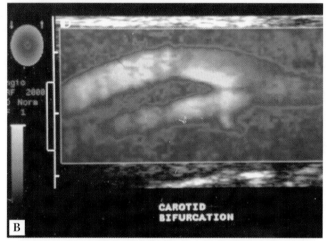

Fig. 6.20 Advantages of discarding velocity information. A: In colour Doppler display the normal vortex at the bifurcation produces a confusing appearance, making it difficult to be confident of the outline of the vessel. **B:** Power Doppler display shows the vessel lumen to be normal.

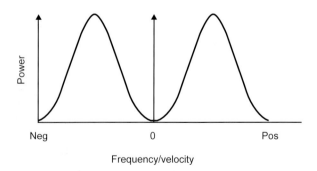

Fig. 6.19 Doppler power distribution. When the number of red cells moving towards and away from the transducer are roughly equal the frequency signals either side of zero will cancel out, giving rise to little if any signal in colour Doppler display. However, both power signals are positive, and when these are added together give a strong signal in power Doppler display.

The second major advantage of power Doppler display derives from its ability to make use of significant signal averaging over time. In conventional colour Doppler display signal averaging is undesirable, as rapid changes in haemodynamic events are best shown by high frame-rate colour Doppler. Signal averaging would defeat this objective. In the power Doppler display mode changes in direction and velocity are not displayed at all and therefore signal averaging becomes a possibility. In view of the fact that the strength of echoes received from moving red cells is extremely feeble, there is a relatively poor signal-to-noise ratio in most Doppler examinations. In power Doppler display mode the signal is merely the amplitude or power of the Doppler signal and remains relatively constant, whereas the noise is essentially random. Fortunately, when information from successive pulses is added and averaged the power signal integrates and therefore

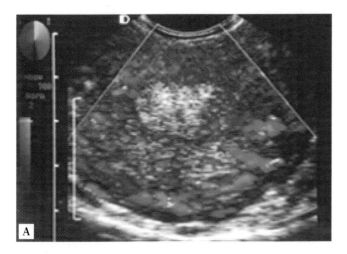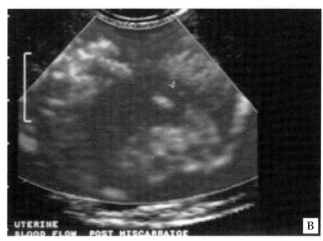

Fig. 6.21 The advantages of frame averaging. Trans-vaginal scans of the uterus. A: Colour Doppler display shows the major intramural vessels. B: Power Doppler display identifies many more areas of blood flow than colour Doppler alone.

improves, whereas the noise tends to be self-cancelling. The degree of noise reduction is approximately proportional to the square root of the number of frames averaged. Clearly, averaging too many frames will give rise to a very slow frame rate and a smeary image if there is significant tissue or vessel movement, but in clinical practice useful degrees of averaging are achieved and can greatly improve the detectability of slow-flowing blood and small vessels (Fig. 6.21).

Continuing technical improvements in power Doppler signal processing and display techniques are now enabling clinically useful information to be obtained from studies in which conventional colour Doppler has failed, and for which it was previously necessary to enhance the Doppler signal by the injection of echo-enhancing agents. It may now be possible to avoid the use of these agents in some cases. However, no doubt the combination of echo-enhancing agents and power Doppler display will further enhance our ability to study small or subtle haemodynamic changes in the future.

Further technical developments

Now that the basic principles of power Doppler display have been well developed a number of manufacturers offer the option to add back into the display some directional information. This offers a hybrid display, with the power Doppler signal showing the presence of moving red cells and the velocity information being added in a contrasting colour. With intelligent use this form of display can benefit from the advantages of both power and colour Doppler display modes, while avoiding many of the disadvantages of colour Doppler. However, in order to obtain the best benefit from this form of display the user must understand the principles involved and make the best possible use of the equipment control settings.

Angle independence

Some manufacturers have claimed that power Doppler display does not suffer from the angle dependence of conventional spectral and colour Doppler imaging. This statement is not strictly true since, if the interrogating beam is at right-angles to the vector of movement of the red cells, no Doppler signal should be obtained. However, in view of the fact that improvements in signal-to-noise ratio enable the detection of lower Doppler shift frequencies, it is possible to obtain a satisfactory signal at much higher beam/vessel angles than with conventional Doppler (Fig. 6.22).

Technical advantages

Sensitivity The most notable advantage in clinical applications is a marked apparent increase in sensitivity, probably of the order of approximately 10 dB. This

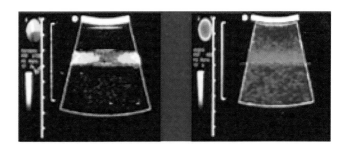

Fig. 6.22 Effective angle independence. The figure on the left is taken from a phantom in which blood substitute is flowing in a straight tube. When viewed with a curvilinear probe the effective change in flow direction with respect to the direction of the pulses gives rise to a confusing flow pattern. In the right-hand image the same Doppler information has been processed in power Doppler mode and shows uniform flow throughout the tube.

improvement is in fact somewhat artefactual, as the information used in power Doppler display is the same as that used for colour Doppler display. However, the ability to identify slower-moving red cells correctly and to improve the signal-to-noise ratio undoubtedly enables the detection of blood flow by this form of display, which cannot be detected by conventional colour Doppler display.

Display stability   The freedom from the need to display velocity information, which may rapidly change in a short space of time, enables a much more stable display which is easier to assimilate and analyse.

Freedom from aliasing   The artefact of aliasing is due to the inability of spectral and colour Doppler systems to identify velocity information correctly. As the power Doppler display mode does not include velocity information there is no aliasing in the display. Similarly, a range of other artefacts related to both velocity and direction ambiguities or changes in colour Doppler display are avoided by the power Doppler display mode (Fig. 6.23).

Border detection   There is an apparent improvement in the ability to define the margins of vessels and the surfaces of plaques and stenoses within those vessels. This arises partly from abandonment of the velocity information, making the display easier to assimilate, especially over irregular or ulcerated plaques. However, there is also a subtle difference in the way in which the information at vessel walls is processed. In colour Doppler display a pixel is completely filled with colour of the appropriate velocity code if any moving red cells are detected at any point within the volume element. This tends to give rise to an irregular and rather pixelated vessel outline. In the power Doppler display mode the hue displayed in a pixel will be significantly reduced if the entire voxel is not filled by moving red cells. There is thus a fall-off in signal amplitude towards the edges of the vessel, giving a more pleasing and apparently less pixelated margin to the vessel (Fig. 6.24).

3D display   Attempts to display conventional colour Doppler information in 3D or pseudo-3D form have led to extremely confusing images, primarily as a result of changes in hue or colour due to vessel geometry rather than actual blood flow velocity.

The relative independence of power Doppler display from the influences of geometry makes this an ideal form of display for volume acquisition of vascular information for 3D reconstruction studies.

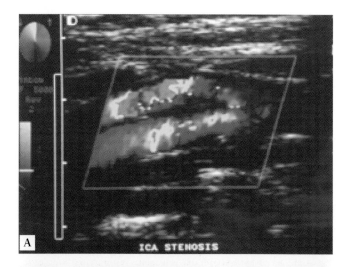

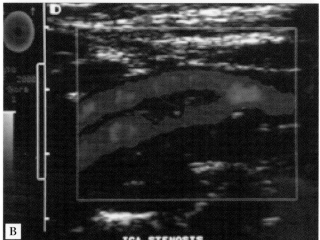

Fig. 6.23 Freedom from aliasing. A: This diseased carotid bifurcation is difficult to evaluate in colour Doppler mode owing to the wide variation in velocities and the presence of aliasing. B: In power Doppler mode the true lumen and irregular plaque become more readily identifiable.

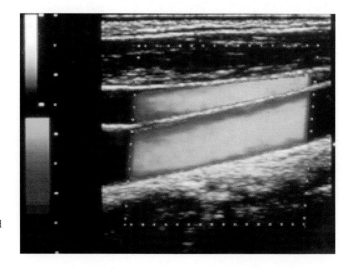

Fig. 6.24 Vessel border detection. Scan of the common carotid artery and jugular vein. The fall-off in signal at the vessel margin results in better vessel wall delineation in power Doppler display.

Technical disadvantages

Loss of velocity and direction information In several clinical situations the presence or absence of disease may be determined by changes in either blood flow velocity or direction. As neither of these features is present in power Doppler display this potentially useful diagnostic information may be lost. However, in the majority of current machines it is possible to switch quickly between conventional colour display and power display, and thus the advantages of both should be available to the prudent user.

Data acquisition time In view of the generally higher degree of frame averaging used for power Doppler display the time taken to collect a full frame of information is increased and the frame rate is therefore considerably reduced compared to colour Doppler display. If the vessel or tissues being examined are moving rapidly this may cause blurring and degradation in the image that would not be apparent in conventional colour display.

Attenuation Because the information used for the power Doppler display is the signal power or amplitude it is subject to the same limitations as conventional grey scale imaging. The signal strength will be reduced in any situation where there is attenuation and will be excessive in areas where attenuation is less than predicted. In clinical practice this has been found to limit severely the application of power Doppler display for the evaluation of areas such as the upper pole of the left kidney and the distal renal cortex, where the signal strength is significantly less than that from the more proximal components of the kidney (Fig. 6.25). Surprisingly, few manufacturers currently offer depth gain compensation in the power Doppler mode and it seems possible that this would at

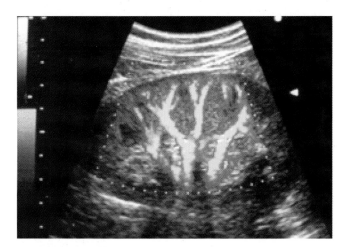

Fig. 6.25 The effect of attenuation. The power Doppler signal from the distal cortex in the upper pole of the kidney is not received, as the amplitude (power) of the signal is attenuated by the greater path length compared to the more superficial cortex.

least partly ameliorate this limitation. Attenuation is less of a problem in paediatric patients and power Doppler has been found to be superior to CFI for the diagnosis of acute focal pyelonephritis.[21,22]

Clinical uses

The main clinical applications for power Doppler derive from the improved detection of flow or from improved ease of image interpretation. To date there are no clinical areas where power Doppler has proved essential for establishing a diagnosis, but it has been shown to be beneficial in a number of investigations, including trans-cranial imaging,[23] musculoskeletal disease,[24] and the differential diagnosis of bowel masses[25] and focal liver lesions.[26,27] There is also some suggestion that it may be superior to colour Doppler display for the detection of testicular torsion.[28,29]

It has also been shown that the number of abnormal new vessels around malignant breast masses demonstrated by power Doppler display is greater than those seen by conventional colour Doppler.[30] This may prove to be advantageous in the differential diagnosis of solid breast lesions.

Improved ability to correctly identify small residual lumina in stenosed arteries[31,32] and partly thrombosed veins is undoubtedly a major advantage.

Its relative freedom from geometrical constraints becomes particularly valuable in certain clinical situations, such as where the vessel is parallel to the surface, or where the window of access is limited. Examples of this include imaging the vertebral artery in the neck, the posterior cerebral artery and sagittal sinus in the neonatal brain, and for determination of the anatomy of the circle of Willis by trans-cranial studies.

Evaluation of plaque surface morphology may be particularly important in patients at risk for emboli from ulcerated or irregular plaques. In this situation colour Doppler display may be extremely confusing owing to local vortices or flow voids in the crevices on the surface of an irregular or ulcerated plaque. Power Doppler gives a much more readily understandable display, with relatively uniform colour throughout the vessel lumen, combined with the ability to detect slower-moving blood within craters on the plaque surface (Fig. 6.26).[32]

Extracting information from the Doppler signal

As discussed above, the Doppler signal contains a spectrum of frequencies which vary to a greater or lesser extent with cardiac or respiratory changes. The range and magnitude of these frequencies and the way in which they change throughout the cardiac cycle embody much information concerning cardiac activity, the proximal vascular

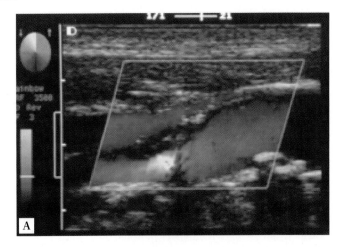

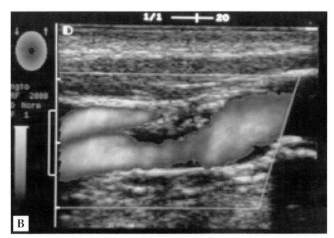

Fig. 6.26 Plaque surface morphology. A: Colour Doppler of this abnormal carotid bifurcation gives a confusing image owing to poor detection of low flow and areas of aliasing. **B:** Power Doppler display gives excellent delineation of the vessel wall and the irregular vessel intima and plaque.

tree, the vessel at the site of interrogation and the state of the vascular bed or vessels distal to the examination site. A wide range of techniques and mathematical computations have been devised in attempts to extract this information,[33] and at present only limited success has been achieved. However, a number of indices are used frequently, all of which are applied to a graphical display of the frequency information. This is termed 'spectral analysis', and the means by which it is achieved should be understood before attempting to interpret any values derived from it.

Spectral analysis

Spectral analysis is the process whereby the frequency content of the ultrasound signal, and the way in which it varies with time, is analysed and displayed. In practice, measurement of the frequency content takes a significant amount of time and there are limitations on both the range of frequencies detectable and the resolution with which the different frequencies can be separated. The way in which the analysis is performed varies somewhat from one make of equipment to another but usually a fast Fourier transform (FFT) is used.[34] It is not necessary to have a technical understanding of the principles of this in order to comprehend and interpret the results it produces.

The spectral analysis display takes the form of a graph of frequency on the vertical axis and time on the horizontal axis (Figs 6.27 and 6.28). Both frequency and time are divided into small but finite increments and the spectral tracing therefore consists of an array of tiny elements or pixels. The amplitude (brightness) of the signal within each pixel of the spectral analysis image is approximately proportional to the number of scatterers giving rise to signals within that particular frequency range during the appropriate time interval. It will therefore be appreciated

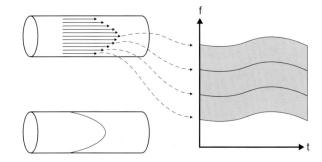

Fig. 6.27 Spectral analysis. Spectral analysis produces a graphic display of frequency (f) on the vertical axis and time (t) on the horizontal axis. The width of the displayed frequency band correlates directly with the range of velocities present within the vessel, the highest velocities corresponding to the highest frequencies, and vice versa.

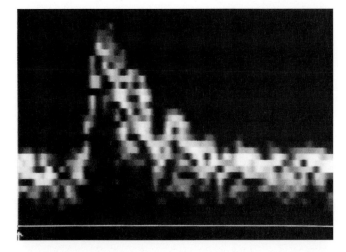

Fig. 6.28 Spectral analysis. Both frequency and time are measured in small increments and give rise to pixelation within the spectral display. In this example the equipment settings have been altered to maximise this effect.

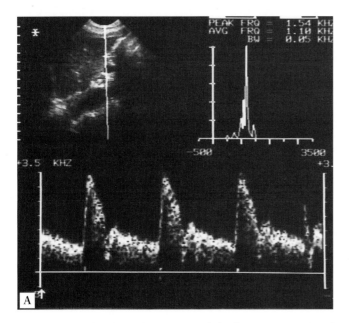
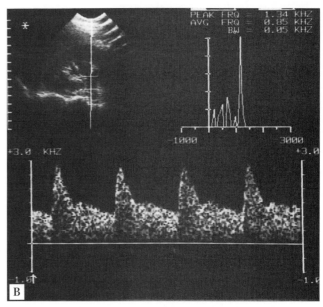

Fig. 6.29 Spectral analysis of plug and parabolic flow. A: During arterial systole, especially during the upstroke, all the blood is moving with a plug profile and a very narrow range of frequencies is displayed. **B:** During diastole in this renal artery there is a uniform spread of frequencies from peak to minimum, indicating a parabolic velocity profile.

that in plug flow, where most of the scatterers are moving with very similar velocities, there is a narrow range of frequencies in the Doppler signal and the spectral display is that of a narrow frequency band (Fig. 6.29A). Conversely, if parabolic flow is present there is a wide frequency range giving rise to a broad spectrum of frequencies in the spectral analysis image (Fig. 6.29B). As a general rule, Doppler shift frequencies from blood flowing towards the transducer are displayed as positive (above the baseline) and those flowing away are displayed as negative. In several physiological and pathological circumstances there may be flow simultaneously towards and away from the transducer, and this can be detected by simultaneous display of both forward and reverse flow in the spectral analysis image (Fig. 6.30).

Evaluation of the spectral Doppler trace is divided into assessment of the waveform shape and analysis of the spectral content and each of these will be considered separately.

Arterial waveform analysis

For the purpose of arterial waveform analysis the spectral content of the waveform is ignored and only the shape of the outline of the tracing is considered (Fig. 6.31).[35] In order to permit analysis of the waveform shape a number of end-points have to be identified (Fig. 6.32).[36] These include peak systole, the peak end-diastolic frequency, the 'mean peak' value and, where relevant, the maximum negative deflection during diastole. From these end-points it is possible to calculate a wide range of values, including sys-

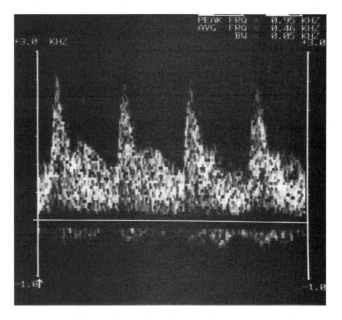

Fig. 6.30 Simultaneous forward and reverse flow. This tracing from an abnormal vessel shows infilling of the systolic frequency window and simultaneous display of flow in both forward and reverse channels, confirming the presence of flow disturbance with vortex formation.

tolic acceleration and deceleration, diastolic deceleration, various ratios of systole to diastole, including the A/B ratio, and numerous simple indices including resistance index and pulsatility index.[33] Many more complex analyses have also been proposed but have not yet found regular clinical application.

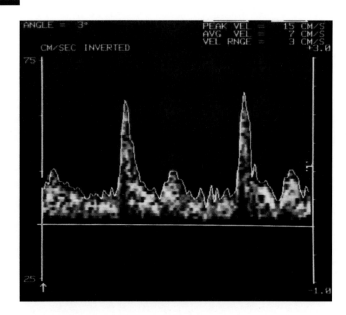

Fig. 6.31 Waveform analysis, peak frequency envelope. In order to permit calculation of the pulsatility index from this complex arterial waveform the equipment has automatically traced the outline of the peak frequency.

Many of these values assume that it is possible to be certain about the exact moment at which diastole begins. This question has received little discussion in the literature, though it is clear that many authors have made assumptions which are not proved by scientific investigation. For unidirectional arterial waveforms (Fig. 6.32A) the point of inflection on the curve from peak systole to end diastole is assumed to indicate the beginning of diastole. For bidirectional flows diastole is assumed to occur at the point where flow changes from forward to reverse (Fig. 6.32B) and for more complex waveforms various notches are assumed to indicate the commencement of diastole (Fig. 6.32C). It is probable that none of these end-points is actually valid and from a purely cardiological point of view diastole actually starts at the point of aortic valve closure, which to all intents and purposes is at peak systole. The subsequent deceleration is therefore not a true systolic deceleration and most, if not all, of the indices that compare or make use of the systolic and diastolic time intervals are probably invalid.

The A/B ratio This was proposed by Gosling in 1976[37] specifically for assessing changes in common carotid and supra-orbital arteries. Spectral analysis of the signals from these vessels shows a secondary peak in early diastole which is termed the B peak and it is the ratio between this and the peak systolic amplitude that is calculated in this index (Fig. 6.32C). This index is not intended for generalised application but it has unfortunately been misquoted, misinterpreted and misused, most commonly by incorrect placement of the point of measurement for

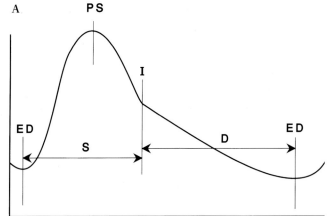
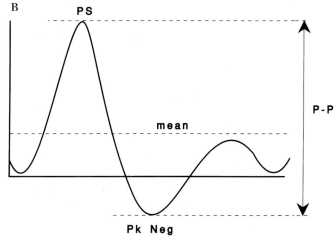
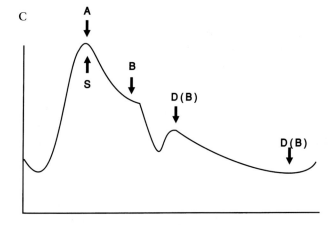

Fig. 6.32 Measurement of arterial waveform shape. A: For measurement of a 'low-resistance' waveform the following values may be measured: end-diastole (ED), peak systole (PS), systolic time interval (S), diastolic time interval (D), systolic/diastolic inflection (I). **B:** For bidirectional waveforms the peak-to-peak interval (P-P) from peak systole (PS) to peak negative deflection (Pk Neg) is measured, together with a computed mean value, throughout at least one (preferably more) cardiac cycles. **C:** For low-resistance waveforms with a 'notch' there is agreement about the position of peak systole (S and A), but the diastolic values (D and B) vary from one author to another.

the B peak in waveforms derived from arteries other than those for which the technique was devised. This ratio has no specific advantages elsewhere for generalised use.

The resistance index   The resistance index (RI)[38] was devised in 1973 for assessment of arterial waveforms where there is no reverse flow component. The value is:

peak systole – end diastole/peak systole

and has the advantage that it is independent of beam/vessel angle (cosine θ) and only requires the measurement of two precisely defined points in the spectral display (see Fig. 6.32A).

There is some confusion about the precise terminology for both this index and the pulsatility index (see below). The resistance index (sometimes incorrectly called the resistive index) was described by Pourcelot and is sometimes referred to as the Pourcelot index and given the abbreviation PI. This leads to confusion with the pulsatility index (also abbreviated to PI), and the situation is further confused by several authors, particularly among North American paediatricians, who use the resistance index but call it the pulsatility index. It is also important to be aware that the waveform is affected by many factors, several of which have nothing whatever to do with resistance to blood flow (see below).

The pulsatility index   This was devised by Gosling in 1971[3] to quantify the energy in the oscillations of the waveform; the full equation is complex and therefore a simplified formula (the PI) is used in clinical practice:

PI = peak systole – end diastole/mean peak value.

It is particularly valuable in arteries in which there is diastolic flow reversal and can be calculated from a frequency trace without the need to know the beam/vessel angle.

The PI requires the computation of the mean peak value throughout the cardiac cycle (see Fig. 6.32B). Manual tracing of complex waveforms may give rise to significant errors and automated tracings from technically inadequate Doppler signals may also give rise to erroneous values. Despite these limitations the PI has gained wide clinical acceptance, particularly in peripheral vascular disease. Again it is important to remember that the waveform shape may be influenced by a wide range of upstream, local and downstream factors and these should always be taken into consideration when using this or any other index.

The systolic/diastolic ratio   The systolic/diastolic (S/D) ratio is effectively a variation of the resistance index and has found particular favour in obstetric applications (Fig. 3.32C).[39–41] The ratio is:

peak systole/end diastole.

Unfortunately, peak systole is frequently referred to as 'A' and end diastole as 'B' and this ratio is therefore also known as the A/B ratio, although it is different from the previously mentioned A/B ratio. If there is also early diastolic flow reduction this is sometimes incorrectly termed the dicrotic notch, or just 'the notch'. Its presence and magnitude may correlate with the severity of vascular disease in the arterial bed of the pregnant uterus.

There is a later version of the S/D ratio which is the D/S ratio. Numerically this is usually indistinguishable from 1 minus the resistance index and is of course the inverse of the S/D ratio.

It is not clear which of the A/B, S/D or D/S ratios is clinically most useful.

There are many other indices that have been devised to assess arterial waveform shapes, particularly in obstetrics.[42] The fact that so many exist tends to suggest that none is entirely satisfactory and this situation is not helped by the confusing terminology, where different indices are given the same name and the same index is given different names. As a general rule it is probably safe to use the PI in peripheral vascular studies and the RI in all carotid and intra-abdominal studies.

Spectral breadth measurement   The Doppler signal contains a spectrum of frequencies and the breadth of this spectrum is a measure of the range of velocities present within the vessel. During systolic flow in normal arteries with a diameter greater than 5–10 mm there is a narrow range of frequencies but this may be increased (broadened) by the presence of vascular disease. The degree to which the spectrum is broadened correlates roughly with the severity of the arterial disease[43] and it is therefore possible to give numerical values to the degree of spectral broadening. In small arteries the velocity profile is closer to parabolic and the normal spectrum is broad.

Unfortunately, as with waveform indices, a number of spectral broadening indices have been devised[44] and the majority are called the 'spectral broadening index' (SBI), although mathematically they are by no means identical. A simple and readily usable SBI compares the range of frequencies displayed at peak systole with the absolute peak systolic value and is expressed as a percentage (Fig. 6.33). The value of the SBI varies widely at different sites, at different phases in the cardiac cycle and with different equipment and control settings. Therefore, normal values are not available and investigators wishing to use this index should assess their own range of normal values on their own patients and equipment and compare them with those obtained in pathological cases.

Velocity information   Using the Doppler formula it is theoretically possible to calculate the instantaneous blood flow velocity, provided that the angle between the ultrasound beam and the direction of blood flow is accurately

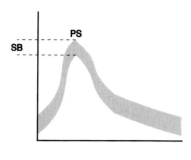

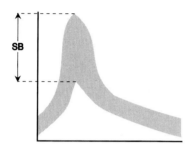

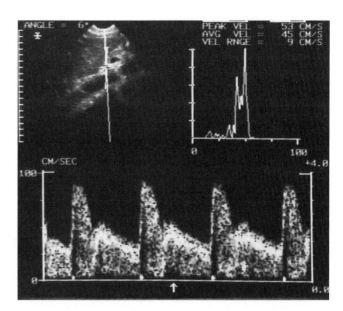

Fig. 6.34 Instantaneous mean velocity. The arrow below the spectrum analysis trace in this example indicates the time interval at which the instantaneous frequency spectrum has been assessed. The grey scale display in the spectrogram indicates that there are many more scatterers travelling with velocities close to the peak, with relatively few low-velocity scatterers at this time. This assessment is confirmed by the histogram (upper right), showing that most scatterers are travelling with velocities between 40 and 55 cm/s. The instantaneous average velocity calculation above the histogram indicates a value of 45 cm/s.

Fig. 6.33 Measurement of spectral breadth. The spectral broadening produced by arterial disease can be assessed by measuring the spectral breadth (SB) during peak systole and comparing this with the peak systolic value (PS).

known and is less than 60°. In clinical practice there is a number of different specific values for velocity which may be useful in different clinical situations,[45] including, peak systole; peak end diastole; mean peak; instantaneous mean; and time-averaged mean. The values for peak systole and end diastole have already been discussed in considering the resistance index.

The mean peak value is the mean of the individual values comprising the peak velocity outline (Fig. 6.31). The instantaneous mean (Fig. 6.34) is difficult (and often impossible) to calculate, but in theory should be the mean value of the velocities of all the red cells moving throughout the vessel cross-section at any instant in time. Unfortunately this information is not generally available but the spectral content of any spectral analysis time interval contains information about both the range of velocities present and the approximate proportion of scatterers travelling with each individual velocity. If there is true plug flow there is, of course, a very narrow band of velocities, with all red cells travelling at almost the same velocity. In true parabolic flow there is a uniform distribution of velocities from the peak down to zero, resulting in an even grey scale in the display throughout the velocity range. In this situation the mean velocity is 50% of the peak, whereas in plug flow the mean is equal to the peak value. In the majority of clinical situations the ratio between the true mean and the peak actually lies somewhere between 50% and 100% and, within arteries, varies throughout the cardiac cycle. It will therefore be appreciated that com-

putation of the true instantaneous mean is both complex and inaccurate and a wide range of different mathematical approaches have been used by different equipment manufacturers.

To compute the volume of blood flowing through a vessel, or to calculate the mean velocity averaged over a significant time interval, it is necessary to calculate the time-averaged mean velocity (Fig. 6.35).[46] Numerically this is simply the mean of a series of instantaneous mean velocities, usually averaged over one or more cardiac cycles. The accuracy of the ultimate value is limited by the same factors that influence the accuracy of the individual instantaneous mean calculations.[47–49] The time-averaged mean velocity is frequently abbreviated to time-averaged velocity (TAV).

Venous waveform analysis

The time-varying waveforms of flow within veins is seldom of clinical significance. It is of course reassuring to see respiratory modulation in the iliac and femoral veins to confirm patency of the IVC and internal iliac veins but no measurements are necessary to confirm this flow pattern.

The only clinical situation in which venous waveform measurement may be of some value is in studying the hepatic veins in patients with liver disease or post-transplantation. A range of different waveform measurement schemes have

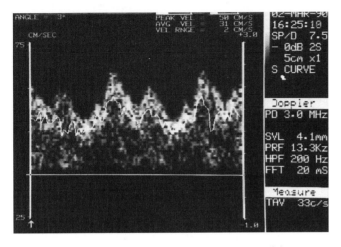

Fig. 6.35 Time-averaged mean velocity. For computation of the time-averaged mean velocity (TAV) the equipment has been set to measure the instantaneous mean velocity for every time interval throughout the trace (indicated by the thin white line) and to calculate the mean of these to give the TAV (33 cm/s).

been suggested,[50-54] all of which aim to assess the degree to which the normal pulsatility of the hepatic vein waveform is reduced and thereby possibly indicate the severity of any liver abnormality that might be present.

Colour flow imaging

Colour flow imaging (CFI) is a rapid and easy to use technique for the detection of flow within the field of view and can be used for the rapid confirmation of vascular patency, for the assessment of the direction of flow and to identify areas of flow disturbance. The precise hues allocated to the colour Doppler overlay are under the user's control and have not yet been standardised, so that it is not possible to draw specific conclusions from the hues seen in the colour display and real velocity information cannot, therefore, be gauged from visual inspection of the display. However, the colour display is a useful 'road map' for identifying specific areas of interest and for guiding placement of the range gate for conventional spectral Doppler analysis to measure the various indices discussed above.

Equipment requirements and selection

The characteristics of the equipment for performing Doppler examinations at different clinical sites vary and can conveniently be divided into four groups: peripheral, deep (abdominal), trans-vaginal and cardiac. Cardiac Doppler requires high PRF, frame rate and high pass filter values. This makes it inappropriate for use outside cardiology and it will not be discussed further.

Peripheral

The majority of vascular surgeons use simple continuous wave (CW) pencil probe systems for assessing the patency of the palpable peripheral arteries (see Vol. 2, Ch. 40) and, with training, simple subjective analysis of the audio signal enables the operator to determine whether a vessel segment is healthy or not. These systems are simple and inexpensive and can be linked to a spectrum analyser to derive the conventional waveform indices. In skilled hands the combination of clinical assessment and CW pencil probe evaluation can predict or exclude clinically significant vascular disease with a high degree of accuracy.

The role of pulsed Doppler and CFI is in the detailed evaluation of the major vessels, particularly the extracranial carotid, iliac, femoral and popliteal arteries (see Vol. 2, Chs 40 and 41). The combination of spectral and colour Doppler probably permits the detection of minor yet haemodynamically significant lesions, and is essential for differentiating between the signals arising from adjacent vessels, e.g. internal from external carotid, or superficial from deep femoral arteries, the signals from which are mixed in the CW Doppler output.

The frequency of the imaging component of a duplex system is determined by the depth of the vessel under investigation, but generally a 7.5 MHz transducer is appropriate.

The frequency of the pulses used to acquire the Doppler information from deep vessels is ideally less than that used for imaging, and is typically between 2 and 3 MHz. Attempts to use a higher frequency generally lead to significant loss in sensitivity and difficulty in acquiring an adequate trace. Equipment for peripheral vascular imaging and Doppler should therefore have the facility for using different frequencies for the imaging and the Doppler pulses.

Unfortunately the carotid and femoral vessels generally run roughly parallel to the skin surface and there may therefore be difficulty in positioning the transducer to give an adequate beam/vessel angle. This problem can to some extent be overcome by using a steerable Doppler beam. Most modern array transducers permit beam steering through an angle of at least 20° (Fig. 6.36); this, together with minor degrees of probe angulation, generally permits a beam/vessel angle of 60° or less to be achieved.

An additional important factor is the range of Doppler shift frequencies the equipment is capable of detecting and displaying. For arterial studies on pathological vessels accurate representation of frequencies above 8 kHz may be necessary to document stenoses adequately, whereas for venous studies in the lower limb frequencies below 50 Hz should be detectable in order to demonstrate spontaneous venous flow.

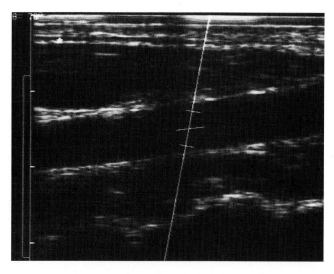

Fig. 6.36 Beam steering. The angle at which the ultrasound beam leaves a straight linear array transducer can be varied by about 20° in most modern machines. This function can be used to improve the beam/vessel angle and is particularly useful when the vessel under investigation lies approximately parallel to the skin surface.

Abdominal and obstetric applications (deep Doppler)

With the exception of fetal heart detection, continuous wave Doppler has no application in abdominal and obstetric applications. Duplex imaging with Doppler and colour flow imaging are essential prerequisites for these deeper investigations. The imaging frequency is determined by the depth of penetration required but is generally from 3.5 to 5 MHz. A transmitted Doppler frequency of 2 MHz is appropriate for the majority of deep investigations, although 3 MHz may be appropriate for more superficial structures, for example in paediatrics and in transplanted kidneys.

Deep Doppler investigations are also compromised by the relationship between pulse repetition frequency and maximum detectable Doppler shift frequency. For imaging deep structures the pulse repetition frequency must be limited to 5 kHz to avoid overlap between consecutive pulses and, because of the way the Doppler information is detected, this prevents the correct identification of Doppler frequencies greater than 2.5 kHz (see aliasing). Although this is not a problem for venous studies, many deep arteries may give rise to Doppler shifts of higher frequency, particularly if the beam/vessel angle is small. There is inevitably a compromise between depth penetration and maximum detectable Doppler frequency, and it is helpful if the equipment has the facility for the operator to directly control the pulse repetition frequency during Doppler investigations.

An alternative approach is to reduce the transmitted ultrasound frequency. Because the Doppler shift frequency is directly proportional to the transmitted frequency this results in a reduction in the Doppler shift frequency and allows a higher PRF to be maintained. Many modern ultrasound scanners allow the operator a choice of several different transmitter frequencies on each transducer.

The range of Doppler frequencies that can be detected and displayed on the spectral analysis must be adequate to cover both portal venous and arterial investigations, though the upper frequency requirement is lower than that required for peripheral vascular work.

Trans-vaginal Doppler

Duplex and/or colour flow imaging are essential for the detection and correct identification of targets from which Doppler spectra are to be obtained.

As with other applications, the imaging frequency is limited by the depth of penetration required and is typically 5–7.5 MHz with a Doppler frequency of 3–5 MHz.

The detectable velocity range need not be as wide as for other applications, as extremely low venous flows and high-velocity arterial flows are unlikely to be encountered in early pregnancy or in gynaecological investigations.

Artefacts, errors and pitfalls

Beam/vessel angle

Problems associated with the angle between the ultrasound beam and the axis of flow within the vessel are probably the commonest source of difficulties and errors with Doppler investigations.[55] If the beam/vessel angle is significantly greater than 60° there is a marked reduction in the Doppler shift frequency and significant uncertainties arise concerning the accuracy of any derived velocity values. As the beam/vessel angle approaches 90° it is unlikely that any useful Doppler trace will be obtained. However, there is occasionally sufficient radial flow during the pulsatile expansion of the vessel in systole for a bidirectional Doppler signal to be detected. The outline of the waveform is obviously arterial in nature but this is valueless for assessing the flow characteristics in the vessel or for measurement of any of the waveform indices.

Aliasing

The phenomenon of aliasing arises from the relationship between the maximum detectable Doppler shift frequency and the pulse repetition frequency (PRF) of the interrogating ultrasound beam. In pulsed Doppler ultrasound, the Doppler shift frequency is compiled from measurements taken from a large number of rapid sequential pulses. As the Doppler shift frequency approaches the PRF there are insufficient samples to enable the waveform to be determined accurately (Fig. 6.37). Any Doppler shift frequency

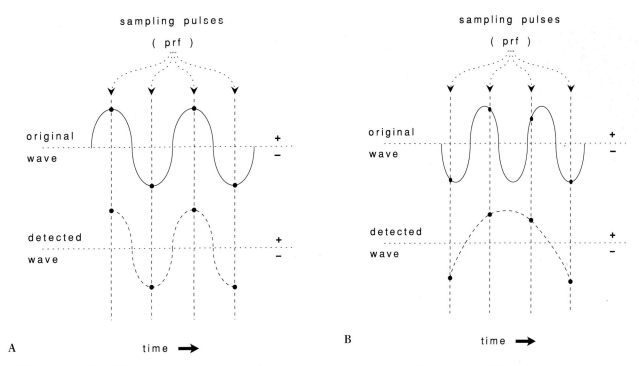

Fig. 6.37 Aliasing. A: The original ultrasound wave is sampled by pulses emitted at the pulse repetition frequency (PRF). In this example the wave is sampled at both the peak positive and peak negative points and the detected wave is an accurate representation of the original wave. **B:** If the frequency of the original wave increases but the PRF remains unchanged the frequency of sampling of the original wave is insufficient for the detected wave to reproduce correctly the frequency of the sampled wave. In this example the detected wave shows a gross artefactual reduction in frequency.

greater than half the PRF is underestimated and interpreted by the equipment as flow in the opposite direction. This situation most commonly occurs where the maximum systolic frequencies fall above the aliasing limit and the peak systolic component of the waveform appears on the wrong side of the baseline (Fig. 6.38A). Provided that the baseline has not been shifted from the middle of the display range the artefact will not be overlooked. However, when studying arteries with high-velocity flow it is often necessary to move the baseline downwards to give a larger area for display of the forward flow component. This may result in the aliased peak information not being displayed in the image and the artefact may therefore go unrecognised (Fig. 6.38B). If any index measurements are taken from the waveform it is essential to be absolutely certain that the peak systolic information is correctly detected and displayed. A similar artefact may occur if the peak systolic frequencies fall above those that can be displayed in the selected frequency range of the equipment.

There are a number of steps that can be taken to attempt to overcome aliasing. First, if the equipment permits it, the PRF may be increased. As this is done, range ambiguities may arise by virtue of the fact that echoes may still be received from one pulse after the subsequent pulse has been transmitted. These echoes will then be misrepresented as appearing from superficial structures. Equipment that permits the operator to increase the PRF

to this level usually includes some indication on the screen to show the sites at which range ambiguities may appear (Fig. 6.39).

If the PRF cannot be raised sufficiently there are a number of alternative approaches and these can be deduced from the Doppler formula. Given that the velocity of ultrasound and the blood flow velocity cannot be changed, the only way in which the Doppler shift frequency can be reduced is for the ultrasound frequency or the value of cosine θ to be reduced. The former can be achieved by using a lower Doppler transmission frequency; the latter may be achieved by increasing the beam/vessel angle and thereby decreasing the effect of cosine θ.

Sample volume size and position

Doppler measurements assume that the vessel is uniformly insonated (p. 88) (see Fig. 6.15) and that the range gate encompasses the whole of its cross-section. In clinical practice these assumptions are seldom true, with the result that the flow is usually undersampled,[43] although occasionally sampling of structures outside the vessel may occur.

Undersampling of the vessel cross-section occurs if the range gate is less than the vessel diameter and is likely to occur if the ultrasound beam width is significantly less

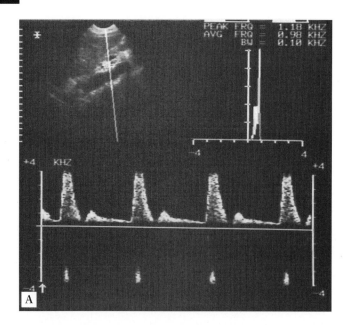

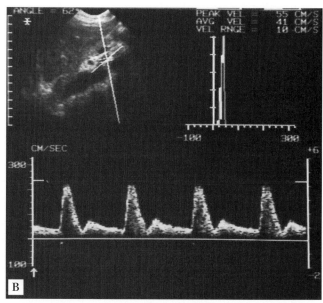

Fig. 6.38 Aliasing. A: The equipment examining this coeliac axis has a PRF of 8.5 kHz. The peak velocity detected exceeds 4.25 kHz and that component above this value is incorrectly displayed in the negative flow channel. **B:** This artefact may be overlooked if the display baseline is shifted downwards, such that the aliased peaks no longer appear in the display. Any waveform indices measured from this display will be incorrect. This problem is overcome in some scanners by repositioning the aliased peak on top of the systolic complex.

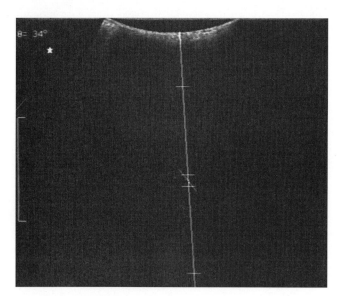

Fig. 6.39 High PRF range ambiguities. In this example the operator has chosen to increase the PRF to 15 kHz. This does not allow sufficient time between pulses for all the echoes from the deepest part of the image to be received before the next pulse is transmitted. Range ambiguities therefore occur and are displayed as additional single lines crossing the Doppler line of sight. Vessels at either of these sites would give rise to a Doppler signal that would be mixed with that from any vessel from within the actual range gate (see Fig. 6.52).

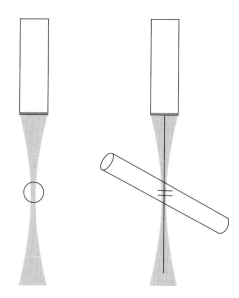

Fig. 6.40 Undersampling. The blood flow within a vessel may be inadvertently undersampled if the vessel diameter is significantly greater than the ultrasound beam width, or if the range gate is narrower than the vessel diameter. Both of these situations lead to an overestimation of mean velocity.

than the vessel width (Fig. 6.40).[56] In array transducers the width of the beam in the scanned plane is variable, and if a large-diameter vessel is being studied it may be prefer-

able to defocus the beam in order to minimise undersampling. Unfortunately, most modern phased array scanners automatically focus the beam at the depth of the range gate position and do not permit the operator to undertake intentional defocusing.

A further and more complex cause of undersampling is vessel movement during the Doppler acquisition process. This is most likely to be a source of difficulty with vessels that undergo significant degrees of translocation during cardiac pulsations, for example the superior mesenteric artery and the umbilical arteries. If the translocatory movements cause the vessel to move in and out of the range gate throughout the cardiac cycle, there may be regular and reproducible loss of Doppler information during a specific phase of the cycle. If this occurs during systole a significant loss in signal strength is noted (Fig. 6.41A), whereas if it occurs during diastole artefactual reduction in diastolic flow is produced, with potentially dangerous clinical consequences (Figs 6.41B and C). This artefact is difficult to identify when the umbilical artery is being studied, and it is therefore advisable to undertake all umbilical artery studies with a range gate that is intentionally longer than the vessel diameter, and to repeat the examination several times, preferably from different segments of the umbilical cord.

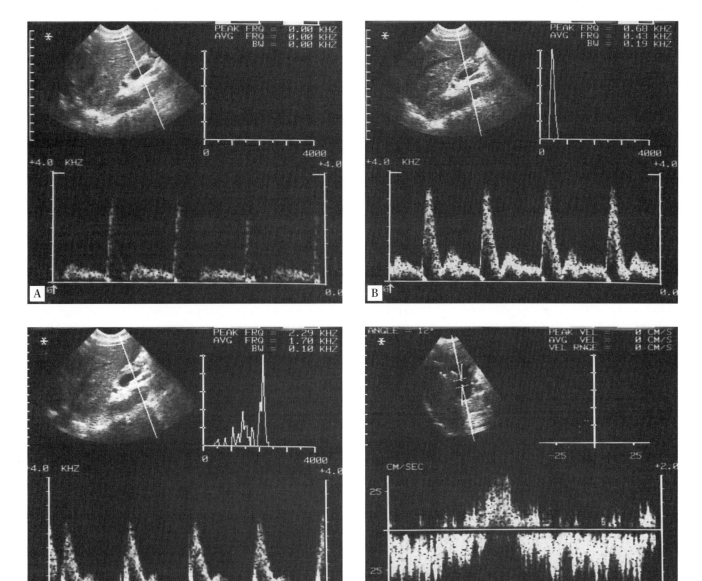

Fig. 6.41 Intermittent undersampling due to vessel movement. A: The range gate has been placed too far posteriorly and the artery is moving out of the sample volume during systole. B: Normal superior mesenteric artery trace. C: The range gate is too proximal, with the artery only entering the sample volume during systole. D: Respiratory movement in a dilated portal vein in which there is a coarse vortex. The flow direction changes from forward to reverse as the vortex moves in and out of the sample volume.

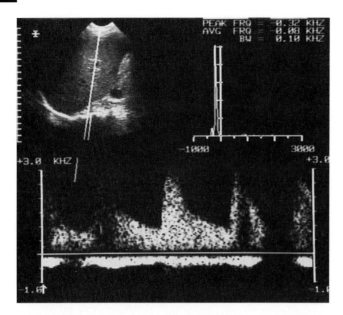

Fig. 6.42 **Oversampling due to large range gate.** A large range gate with consequent oversampling has been employed to advantage in this case with possible portal vein thrombosis to confirm the presence of a low-velocity reversed-flow portal venous signal alongside the intrahepatic arterial branches.

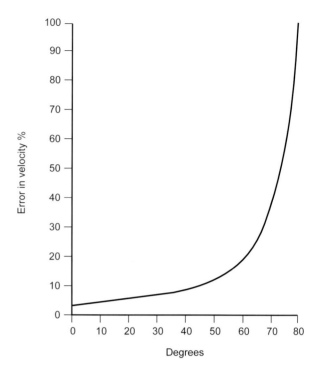

Fig. 6.43 **Change in velocity calculation error with beam/vessel angle.** This graph shows the percentage velocity error that occurs for a 5° error in beam/vessel angle measurement. For angles below 50° the error is insignificant, but there is a very rapid increase for angles greater than 60°.

If a small range gate is placed within a large vein that contains a coarse vortex and the vein moves during respiration, a confusing spectral trace may result (Fig. 6.41D).

If the range gate or beam width is significantly greater than the vessel diameter it is unlikely that problems will arise unless an additional vessel or branch falls within the sample volume. This situation seldom leads to clinical confusion, though in theory it might be possible for a segment of the umbilical vein to pass in and out of the beam width and give a false impression of transitory diastolic flow reversal. More often oversampling gives rise to helpful information, such as simultaneous detection of the renal artery and renal vein at the hilum, confirming the correct location of the range gate when difficulty is experienced in detecting flow in one or other vessel, particularly in suspected renal vein thrombosis. Within the liver, detection of the hepatic artery signal can be used to confirm correct placement of the range gate in the region of the portal vein (Fig. 6.42). If no adjacent venous signal can be detected there is greater confidence in the diagnosis of absence of portal flow.

Velocity calculation

There is an increasing number of clinical applications of Doppler ultrasound in which calculation of one or more aspects of blood velocity is useful. The derived values always depend upon knowledge of the beam/vessel angle and are subject to numerous errors and uncertainties. The degree of error introduced by beam/vessel angle measure-

ment is highly dependent upon the absolute value of the beam/vessel angle.[48] If this is less than 45° a 5° error in measurement gives rise to a velocity error of less than 10% (Fig. 6.43). However, for angles greater than 45° there is a very rapid increase in the error introduced by a 5° uncertainty, such that at 70° the error is 35% and at 80° 100%. This point again emphasises the importance of keeping the beam/vessel angle as small as possible.

In some scanners the spectral display is calibrated in velocity rather than frequency shift, even when no beam/vessel angle information has been entered. These displays assume a beam/vessel angle of 0°; unless a true beam/vessel angle has been indicated the velocity information is totally meaningless, and users of such equipment must be aware of this inadequacy.

The mean peak value (as used for the pulsatility index calculation) should ideally be traced automatically from the waveform outline (see Fig. 6.31).[35] However, the operator must undertake this manually if the machine does not incorporate automatic waveform tracing, or if the automatic tracing fails because of a noisy or interrupted waveform. Minor degrees of error may be introduced by manual tracing, particularly if the waveform is complex in shape. Both the manual and the automatic techniques may also be subject to error if the waveform is inadequate, usually owing to insufficient sensitivity or gain (Fig. 6.44).

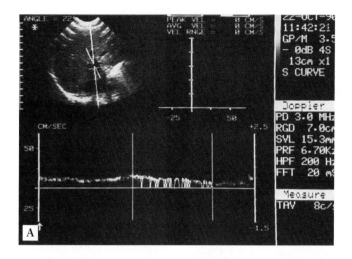

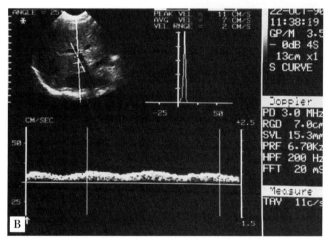
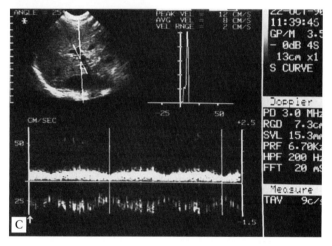

Fig. 6.44 Velocity errors due to incorrect gain settings. A: With the gain too low there are drop-outs in the TAV measurement, giving an inappropriately low value (8 cm/s). B: With correct gain setting a true value of 11 cm/s is obtained. C: With the gain too high there is signal breakthrough into the reverse flow channel, with a resultant apparent decrease in the mean velocity value (9 cm/s) (see also Fig. 6.48).

Measurement of the instantaneous mean velocity and time-averaged mean velocity is influenced by two major factors. The calculation of mean velocity has to make allowance for the different number of scatterers travelling at the different velocities present within the sampled volume. There is no precise way of doing this and different assumptions are made by different equipment manufacturers. Some merely take the mean peak value and multiply this by a constant, usually 0.6–0.7, assuming a standard velocity profile throughout the cardiac cycle in all vessels. Clearly this assumption is invalid. An alternative and common approach is to assess the mode velocity (the most commonly occurring value during any time interval) or to determine the highest frequency detectable with a power level at a predetermined number of decibels less than that of the peak value. Typically this latter measurement may be taken at levels of –3, –6, –9 or –12 dB from the peak value and each of these of course gives rise to a different mean value. There is as yet no uniform agree-

ment concerning the ideal way of calculating the true mean velocity and the results vary by at least 50%. It is therefore essential that in any unit where velocity values are to be used clinically the range of normals must be established using the equipment available in that institution.

Blood flow velocity calculations always assume that the blood is flowing along the long axis of the vessel at the site of measurement but this only applies in the central axis of straight, non-branching vessels. In many clinical situations it may be difficult or impossible to obtain an ideally suited segment of vessel for study, and the consequent distortion of the velocity profile in a suboptimal vessel segment may lead to significant velocity errors. This is particularly marked in the situation illustrated in Figure 6.8B, in which the axis of flow in the left portal vein branch is clearly at approximately 45° to the long axis of the vessel owing to the presence of a coarse vortex within the vessel arising from the bifurcation of the left and right portal veins. It is quite possible for velocity profile distortions and non-axial flow to introduce velocity errors of a further 50%.

An additional significant factor influencing the derived velocity values relates to the relationship between the vessel size and the sample volume size, as discussed above. If the vessel is significantly undersampled this may give rise to loss of low-velocity peripheral flow and a consequent overestimate of the mean velocity, whereas partial or complete movement of the vessel out of the range gate during the sampling period gives rise to loss of information causing a reduction in computed mean velocity.

Volume flow calculation

Volume blood flow is calculated by multiplying the time-averaged mean velocity by the vessel cross-sectional area. The velocity calculation may have an error of at least 50% (see p. 104) and a further major error may be introduced by incorrect assessment of the vessel cross-sectional area.[48,49] In arterial studies the vessel area is usually computed from a one-dimensional diameter measurement and any error in this is squared during the calculation process. In addition, the arterial diameter normally varies by ± 10% through the cardiac cycle, and unless this is taken into account and a mean value obtained, a further potential error of 20% can arise. The vessel diameter must not be measured from a colour Doppler image as the resolution in colour mode is inferior to that in grey scale imaging and the spread of the colour overlays leads to an overestimate of several millimetres.

For veins, computation of the cross-sectional area from a single diameter measurement is not appropriate as very few veins are circular in cross-section. It is therefore essential to measure the cross-sectional area of a vessel directly. However, this must be done on an image at right-angles to the vessel axis in order to prevent geometrical distortion: this is precisely the position in which Doppler information is inadequate, and the Doppler signal must be obtained from a separate study with an appropriate beam/vessel angle. There is therefore often considerable doubt as to whether or not the cross-sectional area and the Doppler information were obtained from the same site. This is especially important where a tributary joins between the sites of the two measurements and in vessels with an irregular cross-sectional area, such as the portal vein.

Waveform analysis

Calculation of the resistance index (RI) depends on measurements of both peak systole and end diastole. Although diastolic flow does decrease with increasing peripheral vascular resistance, the apparent value of the end-diastolic flow is significantly altered by heart rate alone. At fast heart rates the onset of systole encroaches upon diastole, resulting in an apparent rise in the end diastolic value, and

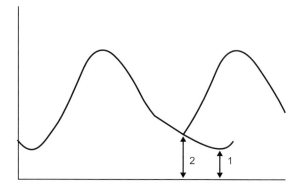

Fig. 6.45 Change in resistance index with heart rate. Measurement of the resistance index depends upon measurement of end diastole. When the heart rate is slow end diastole is late (1) and low. If the heart rate increases, end diastole apparently occurs earlier (2), giving a higher value and corrupting the RI calculation. The effect on PI would be much less.

vice versa (Fig. 6.45). It is theoretically possible to compensate for this by extrapolating the diastolic flow deceleration and normalising the cardiac period to a standardised value. In practice, however, this form of normalisation is almost never undertaken. The significance of the heart rate on RI values must not be overlooked. For example, changes in the RI in the fetal circulation have been attributed to 'circulatory maturation' but are probably a reflection of the changes in heart rate through gestation.

Computation of the pulsatility index (PI) is subject to the same uncertainties if there is continuous forward flow and the diastolic value used in the formula is end diastole. Difficulties in measuring the mean peak value have been discussed (see p. 98) and one piece of equipment has been marketed in which the mean value used in the PI calculation was, in fact, the time-averaged mean and not the mean peak value. Once again it is important to be aware of the way in which the equipment in use calculates the various indices and ideally to establish one's own normal range wherever possible.

A further source of corruption of the RI and PI values is distortion of the waveform due to vessel movement with respect to the sample volume throughout the cardiac cycle. This may lead to significant error in index calculation (see Fig. 6.41).

Finally, when using the waveform indices as diagnostic tools it is essential to remember that the actual waveform is not only determined by the state of the distal vascular tree, but is influenced by a wide range of upstream, local and downstream factors, including cardiac function, aortic valve function, the state of the arterial tree, upstream and downstream stenoses and blocks, and the presence and efficacy of collateral circulations. Changes in any one of these variables may have a significant effect upon the numerical indices, although the source of this effect may not be evident from the Doppler trace alone. Cases of unsuspected right heart disease have been diagnosed by identification of abnormal central venous waveforms, and patent ductus arteriosus has been detected by noting diastolic flow reversal in the renal arteries while undertaking investigations to exclude renal vein thrombosis in neonates.

Spectral information

The range of frequencies present within the Doppler spectrum may be adversely affected by a number of factors, including under and oversampling as discussed above. Undersampling most commonly results from the use of too small a range gate, with consequent loss of low-frequency information, but eccentric placement of a small range gate may also lead to underestimation of the higher velocities present in the centre of the vessel.

An additional artefact that may compromise the quality of the spectral trace is produced by the low-frequency but high-amplitude Doppler signal arising from the pulsating arterial wall. Although the velocity of movement of the wall is low, it is an extremely efficient ultrasound reflector and therefore gives rise to a very low-frequency high-amplitude signal. This appears in the Doppler trace as 'wall thump' (Fig. 6.46A) and its presence corrupts measurements of the peak or mean frequencies. As the wall thump signal is of very low frequency it can be selectively removed by a wall thump filter or 'high pass filter'. This allows the user selectively to reject the low-frequency components of the Doppler signal. For arterial studies it may be necessary to increase the high pass filter to a value of 600 or even 800 Hz, in order to eliminate the wall thump (Fig. 6.46B). However, the filter also removes true low-frequency Doppler shifts and, when such a high filter

frequency is applied, velocity calculations taken from the spectrum show an artefactual apparent increase in velocity. This is seldom of such magnitude to be important in arterial imaging but, if venous studies are performed with a wall filter set at a high value, much of the flow information may be lost, or the presence of flow may even be overlooked.

In addition to the Doppler signal arising from arterial walls, any rapidly moving tissue gives rise to a Doppler shift. This is particularly noticeable with colour flow imaging, when it may be annoying but seldom leads to diagnostic error. When using spectral Doppler, however, errors may easily occur if the operator is unaware of the possible origin of the Doppler trace (Fig. 6.47).

Mirror image artefacts

The mirror image artefact in spectral analysis is seen as a spurious flow signal on the wrong side of the baseline (Fig. 6.48). There are many causes for this effect, the commonest of which is probably related to inadequacies in the scanner's electronics; it is particularly prevalent with multi-element transducers. A similar artefact can be produced if the Doppler gain is too high (Fig. 6.44C) or if the beam/vessel angle is too large. In this case the artefact may be due to radial flow during the systolic expansion of the vessel. An alternative cause in certain circumstances may be the presence of a branch vessel or separate vessel included in the range gate but carrying blood in the opposite direction, in which case the spectrum truly indicates the real flow situation. Care must be taken to differentiate this appearance from that produced from true disturbance with flow reversal, either physiological or due to vessel disease.

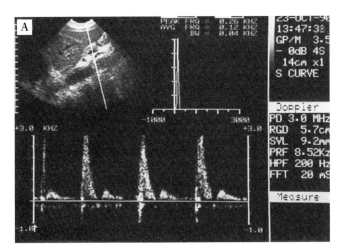
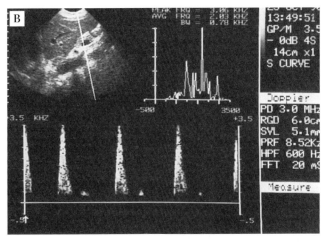

Fig. 6.46 Wall thump. A: The low-velocity excursions of arterial walls give rise to a high-amplitude low-velocity signal, seen in this example as a strong positive and negative peak overlying the beginning of systole. **B:** Increasing the high pass filter (HPF) from 200 to 600 Hz has eliminated the wall thump but also leads to loss of most of the true diastolic flow.

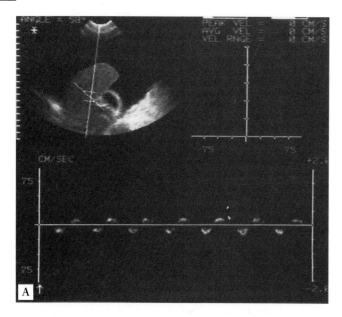

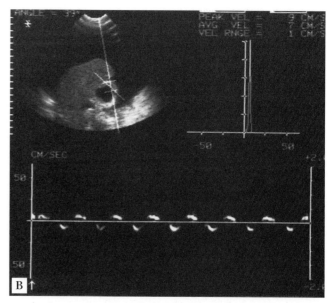

Fig. 6.47 Tissue movement. A: The Doppler trace from the portal vein in this patient with liver disease and ascites shows apparent oscillating flow. **B:** The range gate has been repositioned over the gallbladder wall and gives an identical trace. The Doppler signal is due to tissue movement induced by cardiac contractions, and not to blood flow at all.

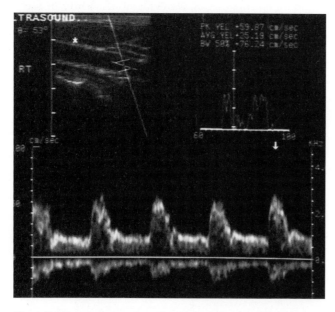

Fig. 6.48 Mirror image artefact. Flow in this common carotid artery is towards the probe and gives rise to the spectral analysis signal above the baseline. The similar low-amplitude waveform below the baseline is a mirror image artefact. The cause is uncertain, but in this case it could be due to simultaneous detection of flow within the superior thyroid artery if the sample volume is greater than that indicated by the range gates (see also Fig. 6.44C).

Colour flow imaging

Colour flow Doppler is subject to the same limitations and artefacts as conventional pulsed Doppler. However, the problem of aliasing is more likely to occur because, in order to prevent range artefacts in the image, the PRF is determined in the normal way by the time necessary to allow all pulses to return from the deepest tissues to be imaged. However, in the majority of colour flow systems some of these pulses are used to produce the conventional grey scale information and the remainder are used for the colour flow Doppler. The effective PRF of the Doppler pulses is thus markedly lower than the imaging PRF and the aliasing limit is therefore lower. As a result even moderate flow velocities present in normal arteries during systole often give rise to aliasing. In the colour flow display this appears as a reversal of the flow colour such that part or all of a vessel may show transient colour reversal during the cardiac cycle. The presence of aliasing can often be inferred from the mosaic mixture of colours in an image (Fig. 6.49). However, there are occasions when the aliased segment of the image gives an appearance almost indistinguishable from true flow reversal (Fig. 6.50). In this situation it can be seen that the colour flips directly from red to blue without passing through black and this provides a clue to the artefactual nature of the appearance. If there is true flow reversal there is almost always a point in the image where the flow passes through a right-angle to the beam as it changes from flow towards the probe to flow away from the probe. At this point there is a brief instant during which no Doppler signal is obtained and this produces a small black gap between the true forward and true reverse flow pixels (Fig. 6.51).

If the operator increases the PRF to the point where range ambiguities occur, the true areas of colour flow

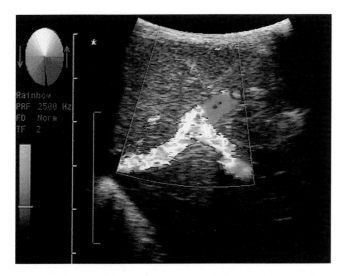

Fig. 6.49 Mosaic artefact due to aliasing. The flow velocity in this patent ductus venosus exceeds the aliasing limit, giving rise to the mosaic artefact. Normal velocity flow within the left branch of the portal vein gives rise to a correctly coded blue signal.

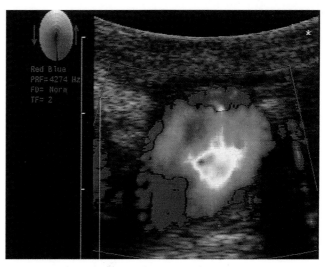

Fig. 6.50 Apparent flow reversal due to aliasing. In this transverse scan of a large vein in which there is parabolic flow the flow velocity in the centre of the vessel exceeds the aliasing limit. The coding passes from blue through white to red without a break, indicating that this is aliasing.

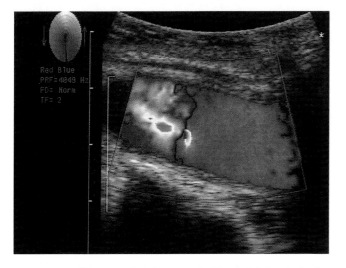

Fig. 6.51 True flow reversal. Same case as in Figure 6.50, longitudinal scan. There is a small area of aliasing within the red flow segment. The radial orientation of the imaging pulses arising from this curvilinear array gives rise to flow effectively towards the transducer in the red segment of the vessel and away from the transducer in the blue segment. At the point where the flow is at right-angles to the beam there is a small black gap between the red and blue segments, confirming true flow reversal at this point.

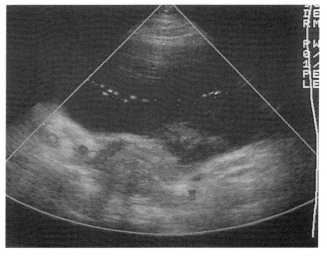

Fig. 6.52 Colour range artefact. Imaging of these deep vessels within the pelvis required a low PRF. In order to overcome aliasing the PRF has been increased, and has resulted in range ambiguities giving rise to artefactual colour signals within the bladder.

may be duplicated at inappropriate sites within the image (Fig. 6.52).

On many colour flow machines the PRF is controlled indirectly by setting the velocity scale. If high-velocity flow is imaged with a low-velocity scale setting, aliasing results (Fig. 6.53A). When this is corrected by choosing a more appropriate velocity scale the aliasing disappears (Fig. 6.53B).

A further and very important artefact in colour flow images results from the relatively poor spatial resolution compared with grey scale imaging. The colour picture elements are fewer and larger than the grey scale imaging elements and the Doppler pulses are often intentionally made longer than imaging pulses to improve the accuracy of frequency measurement. These two factors combine to degrade significantly both the axial and the azimuthal

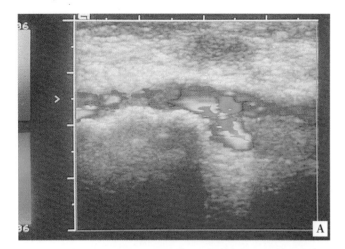
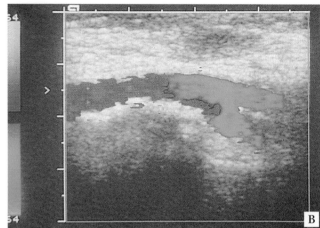

Fig. 6.53 Aliasing and its correction. A: The axillary artery has been examined with an inappropriate velocity range and consequent low PRF. The colour flow image is corrupted by aliasing. **B:** The velocity range, and hence the PRF, has been markedly increased to overcome the aliasing. Note the apparent change in flow direction similar to that seen in Figure 6.51, in this case due to a curved vessel imaged with a straight linear array.

resolution of the colour image. When large vessels are being displayed this is of little importance but with small vessels (a few millimetres in diameter) there is almost always an overestimate of their diameter. This is likely to be of the order of at least 1 mm and for very small vessels may lead to an apparent overestimate approaching 100%! The colour image must therefore never be used for vessel diameter measurements. In addition, many machines permit the colour image to be integrated over a variable period of several seconds. This enhances the resulting 'road map' appearance and may produce attractive colour images but the integrated vessel pulsations lead to yet further artefactual increase in the apparent vessel diameters.

Beam/vessel artefact

The colour coding of blood flow in CDI is determined by the direction of flow 'with respect to the transducer'. If a long vessel segment is examined with a sector scanner, or a curved vessel is examined with a linear array, flow in part of the vessel may be towards the transducer but away from the transducer in another segment. There is thus a sudden reversal in colour coding at the point where the flow is at right-angles to the beam (Fig. 6.53B).

Colour mirror image artefact

In anatomical situations where there is a strong specular reflector in the image (such as the diaphragm or bladder wall) a mirror image artefact may occur, similar to that seen in conventional 2D imaging (see p. 107). This is commonly observed during CDI of the subclavian artery as it crosses the apex of the lung (Fig. 6.54).

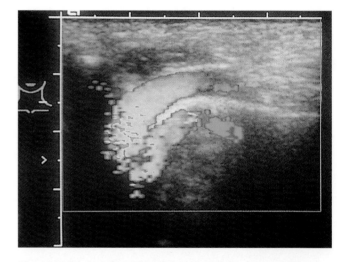

Fig. 6.54 Mirror artefact. The subclavian artery has been imaged as it curves over the apex of the lung. The lung surface acts as a specular reflector and gives rise to a mirror image artefact, with an apparent duplicate vessel lying beneath the lung surface.

Frame rate artefact

The frame rate of CDI may be very low, especially when using a large region of interest or examining deep vessels (see p. 109). If a long vessel segment is being examined it is quite possible for information to be collected from one end of it during systole and from the other end during diastole. This may lead to very confusing and rapidly changing colour hues in the image. This artefact can be simulated by rapid backwards and forwards longitudinal movement of the transducer during scanning (Fig. 6.55).

53 Kardoff R, Klotz M, Melter M et al. Pathological portal and hepatic vein flow patterns – clinical significance in chronic liver diseases of childhood. Eur J Ultrasound 1996; 4: S82

54 Bolondi L, Li Bassi S, Gaiani S et al. Liver cirrhosis: changes of Doppler waveform of hepatic veins. Radiology 1991; 178: 13–16

55 Johnston K W, Maruzzo B C, Cobbold R S C. Errors and artifacts of Doppler flowmeters and their solutions. Arch Surg 1977; 112: 1335–1341

56 Powalowski T, Borodzinski K, Nowicki A. Effect of ultrasonic beam width on blood flow estimation by means of C W Doppler flowmeter. Scripta Medica Univ Brno 1975; 48: 97–103

57 Duck F A, Starritt H C, Anderson S P. A survey of the acoustic output of ultrasonic Doppler equipment. Clin Phys Physiol Meas 1987; 8: 39–49

58 Duck F A. Output data from European studies. Proceedings of the second WFUMB symposium on safety and standardisation in medical ultrasound. Ultrasound Med Biol 1989; 15 (Suppl 1): 61–64

Interventional techniques

*David O Cosgrove,
Hans Henrik Holm,
Jan Fog Pedersen,
Søren Torp-Pedersen,
Steen Karstrup,
Christian Nolsøe and
Anders Glenthøj*

Introduction

Ultrasound-guided interventions are widely used, both as scheduled procedures and as *ad hoc* extensions of the ultrasound examination. Such procedures are therefore discussed in other chapters as appropriate; this chapter focuses on the general principles.[1-3]

Three levels of use of ultrasound for biopsy work may be identified. At the simplest level, suitable only for large or palpable lesions, the scan is used merely to plan the procedure, marking a suitable skin puncture site that avoids penetrating hazardous regions such as major blood vessels and indicates the approximate depth to which the needle needs to penetrate. A common example is in the drainage of a pleural effusion; similarly, in ascites there is usually no need to involve the ultrasound scanner beyond the planning stage, but the importance of avoiding bowel loops adherent to the parietal peritoneum makes a preliminary scan useful.

At the second level the scanner is used not only to plan the procedure but also to monitor the position of the needle in real time throughout. The transducer is simply positioned close to the puncture site so that the needle passes within the scan plane. This is known as the freehand technique, but may be called the 'three hand technique' because it is expedited by having an assistant hold the transducer while the operator uses both hands on the syringe. It is suitable for relatively simple procedures with lesions larger than 1–2 cm not too deeply located, and has the advantage that no special transducer is required. However, the requisite hand–eye coordination makes it a skill-dependent method and not all operators find it easy to learn. Typical situations where freehand guidance is sufficient are in the needling of breast and thyroid masses.

The most precise method, using some form of needle guide, forms the main subject of this chapter.

General principles

In 1969 Kratochwil described a hand-held puncture transducer with a central canal for percutaneous needle insertion under A-scan guided control.[4] A few months later needle puncture guided by B-scanning was introduced in our laboratory using an off-axis puncture transducer mounted on the articulated arm of a static scanner (Fig. 7.1).[5,6] Almost simultaneously, Goldberg and Pollack began performing cyst puncture using A-scan guidance.[7] In 1974 the first dynamic biopsy transducer, a 'homemade' linear array transducer with a needle steering attachment at the end of the transducer, was developed in our laboratory.[8] Today, interventional ultrasound has gained widespread use and the majority of scanner manufacturers supply special transducers or attachments with needle guides.

The basic principle of an ultrasound-guided biopsy is that the complex three-dimensional problem of hitting a

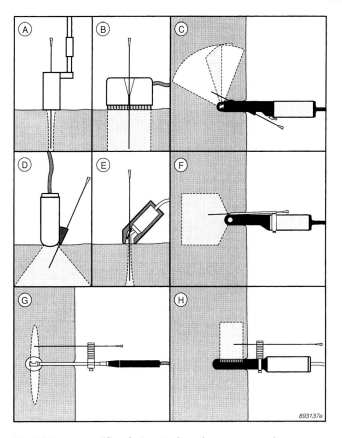

Fig. 7.1 Puncture guiding devices. Dedicated puncture transducers (A–C). Puncture attachments (D–H). **A:** Puncture transducer for static compound scanner. **B:** Linear array puncture transducer which allows perpendicular and oblique needle insertion. **C:** Trans-rectal multiplanar scanner with oblique built-in puncture canal for prostate biopsies. **D:** Sector scanner with needle-steering device attached. **E:** Conventional transducer placed in a puncture adapter, in which the ultrasound field is reflected by an acoustic mirror. The needle is inserted through a puncture canal into the reflected sound field. **F:** Endoscanner with needle-steering device for trans-rectal or trans-vaginal punctures attached (longitudinal scanning). **G:** Trans-rectal scanner with needle-steering device for trans-perineal puncture (transverse scanning). **H:** Trans-rectal scanner with needle-steering device for trans-perineal puncture (longitudinal scanning).

small target is converted to a simpler two-dimensional one by using a two-dimensional imaging technique (Fig. 7.2). A steering device restricts the movement of the needle to a predetermined path in the image plane, so that if inserted when the target is visualised and transected by the electronically generated line that indicates its path, the needle will inevitably cross the target.

Transducers

There are as many puncture-guiding devices as there are transducer types, but they can be divided into two main groups: dedicated puncture transducers which are equipped with an internal canal (Fig. 7.1A to C), and

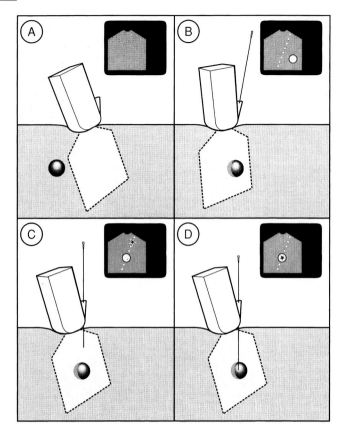

Fig. 7.2 Principle of an ultrasound-guided puncture. A: Target non-visualised, outside image plane. B: Transducer moved and target now visualised in image plane, but not transected by puncture line. C: Transducer tilted, target transected by puncture line. Needle inserted through puncture attachment. Needle-tip echo indicates actual needle position. D: Target hit.

needle attachments which are mounted on ordinary transducers (Fig 7.1D to H); the advantage of a system which enables the examiner to perform the needling with the same transducer as used for the initial scan has led to the predominance of the latter type.

Needle guide systems, which are available from most scanner manufacturers, should fulfil two requirements: the canal must be at least 3 cm long (to prevent the needle from deviating during the procedure) and the examiner must be able to release the needle easily, especially when catheter procedures are to be carried out. As needles of various sizes are used, guides of different calibres must be available, and this can be solved by equipping the attachment with linings of various calibres, e.g. from gauge 14 to gauge 23 (Fig. 7.3) (Table 7.1). Alternatively, a needle guide that can be adjusted for needles of 12–20 gauge may be used.

Endoprobes with a biopsy canal are widely used for prostate and other pelvic biopsies (Figs 7.1C and 7.4).[9] The examination usually starts with transverse scans, which are preferable for the detection of focal lesions, but

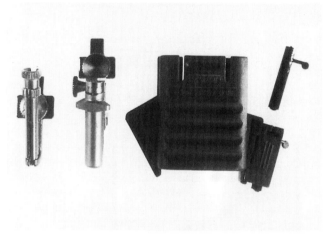

Fig. 7.3 Attachable needle-steering devices. Left: In this version, two U-shaped cylinders which can be rotated independently allow 14 and 18 gauge puncture canals to be selected; they can be opened (Bruel & Kjaer). Centre: Because of the special design the calibre of this puncture canal, which can be opened, is adjustable to any needle size between gauge 14 and gauge 23 (Bruel & Kjaer). Right: Sterile disposable puncture attachment (Acuson).

Table 7.1 Conversion from 'gauge' needle dimension and 'French' catheter dimension to metric system

Needle gauge	Diameter (mm)	Catheter 'French'	Diameter (mm)
25	0.51	5	1.67
24	0.56	6	2.0
23	0.64	7	2.3
22	0.72	8	2.7
21	0.82	9	3.0
20	0.90	10	3.3
19	1.10	11	3.7
18	1.26	12	4.0
17	1.49	13	4.3
16	1.67	14	4.7
15	1.84	15	5.0
14	2.13	16	5.3
13	2.44	17	5.7
		18	6.0
		19	6.3
		20	6.7
		22	7.3
		24	8.0

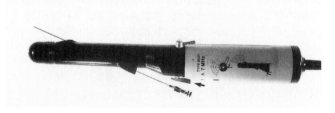

Fig. 7.4 Trans-rectal multiplane scanner with built-in oblique puncture canal (Bruel & Kjaer). The scan plane can be rotated by turning the lever (arrow).

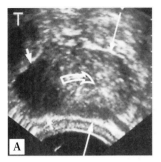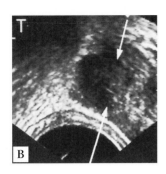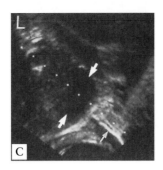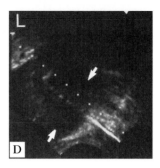

Fig. 7.5 Prostate biopsy with multiplane scanner. A: Transverse rectal scan reveals a suspicious echo-poor lesion in the prostate (short arrows). Axis of image rotation indicated by long arrows. **B:** The probe is rotated to the right until the target area is intersected by the common axis of image rotation (arrows). **C:** By turning the lever the image plane is now shifted through oblique to truly longitudinal. The probe is tilted until the target (arrows) is intersected by the puncture line, which indicates the needle path. The needle (small arrow) is inserted up to the lesion. **D:** Gun biopsy is performed; the needle track is faintly seen within the lesion.

the biopsy is guided by longitudinal scans (Fig. 7.5). Precisely located biopsies can be obtained from suspicious areas.[10] Special puncture devices for trans-perineal treatment of prostatic lesions have been developed and are described later (see Fig. 7.27).

Sterilisation

An ultrasound-guided puncture is a minor surgical procedure and sterilisation of the equipment should be in accordance with the department's normal practice.

Ultrasound transducers do not tolerate autoclaving and gas sterilisation is too time-consuming for routine use. Sterility can, however, be achieved by the use of a sterile cover. Alternatively, provided the transducer and cable junctions are watertight, it can be sterilised by immersion in various fluids, e.g. glutaraldehyde (Cidex) or 70% alcohol. Sterilisation in alcohol takes only a few seconds and is attractive from a practical point of view, but is not effective against fungi, hepatitis or immunodeficiency viruses. Glutaraldehyde is effective against a wide spectrum of bacteria, as well as fungi and viruses: 10 minutes immersion kills vegetative pathogens, including *Pseudomonas*, human immunodeficiency (HIV) and hepatitis B (HBV) viruses, but *Mycobacteria* require 1 hour's immersion. To kill resistant spores 3 hours immersion is needed. Because of the toxicity of glutaraldehyde alternatives are being sought, and superoxidised water is emerging as a promising candidate (see full report of the British Gastroenterology Group on http://www.bsg.org.uk/clinical/data/cdege3.htm). It is important that the equipment is mechanically cleansed of gel and debris before immersion.

Needles

For practical purposes of economy and operator familiarity it is advantageous to restrict the number of different types of needle used to perhaps four or five, maybe in more than one length; most of them will be disposable (Fig. 7.6). A fine needle should be used to reduce the risk of complications.[11] A stylet helps avoid contamination of the needle bore before it reaches the target.

The advancing needle tip is usually visualised clearly as a relatively strong echo, and a missing echo almost always indicates deviation of the needle from the scan plane, but the shaft is sometimes more difficult to locate. The sources of these echoes are rather complex[12] and attempts have been made to improve their visualisation. Roughening the outer surface of the needle enhances its reflectivity in laboratory studies but its clinical value is not as convincing. The contents of the needle can be made more reflective by roughening the stylet, introducing a guidewire, or by filling the needle with air or an air–gel mixture. Needles with special reflective coatings improve visualisation,[13] and an interesting development uses an effervescent coating to highlight the needle track by the presence of gas bubbles (http://www.twi.co.uk/connect/mar99/c991.html).

Almost all fluid collections, even those consisting of thick pus or debris, can be aspirated through an 18 gauge (1.2 mm) needle (Fig. 7.6A), which should contain a stylet to prevent obstruction of the lumen by blood clot or tissue during insertion. An exception to the routine use of an 18 gauge needle is amniocentesis, when a disposable 19 or 20 gauge needle is generally preferable.

Inserting a flexible fine needle through skin can be difficult and the use of an 18 gauge guide needle makes this easier. The guide needle is advanced a few centimetres and hence only one skin puncture is needed to take several samples. For cytology, 22 and 23 gauge (0.7 and 0.6 mm) needles with a non-cutting bevelled tip are commonly used (Fig. 7.6B). A 10 ml syringe, perhaps fitted with an aspiration handle, is used to apply suction. Such fine needles do not need a stylet because the amount of tissue entering the needle during insertion is negligible compared to the amount obtained during aspiration.

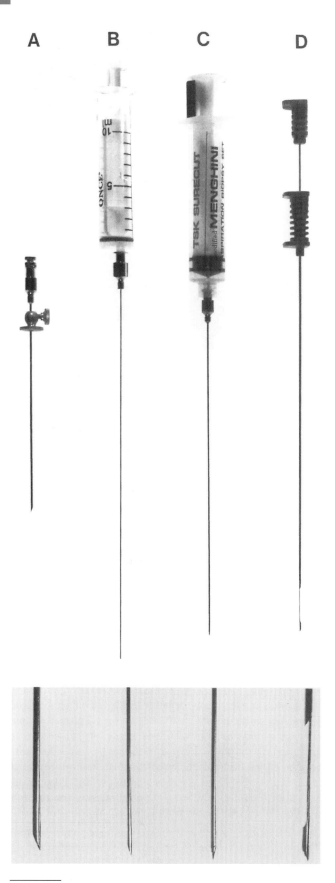

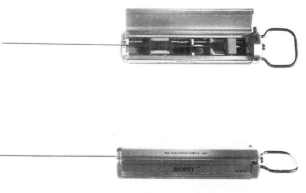

Fig. 7.6 Commonly used needles for interventional ultrasound. A: 18 gauge needle with adjustable stopscrew. Ideal for puncturing fluid collections and as a guide needle for fine needle punctures. **B:** 23 gauge fine needle without stylet mounted on 10 ml syringe for aspiration cytology. **C:** 21 gauge Surecut cutting needle with stylet. The syringe is equipped with a locking device to maintain the vacuum. **D:** Tru-cut type needle especially designed for Biopty-gun.

Cutting needles yield true tissue cores from the target tissue. Two types are commonly used: the Surecut needle (14–25 gauge) is based on the Menghini principle, in which the needle, stylet and syringe are a unit (Fig. 7.6C). The stylet is attached to the plunger of the syringe and, as the plunger is retracted, it moves up in the needle, revealing the cutting tip. A locking device retains the plunger in the retracted position to maintain the negative pressure when the needle is advanced. When the needle is removed the tissue core remains in the distal portion of the needle because of the stylet. The Surecut system can be operated with one hand, which is particularly important for ultrasound-guided biopsy. The most commonly used size for abdominal biopsies is 21 gauge (0.8 mm).

The conventional Tru-cut needle (14 gauge) has a biopsy chamber that can be opened and closed (Fig. 7.6D). After insertion to the correct depth the needle is opened by advancing its inner portion so that the surrounding tissue falls into the biopsy chamber. As the outer part of the needle is advanced with the inner part fixed, the tissue in the chamber is cut by the sharp edge of the outer needle. The closed needle can then be removed with the tissue core in the chamber.

Because conventional Tru-cut needles require two hands, they are not ideal for ultrasound-guided biopsy. Single-handed operation is achieved with an automated system such as the Biopty gun (Fig. 7.7), which uses special disposable Tru-cut type needles (Fig. 7.6D) (gauge 14–20) placed in the spring-loaded gun, which is then closed and

Fig. 7.7 Biopty-gun. Top: The specially designed Tru-cut type needle (Fig. 7.6D) is mounted in the spring loaded gun. **Bottom:** The closed gun ready for biopsy. When triggered, the spring mechanism activates the Tru-cut action and the biopsy is taken instantaneously.

primed for use. When the needle has been guided to the edge of the target, the trigger is activated to take the biopsy sample automatically and instantaneously.

Patient preparation

Fine needle biopsies (i.e. outer needle diameter < 1 mm) can be performed as an outpatient procedure, no tests, preparation or post-biopsy observations being needed. The biopsy can therefore be performed as an extension of the ultrasound study, which saves time for both the patient and the department.

If the patient's clinical condition or biochemical tests suggests a coagulation disorder, special precautions are required. These guidelines are the same as those followed when the patient is to have a large-bore needle biopsy, and are as follows:

1 procedure performed only as an inpatient,
2 INR (International Normalised Ratio) <1.5,
3 thrombocyte count above 40 000 µl (normal range 150 000–400 000),
4 at least 1 unit of blood available for transfusion.

The patient should be informed about the nature and purpose of the procedure and have given consent in advance. However, if the FNA is an integral part of the ultrasound examination consent may not have been given at the time of referral. This has the advantage that the patient is spared anxiety in anticipation. A local anaesthetic is generally used.

Cytology versus histology

Both fine needle aspiration cytology (FNAC) and fine needle aspiration biopsy (FNAB) are reliable methods and complement each other.[14,15] FNAB provides excellent structural information, important in diagnosing both benign and malignant lesions, whereas FNAC provides little structural information (Fig. 7.8). Close collaboration with the pathologist and an understanding of the problems of specimen preparation and interpretation helps optimise the diagnostic information obtainable from a biopsy.

Cytological specimens are obtained by aspiration, which should sample several regions, especially in the periphery of the lesion as central areas are often necrosed and haemorrhagic, leading to non-diagnostic specimens. If Papanicolaou staining is used immediate fixation in 95% alcohol is optimal, but a spray fixative may be used. Air drying is simpler, but in this case May–Grunwald–Giemsa staining will normally be used. Both techniques take about 30 minutes to carry out. If needed, rapid staining techniques on air-dried smears are available and may be useful to check the adequacy of the aspirate and form a preliminary diagnosis. The slides should be restained for the final diagnosis.

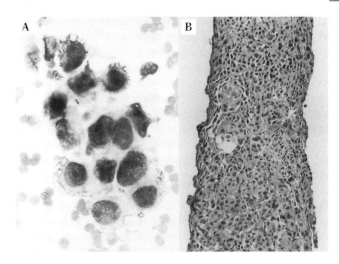

Fig. 7.8 Specimens from a retroperitoneal biopsy. **A:** Cytological fine needle aspiration showing poorly differentiated malignant cells (May–Grunwald–Giemsa stain, ×550). **B:** Histological fine needle biopsy from same lesion showing poorly differentiated carcinoma, probably an epidermoid carcinoma. (Haematoxylin–eosin stain, ×125).

Histological fine needle biopsies are handled in the same way as ordinary biopsies (fixed in formaldehyde, dehydrated, cleared, embedded in paraffin, sectioned and stained).[16] If a 0.6 mm needle is used fragmentation often occurs, and material can easily be lost during embedding; this can be obviated by placing the specimen between two pieces of gauze or on a piece of filter paper. Fragmentation is seldom a problem when the needle diameter is 0.8 mm or larger.

Special stains and immunostaining are more easily performed on FNAB specimens, as many sections can be made from one biopsy. Extra unstained sections should be set aside in case these methods are needed after evaluation of the routinely stained sections. With FNAC only a limited number of smears are available and immunostaining may be difficult to perform, as in a cytological smear the cell membranes remain intact. FNAB evaluation is very fast for a pathologist whose primary training is in histology. On the other hand, FNAC allows a better evaluation of cellular detail, especially for small-cell tumours with fragile cells that are easily crushed during sectioning. The processing of a FNAC specimen is cheaper than that for FNAB and a cytological diagnosis can be made within 1 hour, whereas a histological diagnosis usually has to wait until the following day.

Diagnostic accuracy

The ability of ultrasound to guide the insertion of a needle during a biopsy presumably improves diagnostic accuracy. However, this is not necessarily the case and we need to quantify the diagnostic impact of interventional ultrasound with answers to basic questions, such as: how often is a positive result true? how sensitive is the test? etc. The basic diagnostic accuracies are defined as follows.[17]

The **success rate** is the percentage of biopsy procedures resulting in sufficient material for microscopic evaluation. It is not always easy to classify biopsies into the two simple categories such as 'sufficient' and 'insufficient'. Three tissue cores from a liver lesion may contain only necrotic tissue and the procedure may erroneously be classified as insufficient, lowering the success rate, despite the fact that ultrasound correctly identified a lesion and that the biopsy needle cut three cores without a geographic miss. Likewise, an aspiration biopsy yielding only peripheral blood is not insufficient if the biopsied liver lesion is a haemangioma.

The **sensitivity** of the technique is the percentage of malignancies that are correctly diagnosed. In some series the sensitivity is boosted by excluding inadequate biopsies from the calculation. In these studies sensitivity should be read as the percentage of malignant lesions with an adequate biopsy where the ultrasound-guided biopsy material is evaluated as malignant. The sensitivity of the biopsy procedure is affected by the quality of ultrasound: for example, improved resolution may produce a paradoxical drop in success rate because biopsy of smaller lesions is attempted. Furthermore, the calculated sensitivity is affected by the choice of gold standard, which should be an independent diagnostic technique. The gold standard in a liver biopsy series may be autopsy findings, contrast CT or operative diagnosis within 30 days of the ultrasound-guided fine needle biopsy. This is not always available, and so the calculated sensitivities should be viewed with caution. Furthermore, by using this type of gold standard it becomes impossible to separate the diagnostic abilities of ultrasound and of the guided biopsy, because the gold standard refers to whether or not cancer is present in the liver and not to the nature of the lesion that was biopsied. For the ultrasound-guided biopsy to be correct from a metastatic liver lesion two events must occur:

1) ultrasound must select a malignant lesion for biopsy,
2) the subsequent biopsy must be evaluated as malignant.

Figure 7.9 illustrates that autopsy does not necessarily provide the truth.

The **specificity** of the technique is the percentage of benign lesions where the ultrasound-guided biopsy material is evaluated as benign; sensitivity is the ability to diagnose cancer, specificity is the ability to diagnose non-cancer. Specificity seems to be more at the mercy of the gold standard than is sensitivity, because negative biopsy results are not as likely to be followed by CT, operation or autopsy as are malignant results. A false-positive result often leads to surgery, whereas a true negative result usually will not.

Sensitivity and specificity are useful in comparing different procedures, but the predictive values are more

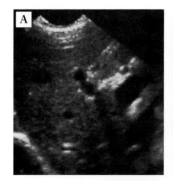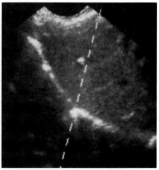

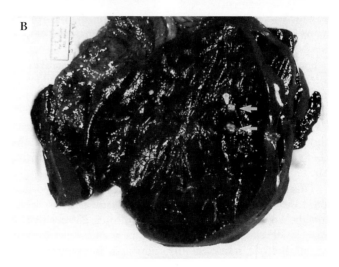

Fig. 7.9 Ultrasound image of fine needle biopsy. A: An echo-poor lesion in the right lobe of the liver (left). The needle tip is seen on the puncture line inside the lesion (right). The patient had a primary lung cancer and the biopsy was positive. B: Fourteen days later the patient died and autopsy was performed. Surprisingly, no metastasis was found and the pathologist speculated that perhaps the needle had passed through the liver into the right-sided lung tumour, thereby explaining the positive result. The ultrasound department disagreed with this explanation and insisted that the liver be sliced more finely; eventually the metastasis was found (the two halves are indicated by arrows).

useful in the diagnostic situation, where we wish to know the reliability of a biopsy result.

The **positive predictive value** (PV-positive) is the percentage of malignant biopsy results that are true positives. A PV-positive of 90% tells us that a malignant biopsy result has a 90% probability of being correct. Because cancer is defined histologically, the PV-positive of a histological biopsy is 100%. Therefore, analysis of PV-positive is only meaningful in cytological biopsies. A cytological diagnosis of cancer is an indirect diagnosis and not necessarily correct, inflammation, for example, sometimes giving cellular changes which are misinterpreted as cancer. The PV-positive is affected by the prevalence of malignant lesions in the biopsy series, which again is determined by the quality of ultrasound (ability to find subtle lesions) and the patient population. If the only lesions biopsied are those with a high clinical and ultrasound suspicion of malignancy, there will be very few benign lesions to create false positives and the PV-positive will be high. On the other hand, if even regions with only slightly suspicious changes in echo pattern are sampled, there will be a larger fraction of benign lesions, increasing the number of false positives and giving a lower PV-positive result.

PV-positive is one of the few diagnostic indices that can be measured reliably because a positive biopsy result will normally be verified by other means. It is an important index because it denotes the patient's risk of cancer when the biopsy is positive, and is therefore a measure of the diagnostic impact of the ultrasound-guided biopsy. This can be illustrated by a clinical example. A patient on chemotherapy for colonic cancer develops elevated liver enzymes (the risk for liver metastases may be 50%). Ultrasound shows a solid lesion in the liver (the risk for metastasis now increases to 90%). A cytological biopsy is positive (the risk for cancer is now 98%). As long as the PV-positive increases above the patient's risk before biopsy, there is a diagnostic impact.

The **negative predictive value** (PV-negative) is the percentage of non-malignant biopsy results that are true negatives. Its significance is parallel to a PV-positive, signifying the trustworthiness of a negative biopsy result. However, it is difficult to quantify as a negative biopsy result is rarely verified by the gold standard.

Sensitivity, specificity, PV-positive and PV-negative are intertwined, as can be seen from Table 7.2. Sensitivity and specificity are the true characteristics of a test and do not change with changing prevalence of disease. PV-positive and PV-negative are the diagnostic outcomes and do change with prevalence. Problems with the gold standard are often so great that only PV-positive can be calculated.

This synopsis of the basic diagnostic indices is important as they are used to compare procedures. It must therefore be kept in mind that, for instance, a PV-positive of 98% is determined by the sensitivity and specificity of

ultrasound (do we select the right area for biopsy?), the geographic accuracy of the biopsy procedure (do we actually sample what we think we are sampling?), the success rate of the procedure (how good is the needle or the person manipulating it?), and the sensitivity and specificity of the microscopic evaluation (how good is the pathologist?).

Safety and complications

A number of papers have been published on the risks of ultrasound-guided percutaneous procedures. In a large questionnaire, including 63 108 cases of fine needle aspiration biopsy, Smith[18] found a total of 101 complications (0.16%). There were four deaths, giving a mortality rate of 0.006%. In a literature survey of 11 700 cases Livraghi et al.[19] found a rate of major complications of 0.05% and a mortality rate of 0.008%. These data suggest that ultrasound-guided interventional procedures carry a very low risk; however, in these surveys it was not specified to what extent ultrasound was the guiding modality.

In a series of approximately 8000 ultrasound-guided interventional procedures, 3500 were needle biopsies for cytology or histology and three passes with each needle type were used routinely in each case[20] (Table 7.3, Fig. 7.10); 700 were large-bore biopsies (needle diameter between 1.2 and 2.1 mm) from the liver, kidney or prostate; 2800 were punctures of fluid collections, mainly in the abdomen, using a 1.2 mm spinal needle or a one-step 5.7 Fr (1.8 mm) pigtail catheter. There were also 1000 percutaneous nephrostomies with insertion of either a one-step 5.7 Fr (1.8 mm) pigtail catheter or a 10 Fr (3.2 mm) Foley catheter using the Seldinger technique, with dilation to 14 Fr (4.5 mm). Unless the patient's clinical condition suggested a coagulation disorder, all fine needle procedures, including those done on an outpatient basis, were performed without any preparation or laboratory test. Biopsies with larger needles were performed following the guidelines routinely used by the referring department.

Complications are defined as post-procedure conditions that required treatment. This means that transient pyrexia, haematuria or pain which did not require treatment (except for simple analgesics and observation) were not included. Patients who have abscess drainage often develop a fever after needling, and consequently receive

Table 7.2 Diagnostic indices. The relationship between sensitivity, specificity, PV-positive, PV-negative and prevalence. The bottom equation illustrates that a given test, i.e. constant S and SP, will have increasing PV-positive with increasing prevalence. Likewise, in a given population, i.e. constant prevalence, any increase/decrease in S or SP will result in an increase/decrease in PV-positive.

	Cancer	Non-cancer
Positive test	True positive (TP)	False positive (FP)
Negative test	False negative (FN)	True negative (TN)

Sensitivity (S): TP/(TP+FN)
Specificity (SP): TN/(TN+FP)
PV-positive: TP/(TP+FP)
PV-negative: TN/(TN+FN)
PV-positive = $(S \times p)/((S \times p) + ((1-SP) \times (1-p)))$,
p = prevalence.

Table 7.3 Distribution of punctures for the entire material

Type of puncture	Number
Fine needle biopsy (0.6–0.8 mm)	3500
Large-bore biopsy (1.2–2.1 mm)	700
Puncture or catheter drainage (1.2–1.8 mm)	2800
Nephrostomy (1.8–3.2 mm)	1000
Total	8000

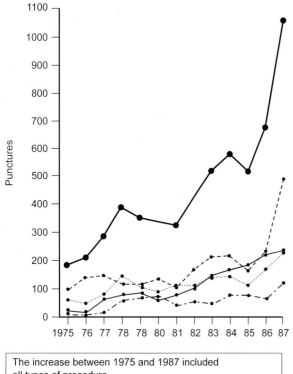

The increase between 1975 and 1987 included all types of procedure.

——— = Total number of punctures
----- = Fine needle biopsies (0.6 to 0.8 mm)
-·-·- = Large bore biopsies (1.2 to 2.1 mm)
——— = Catheter drainage or nephrostomy (1.8 to 3.2 mm)
········· = Puncture of fluid collections (1.2 mm)

Fig. 7.10 Annual changes in different types of punctures. The increase between 1975 and 1987 included all types of procedure.

antibiotic treatment to prevent severe septicaemia. In this group, therefore, fever and antibiotic treatment were not considered to be a complication.

A total of 15 complications were registered (Table 7.4), of which three were fatal (numbers 3, 7 and 14). This gave an overall complication rate of 0.19% and a mortality rate of 0.04%. Patients having only fine needle aspiration had approximately the same rates of complications and mortality, 0.20% and 0.03%, respectively. It must be admitted that these rates are minimum estimates, as the data are based upon information from clinical departments, though in practice complications are usually notified immediately.

Three of the complications were intraperitoneal bleeding in patients who had hepatomegaly caused by multiple metastases, and the only death after fine needle biopsy was in this group. Based on this, the guidelines have been changed and this group of patients should not be biopsied routinely. If it is considered essential to obtain microscopic diagnosis, the biopsy should be performed using special precautions such as plugging the needle track.[21]

It is debatable whether FNA of liver haemangiomas carries a high risk.[19] In this series, which included many haemangiomas, there was only one complication, a patient who developed intraperitoneal bleeding after biopsy with a 1.2 mm cutting needle; blood transfusion was required but recovery was complete.

The possibility of spreading tumour cells, either along the needle track or into the blood or lymph, is of major importance when biopsy of a malignancy is performed. Malignant cells have been found in the circulation after needle biopsy,[22] but this does not necessarily mean that metastases will occur and circulating cells probably do not worsen the prognosis.[23-27] In clinical practice, tumour seeding attributable to needle biopsy is extremely rare. In a series of 469 patients with prostatic cancer there was no evidence of local tumour growth at the biopsy site.[22] In only one of almost 4000 fine needle biopsies of cancers of the lung was tumour growth from the needle track demonstrated.[28] Livraghi *et al.*[19] found two cases of needle track seeding in their literature search of 11 700 fine needle biopsies, and Smith, in his large questionnaire, found three cases of cancer seeding along the needle track among 63 108 fine needle biopsies,[18] although rates of up to 3% have been reported after three-pass biopsies of hepatocellular carcinomas using 18–20 G needles.[27] In our own material of 3500 fine needle biopsies with six needle

Table 7.4 Registered complications after 8000 ultrasound guided punctures

Case	Complication	Target	Needle	Treatment
1	Bleeding	Renal cyst	1.2 mm	1000 ml blood transfusion
2	Bleeding	Liver haemangioma	1.2 mm	1000 ml blood transfusion
3	Bleeding	Aneurysm (misinterpreted as pancreatic cyst)	1.2 mm	Patient died
4	Bleeding (haematoma)	Pancreatic cancer		Laparotomy
5	Bleeding	Liver metastasis	FNAB	2500 ml blood transfusion
6	Bleeding	Liver metastasis	FNAB	1500 ml blood transfusion
7	Bleeding	Liver metastasis	FNAB	Patient died
8	Abscess	Pyonephrosis	Catheter	Surgery for ureteric stricture
9	Septic shock	Renal abscess	Catheter	Antishock treatment
10	Bile leak	Gallbladder	1.2 mm	Laparotomy (1500 ml bile)

passes per case we have never experienced seeding of cancer into the track. Thus, it seems reasonable to conclude that there is little risk of spreading tumour cells by a fine needle biopsy.[29]

Diagnostic procedures

Cytological fine needle aspiration biopsy (FNAC)

A 0.6–0.8 mm fine needle without a stylet is used with a 10 cm long 1.2 mm guide needle and a 10 ml syringe and needle guide, all on a sterile tray. A sterile cover for the transducer is needed unless the transducer can be sterilised, and sterile scanning gel is required. The skin is surprisingly resistant to a fine needle, and if the guide needle is not to be used a minute incision is recommended. One benefit of using a guide needle is that there is only one skin puncture, even when multiple needle insertions are made.

The transducer is positioned with the electronic needle line on the scanner screen traversing the target and the entry point of the needle is marked on the skin. The scanning gel is then wiped off, the skin sterilised, local anaes-

thetic administered and the area draped as for minor surgery (Fig. 7.11). The needle guide is mounted on the sterilised or draped transducer and sterile scanning gel is applied. The transducer is again positioned so that the needle line traverses the target and the guide needle is inserted through the guide: it need only be inserted 1 or 2 cm, depending on the thickness of the skin (Fig. 7.11B). If a sector scanner is used the guide needle is rarely visualised because of the blind region alongside the probe.

The fine needle attached to the 10 ml syringe is then passed through the guide needle: it is seen moving along the puncture line as a bright spot indicating the position of the needle tip. Not uncommonly the needle deviates (indicated by loss of visualisation of the tip) and, if the pass seems likely to miss the target, is retracted and reinserted. When the needle echo is seen inside the target full suction is applied with the syringe. The needle is then moved in and out of the lesion several times and the suction gently released, before removing the needle and handing it to an assistant who separates the needle from the syringe, fills the syringe with air, reconnects needle and syringe, and expels the contents on to a glass slide. This is then smeared with another glass slide. One needle pass thus produces

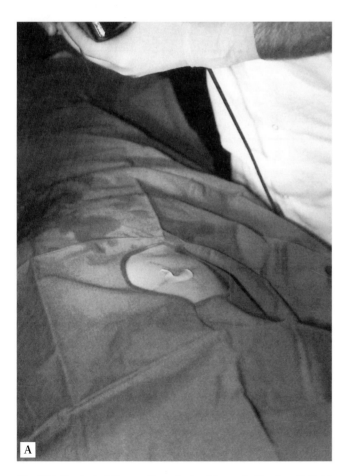
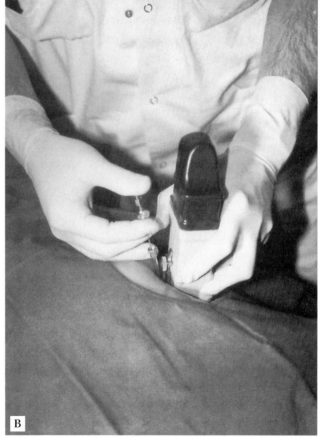

Fig. 7.11 Cytological fine needle aspiration biopsy. A: Draping. **B:** Guide needle inserted.

two slides for microscopic evaluation. The procedure is repeated sampling different areas of the target; three needle passes are normally performed.

Histological fine needle aspiration biopsy (FNAB)

The equipment required and the overall approach are the same as for cytological FNA, except that a cutting needle with an outer diameter of 0.6–0.8 mm is used and a sterile piece of paper is needed. When the tip of the cutting needle is seen just outside the target, the plunger is retracted. A locking device holds the plunger retracted, the needle is advanced into the target and a tissue core cut into the needle. If the target is small the needle can be retracted and readvanced, as there is room for a 3 cm tissue core in the needle. The needle is then removed and the tip placed on the sterile paper, the locking device is deactivated and the tissue core dislodged on to the paper. Typically three needle passes are performed. The tissue cores can be seen with the naked eye, so the adequacy of the samples can be evaluated immediately. The cores are placed in formalin and undergo routine histological processing.

In choosing a fine needle system an important practical consideration is that it can be operated with one hand. Systems that require the removal of a stylet and mounting of a syringe are awkward. Because it may be difficult to manipulate the syringe with one hand, we recommend an unorthodox grip or the use of an aspiration handle (Fig. 7.12).

Some investigators advocate the use of a quick stain performed in the biopsy room for immediate evaluation by a pathologist to ensure that representative material has been obtained. The biopsy can then be repeated immediately if necessary. This approach depends on skilled interpretation of the slides, and therefore usually demands that a pathologist be present, and so the procedure must be planned ahead.

Comparison of fine needle techniques

The two types of needle have the same outer diameter and probably carry the same complication rate. The cutting needle samples a smaller volume of the lesion and so a slightly lower sensitivity might be expected, but histological diagnosis is more reliable as false positives theoretically do not occur. Furthermore, tumour typing is easier with tissue specimens.

The choice of needle depends on the clinical situation and the target organ. If the patient has a known primary cancer and a lesion in the liver is identified, only FNAC is needed. If a patient without a known primary has a lesion in the liver both FNAC and FNAB are performed, the latter to help in deciding the primary site. In these cases an extra tissue core for electron microscopy may be added.

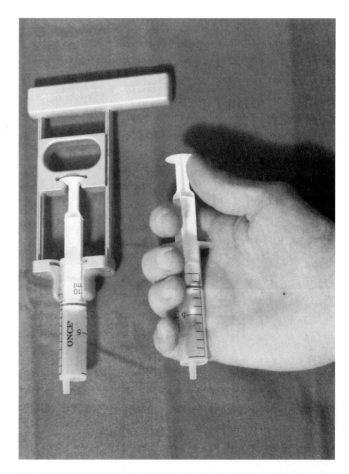

Fig. 7.12 Aspiration handle. Left: Aspiration handle for a 10 ml syringe. **Right:** If a handle is not available an unorthodox grip will allow the thumb to retract the plunger.

The liver is one of the easiest organs to biopsy: both FNAC and FNAB carry a success rate of 95%.[30-32] Furthermore, interpretation of the material is not difficult as the demonstration of extrahepatic cells or tissue alone indicates the presence of tumour. Cytology alone will not usually permit differentiation between primary and secondary liver tumours. Ultrasound-guided FNAB also improves the success rate in diffuse liver diseases.[33]

Other organ systems are more difficult to biopsy. Table 7.5 shows the results of a series of gynaecological fine needle biopsies where both needle types have a success rate of approximately 80%. Fortunately the two techniques are complementary and, when performed together, the success rate rises to 96%. The explanation for this is probably that soft tumours are easy to biopsy with FNAC (the tissue is easily dislodged into the needle), whereas it is difficult to cut a core; hard tumours such as uterine fibromyomas, however, give meagre cytological specimens but excellent cores. For the pancreas both methods give good results.[35]

Table 7.5 Results of 0.6 mm cytological and 0.8 mm histological biopsies in 91 operated cases of solid or solid/cystic pelvic masses

	Positive	Negative	Insufficient	Total
Cytological diagnosis				
Malignant tumour	27	1	3	31
Benign condition	2	38	20	60
Total	29	39	23	91

Success rate: 68/91 – 75%
PV-positive: 27/29 – 93%
PV-negative: 38/39 – 97%

	Positive	Negative	Insufficient	Total
Histological diagnosis				
Malignant tumour	23	3	5	31
Benign condition	0	45	15	60
Total	23	48	20	91

Success rate: 71/91 – 78%
PV-positive: 23/23 – 100%
PV-negative: 45/48 – 94%

Table 7.6 Results of 0.6 mm cytological biopsies in 301 cases of solid renal masses on ultrasound (first series)

	Positive	Negative	Insufficient	Total
Cytological diagnosis				
Malignant tumour	185	25	8	218
Benign condition	14	61	8	83
Total	199	86	16	301

Success rate: 285/301 – 95%
PV-positive: 185/199 – 93%
PV-negative: 61/86 – 71%

Table 7.7 Results of 0.6 mm cytological and 0.8 mm histological biopsies in 138 cases of solid renal masses on ultrasound (second series)

	Positive	Negative	Insufficient	Total
Cytological diagnosis				
Malignant tumour	78	7	2	87
Benign condition	7	43	1	51
Total	85	50	3	138

Success rate: 133/138 – 96%
PV-positive: 78/85 – 92%
PV-negative: 43/50 – 86%

	Positive	Negative	Insufficient	Total
Histological diagnosis				
Malignant tumour	63	8	16	87
Benign condition	0	39	12	51
Total	63	47	28	138

Success rate: 110/138 – 80%
PV-positive: 63/63 – 100%
PV-negative: 39/47 – 83%

Fine needle biopsy of the kidney is a special problem (Table 7.6): initial experiences gave a PV-positive of 93%,[36] but subsequent studies indicated an unacceptable false-positive rate for FNAC and therefore FNAB is recommended (Table 7.7).[37] Unfortunately, renal tumours are often necrotic and soft, so the success rate of FNAB in the kidney is not impressive. Repeated biopsies are therefore sometimes necessary.

Coarse needle biopsy

Needles with an outer diameter equal to or larger than 1 mm are termed 'coarse'. The Biopty system is the first of a series of simple and effective devices for using such needles, which have outer diameters of 1.2 and 2.0 mm (see Fig. 7.6D).

The patient is prepared in the same way as for a fine needle biopsy and the needle is mounted in the sterile firing device (see Fig. 7.7). A small skin incision is made for the needle guide and the needle observed moving along the puncture line. The gun is fired when the needle tip is at the surface of the target. The action advances the inner needle, revealing the biopsy chamber; immediately afterwards the outer cutting needle advances, cutting a tissue core into the biopsy chamber. The two movements are so fast that they are perceived as one. Typically a 23 mm sample is taken, but some systems allow a choice of sample lengths, the shorter ones being useful for small lesions lying close to structures that must be avoided. Because the system is automatic the cutting action is always performed correctly, ensuring a success rate close to 100%. A large-bore needle is required when the samples from a fine needle are not adequate. This is especially the case in non-neoplastic diseases in the liver and kidney.

For many years prostate biopsies have been performed with the 2.1 mm Tru-Cut needle via the trans-perineal or the trans-rectal approach, the latter being preferred because it is less painful and can be performed without anaesthesia.[38] Antibiotic cover is routinely used, despite which some 5% of men develop post-biopsy pyrexia requiring treatment.[39] A few units do not use an antibiotic at all.[40]

Cyst puncture

The equipment needed is a 1.2 mm needle (with stylet, long enough to reach the target), a syringe (10, 20 or 60 ml, depending on the size of the cyst), a needle guide (with a slot for a 1.2 mm needle) and sterile gel, all on a sterile tray. The procedure is as for fine needle biopsy. The skin puncture site is identified, local anaesthesia applied and the area cleansed and draped. No skin incision is necessary.

The needle is inserted and the tip is seen moving along the puncture line. Needle deviation is seldom a problem as the needle does not bend as easily as a fine needle. The tip

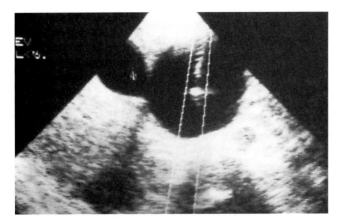

Fig. 7.13 Puncture of pancreatic cyst. Transverse scan shows pancreatic pseudocyst in the midline close to the gallbladder. The needle is seen in the cyst. Note the guide line.

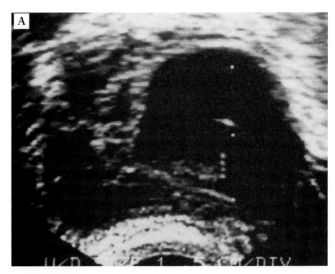

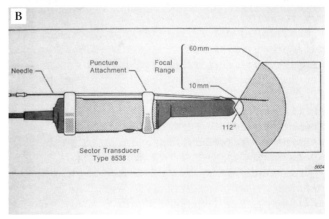

Fig. 7.14 Trans-vaginal puncture of an ovarian cyst. A: The echo from the needle tip is seen centrally in the cyst. **B:** The trans-vaginal scanner is a sector scanner at the tip of a finger-shaped probe. The needle leaves the needle guide immediately outside the image.

of the needle is positioned in the cyst (Fig. 7.13), the stylet removed and the syringe attached. Evacuation of the cyst is then monitored on ultrasound. As the cyst shrinks the needle is repositioned so that the tip remains in the fluid. The needle is then removed and the fluid sent for appropriate analysis. Even multiloculated cysts can usually be emptied. It is common for the compartments to communicate, so that evacuation can be accomplished with a single puncture. Where the loculi do not communicate the needle is repositioned until all compartments have been evacuated.

The standard technique must be modified for the aspiration of three commonly encountered cysts, ovarian, breast and thyroid.

Ovarian cysts may be approached via the trans-vaginal route. The tip of the probe can almost always be brought into contact with the cyst, separated from it only by the vaginal wall at the fornix. When a trans-vaginal needle guide is used needle deviation is not a problem, as the distance from the scanner to the cyst is usually only 1 cm (Fig. 7.14).

Breast and thyroid cysts are very superficial and a free-hand technique is recommended as they are easily accessed. A 5 cm intramuscular needle (0.6 mm outer diameter, no stylet) mounted on a syringe is appropriate.

When large cysts are being aspirated it may be cumbersome to manipulate a large syringe at the same time as ensuring correct needle placement. This difficulty can be overcome by fitting a connecting tube between the needle and the syringe. An assistant can then apply suction while the examiner only has to handle the needle and transducer.

Occasionally what was thought to be a cyst turns out to be solid. When this happens the procedure is easily converted into a fine needle biopsy, using the 1.2 mm needle positioned in the lesion as a guide needle for the fine biopsy needle.

Generally there is no need to puncture a cyst simply to verify its cystic nature, as this can almost always be reliably established from ultrasound criteria. The most important indication for abdominal cyst puncture is to rule out an abscess.

Cytological examination of cyst fluid seldom reveals important information as the contents are nearly always acellular. Cyst puncture will therefore rarely distinguish malignant from benign pathology, although elevated lipid contents in renal cysts have been reported as an indirect sign of malignancy.[41]

Because the diagnosis of hydatid disease is primarily serological, diagnostic puncture, though not contraindicated, is seldom needed. However, ultrasound can be used to guide the therapeutic instillation of 0.5% silver nitrate solution or antihelminthic agents or simply for repeated emptying in the management of persistent disease.[42,43] Where the origin of a cyst is unknown, puncture may be carried out simply to establish which organ system it belongs to. Amylase in the fluid establishes a pancreatic origin, just as appropriate hormone analyses establish a gynaecological origin.

Therapeutic cyst puncture is undertaken in the hope that the cyst will not recur after evacuation. This raises the question of whether to inject substances that will reduce the recurrence rate: so far, no controlled trial in any organ system has shown that this is effective. For instance, a controlled trial comparing tetracycline and saline as sclerosing agents in thyroid cysts showed no difference and established that the benefit was in the puncture and flushing, and not in the tetracycline.[44]

The indication for cyst puncture varies from organ to organ:

1   liver: therapeutic puncture is rarely indicated,
2   kidney: cyst puncture is only indicated if the patient has pain from the cyst or if it is causing obstruction. Both are very rare, and the relevance of using various sclerosing agents, e.g. 96% alcohol, is not obvious,
3   pancreas: there are many optimistic reports of high cure rates after pancreatic pseudocyst puncture. They share one common weakness, namely a very short follow-up time. Reaccumulation during the first year brings the cure rate down to the spontaneous regression rate of approximately 7%,[45]
4   ovaries: the fear of overlooking neoplasm is the main reason for gynaecological cyst puncture. Some patients referred for puncture have previously undergone surgery where a cyst of non-epithelial origin was removed. A prudent approach in non-operated patients is to select those under the age of 40 with a simple unilocular cyst. Granberg reports a cure rate of 70% in such patients,[46]
5   breast: provided the typical features are unequivocally demonstrated, diagnostic aspiration is not needed. However, cysts that concern the patient because they cause pain or are readily palpable are easily aspirated, though they may recur,
6   thyroid: these cysts are almost always cystic degeneration in an adenoma, and the main problem for the patient is cosmetic. Hegedüs reports a cure rate of around 45% in these patients.[44]

The clinical history will often limit the likely diagnoses of a fluid collection found on ultrasound to one or two, and diagnostic aspiration is useful when management depends upon the nature of the fluid. Many collections are large or superficially located, and therefore easily punctured with a free-hand technique. However, if the collection is more deeply located or lies close to a structure that must not be punctured, guided aspiration may be simpler. Inspection of the fluid will reveal the presence or absence of blood, bacteria and bile, and the sample may be sent for laboratory analysis (Table 7.8).

Table 7.8 Biochemical tests on cyst fluid

Test	Elevated in
Creatinine	Urinoma
Amylase	Pancreatic cyst
Protein (†)	Exudate, lymphocele
Protein, glucose (†) Urea	Renal cyst
Bilirubin (†)	Biloma
Potassium; chloride	Hydatid cyst

(†) Labstix

Contrast studies

As described in the following section under nephrostomy and abscess drainage, a catheter can serve not only a therapeutic but also a diagnostic purpose. Antegrade pyelography is frequently used to delineate a ureteric obstruction.[47] Fistulography is a simple and effective way to monitor abscess cavity size and to disclose a communication between an abscess cavity and a hollow organ, and can be performed with ultrasound using hydrogen peroxide as the contrast agent.[48]

Two further diagnostic applications are ultrasound-guided percutaneous trans-hepatic cholangiography (PTC) and ultrasound-guided percutaneous pancreatography.[49] The typical indication for performing a PTC is to differentiate between a stone in the common bile duct and cancer or chronic pancreatitis of the head of the pancreas. Rather than relying on presumed normal anatomy, it is an obvious advantage to perform the PTC under ultrasound guidance to delineate the actual anatomy. Usually only one puncture is needed and, if only part of the intrahepatic bile duct system is dilated, a selective PTC can be performed. Percutaneous injection of contrast directly into a pancreatic duct is not possible without ultrasound guidance. This technique can be very useful in patients in whom ERCP is impossible, where biopsy of a suspected pancreatic mass is negative, or for pre-operative staging of a malignancy.

Therapeutic procedures

Nephrostomy

Since the introduction of ultrasound-guided percutaneous nephrostomy in 1974[50] this technique has gained widespread use.[47] Using ultrasound it is possible both to visualise the interventional procedure and subsequently to control the correct placement of the inserted catheter. However, the majority of centres use a combined approach, ultrasound to guide the fine needle and radiological fluoroscopy for placement of the guidewire and catheter.

Two different nephrostomy techniques are generally used: a Seldinger technique with tract dilatation and subsequent balloon catheter placement (Fig. 7.15), and a one-step technique in which a pigtail catheter is introduced with a trocar inserter (Fig. 7.16).

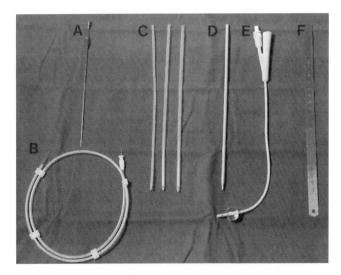

Fig. 7.15 Foley balloon catheter nephrostomy kit. A: 1.2 mm lumbar puncture needle with stylet. **B:** Soft-tip Lunderquist guidewire. **C:** 10, 12 and 14 Fr dilators for three-step dilatation technique. **D:** 14 Fr one-step screw dilator. **E:** 10 Fr Foley balloon catheter with 3 ml sterile water in balloon. **F:** Ruler for measuring the distance to the calyx.

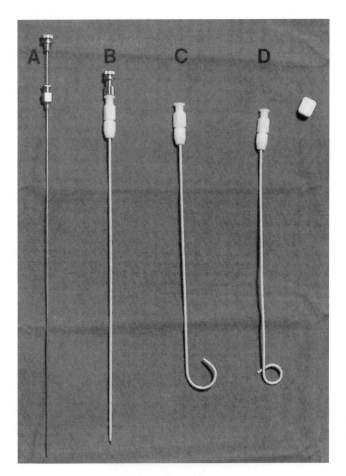

Fig. 7.16 Trocar nephrostomy catheters. A: Trocar with stylet. **B:** Trocar with catheter pulled over it. **C:** 5.7 Fr pigtail catheter. **D:** 5.7 Fr loop catheter.

If the nephrostomy is primarily for antegrade pyelography, or if the nephrostomy tube is expected to be left in place for only 2 or 3 days, a 5 to 7 Fr one-step pigtail catheter can be used, as the relatively small diameter of the catheter and the speed of the procedure are easier for the patient. If a prolonged or permanent nephrostomy is planned a 10 Fr Foley balloon catheter is required. The soft silicone material causes less skin irritation than the rigid polyethylene of the one-step catheter. If the drainage lasts longer than 2 months the catheter should be exchanged to avoid concretions on the balloon and inside the catheter. This can be done without any imaging technique, as the tract is mature.

Recently, a third type of catheter, the pigtail loop, has been introduced. This combines the one-step technique with internal fixation (Fig. 7.17).

The patient is placed in the lateral decubitus or prone position to permit a retroperitoneal needle route. A sector scanner should be used to provide a small footprint with a large field of view. The transducer is placed over the region of interest and the skin site is carefully chosen in order to keep the needle path perpendicular to the renal capsule. A lower or middle calyx is selected for catheterisation and the depth of the calyx is measured to ensure that the dilators will be inserted far enough. Local anaesthesia is applied, preferably under ultrasound guidance to ensure that it is placed correctly. If the procedure is an elective balloon catheter nephrostomy it is recommended that the patient be given systemic analgesics, as the dilatation can be painful.

The procedure must be performed under sterile conditions. After skin disinfection, an incision is made in order to allow the passage of dilators and catheter. An 18 gauge spinal needle is introduced through the steering device along the electronic needle line to the centre of the renal

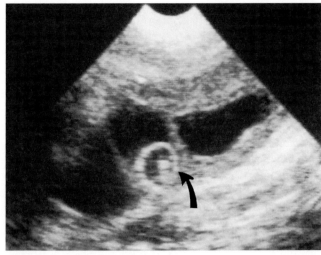

Fig. 7.17 Kidney with dilated pelvis and 10 Fr balloon catheter in the middle calyx. Arrowhead points at inflated balloon.

pelvis. The stylet is removed and, if the needle has been correctly placed, urine escapes. A soft-tip Lunderquist guidewire is introduced through the needle, which is then removed. From this stage on fluoroscopy is often a better means of monitoring the procedure. The dilator is inserted over the guidewire and passed through the tissue: penetration is easier if the dilator is rotated as it is inserted. A three-step serial dilatation technique with 7, 10 and 14 Fr dilators has proved effective (Fig. 7.15C). Recently a screw dilator that dilates to 14 Fr in one step (Fig. 7.15D) has been developed.[51] Regardless of the type of dilator, it is mandatory to ensure that the length of the inserted part corresponds to the previously measured distance to the centre of the calyx. If the dilatation has been performed thoroughly the soft 10 Fr silicone Foley catheter can easily be introduced and the balloon inflated with 3 ml sterile saline (Fig. 7.17). If any doubt remains concerning the correct placement of the catheter, sterile saline can be injected through it while observing the kidney with ultrasound: if the catheter is correctly placed bubbles in the saline will 'light up' the pelvis.

For the one-step method, the trocar with the pigtail catheter pulled over it is introduced via the needle steering device. When the needle tip is seen inside the calyx the needle is held in position while the catheter is advanced and curls up inside the calyx; urine will then flow through it. Simple catheters must be fixed to the skin with a suture, but loop catheters need no skin fixation. Confirmation of the catheter position is obtained with an antegrade pyelogram.

Abscess drainage

Ultrasound-guided percutaneous aspiration of fluid collections in the upper abdomen and pelvis is an effective tool for diagnosis and treatment, to the extent that surgical drainage of intra-abdominal abscesses has been almost completely replaced by percutaneous drainage in many centres. The technique differs from radiologist to radiologist and has been extensively described.[52,53] In principle two different methods may be used:[52]

1   needle drainage. The pus is aspirated through a 1.2 mm needle and the abscess is irrigated with sterile saline until the returning fluid is clear. Follow-up scanning is performed after approximately 2 days and the procedure is repeated if necessary,
2   continuous catheter drainage. A catheter is placed into the abscess cavity and is secured in place for drainage and daily irrigation until the infection has resolved (Fig. 7.18).

The catheter can be introduced via a trocar or via the Seldinger technique. The type usually used is a multihole soft pigtail of 6–10 Fr. Radiography is used to demonstrate correct catheter placement and to reveal fistulae.

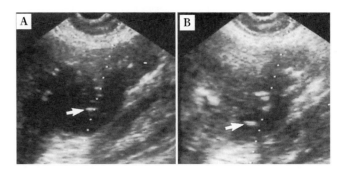

Fig. 7.18 **Percutaneous drainage of a liver abscess. A:** The echo from the tip of the trocar is seen inside the abscess (arrow). **B:** The pigtail catheter is seen inside the almost empty abscess (arrow).

Catheters should not be inserted through the gastrointestinal tract or urinary bladder: where this is unavoidable needle drainage should be performed instead. Antibiotics can be instilled into the abscess cavity, but the value of this has not been proven. Many antibiotics are prodrugs which need to be metabolised before they are effective, and they may be locally irritant if used in high concentration. Cure rates of over 80% have been reported for intra-abdominal abscesses, and a marked clinical improvement can usually be observed a few hours after the drainage.

The most common complication, seen in less than 5% of patients, is rigors a few hours following the treatment, caused by bacteraemia, which can be avoided by giving antibiotic cover.[52,54] Bleeding following catheter insertion has been reported in a few patients.[53,55]

Pelvic abscesses may be more difficult to access and a trans-rectal, trans-vaginal, trans-perineal or trans-gluteal approach may be required.[56] Ultrasound-guided percutaneous drainage has also been described from the thorax, neck, brain, skin and breast.[55,57]

Pleural effusions

Pleural effusions are common in patients with malignancies and their effective control can improve the quality of life of the cancer patient.[58] Ultrasound is most often used to determine whether a radiographic opacity is due to consolidation or a pleural effusion, and to locate the best site for thoracocentesis, either for diagnostic or for therapeutic purposes.[59] If possible, the patient is examined in the sitting position using a small sector transducer to facilitate intercostal scanning. For a diagnostic puncture, a short 19 or 21 G needle can be used and a pigtail catheter, inserted via a trocar, can be connected to a sealed system for continuous drainage.[60]

Gastrostomy

Ultrasound-guided percutaneous gastrostomy can be performed for nutritional support, for example in patients

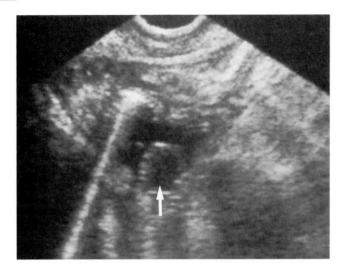

Fig. 7.19 Percutaneous gastrostomy. A soft balloon catheter (arrow) has been inserted into the antrum of the stomach.

with oesophageal or oropharyngeal malignancy. The procedure is performed under local anaesthesia and can be facilitated by distending the stomach with air or fluid through a nasogastric tube. Under ultrasound guidance the safest access is chosen, special care being taken to avoid traversing the liver, retroperitoneal vessels or the spleen. Both Seldinger and trocar methods have been described.[61,62] When the Seldinger technique is used a soft balloon catheter is inserted via the dilated track into the lumen of the stomach (Fig. 7.19).

Cholecystostomy

The gallbladder is readily accessible for needle puncture and catheterisation and several reports have documented the usefulness and safety of ultrasound-guided percutaneous cholecystostomy for both diagnosis and treatment.[63,64] Percutaneous cholecystostomy may replace surgery in the treatment of patients with acute cholecystitis who are a poor operative risk (Fig. 7.20). The technique has also proved useful in the diagnosis and treatment of patients with distal common bile duct obstruction.

Theoretically the safest approach is via a trans-hepatic puncture, entering the gallbladder where it is adherent to the liver to avoid bile leaks, but the trans-peritoneal route has also been used safely.[65] Both the trocar and the Seldinger techniques can be used, with either a soft pigtail or a balloon catheter (Fig. 7.20E).

Other indications for ultrasound-guided puncture of the gallbladder include diagnostic aspiration of fluid for chemical or bacteriological examination, diagnostic cholecystocholangiography and fine needle biopsy. Gallstones can be removed or solvents infused for dissolution via a percutaneous cholecystostomy.

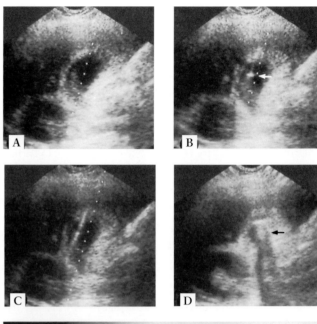

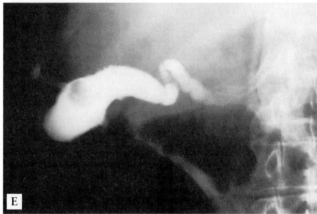

Fig. 7.20 Ultrasound-guided percutaneous cholecystostomy. A: Infected gallbladder with thick wall. A trans-hepatic puncture route has been chosen. **B:** The echo from the tip of a puncture needle (arrow) is seen in the lumen of the gallbladder. **C:** The echo from a guidewire in the lumen of the gallbladder. **D:** An air-filled balloon is seen inside an emptied gallbladder (arrow). **E:** Cholecystogram showing the catheter with the balloon centrally in the fundus of the gallbladder.

Pancreatic pseudocysts

Pancreatic pseudocysts that develop in patients with pancreatitis (see Ch. 16) can be punctured for either diagnostic or therapeutic purposes (Fig. 7.21).[66,67] For diagnostic aspiration a 0.9 or 1.2 mm needle is appropriate, depending on the size of the cyst and the amount of debris. The aspirate is routinely sent for amylase levels, culture and cytology. If the aspirate is purulent, percutaneous drainage should be undertaken. Other common indications for therapeutic drainage include pain, biliary and gastric outlet obstruction, and large cysts which are not resolving spontaneously.

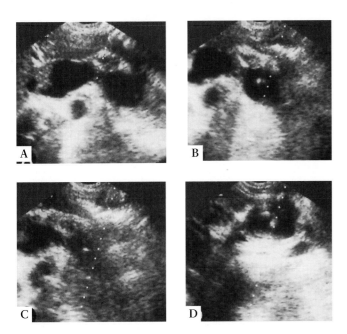

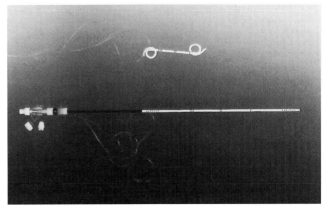

Fig. 7.22 Internal drainage of pancreatic pseudocyst. **Top:** Double-pigtail catheter for pancreatic cystogastrostomy. **Bottom:** Catheter mounted on trocar needle.

Fig. 7.21 Puncture drainage of two pancreatic pseudocysts. **A:** Cysts are seen in the head and body of the pancreas. **B:** A needle has been inserted into the cyst in the body, traversing the stomach. **C:** The cyst has been emptied. **D:** Puncture drainage of the cyst in the pancreatic head.

A pseudocyst may be drained using either repeated needling or long-term continuous catheter placement. Short-term needle drainage is indicated in acutely ill patients, with the intention of avoiding spontaneous rupture of the cyst, and can also be performed in non-acute cysts for pain relief. Unfortunately, cysts often recur following drainage, even after repeated needling.

Long-term catheter drainage is indicated in patients with cysts that cannot be controlled by repeated needling, and is most simply performed using the trocar technique with 6–10 Fr pigtail catheters. The trans-peritoneal route is generally preferred, but retroperitoneal or trans-gastric routes can also be used, and a combined ultrasound and gastroscopic technique using a special double-pigtail catheter (Fig. 7.22) introduced percutaneously and trans-gastrically into the cyst cavity has been described. Under gastroscopy the catheter is positioned with one curved end in the cyst and the other in the stomach.[68,69] Overall success rates of 70–90% have been reported; on average drainage takes about 3 weeks but may take as long as 3 months.[66,67] A potential risk of long-term catheter drainage is infection of a previously sterile cyst, but complications such as pneumothorax and pleural effusion are rare.

Tumour therapy

Ultrasound-guided percutaneous destruction of tumours seems to be an obvious approach as a needle can be placed in any tumour visible on the scan for accurate interstitial delivery of therapeutic agents.[70] Several different means of tissue destruction have been described, including chemical, ionising radiation, heat and high-intensity focused ultrasound.[71]

Chemical agents

Chemical tissue destruction is an accepted treatment in selected patients. Ultrasound-guided ethanol injection of parathyroid adenomas is widely used in patients who are unfit for surgery (see below).[72] In the same way, liver tumours have been treated with some success.[73] Injection of caustic and antineoplastic drugs is another possibility, although its role is not established.[74]

Adhesive agents can be used to treat cysts in various sites, e.g. kidney, liver, thyroid. Alcohol has been used with limited success; fibrin seems to be a promising possibility for accelerating thrombosis of femoral artery pseudo-aneurysms treated by ultrasound-guided compression.[75]

Radiotherapy

Interstitial radiotherapy (brachytherapy) provides an alternative to external radiation in selected tumours, especially in the prostate.[76–78] The advantages over conventional external radiotherapy are that radiation can be confined to the tumour, thereby limiting damage to normal tissue, and the precise control of the radiated volume allows a higher dose to be delivered. Radioactive seed implantations have occasionally been used in the treatment of otherwise untreatable abdominal cancers,[79] but the results have not been promising.

Heat

Hyperthermia as a treatment for cancer has been applied both systemically and locally, with limited success.[80]

Reaching a sufficiently high temperature inside the tumour without damaging the surrounding healthy tissue is most easily achieved by interstitial or local hyperthermia using implantable energy sources, such as microwave antennae, coils and filaments. For percutaneous treatment the device must be small enough to pass through a small needle.

An approach to this uses a low-power neodynium yttrium aluminium garnet (Nd-YAG) laser, which destroys tumour tissue by means of phototoxicity and thermoradiation.[81,82] The fibreoptics used to deliver the light are introduced through a needle and arranged to spread the light in a sphere.[82] The size of the lesion created depends on the energy delivered, with a maximum diameter of 44 mm (4 W for 30 min). The lesions have a central cavity delineated by a charred rim of tissue and a peripheral zone of coagulation (Fig. 7.23A): on ultrasound they appear as highly reflective circles (Fig. 7.23B).

A very promising way to heat tissue uses high-intensity focused ultrasound (HIFU). Heating of surrounding tissues is minimal and tissues that do not reach the critical temperature for coagulation (around 50°C) recover completely, so that the ablation can be precisely controlled. The lesions produced are around 1 mm in diameter and some 20 mm in length; a raster sonication pattern is developed in the HIFU plan to cover the tumour volume. Clinical trials have included prostate, bladder and liver tumours.[71]

Prostate cancer

Trans-perineal insertion of ^{125}I seeds into the prostate, guided by trans-rectal ultrasound, was described in 1983[76] and is a modification of the method described by Whitmore.[83,84] The rationale is that radioactive sources distributed uniformly throughout the prostate deliver a radiation dose sufficient to destroy all tumour tissue, a dose higher than can be safely administered by external beam therapy. [125]I has ideal physical characteristics for the treatment of prostatic cancer as its half-life of approximately 60 days is well suited for a slow-growing cancer, but other radionuclides such as [103]paladium have also been used.[85,86]

A trans-rectal transducer is used for radiation planning and to guide seed insertion (Fig. 7.24). The probe is mounted in a rigid holder that can be manipulated in the x, y and z planes. A needle guide matrix with multiple channels is mounted on the rectal tube outside the patient. Needles inserted through the canals cross the sound field at specific points, which are indicated on the ultrasound image by an electronically generated grid.

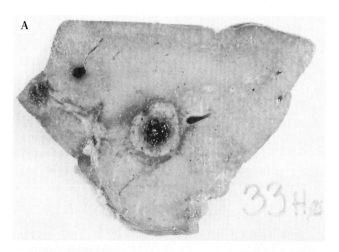

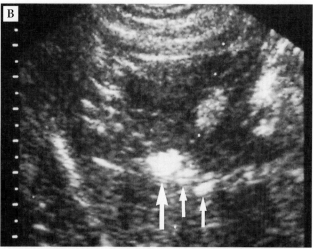

Fig. 7.23 Laser therapy. A: Section of pig liver 8 days after interstitial laser coagulation with 4 W for 600 s. The charred wall of the central cavity is seen surrounded by a light zone of heat necrosis. **B:** *In vivo* ultrasound scan of pig liver following laser coagulation (large arrow). Two microthermocouples are seen close to the lesion (small arrows).

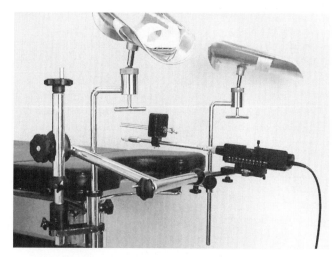

Fig. 7.24 Equipment for trans-perineal seed implantation. The rectal transducer is mounted in a fixture that can be positioned accurately in the x, y and z planes. The multichannel puncture guide is mounted on the rectal tube. For illustration purposes needles are inserted in the guide.

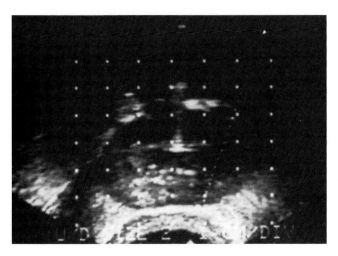

Fig. 7.25 **Transverse image of the prostate** with superimposed electronic needle matrix. Each dot corresponds to a canal in the puncture guide. The bottom row of dots is a constant distance from the rectal wall as the scanner is moved in and out.

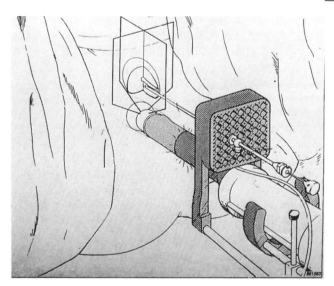

Fig. 7.27 **Apparatus for trans-perineal seed implantation** guided by multiplanar imaging. The multiplanar probe is mounted in a fixture which allows the transducer to be rotated. When the transducer is locked, the electronic matrix corresponds to the multichannel needle guide. When the transducer is rotated away from the locked position the needle guide does not follow the movement. Any needle can thus also be visualised longitudinally.

At a planning session the patient is placed in the lithotomy position and the fixture is manipulated until the lower row of needle canals is a constant and preselected distance from the rectal wall as the transducer is moved in and out of the rectum (Fig. 7.25). In this position needle insertion is parallel to the rectum and the position of the transducer is well defined and can be reproduced on the day of actual insertion. The prostatic volume is calculated from serial planimetry,[87] and the appropriate number and activity of seeds calculated to produce a uniform distribution. The loaded needles are implanted under direct ultrasound vision using a multiplanar probe system, so that both the position and the depth of the seeds can be controlled (Figs 7.26 and 7.27).

Good immediate and long-term results have been reported.[85,88–90]

Liver cancer

The increasing use of ultrasound liver screening has resulted in the detection of more and more early-stage hepatocellular carcinomas (HCC). Non-surgical treatment of HCC, such as trans-catheter arterial embolisation, chemotherapy and radiotherapy, have not proved curative and liver resection has become the method of choice. However, a high proportion of patients with HCCs are not candidates for surgery because of either severe cirrhosis, age, multifocal disease or tumour site. For these patients, as well as those with a limited number of liver metastases, ultrasound-guided percutaneous treatment is an alternative form of therapy.

A number of authors have injected 96% alcohol in HCC.[73,91,92] Their techniques have only differed slightly, and in the largest series of over 100 lesions good results were obtained.[29,93,94] Depending upon the lesion diameter, the extent of necrosis and the compliance of the patient, 1–4 ml of 96% alcohol is injected under ultrasound control once or twice weekly on an outpatient basis. For large lesions the one-stop approach has been used, delivering larger volumes of ethanol under general anaesthetic. The echo pattern of the HCC changes considerably during the injection, generally becoming increasingly reflective (Fig. 7.28). The only significant complication is intraperitoneal haemorrhage, which is uncommon.[95] Moderate

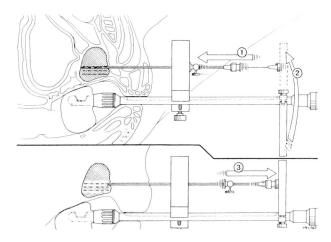

Fig. 7.26 **Needle insertion. Top:** When the needle is correctly positioned the seeds and spacers are correctly positioned in the prostate but are still in the needle. **Bottom:** As the needle is withdrawn over the immobile stylet, the row of seeds and spacers is left in the prostate.

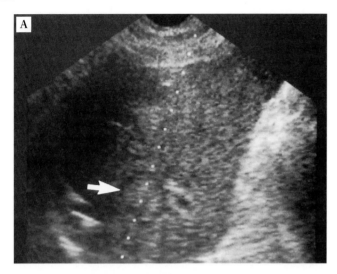
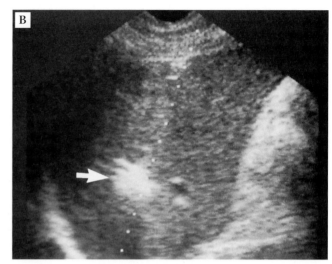

Fig. 7.28 Ultrasound-guided alcohol injection in liver cancer. A: A 2 cm isoechoic liver lesion proved on histological fine needle biopsy to be an HCC. B: A fine needle has been inserted along the puncture line and 4 ml of 96% alcohol injected. The lesion has become highly reflective, corresponding to the distribution of the alcohol.

pain is usual, as is a transient fever and a slight increase in liver enzyme levels.

Ensuring that the entire lesion has been alcoholised is assisted by using colour Doppler to check for vascularised remaining tumour, and this can be improved using a microbubble contrast agent: if flow signals are seen further treatment can be performed immediately, an advantage over the standard enhanced CT technique.[96] At present there are no randomised studies available but the results are promising. In Livraghi's series all lesions were smaller after 6–27 months follow-up, and no evidence of HCC was present on fine needle biopsy or dynamic CT.

Parathyroid adenomas

Ultrasonography is a useful technique for localising enlarged parathyroid glands in the neck and, despite occasional confusion with exophytic thyroid nodules and with lymph nodes, is usually straightforward; confusion with thyroid nodules can be avoided by using colour Doppler to demonstrate the high vascularity of the parathyroid.[97,98] When there is doubt, ultrasound-guided fine needle biopsy can be used, although the cytological distinction between thyroid and parathyroid cells may be difficult.[99,100] Immunochemical measurement of the parathyroid hormone content in the aspirate is a useful supplement to cytology, as is the use of small-core biopsies.[101–103] The precision with which a needle can be sited is the basis of ultrasound-guided percutaneous inactivation of parathyroid adenomas by ethanol injection, which can be performed on an outpatient basis under local anaesthesia.[104,105] The optimal dose of ethanol is half of the volume of the tumour and its dispersion is marked by the appearance of fine, dotted echoes spreading through the gland (Fig. 7.29).

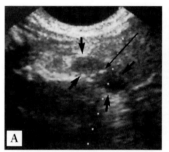
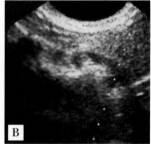

Fig. 7.29 Longitudinal scan of the neck. A: A parathyroid tumour (short arrows) is seen close to the thyroid gland. The echo from a fine needle is seen centrally in the parathyroid tumour (long arrow). B: The parathyroid tumour has become of increased reflectivity following injection of ethanol.

In a prospective study including treatment of 18 patients with primary hyperparathyroidism, a significant biochemical improvement was observed in 12 and obvious clinical improvement in eight.[106] Similar results were found in a later study in which eight of 12 patients with primary hyperparathyroidism and a high surgical risk became normocalcaemic after treatment.[105] A rare complication is vocal cord paralysis from damage to the recurrent laryngeal nerve.[105,106] Ultrasound-guided chemical parathyroidectomy is an attractive alternative to surgery but should be limited to patients with severe or life-threatening hypercalcaemia who are poor surgical candidates (Fig. 7.30).

Coeliac plexus block

Severe chronic upper abdominal pain, most often caused by pancreatic cancer, may be relieved by blocking the coeliac plexus using alcohol injection under ultrasound

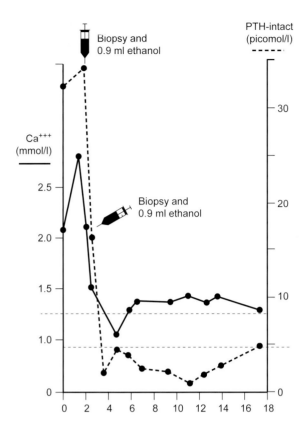

Fig. 7.30 **Example of the value of ultrasonically guided chemical parathyroidectomy** in a patient in hypercalcaemic crisis. The serum concentration of ionised calcium (continuous line) is normalised following injections of ethanol (syringes). The serum concentration of intact parathyroid hormone (PTH-intact) (dotted line) decreases dramatically after injections (same patient as in Fig. 7.29).

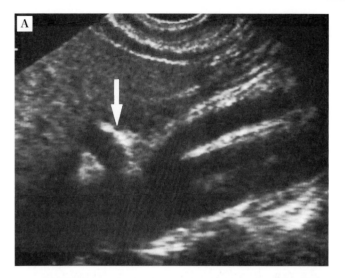

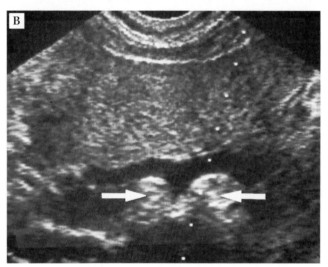

Fig. 7.31 **Localisation of the coeliac trunk prior to coeliac block.** A: Longitudinal scan through the aorta. Arrow indicates coeliac trunk. Anteriorly to the trunk is the superior mesenteric artery. B: Transverse scan through the coeliac trunk. Arrows indicate the two locations where 10 ml of 96% alcohol are injected to inactivate the coeliac plexus.

control[107,108] (Fig. 7.31). Under ultrasound guidance, a fine needle is placed as close as possible on each side of the origin of the coeliac axis. A test injection of 10 ml local anaesthetic on each side may be attempted. If the test block proves effective, permanent coeliac ganglion neurolysis by injection of 10 ml 96% alcohol on each side is performed. Good results can be expected in about one-third of patients.[107,108]

Subclavian vein catheterisation

Subclavian vein catheterisation is commonly used for administering fluid, blood and drugs, as well as for monitoring central venous pressure, but the conventional technique is quite frequently associated with complications, some of which can be serious and even lethal.[109,110] These include pneumothorax, arterial puncture, haemothorax and pneumomediastinum; ultrasound guidance reduces these problems[111,112] (Fig. 7.32).

With the patient in the Trendelenburg position, the transducer is placed lateral to the costoclavicular ligament and the vein identified by the fact that it is compressible with the transducer (Fig. 7.33A). A spinal needle with the guidewire inserted as a stylet (Fig. 7.32) is introduced and will follow the electronically displayed puncture line. When the needle tip is seen inside the vein (Fig. 7.33B) the guidewire is gently pushed forward by the hand holding the needle; its echoes confirm correct placement (Fig. 7.33C). The needle is then withdrawn and the catheter threaded over the guidewire (Figs 7.32 and 7.33D).

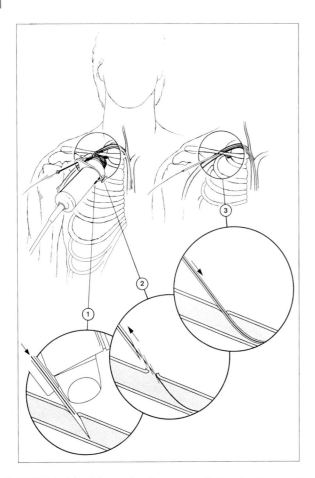

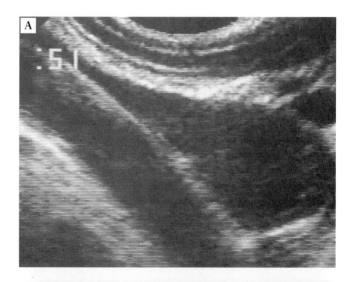

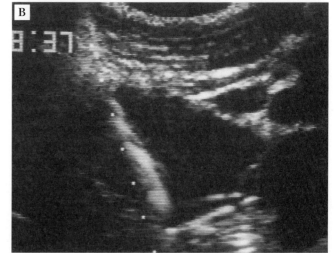

Fig. 7.32 Principle of the one-hand one-step technique for ultrasound-guided subclavian vein catheterisation. (1) The spinal needle with the guidewire serving as a stylet punctures the vein. (2) The needle is withdrawn, leaving the guidewire inside the vein. (3) The catheter is inserted over the guidewire.

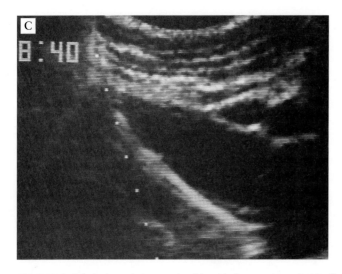

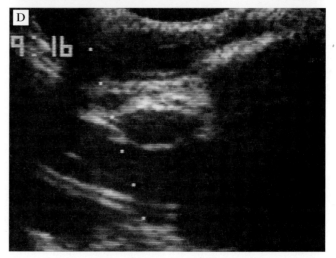

Fig. 7.33 A: Subclavian vein is compressible with the transducer. **B:** Needle is seen inside the vein. **C:** Highly reflective guide wire is clearly visible inside the vein. **D:** Catheter correctly placed in subclavian vein.

REFERENCES

1 Holm H H, Skjoldbye B. Interventional ultrasound. Ultrasound Med Biol 1996; 22: 773–789

2 Holm H H. Interventional ultrasound in Europe. Ultrasound Med Biol 1998; 24: 779–791

3 Takes R P, Righi P, Meeuwis C A et al. The value of ultrasound with ultrasound-guided fine-needle aspiration biopsy compared to computed tomography in the detection of regional metastases in the clinically negative neck. Int J Radiat Oncol Biol Phys 1998; 40: 1027–1032

4 Kratochwil A. Presentation: First World Congress on Ultrasonic Diagnostics in Medicine. Vienna: 1969

5 Gammelgaard P A, Holm H H, Kristensen J K, Rasmussen S N. Ultrasound in renal diagnosis. Film presented at the American Institute of Ultrasound in Medicine, Annual meeting. Cleveland, 1970

6 Holm H H, Kristensen J K, Rasmussen S N, Northeved A, Barlebo H. Ultrasound as a guide in percutaneous puncture technique. Ultrasonics 1972; 10: 83–86

7 Goldberg B B, Pollack H M. Ultrasonic aspiration transducer. Radiology 1972; 102: 187–190

8 Pedersen J F. Percutaneous puncture guided by ultrasonic multitransducer scanning. JCU 1977; 5: 175–177

9 Rifkin M. Biopsy techniques of the prostate. Ultrasound Q 1999; 15: 162–183

10 Holm H H, Gammelgaard J. Ultrasonically guided precise needle placement in the prostate and the seminal vesicles. J Urol 1981; 125: 385–387

11 Menghini G. One-second biopsy of the liver: problems of its clinical application. N Engl J Med 1970; 283: 582–584

12 Hjelmroth H E. Puncture needles and ultrasonic wave propagation in ultrasonically guided puncture. In: Holm H H, Kristensen J K, eds. Ultrasonically guided puncture technique. Copenhagen: Munksgaard, 1980: 25–28

13 Lees W, Gillams A, Slater B. Trials of a new reflective coating for ultrasound-guided needles. Radiology 1999; 213: 281

14 Glenthøj A, Sehested M, Torp-Pedersen S. Diagnostic realiability of cytological and histological fine needle biopsies from focal liver lesions. Histopathology 1989; 15: 375–383

15 Glenthøj A, Sehested M. Histological and cytological fine needle biopsies from focal liver lesions. Intra- and interobserver reproducibility of diagnoses. Acta Pathol Microbial Scand 1989; 97: 611–618

16 Torp-Pedersen S, Juul N, Vyberg M. Histological sampling with a 23 gauge modified Menghini needle. Br J Radiol 1984; 57: 151–154

17 Wulff H R. Rational diagnosis and treatment. Oxford: Blackwell, 1986

18 Smith E H. The hazards of fine needle aspiration biopsy. Ultrasound Med Biol 1984; 10: 629–634

19 Livraghi T, Damascelli B, Lombardi C, Spagnoli I. Risk in fine needle abdominal biopsy. JCU 1983; 11: 77–81

20 Nolsøe C, Nielsen L, Torp-Pedersen S, Holm H H. Major complications and deaths due to interventional ultrasound: a review of 8000 cases. JCU (in press)

21 Drinkovic I, Brkljacic B. Two cases of lethal complications following ultrasound-guided percutaneous fine-needle biopsy of the liver. Cardiovasc Intervent Radiol 1996; 19: 360–363

22 Engzell V, Esposti P L, Rubio C et al. Investigation on tumor spread in connection with aspiration biopsy. Acta Radiol Ther Phys Biol 1971; 10: 385

23 Engell H C. Cancer cells in the circulating blood. Acta Chir Scand 1955; (Suppl 201): 1–70

24 Main M E, Dunning W F. Is the biopsy of neoplasms dangerous? Surg Gynecol Obstet 1946; 82: 567

25 Robbins G F. Is aspiration biopsy of breast cancer dangerous to the patient? Cancer 1954; 7: 774

26 von Schreeb T, Arner O, Skovsted G. Renal adenocarcinoma: is there a risk of spreading tumour cells in diagnostic puncture? Scand J Urol Nephrol 1967; 1: 270–276

27 Chapoutot C, Perney P, Fabre D et al. Needle-tract seeding after ultrasound-guided puncture of hepatocellular carcinoma. A study of 150 patients. Gastroenterol Clin Biol 1999; 23: 552–556

28 Nordenstrom B, Björk V O. Dissemination of cancer cells by needle biopsy of lung. J Thorac Cardiovasc Surg 1973; 65: 671

29 Livraghi T, Benedini V, Lazzaroni S, Meloni F, Torzilli G, Vettori C. Long term results of single session percutaneous ethanol injection in patients with large hepatocellular carcinoma. Cancer 1998; 83: 48–57

30 Stotland B R, Lichtenstein G R. Liver biopsy complications and routine ultrasound [editorial; comment]. Am J Gastroenterol 1996; 91: 1295–1296

31 Pasha T, Gabriel S, Therneau T, Dickson E R, Lindor K D. Cost-effectiveness of ultrasound-guided liver biopsy [see comments]. Hepatology 1998; 27: 1220–1226

32 Smith C I. Cost-effectiveness of ultrasonography in percutaneous liver biopsy [letter; comment]. Hepatology 1999; 29: 610

33 Caturelli E, Giacobbe A, Facciorusso D et al. Percutaneous biopsy in diffuse liver disease: increasing diagnostic yield and decreasing complication rate by routine ultrasound assessment of puncture site [see comments]. Am J Gastroenterol 1996; 91: 1318–1321

35 Di Stasi M, Lencioni R, Solmi L et al. Ultrasound-guided fine needle biopsy of pancreatic masses: results of a multicenter study. Am J Gastroenterol 1998; 93: 1329–1333

36 Juul N, Torp-Pedersen S T, Grønvall S, Holm H H, Kock F. Ultrasonically guided fine needle aspiration biopsy of renal masses. J Urol 1985; 133: 579–581

37 Juul N, Torp-Pedersen S, Glenthøj A. US-guided biopsy of solid renal masses. 5th International Congress on Interventional Ultrasound. Herlev, Denmark, August 1989

38 Price R, Dewbury K, Wedderburn A. Transrectal ultrasound in the diagnosis of prostate carcinoma [letter; comment]. Clin Radiol 1997; 52: 402–403

39 Crundwell M C, Cooke P W, Wallace D M. Patients' tolerance of transrectal ultrasound-guided prostatic biopsy: an audit of 104 cases. Bju Int 1999; 83: 792–795

40 Enlund A I, Varenhorst E. Morbidity of ultrasound-guided transrectal core biopsy of the prostate without prophylactic antibiotic therapy. A prospective study in 415 cases. Br J Urol 1997; 79: 777–780

41 Kleist H, Jonsson O, Lundström S, Naucler J, Nilson A E, Petterson S. Quantitative lipid analysis in the differential diagnosis of cystic renal lesions. Br J Urol 1982; 54: 441–445

42 Dilsiz A, Acikgozoglu S, Gunel E, Dagdonderen L, Koseoglu B, Gundogan A H. Ultrasound-guided percutaneous drainage in the treatment of children with hepatic hydatid disease. Pediatr Radiol 1997; 27: 230–233

43 Felice C, Brunetti E, Crippa F, Bruno R. Treatment of echinococcal abdominal cysts. Ultrasound Q 1999; 15: 223–233

44 Hegedüs L, Hansen J M, Karstrup S, Torp-Pedersen S T, Juul N. Tetracycline for sclerosis of thyroid cysts. A randomised study. Arch Intern Med 1988; 148: 1116–1118

45 Hancke S, Holm H H, Koch F. Ultrasonically guided puncture of pancreatic mass lesions. In: Holm H H, Kristensen J K, eds. Interventional ultrasound. Copenhagen, Munksgaard, 1985: 100–105

46 Granberg S. Ultrasound in the diagnosis and treatment of ovarian tumors. Thesis. Gothenburg, Sweden: Kompendiet Lindome, 1989

47 Montanari E, Serrago M, Esposito N et al. Ultrasound–fluoroscopy guided access to the intrarenal excretory system. Ann Urol 1999; 33: 168–181

48 Maconi G, Parente F, Bianchi Porro G. Hydrogen peroxide enhanced ultrasound-fistulography in the assessment of enterocutaneous fistulas complicating Crohn's disease. Gut 1999; 45: 874–878

49 Makuuchi M, Bandai Y, Ito T, Wada T. Ultrasonically guided percutaneous transhepatic cholangiography and percutaneous pancreatography. Radiology 1980; 134: 767–770

50 Pedersen J F. Percutaneous nephrostomy guided by ultrasound. J Urol 1974; 112: 157–159

51 Nielsen L. Quick step screw dilatator. WFUMB meeting, Washington DC: October 1988

52 Gronvall S. Diagnostic and therapeutic puncture of intraabdominal fluid collections. In: Holm H H, Kristensen J K, eds. Interventional ultrasound. Copenhagen: Munksgaard, 1985: 154–159

53 Pruett L T, Simmons I. R. Status of percutaneous catheter drainage of abscesses. Surg Clin North Am 1988; 68: 89–105

54 Bagi P, Dueholm S, Karstrup S. Percutaneous drainage of appendiceal abscess. Dis Colon Rectum 1987; 30: 532–535

55 Casola G, vanSonnenberg E. Sonographic guidance for percutaneous drainage of abscesses and fluid collections. In: vanSonnenberg E, ed. Interventional ultrasound. New York: Churchill Livingstone, 1987

56 Nosher L J, Winchman K H, Needell S G. Transvaginal pelvic abscess drainage with US guidance. Radiology 1987; 165: 872–873

57 Karstrup S, Nolsøe C, Branrand K, Nielsen K R. Ultrasonically guided percutaneous drainage of breast abscesses. Acta Radiol 1990; 31(2): 157–159

58 Austin H E, Wayne F. The treatment of recurrent malignant pleural effusion. Ann Thorac Surg 1979; 28: 190–203

59 Marks M W, Filly A R, Callen W P. Real-time evaluation of pleural lesions: new observations regarding the probability of obtaining free fluid. Radiology 1982; 142: 162–164

60 Simeone F J. Interventional ultrasound of the thorax. In: vanSonnenberg E. ed. Interventional ultrasound. New York: Churchill Livingstone, 1987

61 vanSonnenberg E, Wittich G R, Cabera O A et al. Percutaneous gastrostomy and gastroenterostomy. II. Clinical experience. AJR 1986; 146: 581–586

62 Ho C S, Gray R R, Goldfinger M, Rosen I E, McPerson R. Percutaneous gastrostomy for internal feeding. Radiology 1985; 156: 349–351

63 Lohela P, Soiva M, Suramo I, Taavitsainen M, Holopeinen O. Ultrasound guidance for percutaneous puncture and drainage in acute cholecystitis. Acta Radiol 1986; 27: 543–546

64 Bandai Y. Percutaneous transhepatic gallbladder drainage (PTGBD). In: Watanabe H, Makuuchi M, eds. Interventional real-time ultrasound. Tokyo: lgaku-Shoin, 1985

65 Gronvall S, Stage G J, Boesby S, Sobye A. Transperitoneal US-guided cholecystostomy in acute cholecystitis. Abstract. 5th International Congress on Interventional Ultrasound, Copenhagen, 1989

66 vanSonnenberg E, Wittich R G, Casola G et al. Percutaneous drainage of infected and noninfected pancreatic pseudocysts: experience in 101 cases. Radiology 1989; 170: 757–761

67 Torres E W, Evert B M, Baumgartner R B, Bernardino E M. Percutaneous aspiration and drainage of pancreatic pseudocysts. AJR 1986; 147: 1007–1009

68 Hancke S, Henriksen W F. Percutaneous pancreatic cystogastrostomy guided by ultrasound scanning and gastroscopy. Br J Surg 1985; 72: 916–917

69 Sacks B, Greenberg J J, Porter H D et al. An internalised double-j catheter for percutaneous transgastric cystogastrostomy. AJR 1989; 152: 523–526

70 Holm H H, Juul N. Interventional ultrasound in cancer therapy. In: Holm H H, Kristensen J K, eds. Interventional ultrasound. Copenhagen: Munksgaard, 1985: 178–184

71 Chapelon J Y, Ribault M, Vernier F, Souchon R, Gelet A. Treatment of localised prostate cancer with transrectal high intensity focused ultrasound. Eur J Ultrasound 1999; 9: 31–38

72 Karstrup S, Holm H H, Torp-Pedersen S, Hegedüs L. Ultrasonically guided percutaneous inactivation of parathyroid tumours. Br J Radiol 1987; 60: 667–670

73 Livraghi T, Festi D, Manti F, Salmi A, Vettori C. US-guided percutaneous alcohol injection of small hepatic and abdominal tumors. Radiology 1986; 161: 309–312

74 Guarnieri A, Canale M. Ultrasonically guided fine needle drug-infiltration of liver metastases. Third Interventional Congress on Interventional Ultrasound, Copenhagen, 1983

75 Chatterjee T, Do D D, Kaufmann U, Mahler F, Meier B. Ultrasound-guided compression repair for treatment of femoral artery pseudoaneurysm: acute and follow-up results. Cath Cardiovasc Diagn 1996; 38: 335–340

76 Holm H H, Juul N, Pedersen J F, Hansen H, Strøyer I. Transperineal 125I seed implantation in prostatic cancer guided by transrectal ultrasonography. J Urol 1983; 130: 283–286

77 Hilaris B S. Brachytherapy in cancer of the prostate: an historical perspective. Semin Surg Oncol 1997; 13: 399–405

78 Ragde H. Prostate cancer brachytherapy [editorial]. Semin Surg Oncol 1997; 13: 389–390

79 Holm H H, Strøyer I, Hansen H, Stadil F. Ultrasonically guided percutaneous interstitial implantation of iodine-125 seeds in cancer therapy. Br J Radiol 1981; 54: 665–670

80 Bleehen N M. Hyperthermia in the treatment of cancer. Br J Cancer 1982; 45: 96–100

81 Matthewson K, Coleridge-Smith P, O'Sullivan J P, Northfield T C, Bown S G. Biological effects of intrahepatic neodynium:yttrium-aluminium-garnet laser photocoagulation in rats. Gastroenterology 1987; 93: 550–557

82 Nolsøe C, Torp-Pedersen S, Oldag E, Holm H H. Nedynium-YAG laser induced interstitial hyperthermia. Development of a diffuser tip. Comparison of ultrasonic and macroscopic measurement of the thermal lesions produced. 8th Congress of Interventional Society for laser surgery and medicine, Taipei, 1989

83 Whitmore W F, Hilaris B, Grabstald H. Retropubic implantation of iodine-125 in the treatment of prostatic cancer. J Urol 1972; 108: 918–920

84 Holm H H. The history of interstitial brachytherapy of prostatic cancer. Semin Surg Oncol 1997; 13: 431–437

85 Ragde H, Blasko J C, Grimm P D et al. Brachytherapy for clinically localized prostate cancer: results at 7- and 8-year follow-up. Semin Surg Oncol 1997; 13: 438–443

86 Sharkey J, Chovnick S D, Behar R J et al. Outpatient ultrasound-guided palladium 103 brachytherapy for localized adenocarcinoma of the prostate: a preliminary report of 434 patients [see comments]. Urology 1998; 51: 796–803

87 Hastak S M, Gammelgaard J, Holm H H. Transrectal ultrasonic volume determination of the prostate: A preoperative and postoperative study. J Urol 1982; 127: 1115–1118

88 Blasko J C, Ragde H, Luse R W, Sylvester J E, Cavanagh W, Grimm P D. Should brachytherapy be considered a therapeutic option in localized prostate cancer? Urol Clin North Am 1996; 23: 633–650

89 Prestidge B R, Prete J J, Buchholz T A et al. A survey of current clinical practice of permanent prostate brachytherapy in the United States. Int J Radiat Oncol Biol Phys 1998; 40: 461–465

90 Walsh P C. Ten-year disease free survival after transperineal sonography-guided iodine-125 brachytherapy with or without 45-gray external beam irradiation in the treatment of patients with clinically localized, low to high gleason grade prostate carcinoma. J Urol 1999; 161: 357–358

91 Shinagawa T, Ukaji H, Iino Y et al. Intratumoral injection of absolute ethanol under ultrasound imaging for treatment of small hepatocellular carcinoma: attempts in three cases. Acta Hepatol Jpn 1985; 26: 99–103

92 Sheu J C, Huang G T, Chen D S et al. Small hepatocellular carcinoma: Intratumor ethanol treatment using new needle and guidance system. Radiology 1987; 163: 43–48

93 Livraghi T. Percutaneous ethanol injection in hepatocellular carcinoma. Digestion 1998; 59 (Suppl 2): 80–82

94 Livraghi T. Percutaneous ethanol injection in the treatment of hepatocellular carcinoma in cirrhosis. Hepatogastroenterology 1998; 45(Suppl 3): 1248–1253

95 Shina S, Yasuda H, Muto H et al. Percutaneous ethanol injection in the treatment of liver neoplasms. AJR 1987; 149: 949–952

96 Solbiat L, Goldberg S N, Ierace T, Dellanoce M, Livraghi T, Gazelle G S. Radio-frequency ablation of hepatic metastases: postprocedural assessment with a US microbubble contrast agent – early experience. Radiology 1999; 211: 643–649

97 Butch R J, Simeone J F, Mueller P R. Thyroid and parathyroid ultrasonography. Radiol Clin North Am 1985; 23: 57–71

98 Chen M H, Chang T C, Hsiao Y L, Chang T J, Huang S H. Combination of color Doppler ultrasonography and ultrasound-guided fine-needle aspiration cytology for localization of parathyroid lesions. J Formosan Med Ass 1999; 98: 506–511

99 Söderström N. Identification of normal tissue by aspiration cytology. In: Linsk J A, Franzen S, eds. Clinical aspiration cytology. Philadelphia: J B Lippincott, 1983: 1–24

100 Glenthøj A, Karstrup S. Parathyroid identification by ultrasonically guided aspiration cytology. Is a correct cytological identification possible? Acta Pathol Microbiol Scand 1989; 97: 497–502

101 Doppman L J, Krudy A G, Marx J S et al. Aspiration of enlarged parathyroid glands for parathyroid hormone assay. Radiology 1983; 148: 32–35

102 Karstrup S, Glenthøj A, Torp-Pedersen S, Hegedüs L, Holm H H. Ultrasonically guided fine needle aspiration of suggested enlarged parathyroid glands. Acta Radiol 1988; 29: 213–216

103 Karstrup S, Glenthøj A, Hainau B, Hegedüs L, Torp-Pedersen S, Holm H H. Ultrasound-guided, histological, fine-needle biopsy from suspected parathyroid tumours: Success-rate and reliability of histological diagnosis. Br J Radiol 1989; 62: 981–985

104 Solbiati L, Giangrande A, De Pra L, Bellotti E, Cantu P, Ravetto C. Percutaneous ethanol injection of parathyroid tumours under US guidance: treatment of secondary hyperparathyroidism. Radiology 1985; 155: 607–610

105 Karstrup S, Holm H H, Glenthøj A, Hegedüs L. Nonsurgical treatment of primary hyperparathyroidism with sonographically guided percutaneous injection of ethanol: results in a selected series of patients. AJR 1990; 154: 1087–1090

106 Karstrup S, Transbøl I, Holm H H, Glenthøj A, Hegedüs L. Ultrasound-guided chemical parathyroidectomy in patients with primary hyperparathyroidism: a prospective study. Br J Radiol 1989; 62: 1037–1042

107 Gammelgaard J, Jensen F. Ultrasonically guided celiac plexus block in intractable pain. Abstract: 4th European Congress on Ultrasonics in Medicine. Dubrovnik, Yugoslavia, 1981

108 Greiner L, Ulatowski L, Prohm P. Sonographisch gezielte und intraoperative alkoholblockade bei der z liakalganglien bei konservativ nicht beherrschbaren malignombedingten oberbauchschmerzen. Ultraschall Med 1983; 4: 57–59

109 Eerola R, Kaukinen L, Kaukinen S. Analysis of 13 800 subclavian vein catheterisations. Acta Anaesthesiol Scand 1985; 29: 193–197

110 Mitchell E S, Clark A R. Complications of central venous catheterisation. AJR 1979; 133: 467–476

111 Machi J, Takeda J, Kakegawa T. Safe jugular and subclavian venipuncture under ultrasonographic guidance. Am J Surg 1987; 153: 321–323

112 Fry W R, Clagett G C, O'Rourke P T. Ultrasound-guided central venous access. Arch Surg 1999; 134: 738–740; discussion 741

Intra-operative ultrasound

Robert A Kane

Introduction

Intra-operative ultrasound (IOUS) is one of the most rapidly growing areas in ultrasonography and diagnostic imaging. The demand for IOUS imaging in the abdomen has grown steadily over the past 10–15 years because of the recognition that it provides consistent high-quality information to the surgeon at the time of the operative procedure, and that this is useful in selecting the appropriate surgical approach.[1-4] A prospective study of the impact of IOUS on surgical decision making at the time of planned liver resection for primary or secondary neoplasms demonstrated it to be highly efficacious, with a direct influence on surgical management in nearly 50% of cases.[1]

Nevertheless, many radiologists are still reluctant to become involved in intra-operative studies because of the time required; as a result, the majority of IOUS studies are performed by surgeons themselves, either with or (frequently) without consultation with radiologists. Although surgeons certainly can learn to scan and interpret IOUS studies, very few are specifically trained in these techniques and many do not have the time to acquire sufficient experience to ensure consistent high-quality examinations. The inexperienced tend to move the probe too rapidly across the targeted field, may have less awareness of ultrasound artefacts and techniques to optimise image quality, and probably also have less appreciation of subtle abnormalities than do experienced ultrasonologists.

For these reasons, radiologists should be willing to scrub up and perform the intra-operative ultrasound examination, and strategies to improve their efficiency in IOUS have been evolved. The radiologist can learn to change and scrub, perform the scan and return to the radiology department within 30 minutes. The actual time required to scan a liver or other intra-abdominal organs is generally only 5–10 minutes. Strategies for maximising efficiency are listed in Table 8.1. This efficient approach should encourage radiologists to be more willing to perform as well as interpret IOUS scans, and should result in better-quality examinations. An alternative, although less satisfactory, approach is for the surgeon to perform the scan with the radiologist available for consultation when the findings are perplexing. This could be remote (via PACS or other tele-radiology link), but more commonly would require the radiologist to observe the scans in the operating suite, though not actually to scrub up. Although this approach is practical, the lack of hand-to-eye information obtained during the scanning process makes it less effective.

As with many seemingly new and innovative techniques, the history of IOUS is surprisingly long. One of the earliest reports of intra-operative ultrasound was in the 1960s, when A-mode ultrasound was used to detect renal calculi during nephrolithotomy; subsequently reports of B-mode ultrasound for this use were published.[5] Similarly there were early publications describing the use of ultrasound for the detection of biliary calculi.[6] It was not until the 1980s, however, with the development of specific probes for IOUS applications, that the field began to develop rapidly, and there are now numerous reports describing its applications in neuro- and abdominal surgery.[7-11]

Equipment

Although standard ultrasound probes with sterile coverings can be used for intra-operative scanning, in most instances their size and configuration make it difficult to access the targeted organs. Consequently, specifically designed small probes have been developed for various intra-operative uses (Fig. 8.1). These can be linear, curvilinear or phased

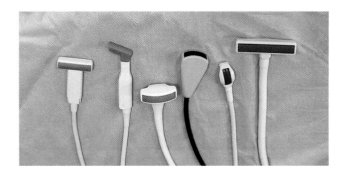

Fig. 8.1 End-fire and side-fire IOUS probes, both curvilinear and linear arrays.

Table 8.1 Strategies for efficient intra-operative ultrasound scanning

Strategy	Notes
1. Book scan in advance	Allows scheduling to help clash of commitment
2. Take scanner to theatre in advance	Minimises time spent
3. Radiologist in interventional	No need to change again
4. Presterilise probe	Saves time applying probe covers
5. Liaise with surgeons	Cooperation reduces time commitment
	Surgeon calls radiologist 10–15 min before scan needed

array probes, usually with spectral and colour Doppler, as well as grey scale modes. Because many of the barriers to ultrasound imaging, such as skin, subcutaneous fat and gas, do not present a problem for intraoperative imaging, the transducer frequency can be higher than for standard abdominal ultrasound studies. Typically, frequencies ranging from 5 to 10 MHz are appropriate, depending on the target organ.

For the liver 5 MHz is usually a good choice to allow complete penetration to the back of the right lobe, which may be up to 12 cm deep.[12] Organ systems such as the gall-bladder, common bile duct, pancreas and vascular structures can be scanned with higher frequencies of 7–10 MHz, as penetration of only a few centimetres is required. The optimum probe configuration also depends on the target organ: end-fire probes are suitable for the pancreas, common bile duct and gallbladder, kidneys and vascular structures, but scanning of the liver is much easier with a side-fire probe. Using an end-fire probe may result in incomplete scanning of the dome and right lateral aspects of the liver, particularly if the liver has not been fully mobilised or lies high under the diaphragm. A side-fire probe can be cradled in the hand and scanned across the liver surface even in the tightest areas, such as the dome of the liver or between the ribcage and lateral liver margin.[13]

Special probes are also required for laparoscopic ultrasound (LUS). These systems require miniaturised linear or curvilinear array probes mounted on a shaft, typically some 30 cm or more in length. Although the initial systems were entirely rigid, it rapidly became evident that some degree of flexibility of the scanning tip improved contact with the target organs (Fig. 8.2). Most commercially available systems operate at frequencies between 5 and 7.5 MHz, and many allow multiple frequencies to be selected for the same probe. The system must be small enough to fit through a standard 10–11 mm laparoscope port and the transducer tip can usually be flexed in the plane of the transducer shaft. Some systems also allow a left/right deflection of the transducer tip. Doppler is routinely available, but most systems do not as yet have biopsy guidance devices.[14]

Methods of probe sterilisation vary according to the manufacturers' specifications and individual institutional protocols. Ethylene oxide gas sterilisation avoids the need to use probe covers and can save a few minutes time in theatre, but requires overnight aeration and therefore limits the use of a gas-sterilised probe to once a day. However, many ultrasound manufacturers do not allow gas sterilisation of their probes for fear that the high aeration temperatures might damage the transducer.[15] Most manufacturers recommend sterilisation in liquid glutaraldehyde, but this also requires prolonged immersion for several hours, which again may limit probe utilisation to one procedure each day.[16] In addition, in many operative suites the use of glutaraldehyde is prohibited on any

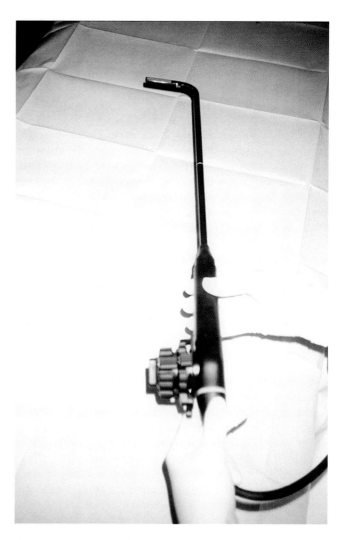

Fig. 8.2 Laparoscopic probe. This linear-array configuration allows left/right deflection as well as flexion and extension of the transducer tip.

instruments that contact organs or structures within the body cavity, and environmental concerns have led some hospitals to prohibit the use of glutaraldehyde completely. Consequently, in most operating theatres sterile sheaths are used: these should be large enough to cover not only the scanning surface but also the entire probe handle and cable. Specially designed covers that fit snugly over the transducer are optimal; some of these include a long sheath which can cover the entire cable, but if not, a conventional arthroscopic camera drape can be used. A small amount of sterile gel or saline should be used inside the probe cover to ensure good acoustic coupling. Specially designed covers minimise problems with wrinkles, which produce air pockets over the scanning surface, and thus reduce artefacts that limit the scan quality.[17] One of the important advantages of using sterile probe covers is the ability to use the same probe more than once a day.

Techniques

Scanning technique varies according to the target organ. In general, for right-handed sonologists it is easiest to scan from the patient's right side, and it is important to position the scanner so that the screen can be viewed comfortably; this can usually be achieved by positioning the scanner towards the patient's head. Usually there is sufficient moisture in the body cavity to afford good acoustic coupling but, if needed, sterile saline can be applied over the surface of the target organ to provide better contact. Gel should not be applied to the abdominal cavity, although sterile gel may be used as a couplant inside the sterile transducer sheath.

For the liver, the transducer is preferably orientated in the transverse or the axial plane. With the probe on the left-most edge of the liver at the dome, a scan is made downward to the caudal edge of the liver. The transducer is then moved towards the patient's right, by approximately the width of the transducer footprint, and a second scan is obtained from dome to caudal edge. In this fashion, by slightly overlapping the scanning fields, the entire liver can be studied in approximately 5 minutes.[13] A 5 MHz probe should give complete penetration to the posterior part of the liver in nearly all cases, thereby decreasing the amount of scanning time required and simplifying the procedure.

Scans of the gallbladder and common bile duct can usually be performed by placing an end-fire probe directly on the surface of the structure. At times portions of the gallbladder neck and cystic duct may be best visualised by scanning through the liver parenchyma and, likewise, portions of the distal-most common bile duct will be best seen by scanning through the pancreas. If reverberation artefacts limit visualisation, sterile saline may be used to provide an acoustic stand-off. When a complete evaluation of the bile ducts is necessary it may be preferable to change to a side-fire probe for best visualisation of the intrahepatic ducts.[18]

Similarly, imaging the pancreas is best performed with an end-fire probe in direct contact with its surface. The pancreas can also be visualised through the overlying stomach and duodenum by compressing these structures with the ultrasound probe, and portions of the pancreas may also be visualised by scanning through the liver substance. If access to the pancreas is limited the peritoneal cavity can be filled with degassed saline and scans obtained by placing the transducer in the saline puddle, using the fluid as an acoustic stand-off. Complete evaluation of patients with malignant pancreatic neoplasms should also include scans of the liver for metastases, again usually requiring a side-fire liver probe. Scans of intra-abdominal vascular structures and other organs, such as the kidneys or spleen, can be readily accomplished with end-fire probes.

When using laparoscopic probes it is important to decide which port provides best access to the target organ. Because the probe is mounted on a long, rigid shaft, choosing a port too close to the target organ may be awkward and present mechanical difficulties in siting the transducer adequately on the appropriate surface. For instance, a relatively high right subcostal port might be too close to image the gallbladder and common bile duct adequately, and using a peri-umbilical port will often provide more satisfactory access. For complete assessment of the liver using laparoscopic ultrasound it is frequently necessary to use more than one port, as the lateral part of the left lobe may be inaccessible from a right subcostal port, but the dome or right lateral aspects of the liver might be poorly visualised from a midline or left-sided port.[17] Once again it may be useful to fill the abdominal cavity with degassed sterile saline to provide an acoustic stand-off medium.

It is also very important during laparoscopic ultrasound scanning to visualise the transducer via the laparoscope during the procedure, because the probe operator experiences very little tactile sensation and tissues can be damaged if the probe is not continuously visualised. This can be facilitated by use of a simple video mixer, which allows simultaneous display of the ultrasound and the laparoscopic images on the same viewing screen, the latter as a smaller 'picture within the picture'.[14]

Applications

Gallbladder and biliary tract

Pre-operative ultrasound imaging of the gallbladder is excellent and consequently requests for IOUS of the gallbladder are uncommon. Patients undergoing gastric stapling procedures or other forms of gastric exclusion for the treatment of morbid obesity are routinely screened pre-operatively for the presence of gallstones, because of the high incidence of acute cholecystitis in patients with gallstones who lose weight. Therefore, if pre-operative imaging demonstrates gallstones the patient undergoes cholecystectomy at the time of gastric bypass procedure. Because these patients are markedly obese, there may be difficulty in obtaining adequate pre-operative ultrasound images. In this rare instance IOUS imaging of the gallbladder can be performed rapidly (Fig. 8.3) and can identify small stones which may not have been visualised pre-operatively or, alternatively, confirm the gallbladder to be normal.[19]

IOUS can play a role in evaluating gallbladder masses, whether found incidentally during surgical inspection and palpation, or to assess the extent of a known gallbladder carcinoma prior to resection (Fig. 8.4). In this setting one would look carefully for signs of hepatic and lymph node metastases, which might make radical resection impossible. Direct invasion of gallbladder carcinoma into the adjacent liver bed occurs frequently (stage T3), and in this

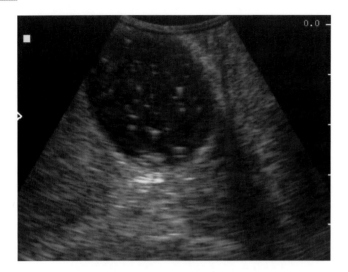

Fig. 8.3 **IOUS of gallbladder.** The gallbladder contains sludge and numerous tiny stones, poorly visualised on pre-operative imaging.

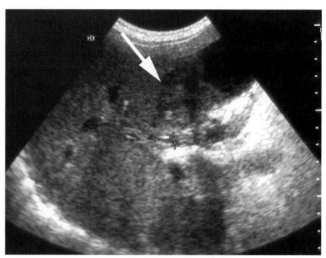

Fig. 8.4 **Carcinoma of the gallbladder.** The arrow points to an area of direct invasion through the gallbladder wall into the bare area of the liver.

case most surgeons advocate a wedge resection of adjacent normal liver parenchyma in order to obtain a tumour-free margin.[20]

IOUS evaluation of the bile ducts for stones has been regarded as competitive or even superior to radiographic intra-operative cholangiography by several groups.[21] As most gallbladder surgery is now performed laparoscopically, there has been a renewed interest in the use of LUS imaging for assessment of the bile ducts for choledocholithiasis. Although laparoscopically assisted intra-operative cholangiography is technically challenging, the extrahepatic common duct, as well as the intrahepatic bile ducts, can be well visualised[22] and common duct stones identified.[23] Jakimowicz *et al.*[24] reported a large consecutive series of patients in whom LUS imaging of the common bile duct was very successful, but unsuspected pathology was demonstrated in fewer than 4%. A similar study by Rothlin *et al.*[25] also found unsuspected common duct stones in only 3% of 100 consecutive patients.

Whenever the patient's history, clinical findings or laboratory assessment suggests the possibility of choledocholithiasis a pre-operative endoscopic retrograde cholangiographic study is usually performed, both for diagnostic assessment and for therapeutic intervention when positive, via endoscopic sphincterotomy and stone extraction. This aggressive use of the endoscopic approach means that intra-operative bile duct assessment for stones is rarely needed.

IOUS imaging frequently provides valuable information in patients undergoing surgical procedures for both benign and malignant lesions of the biliary tract (Fig. 8.5). It can define the site and extent of the obstruction precisely, as well as identify the presence of metastatic disease in the liver and lymph nodes, and thereby help to plan the

optimal type of biliary bypass procedure or surgical resection. The detection of metastatic disease or the demonstration of tumour boundaries that are too extensive for resection may even result in the surgical approach being cancelled in favour of endoscopic or percutaneous transhepatic procedures.[26]

IOUS and LUS are very valuable in patients with segmental Caroli's disease in helping to define normal and abnormal duct segments and guide surgical resection (Fig. 8.6). In patients with more diffuse Caroli's disease, as well as those with oriental cholangiohepatitis, IOUS is helpful in defining the extent of disease and the presence of occult stones and sludge, which frequently are incompletely imaged by pre-operative studies. Intra-operative imaging is also useful in planning the surgical approach to resection of choledochal cysts (Fig. 8.7) by demonstrating the full extent of disease and defining areas that are unaffected. Although these latter conditions are rare, the information obtained by intra-operative or laparoscopic ultrasound is of critical importance and unobtainable by other methods.

Pancreas

One of the earliest successful applications of intra-operative ultrasound imaging was in the identification and localisation of islet cell tumours. Functioning neuroendocrine tumours are often quite small when discovered because the effects of their hormones lead to early investigation. Many pre-operative imaging modalities have been used to detect these neoplasms, including ultrasonography, CT, MRI, superselective angiography, radionuclide scanning and selective portal venous sampling. The sheer number of techniques recommended for the work-up attests to

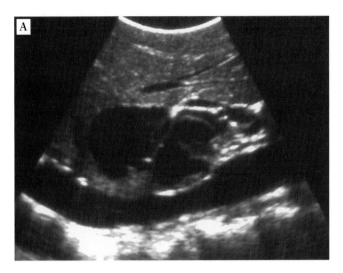
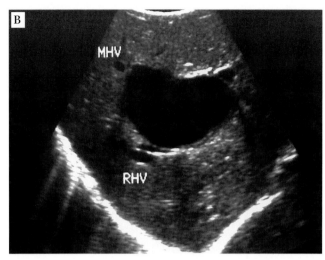

Fig. 8.5 **Biliary cystadenoma. A:** The medial component demonstrates a typical multiloculated configuration with relatively thin septa. The mass insinuates between the right portal vein and the inferior vena cava. **B:** Laterally a unilocular component of the mass is seen and its relationships to the middle hepatic vein (MHV) and right hepatic vein (RHV) are demonstrated.

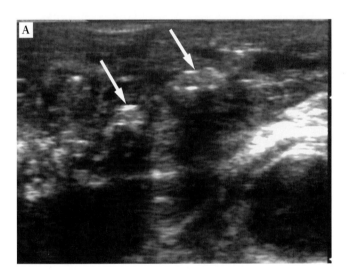
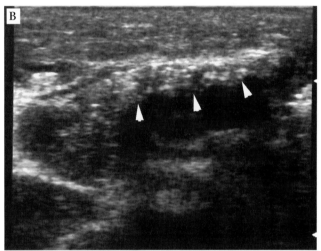

Fig. 8.6 **Segmental Caroli's disease. A:** Discrete 5 mm stones (arrows) are visualised in the ducts of segment III, corresponding to the pre-operative cholangiogram. **B:** A segmental duct is seen to be filled with sludge and crystalline material (arrowheads). The subtle acoustic shadowing could only be demonstrated on IOUS because of the higher-frequency transducers used.

the difficulties in detection of these very small lesions. Indeed, many are too small to be palpable in the operating suite and, in the past, blind resection of portions of the pancreas was performed when the tumour site could not be localised adequately.

Intra-operative ultrasound, however, is the method of choice for the detection of functional pancreatic islet cell tumours, as high-resolution probes of 7–10 MHz can be used. Most islet cell tumours are homogeneous and therefore relatively echo-poor compared to the surrounding pancreas.[27] They are also hypervascular, and velocity and power colour Doppler may be helpful in their detection.

Intra-operative ultrasound is clearly the most accurate technique for localising islet cell tumours of the pancreas, and its routine use can obviate the necessity for an overly extensive pre-operative work-up.[28,29]

Most insulinomas are solitary and echo-poor,[30] although in one series 10% were described as being of increased reflectivity.[31] This apparent increase in reflectivity may be a relative phenomenon, particularly in young patients in whom the pancreas itself is less reflective than is typically seen in older age groups (Fig. 8.8). A complete IOUS study should include a search for metastatic peripancreatic and portal lymphadenopathy and liver metastases, but these are

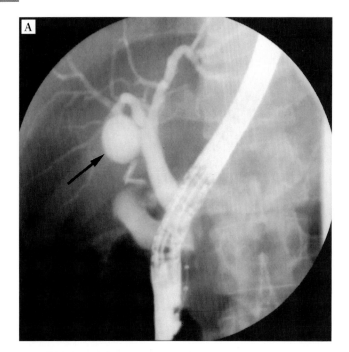

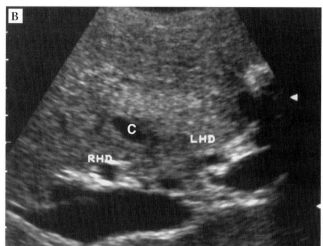

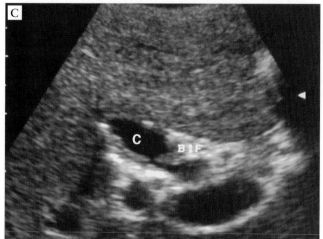

Fig. 8.7 Intrahepatic choledochal cyst. A: An ERCP shows normal extrahepatic and intrahepatic bile ducts and a diverticulum (arrow) representing the choledochal cyst. The site of origin is not visualised. **B:** The IOUS scan demonstrates a portion of the choledochal cyst (C) and the right (RHD) and left (LHD) main intrahepatic ducts. **C:** Just caudal, the communication of the choledochal cyst (C) to the right and left hepatic duct bifurcation (BIF) is well demonstrated.

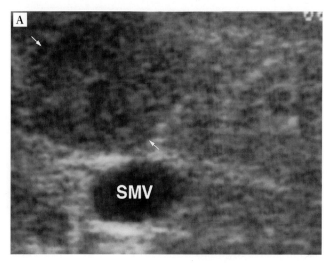

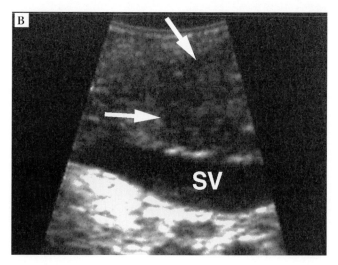

Fig. 8.8 Insulinomas. A: A transverse view shows a solid, slightly echo-poor rounded mass (arrows) in the neck of the pancreas just anterior to the superior mesenteric vein (SMV). **B:** An isoechoic insulinoma (arrows) is shown lying anterior to the splenic vein (SV).

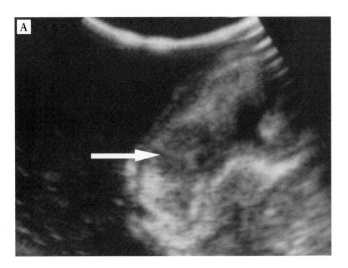
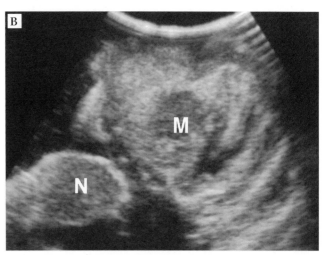

Fig. 8.9 **Gastrinoma. A:** The arrow points to a 6 mm gastrinoma in the wall of the duodenum. Imaging was facilitated by filling the abdomen with saline to provide an acoustic stand-off. **B:** Further scanning demonstrates the primary tumour (M) in the duodenal wall, as well as a larger metastatic lymph node (N).

infrequently seen with insulinomas, which are usually benign. Patients with multiple endocrine neoplasia syndrome (MEN type I), in which there are tumours of the pancreas, pituitary gland, thyroid and parathyroid glands and adrenal cortex, often have multifocal pancreatic islet cell tumours. A very careful search of the entire pancreas is essential to detect these numerous small adenomas.[32]

Gastrinomas are also often multiple and are frequently found outside the pancreas,[33] although most occur in the so-called 'gastrinoma triangle', which extends from the head and neck of the pancreas to the junction of the cystic duct and common bile duct superolaterally, and to the second and third portions of the duodenum caudally.[34] They are frequently found in the wall of the duodenum (Fig. 8.9), as well as in extraluminal soft tissues and adjacent lymph nodes (Fig. 8.10). Gastrinomas are multiple in 20–40% of cases and most are malignant, so that careful scanning of the liver is recommended to search for metastases. Other types of islet cell neoplasms, such as glucagonoma and somatostatinoma, are also frequently malignant and require a careful search for metastatic disease.

IOUS imaging is infrequently required for patients with ductal adenocarcinoma of the pancreas because this scirrhous lesion is usually easily palpated. However, pancreatic adenocarcinomas may be associated with extensive chronic pancreatitis (Fig. 8.11), and in this setting palpation may not distinguish the cancer from the adjacent chronic inflammation (Fig. 8.12); here IOUS may be useful in defining the 'mass within a mass'. Pancreatic adenocarcinoma is typically seen as a solid, echo-poor and fairly discrete mass. IOUS can be used for staging of pancreatic neoplasms, although pre-operative CT angiography or MRI are highly accurate in staging vascular invasion. However, these studies are still relatively insensitive to

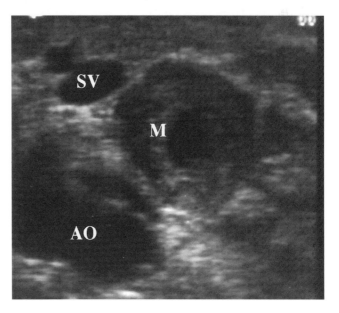

Fig. 8.10 **Gastrinoma.** In this patient no lesion was identified within the pancreas or duodenal wall, but a mass (M) was seen adjacent to the third part of the duodenum between the aorta (AO) and splenic vein (SV), representing extrapancreatic and extraduodenal gastrinoma, presumably a lymph node metastasis.

metastatic disease involving the peritoneal surfaces and mesentery, as well as small metastases on the liver surface and lymph node metastases. Consequently many surgeons routinely use laparoscopy prior to open laparotomy, in order to detect occult metastatic disease. In this setting the addition of laparoscopic ultrasound has been advocated, both to assess resectability by evaluation of critical adjacent vasculature (Fig. 8.13), such as the superior mesenteric vein, splenic vein, superior mesenteric and coeliac

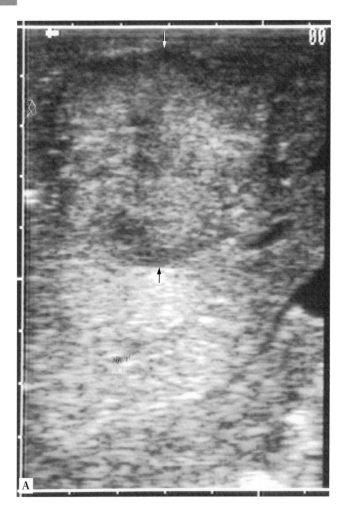

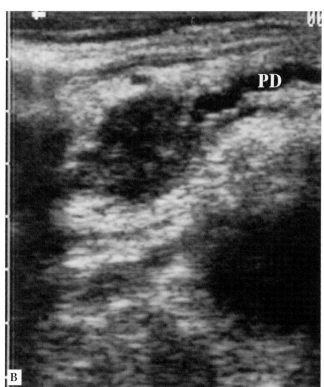

Fig. 8.11 Pancreatic cancer. A: A 4 cm hepatic metastasis (arrows).
B: The primary adenocarcinoma in the head of the pancreas could not
be palpated because of surrounding inflammation, but is well visualised
on IOUS. Pancreatic duct (PD) dilatation is seen proximal to the mass.

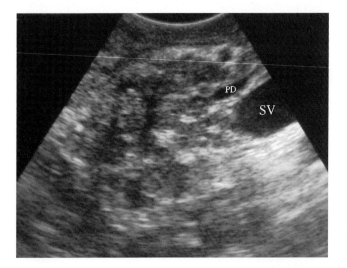

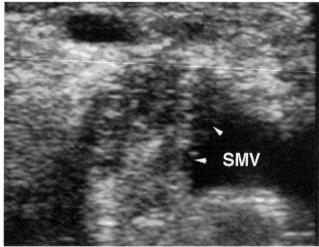

Fig. 8.12 Calcific pancreatitis. IOUS image of a large heterogeneous
pancreatic head with scattered foci of calcification. No discrete
echo-poor mass was demonstrated within this enlarged head and
biopsies confirmed only chronic pancreatitis. PD – pancreatic duct,
SV – splenic vein.

Fig. 8.13 Unresectable pancreatic carcinoma. There is invasion of the
wall of the superior mesenteric vein (SMV) (arrowheads), rendering
this mass unresectable.

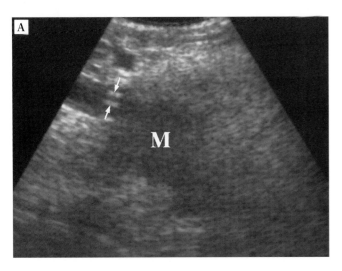

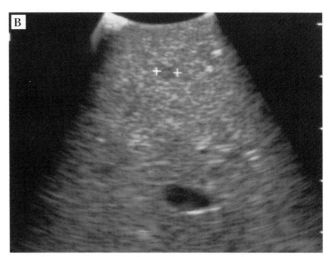

Fig. 8.14 **Metastatic pancreatic adenocarcinoma. A:** The common bile duct and biliary stent (arrows) are demonstrated close to a small solid mass (M) in the head of the pancreas. **B:** Laparoscopic scan of the liver demonstrates a 4 mm metastasis (between calipers) from this pancreatic adenocarcinoma.

arteries, and to look for metastatic lymphadenopathy and metastatic disease in the liver (Fig. 8.14).[35,36] In a prospective series by Hann *et al.*, LUS provided additional information in 33% of patients with pancreatic carcinoma and altered surgical management in 17%.[37]

Cystic neoplasms of the pancreas can be evaluated with IOUS. Microcystic serous adenomas of the pancreas

(Fig. 8.15) are almost invariably benign and typically appear as multiple, very small, thin-walled cysts, most of which are only a few millimetres in diameter, the largest cystic components usually being less than 1–2 cm in diameter. When larger cystic cavities are identified, or when there is evidence of thickening and irregularity of the septa, mural nodularity, or solid components to the lesion (Fig. 8.16), the findings suggest mucinous cystadenoma or cystadenocarcinoma.[13] It is impossible to distinguish benign from malignant versions of this tumour and, as the benign version is considered to be premalignant, surgical

Fig. 8.15 **Microcystic (serous) cystadenoma of the pancreatic head (C).** IOUS image shows a single thin septation and no nodularity. SV – splenic vein, AO – aorta, IVC – inferior vena cava.

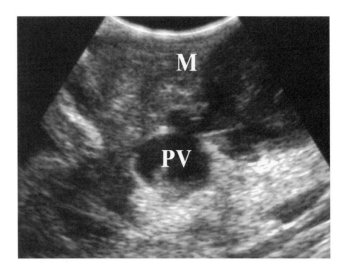

Fig. 8.16 **Mucinous cystadenocarcinoma of the pancreas.** IOUS scan shows a large mass (M) with an echo-poor complex cystic portion as well as a more solid portion extending out of the pancreas anterior to the portal vein (PV). This complex solid and cystic appearance is indicative of a mucinous tumour, either premalignant or malignant.

resection is needed. IOUS imaging may be useful for patients who are undergoing surgery for complications of chronic pancreatitis, such as biliary or pancreatic drainage procedures. The pancreatic duct can be seen, whether normal or dilated (Fig. 8.17), as well as pseudocysts of the pancreas and any communications between the pseudocyst cavity and the pancreatic duct.[38,39] This information can be useful in guiding the choice of drainage procedure, as communication between an obstructed pancreatic duct and a pseudocyst cavity may require separate drainage of the pancreatic duct itself (Fig. 8.18). Colour Doppler should be used when evaluating focal peripancreatic fluid collections in order to exclude an aneurysm or pseudo-aneurysm as a complication of acute pancreatitis.[13] As mentioned above, pancreatic cancer may arise in a gland involved with chronic pancreatitis, or the pancreatic cancer itself may result in pancreatitis. In this setting it is difficult to assess the presence of pancreatic cancer by palpation, and IOUS can be employed to search for a focal mass and to guide intra-operative biopsies.[40]

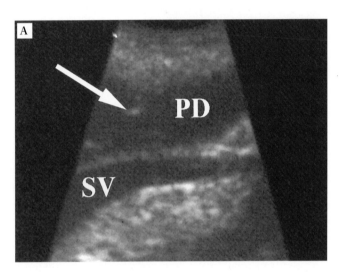
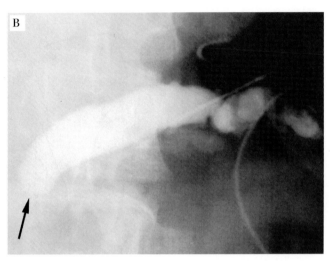

Fig. 8.17 Obstructed pancreatic duct. A: IOUS demonstrates a dilated pancreatic duct (PD) immediately anterior to the splenic vein (SV). The arrow indicates a needle which was passed under real-time guidance into the dilated duct for pancreatography. **B:** Pancreatogram demonstrates complete obstruction of the pancreatic duct (arrow) caused by a carcinoma in the head of the pancreas. Dilatation and changes of chronic pancreatitis are seen in the duct.

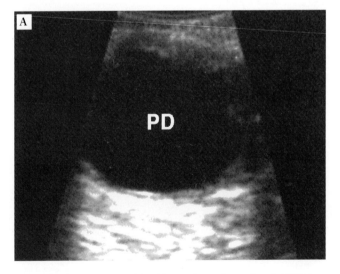
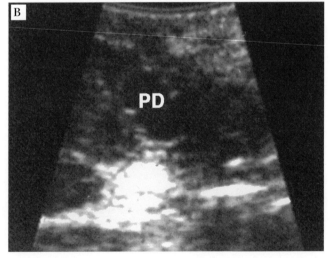

Fig. 8.18 Chronic pancreatitis with pseudocyst formation. A: IOUS image of a pseudocyst of the pancreatic duct (PD). **B:** Proximal to the pseudocyst there is an irregular dilated and tortuous pancreatic duct (PD) which communicated with the pseudocyst.

Liver

IOUS of the liver is most frequently performed in patients with primary and metastatic malignancies for whom surgical resection is planned. It affords the most complete detection of both primary and metastatic tumours within the liver, detecting 20–30% more lesions than conventional pre-operative imaging techniques and 10–15% more than CT arterial portography. Real-time demonstration of lobar and segmental liver anatomy allows accurate tumour localisation and facilitates planning of the most appropriate type of lobar or segmental resection. It can also provide guidance for non-segmental wedge resections in order to ensure adequate surgical margins. Assessment of the vascular supply and drainage, particularly accessory or aberrant vasculature, as well as assessment of vascular invasion, helps plan surgery, particularly in patients with primary hepatocellular carcinoma. Real-time guidance for biopsy procedures and aspiration and drainage of fluid collections is simple and precise. IOUS can also be used for real-time guidance for tumour ablations, such as cryosurgery, or alcohol or radiofrequency ablations (see Chapter 7).

There are two particular advantages to the use of IOUS for liver imaging. First, the direct application of the probe to the liver surface avoids both the attenuation of sound and the noise production generated by the superficial tissues. Secondly, higher-frequency transducers can be used routinely, producing better spatial resolution. IOUS can routinely demonstrate cysts as small as 1–3 mm in diameter (Fig. 8.19) and solid lesions as small as 3–5 mm (Fig. 8.20), and this spatial resolution is superior to all methods of pre-operative imaging. IOUS consistently detects many more liver lesions than predicted by pre-

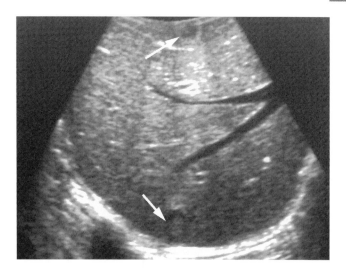

Fig. 8.20 Colorectal metastases. Arrows point to two non-palpable metastatic lesions, each less than 1 cm in diameter.

operative imaging techniques and, because the spatial resolution is improved (Fig. 8.21), the majority of additional lesions are 1 cm or less in diameter.[41,42] Although CT arterial portography (CTAP) has a high sensitivity for the detection of focal liver lesions, IOUS detects 10–15% more lesions.[43] In addition, the push to increase the sensitivity of CTAP results in a decrease in specificity, with false-positive findings resulting from small hepatic cysts, haemangiomas and other pseudolesions caused by perfusion anomalies (Fig. 8.22).[44,45]

Even with the best pre-operative imaging techniques, identification of metastatic disease outside the liver, including peritoneal and mesenteric implants and lymphadenopathy, is difficult. Because extrahepatic metastatic disease is generally considered a contraindication to liver resection, laparoscopy is often performed at the beginning of the procedure (Fig. 8.23).[46] Although laparoscopy may detect small surface liver metastases, the addition of laparoscopic ultrasound may allow the detection of deeper occult metastases undetectable by routine laparoscopy. The spatial resolution of LUS is similar to that of open IOUS, and the impact could be even greater as palpation of the liver is not possible during laparoscopy. However, there are more technical challenges in performing LUS, and the overall detection rate may be slightly less than with IOUS.[47,48] Nevertheless, it seems logical to use laparoscopic ultrasound in this setting in order to avoid unnecessary laparotomy incisions in patients who ultimately prove unresectable.

Both grey scale and colour Doppler imaging should be used to assess hepatic vascular supply and drainage, particularly to identify anomalous or accessory vessels. A replaced or accessory left hepatic artery is well seen, arising from the left gastric artery and entering the liver

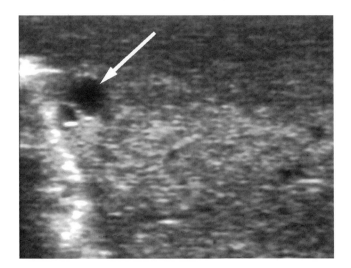

Fig. 8.19 Simple cyst. IOUS image of a palpable 'nodule' demonstrates a 5 mm simple hepatic cyst (arrow). Two metastases were located elsewhere in the liver.

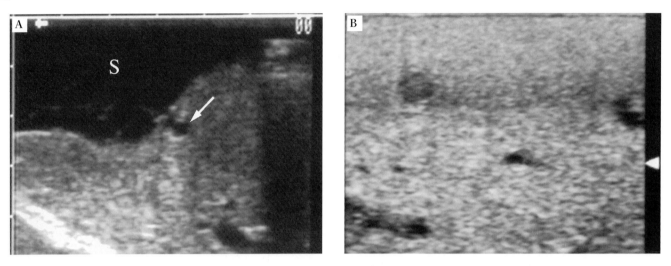

Fig. 8.21 High-resolution IOUS. A: A 3 mm simple cyst (arrow) was felt as a palpable abnormality in this cirrhotic liver. Image obtained through saline (S) allows confident exclusion of a possible small hepatoma. **B:** A 4 mm colorectal metastasis. Pre-operative imaging had predicted a solitary 4 cm metastasis but IOUS demonstrated an additional six metastatic sites, all 5 mm or less in size.

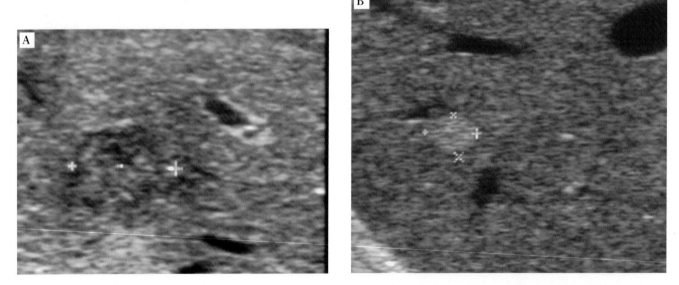

Fig. 8.22 Metastases and haemangiomas. A: A 2 cm colorectal metastasis (between calipers). There were three such lesions present. **B:** 8 mm haemangioma (between calipers). Five additional tiny haemangiomas were identified on IOUS imaging in this same patient.

along the fissure for the ligamentum venosum (Fig. 8.24). A replaced or accessory right hepatic artery usually arises from the superior mesenteric artery and courses into the liver posterior to the main portal vein.[49] The presence of these accessory or replaced arterial vessels may influence the resectability (or lack thereof) of certain tumours (Fig. 8.25). There are numerous variations in the anatomy of the hepatic veins and these vessels should therefore be carefully evaluated during IOUS. For instance, most typically, the left and middle hepatic veins share a common trunk. An inferior accessory right hepatic vein is occasion-ally encountered as a vessel which drains into the inferior vena cava several centimetres caudal to the hepatic venous confluence (Fig. 8.26). This is an important structure to identify on IOUS, not only because it could be torn during mobilization of the liver, but also because this additional drainage route might allow a more extensive left triseg-mentectomy to be performed when needed.[13]

Metastastic lymphadenopathy in the porta hepatis, peripancreatic and coeliac nodal regions can be assessed while performing IOUS of the liver. If enlarged nodes are detected, ultrasound-guided core biopsies can be per-

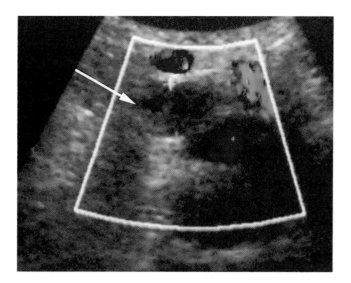

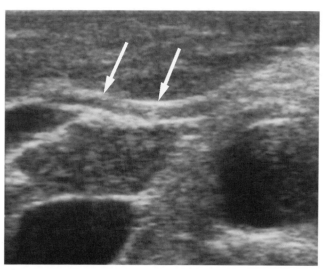

Fig. 8.23 Periportal metastatic lymphadenopathy. LUS with colour flow imaging demonstrates a solid 1.2 cm metastatic lymph node (arrow) between the hepatic artery and the portal vein.

Fig. 8.24 Replaced left hepatic artery. Arrows indicate the replaced left hepatic artery arising from the left gastric artery and coursing into the liver along the fissure for the ligamentum venosum.

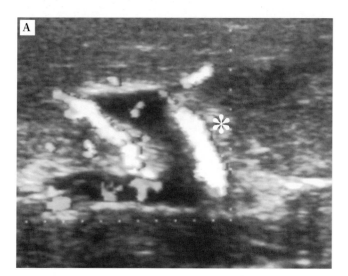

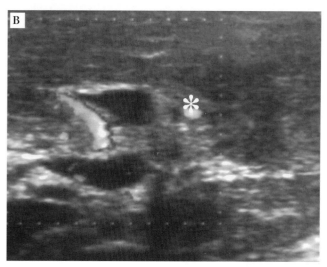

Fig. 8.25 Dual blood supply to left lobe. A: A patient with a solitary left lateral segment breast metastasis was noted to have two large arterial feeders to the left lobe. The tumour is seen just lateral to the asterisk and arterial flow is seen on both medial and lateral sides of the left portal vein. **B:** After clamping the early branching left hepatic artery, arterial flow is diminished to segment 2 but unaltered to segment 3, which was supplied separately from the proper hepatic artery. This anomalous blood supply allowed for a successful segmentectomy, without compromising blood flow to the remainder of the left lobe.

formed and frozen sections obtained to confirm metastatic disease. Confirmation of malignant lymphadenopathy would result in the cancellation of any liver resection, as a curative resection is not possible in the presence of extrahepatic metastatic disease.

Careful imaging of the portal and hepatic veins is particularly important in patients with hepatocellular carcinoma (Fig. 8.27) as this tumour has a marked propensity to invade veins.[50] Portal venous invasion was once consid-

ered a complete contraindication to surgical resection, but surgical extraction of the intravascular portion of the neoplasm is sometimes possible, thereby allowing the resection to proceed (Fig. 8.28). Hepatic venous invasion may extend into the inferior vena cava and even into the right atrium; correct assessment of the full extent of this venous invasion is important in order to avoid fragmentation of tumour thrombus, which could result in life-threatening pulmonary embolisation.

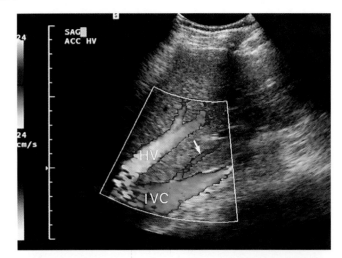

Fig. 8.26 Inferior accessory right hepatic vein. Colour flow IOUS image shows a small accessory inferior right hepatic vein (arrow) between the inferior vena cava (IVC) and main right hepatic vein (HV).

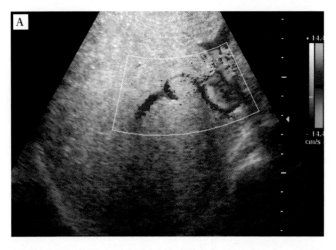
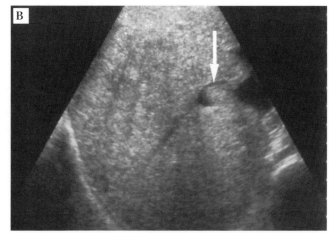

Fig. 8.27 Hepatoma invading right hepatic vein. A: Colour flow IOUS image shows bowing and near occlusion of the right hepatic vein near its junction with the inferior vena cava. **B:** Grey scale IOUS shows tumour growing in the right hepatic vein lumen (arrow) and gross distortion of the hepatic architecture caused by a diffusely infiltrating hepatoma.

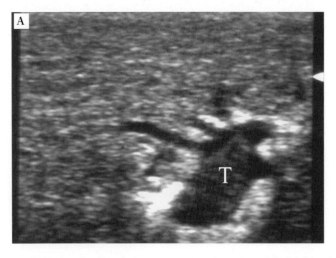
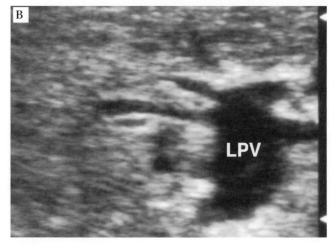

Fig. 8.28 Tumour thrombus. A: Transverse IOUS image of the left lobe shows hepatoma with tumour thrombus (T) growing in the lumen of the left portal vein. **B:** Repeat imaging after incision of the portal vein and extraction of the tumour shows a clear lumen in the left portal vein (LPV).

IOUS-guided procedures are generally performed free-hand, although there are some real-time guidance systems that can provide electronic screen markers for needle or probe placement. However, the freehand technique is usually satisfactory. Laparoscopic interventional procedures, such as laparoscopic ultrasound-guided biopsy, are more difficult because of the distances involved. Typically, an LUS-guided biopsy would be performed using an extra long biopsy needle, puncturing through the anterior abdominal wall and penetrating the liver adjacent to the probe. This can be quite arduous and difficult to perform for small deep-seated lesions, and biopsy guidance devices would be useful to assist LUS-guided interventional procedures. However, most manufacturers do not as yet provide such devices.[14] Tumour ablation techniques require the use of IOUS, for placement of the cryoprobe or RF probe, or the introduction of a needle when performing ethanol ablation (Fig. 8.29), and to provide continuous real-time monitoring of the actual ablation procedure, to ensure adequate treatment margins.[49,51] In cryosurgery the goal is to extend the freeze front into the normal adjacent liver parenchyma for a distance of 5–10 mm beyond the tumour margin (Fig. 8.30).

Vascular

Intra-operative vascular ultrasonography is most often used for the immediate assessment of vessels following

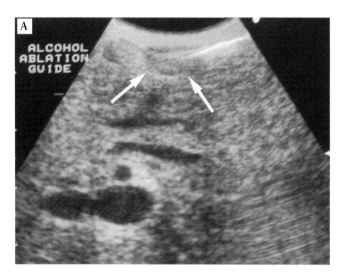
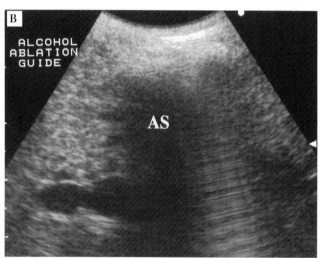

Fig. 8.29 **Alcohol ablation of small hepatoma. A:** IOUS image shows a 20-gauge needle entering a 1 cm hepatoma (arrows). **B:** After injection of absolute alcohol, the lesion is lost in an area of increased reflectivity with posterior acoustic shadowing (AS).

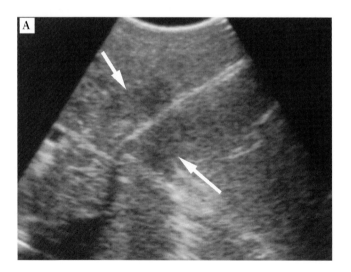
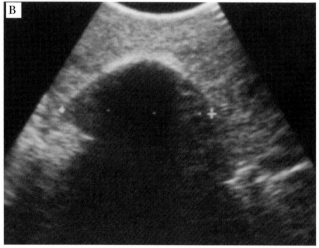

Fig. 8.30 **Cryosurgery of colorectal metastasis. A:** A 5 mm cryoprobe is seen bisecting a colorectal metastasis (outlined by arrows). **B:** After 7 minutes of freezing, the iceball (indicated by calipers) has completely encompassed the metastasis and extended beyond into the normal liver.

endarterectomy or arterial bypass grafting, to assess the adequacy of the reconstructed lumen, to exclude significant residual stenosis and to search for intimal flaps and dissections. The detection of such defects intra-operatively allows for immediate surgical correction and hence a reduction in postoperative thrombosis/occlusion and early postoperative restenosis. As most surgical reconstructions are performed to relieve stenoses in peripheral vessels, such as the carotid and femoral arteries, the most frequent applications of vascular IOUS are extra-abdominal; examples of intra-abdominal uses are in patients undergoing renal artery bypass grafting or endarterectomy.

The technique is demanding and requires experience and knowledge of ultrasound artefacts to avoid misinterpretations. Scans are generally performed using high-resolution linear-array end-fire probes ranging from 7 to 10 MHz in frequency. Acoustic coupling is achieved by filling the surgical site with degassed sterile saline, which provides an acoustic window and allows the transducer to stand off from the target vessel, thereby avoiding near-field artefacts. Using a saline waterbath also allows scanning in multiple planes, so that the optimal transducer position can be found to achieve proper Doppler angulation of 60° or less.[52] The vessel is imaged both in grey scale, which is useful for visualising intimal flaps, and with colour and spectral Doppler to assess localised areas of flow disturbance.

Some judgement and experience is required to assess very small postoperative defects, which are frequent but may not be sufficiently severe to require surgical re-intervention. In one study of 96 vascular reconstructions in the abdomen, 28% of cases had minor defects which did not require surgical repair, and only 4% had major defects.[53]

These major problems included occlusion and flaps or thrombi which narrowed the lumen more than 50%. In another study focusing only on renal artery revascularisation, vascular IOUS identified 11% of the total of 64 revascularisations which had technical defects requiring surgical revision.[54] Vascular IOUS also plays a role in the evaluation of patients with portal hypertension undergoing surgical portosystemic shunting (Fig. 8.31). In patients with abdominal tumours undergoing surgical resection, vascular ultrasound is important in detecting venous invasion from tumours such as hepatocellular carcinoma and renal cell carcinoma. In patients undergoing a liver transplantation vascular IOUS may be important in the evaluation of anomalous vascular supply or drainage, as well as confirmation of the patency of vascular anastomoses, particularly of the hepatic artery (Fig. 8.32), which is the most vulnerable to post-surgical complications, including stenosis or thrombosis.

Renal

One of the earliest applications of intraoperative ultrasound was in the identification of renal stones in patients undergoing nephrolithotomy.[5] However, extracorporeal shockwave lithotripsy and percutaneous stone extraction techniques have almost completely replaced open surgical nephrolithotomy. Surgery is still occasionally required for the treatment of large staghorn calculi, and Doppler ultrasound has been advocated to help define an avascular inter-segmental plane for the incision in an attempt to avoid damaging segmental end-arteries during nephrotomy, and thereby minimise renal parenchymal loss.[55,56]

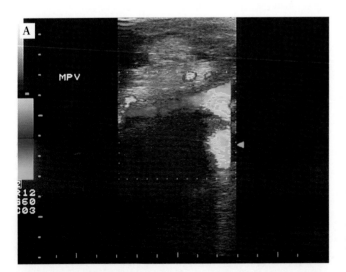
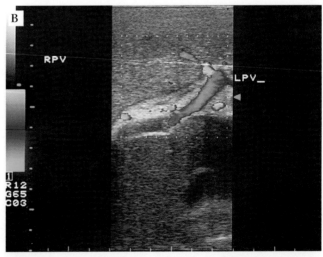

Fig. 8.31 Portosystemic shunt. A: After completion of a portocaval shunt using a portion of the renal vein as a conduit, flow in the main portal vein is seen as hepatofugal (red), leaving the liver and communicating with the inferior vena cava (mixed yellow and blue). **B:** Intrahepatic scan through the left lobe confirms hepatofugal flow (blue) in the left portal vein, consistent with a successful portosystemic shunt.

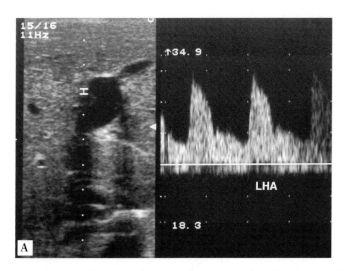
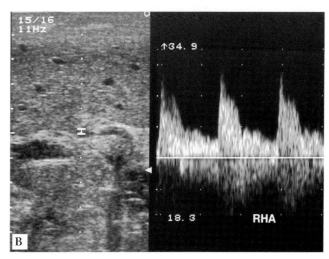

Fig. 8.32 Arterial supply to liver transplant. Grey scale and spectral Doppler confirmation of excellent arterial flow in **A:** the left and **B:** the right hepatic arteries.

Probably the most significant use of renal IOUS at present is in patients undergoing partial nephrectomy for neoplasms. This situation may occur when bilateral renal tumours present synchronously; when patients have undergone radical nephrectomy and developed a metachronous tumour in the remaining kidney and in patients with syndromes associated with multiple renal neoplasms, such as von Hippel–Lindau syndrome or tuberous sclerosis. In this setting, complete definition of the extent of the renal tumour is most important in order to remove the entire tumour and achieve adequate surgical margins (Fig. 8.33). Local recurrence after partial nephrectomy for tumour may occur in 3–13% of patients[57] as some lesions may be completely invisible and impalpable and others may be detectable by the surgeon but their deep intraparenchymal extent may still remain poorly defined. Renal IOUS could play a significant role in guiding adequate partial nephrectomy and thereby minimise recurrences.[58]

The propensity for renal cell carcinoma to invade into the renal vein and inferior vena cava is well known. Venous invasion by itself does not contraindicate surgical resection, but the extent of invasion must be carefully defined, particularly when it extends into the inferior vena cava (Fig. 8.34). The proximal extent of the tumour must

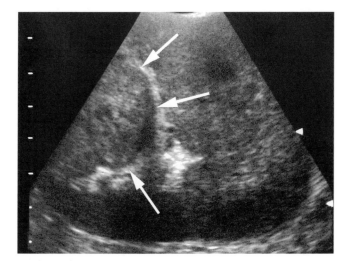

Fig. 8.33 Recurrent renal cell carcinoma. This patient had undergone previous left radical nephrectomy for cancer and developed a metachronous tumour in the right kidney. IOUS demonstrates the deep boundaries of the tumour (arrows), thereby allowing a successful partial nephrectomy.

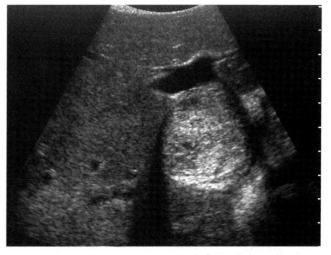

Fig. 8.34 Renal cell carcinoma invading the inferior vena cava. Extensive tumour thrombus is seen distending the lumen of the inferior vena cava in its intrahepatic portion, just posterior to the portal vein.

be visualised and control of the inferior vena cava above the tumour is important to avoid fragmentation and embolisation of thrombus into the lungs, which could result in potentially lethal embolus. IOUS can be extremely important in the real-time demonstration of the full extent of venous invasion at the time of resection.

Other applications

The more experience is gained with the uses of intra-operative ultrasonography, the more applications can be found for this highly efficacious technique. The neurosurgical applications are extensive and are covered in Chapter 44. IOUS has been advocated to help locate parathyroid tumours in patients who have failed a primary resection and who are scheduled for re-exploration. The scarring and disruption of anatomical planes from the initial surgery make inspection and palpation difficult and IOUS can be useful in limiting the re-exploration.[59] IOUS has been advocated for patients undergoing surgery for non-palpable breast masses.[60] Some lesions can be localised with a mark on the skin directly over the lesion, but deeper lesions require the use of breast localising needles or dye injection. The surgical specimen can be scanned immediately after resection to confirm that the mass has been removed; if the nodule is not identified, the surgical site can be rescanned and the lesion relocalised for immediate resection.

In the genitourinary system, in addition to renal IOUS, intra-operative ultrasound is frequently used in prostate surgery, particularly to monitor cryoablation for prostate cancer.[61] Prostate IOUS is also utilised to guide radioactive seed placement for prostate brachytherapy.[62] In gynaecology, IOUS can help guide intra-uterine endoscopic procedures or real-time placement of instruments in the endocervical and endometrial canal where there is difficulty in instrumentation owing, for example, to cervical stenoses, the presence of large fibroids or hyperflexion of the uterus. IOUS can also be helpful in guiding the placement of radioactive devices for the treatment of uterine tumours[63] as well as assisting with difficult dilatation and curettage procedures.[64]

Trans-rectal ultrasound scanning (TRUS) can be performed in the operating room to assist in the incision and drainage of perirectal abscesses by demonstrating their full extent. Intra-operative staging of anal and rectal neoplasms using TRUS may be useful in patients with such tight stenotic lesions that pre-operative staging procedures could not be performed successfully. Occasionally there may be unexpected findings during inspection and palpation of the abdomen and IOUS may prove helpful in defining the underlying abnormality (Fig. 8.35).

Perhaps somewhat surprisingly, intra-operative ultrasound has a role in chest surgery in the resection of pulmonary nodules. Although ultrasound does not propagate

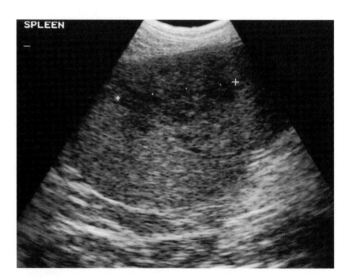

Fig. 8.35 Splenic infarct. IOUS image of the spleen reveals a poorly defined, slightly echo-poor area within the splenic parenchyma (between calipers). This was avascular and relatively soft, consistent with a splenic infarction.

through air, during video-assisted thoracoscopic surgery (VATS) the lung is carefully deflated; the collapsed lung has an ultrasound appearance similar to that of liver, so that IOUS can be successful in localising pulmonary nodules. This has been successfully performed using a variety of approaches, including the use of a flexible endorectal probe,[65] as well as probes designed for laparoscopic ultrasound.[66]

Conclusion

Undoubtedly, as experience with IOUS grows, further innovative and useful applications for this technology will be developed. The linkage of intra-operative ultrasound images to a virtual reality depiction of underlying anatomy and pathology is an exciting potential application which is already being developed for neurosurgical uses and which may have wider applications. Further improvements in miniaturisation, probe design and computer power can be expected. The trend to minimally invasive surgery will undoubtedly continue, and one can therefore expect increasing demands for ultrasound assistance.

REFERENCES

1 Kane R A, Hughes L A, Cua E J et al. The impact of intraoperative ultrasonography on surgery for liver neoplasms. J Ultrasound Med 1994; 13: 1–6
2 Boldrini G, deGaetano A M, Giovanni I et al. The systematic use of operative ultrasound for detection of liver metastasis during colorectal surgery. World J Surg 1987; 11: 622–627
3 Jakimowicz J J, Rutten H, Jurgens P J et al. Comparison of operative ultrasonography and radiography in screening of the common bile duct for calculi. World J Surg 1987; 11: 628–634

4 Bottger T C, Junginger T. Is preoperative radiographic localization of islet cell tumors in patients with insulinoma necessary? World J Surg 1993; 17: 427–432

5 Sigel B, Coelho J C U, Sharifi R et al. Ultrasonic scanning during operation for renal calculi. J Urol 1982; 127: 421–424

6 Knight P R, Newell J A. Operative use of ultrasonics in cholelithiasis. Lancet 1963; i: 1023–1025

7 Knake J E, Chandler W F, McGillicuddy J E et al. Intraoperative sonography for brain tumor localization and ventricular shunt placement. AJR 1982; 139: 733–738

8 Rubin J M, Dohrmann G J. Intraoperative ultrasonography of the spine. Radiology 1983; 146: 173–175

9 Sigel B, Coelho J C U, Nyhus L M et al. Comparison of cholangiography and ultrasonography in the operative screening of the common bile duct. World J Surg 1982; 6: 440–444

10 Gorman B, Charboneau J W, James E M et al. Benign pancreatic insulinoma: preoperative sonographic localization. AJR 1986; 147: 929–934

11 Clarke M P, Kane R A, Steele G Jr et al. Prospective comparison of preoperative imaging and intraoperative ultrasound in the detection of liver tumors. Surgery 1989; 106: 849–855

12 Kane R A. Intraoperative ultrasound. In: Wilson S R, Charboneau J W, Leopold G R, eds. Ultrasound: categorical course syllabus. Presented at the American Roentgen Ray Society 93rd Annual Meeting, San Francisco, 1993: 241–250

13 Kane R A. Intraoperative ultrasound: a call from the operating room. RSNA Special Course in Ultrasound 1996; 339–349

14 Kane R A. Laparoscopic ultrasound. In: Kane R A, ed. Intraoperative, laparoscopic and endoluminal ultrasound. Philadelphia: Churchill Livingstone, 1999: 90–105

15 Lee R A, Kane R A, Lantz E J, Charboneau J W. Intraoperative and laparoscopic sonography of the abdomen. In: Rumack C M, Wilson S R, Charboneau J W, eds. Diagnostic ultrasound, Vol. 1. St. Louis: Mosby, 1998: 671–699

16 Kruskal J B, Kane R A. Intraoperative ultrasonography of the liver. Crit Rev Diagn Imag 1995; 36(3): 175–226

17 Sammons L G, Kane R A. Technical aspects of intraoperative ultrasound. In: Kane R A, ed. Intraoperative, laparoscopic and endoluminal ultrasound. Philadelphia: Churchill Livingstone, 1999: 1–11

18 Kane R A. Intraoperative ultrasound. In: Yamada T et al., eds. Atlas of gastroenterology, 2nd edn. New York: Lippincott Williams & Wilkins, 1999: 758–772

19 Herbst C A, Mittlestaedt C A, Staab E V et al. Intraoperative ultrasonography evaluation of the gallbladder in morbidly obese patients. Ann Surg 1984; 200: 691–692

20 Machi J, Sigel B, Zaren H A, Kurohiji T, Yamashita Y. Operative ultrasonography during hepatobiliary and pancreatic surgery. World J Surg 1993; 17: 640

21 Sigel B, Machi J, Beitler J G et al. Comparative accuracy of operative ultrasonography and cholangiography in detecting common duct calculi. Surgery 1983; 94: 715–720

22 Stiegmann G V, McIntyre R, Yamamoto M, Durham J, Berguer R, Oba Y. Laparoscopy-guided intracorporeal ultrasound accurately delineates hepatobiliary anatomy. Surg Endosc 1993; 7: 325–330

23 Liu J B, Feld R I, Goldberg B B et al. Laparoscopic gray-scale and color Doppler US: preliminary animal and clinical studies. Radiology 1995; 194: 851–857

24 Jakimowicz J. Laparoscopic intraoperative ultrasonography, equipment, and technique. Semin Laparosc Surg 1994; 1(1): 52–61

25 Rothlin M A, Schlumpf R, Largiader F. Laparoscopic sonography. Arch Surg 1994; 129: 694–700

26 van Delden O M, de Wit L T, van Dijkum E J M N et al. Value of laparoscopic ultrasonography in staging of proximal bile duct tumors. J Ultrasound Med 1997; 16: 7–12

27 Gorman B, Charboneau J W, James E M et al. Benign pancreatic insulinoma: preoperative sonographic localization. AJR 1986; 147: 929–934

28 Zeiger M A, Shawker T H, Norton J A. Use of intraoperative ultrasonography to localize islet cell tumors. World J Surg 1993; 17: 448–454

29 van Heerden J A, Grant C S, Czako P F et al. Occult functioning insulinomas: which localizing studies are indicated? Surgery 1992; 112(6): 1010–1014

30 Gorman B, Reading C. Imaging of gastrointestinal neuroendocrine tumors. In: Freeny P C et al., eds. In: Radiology of the liver, biliary tract, and pancreas. Categorical course syllabus. American Roentgen Ray Society, 1996: 191–198

31 Charboneau J W, Gorman B, Reading C C et al. Intraoperative ultrasonography of pancreatic endocrine tumors. In: Rifkin MD, ed. Clinics in diagnostic ultrasound – intraoperative and endoscopic ultrasound 1987; 7(22): 123–134

32 Davies P F, Shevland J E, Shepherd J J. Ultrasonography of the pancreas in patients with MEN I. J Ultrasound Med 1993; 12(2): 67–72

33 Sugg S L, Norton S L, Fraker D L et al. A prospective study of intraoperative methods to diagnose and resect duodenal gastrinomas. Ann Surg 1993; 218(2): 138–144

34 Stabile B E, Morrow D J, Passaro E Jr. The gastrinoma triangle: operative implications. Am J Surg 1984; 147: 25–31

35 Bemelman W A, de Wit L T, van Delden O M et al. Diagnostic laparoscopy combined with laparoscopic ultrasonography in staging of cancer of the pancreatic head region. Br J Surg 1995; 82: 820–824

36 John T G, Greig J D, Carter D C, Garden O J. Carcinoma of the pancreatic head and periampullary region: tumor staging with laparoscopy and laparoscopic ultrasonography. Ann Surg 1995; 221(2): 156–164

37 Hann L E, Conlon K C, Dougherty E C et al. Laparoscopic sonography of peripancreatic tumors; preliminary experience. AJR 1997; 169(5): 1257–1262

38 Sigel B, Machi J, Ramos J R et al. The role of ultrasound imaging during pancreatic surgery. Ann Surg 1984; 200: 486–493

39 Printz H, Klotter J H, Nies C et al. Intraoperative ultrasonography in surgery for chronic pancreatitis. Int J Pancreatol 1992; 12(3): 233–237

40 Serio G, Fugazzola C, Iacono C et al. Intraoperative ultrasonography in pancreatic cancer. Int J Pancreatol 1992; 11(1): 31–41

41 Clarke M P, Kane R A, Steele D G et al. Prospective comparison of preoperative imaging and intraoperative ultrasonography in the detection of liver tumors. Surgery 1989; 106: 849–855

42 Kane R A, Longmaid H E, Costello P, Finn J P, Roizental M. Noninvasive imaging in patients with hepatic masses: a prospective comparison of ultrasound, CT and MR imaging (abstr). AJR 1993; 160(Suppl): 133

43 Soyer P, Levesque M, Elias D, Zeitoun G, Roche A. Detection of liver metastases from colorectal cancer: comparison of intraoperative US and CT during arterial portography. Radiology 1992; 183: 541–544

44 Nelson R C, Thompson G H, Chezmar J L, Harned R K, Fernandez M P. CT during arterial portography; diagnostic pitfalls. Radiographics 1992; 12: 705–718

45 Matsui O, Takahashi S, Kadoya M et al. Pseudolesion in segment IV of the liver at CT during arterial portography: correlation with aberrant gastric venous drainage. Radiology 1994; 193: 31–35

46 Babineau T J, Lewis W D, Jenkins R J et al. Role of staging laparoscopy in the treatment of hepatic malignancy. Am J Surg 1994; 167: 151–155

47 Kane R A, Roizental M, Kruskal J B et al. Preliminary investigation of liver and biliary imaging with a dedicated laparoscopic US system (abstr). Radiology 1994; 193(P): 287

48 John T G, Greig J D, Crosbie J L, Miles W F, Garden O J. Superior staging of liver tumors with laparoscopy and laparoscopic ultrasound (comments). Ann Surg 1994; 220: 709–711

49 Kruskal J B, Kane R A. Intraoperative ultrasound of the liver. In: Kane R A, ed. Intraoperative, laparoscopic and endoluminal ultrasound. Philadelphia: Churchill Livingstone, 1999: 40–67

50 Kruskal J B, Kane R A. Correlative imaging of malignant liver tumors. Semin Ultrasound CT MRI 1992; 13: 336–354

51 Kane R A. Ultrasound-guided hepatic cryosurgery for tumor ablation. Semin Interv Radiol 1993; 10: 132

52 Lee R A, Reading C C. Intraoperative vascular ultrasound. In: Kane R A, ed. Intraoperative, laparoscopic and endoluminal ultrasound. Philadelphia: Churchill Livingstone, 1999: 106–129

53 Okuhn S P, Reilly L M, Bennett J B et al. Intraoperative assessment of renal and visceral artery reconstruction: the role of duplex scanning and spectral analysis. J Vasc Surg 1987; 5: 137

54 Dougherty M J, Hallett J W Jr, Naessens J M et al. Optimizing technical success of renal revascularization: the impact of intraoperative color-flow duplex ultrasonography. J Vasc Surg 1993; 17: 849

55 Riedmiller H, Thuroff J, Alken P et al. Doppler and B-mode ultrasound for avascular nephrotomy. J Urol 1983; 130: 224–227

56 Walther M M, Choyke P L, Hayes W et al. Evaluation of color Doppler intraoperative ultrasound in parenchymal sparing renal surgery. J Urol 1994; 152: 1984–1987

57 Topley M, Novick A C, Montie J E. Long-term results following partial nephrectomy for localized renal adenocarcinoma. J Urol 1984; 131: 1050–1052

58 Gilbert B R, Russo P, Zirinsky K et al. Intraoperative sonography: application in renal cell carcinoma. J Urol 1988; 139: 582–584

59 Kern K A, Shawker T H, Doppman J L et al. The use of high-resolution ultrasound to locate parathyroid tumors during reoperations for primary hyperparathyroidism. World J Surg 1987; 11: 579–585

60 Fornage B D. Intraoperative ultrasound of the breast. In: Kane R A, ed. Intraoperative, laparoscopic and endoluminal ultrasound. Philadelphia: Churchill Livingstone, 1999: 142–147

61 Onik G M, Cohen J K, Reyes G D et al. Transrectal ultrasound-guided percutaneous radical cryosurgical ablation of the prostate. Cancer 1993; 72: 1291–1299

62 Edmundson G K, Yan D, Martinez A A. Intraoperative optimization of needle placement and dwell times for conformal prostate brachytherapy. Int J Radiat Oncol Biol Phys 1995; 33(5): 1257–1263

63 Letterie G S, Kramer D J. Intraoperative ultrasound guidance for intrauterine endoscopic surgery. Fertil Steril 1995; 64: 664–665

64 Letterie G S, Case K J. Intraoperative ultrasound guidance for hysteroscopic retrieval of intrauterine foreign bodies. Surg Endosc 1993; 7: 182–184

65 Mack M J, Shennib H, Landreau R J et al. Techniques for localization of pulmonary nodules for thoracoscopic resection. J Thorac Cardiovasc Surg 1993; 106: 550–553

66 Greenfield A L, Steiner R M, Liu J B et al. Sonographic guidance for the localization of peripheral pulmonary nodules during thoracoscopy. AJR 1997; 168: 1057–1060

Liver anatomy

David O Cosgrove

Anatomy

The liver, the largest abdominal organ weighing 1.5 kg, lies in the upper abdomen, predominantly on the right side (Fig. 9.1).[1–3] It has an overall wedge shape, tapering from right to left with a domed upper surface that fits under the cupola of the right hemidiaphragm. The flatter inferior surface is actually tilted quite markedly so that it faces posteriorly and to the left, thus it is more informatively described as the visceral surface.

The superior surface is relatively featureless but, by contrast, the visceral surface is complex because it contains the liver hilum (the porta hepatis) and also is indented by the shallow fossae that accommodate the organs that are in direct contact with the liver. These are the stomach on the left and, moving to the right, the duodenum and gallbladder, the inferior vena cava and the right kidney. In addition, the visceral surface is marked by fissures that separate some of the liver segments (see below). Posteriorly the superior and visceral surfaces continue smoothly into each other, while the infero-anterior border is sharp and is indented by the ligamentum teres and the gallbladder.

The porta lies approximately transversely; through it pass the portal vein, the hepatic artery and the bile duct (Fig. 9.2). The portal vein usually divides into left and right branches before actually penetrating the liver substance though, like so many anatomical features of the liver vasculature, this is subject to some variation. However, the vein always lies posterior to the artery and duct, with the duct lying laterally and deviating further to the right as it passes down to enter the duodenum. The medial position of the hepatic artery can be remembered from the fact that it originates in the midline from the

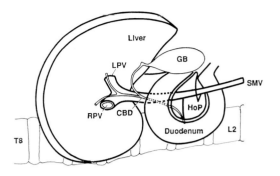

Fig. 9.2 The hepatic pedicle. The relations of the vessels in the hepatic pedicle are illustrated in this cutaway diagram in which the porta is viewed from the right. Those portions of the bile duct that are overlain by duodenum are shown dotted to indicate the difficulty of imaging these parts with ultrasound. CBD – common bile duct, GB – gallbladder, HoP – head of pancreas, LPV – left portal vein, RPV – right portal vein, SMV – superior mesenteric vein.

coeliac axis; it retains this relatively medial position throughout its course. The right branch of the portal vein passes transversely within the liver substance for a few centimetres before dividing into anterior and posterior branches, while the left branch curves anteriorly, giving branches to the parts of the liver it traverses. The hepatic arterial branches follow the same pattern.

The overall arrangement of the bile ducts is similar, the smaller ducts joining to form right and left ducts which generally lie anterior to the associated portal vein branches. As it passes inferomedially to the porta, the right hepatic duct crosses over the right portal vein with the right hepatic artery lying between them (though the artery is more variable and lies anterior to the duct in some 10% of subjects). The right and left hepatic ducts emerge from

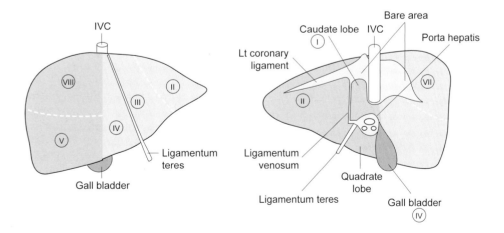

Fig. 9.1 Anatomy of the liver. Two views of the liver are shown in diagrammatic form. The diaphragmatic surface is much simpler than the visceral surface which contains the porta hepatis. Note that *in vivo* the visceral surface is tilted to face inferomedially. Coinaud's segmental numbering system is indicated.

the liver substance before joining to form the common hepatic duct which passes down anterolateral to the main portal vein, posterior to the duodenum (first part) and across the posterior surface of the pancreas before turning laterally (to the right) to enter the second part of the duodenum at the papilla (ampulla) of Vater. At some point along this course, most often in the porta itself, the common hepatic duct is joined by the cystic duct; below this it is referred to as the common bile duct. The overall lie of the bile duct is inferolateral, approximately at right angles to the costal margin, but this also is variable, depending mainly on the level of the pancreas, so that in some subjects the common bile duct runs almost transversely while in others it lies in a sagittal plane.

Three main hepatic veins drain the liver; they empty into the upper part of the inferior vena cava. The right hepatic vein lies in the coronal plane and empties separately into the inferior vena cava. The middle passes from the position of the gallbladder fossa and joins the left to form a short common trunk of a centimetre or so in length, so that both empty together into the anterior aspect of the inferior vena cava just below the diaphragm. The left hepatic vein is often found in the mid-sagittal plane but may lie to one or other side. In addition, a series of smaller, short hepatic veins drain the portions of the liver that are in direct contact with the inferior vena cava, i.e. the superomedial part of the right lobe and the caudate lobe; these are known as the inferior hepatic veins (see below).

The liver is divided into segments based on its vasculature (Fig. 9.3). The supply vessels separate the right from the left parts of the liver along a line joining the gallbladder fossa inferiorly with the fossa for the inferior vena cava superiorly; this virtual line passes through the porta

and demarcates the equal sized parts of the liver supplied by the right and left portal veins and hepatic arteries and drained by the right and left bile ducts. The middle hepatic vein lies in this plane but the line of demarcation is not obvious on the surface of the liver (this is why, despite its significance, this major division was not recognised until the importance of the vascularisation of the liver emerged with the development of hepatic surgery). The two lobes are approximately equal in size and so their veins, arteries and bile ducts are of similar diameters. While generally their designations are appropriate to their position in the upper abdomen, the plane separating the right and left livers is usually tilted to face anteriorly and to the left, so that the portions of the left liver near the porta overlie the medial portions of the right liver.

An important, though small, additional segment of the liver is the caudate, which may be considered as a finger-like extension from the upper posterior part of the right lobe.[4,5] It passes as the caudate process to the left across the subdiaphragmatic portion of the inferior vena cava and then expands into a variable sized lobe that commonly extends inferiorly. Here it lies immediately posterior to the left lobe, the two being separated by a fissure in which the ligamentum venosum is buried.

Coinaud's numbering system for the liver segments has become widely accepted and is particularly useful when a precise description of the position of a lesion is required, for example for planning liver surgery[6-8] (Fig. 9.3). The segments are numbered clockwise, starting with the caudate as segment I, segments II and III being the left and right portions of the lateral part of the left lobe while segment IV corresponds with the quadrate lobe, which is often subdivided into superior (IVA) and inferior (IVB) portions. Segments V and VI are the anterior and posterior portions of the inferior parts of the right lobe, while VII and VIII are the posterior and anterior portions of the superior part of the right lobe. The anatomical relationships are based on the fetal circulation (Fig. 9.4) which differs significantly from the mature pattern.

The liver is almost entirely covered by peritoneum which is folded in a rather complex way, especially around the porta and the caudate lobe (Fig. 9.1). Over the superior (diaphragmatic) surface the peritoneum is drawn into transverse folds, triangular in shape with their apices laterally where the visceral layer (on the liver capsule) folds over to continue as the parietal layer on the inferior surface of the diaphragm. These so-called 'coronary ligaments' leave a 'bare' area where the liver is in direct contact with the diaphragm (mainly its central tendinous portion). Anteriorly the peritoneal folds continue into the falciform ligament, a crescentic double peritoneal layer that passes toward the inferior border of the left lobe. Here it folds over the ligamentum teres which lies in its free edge (Fig. 9.4). Posteriorly the peritoneal folds continue into the fissure for the ligamentum venosum.

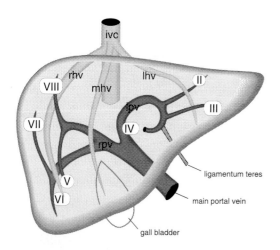

Fig. 9.3 Blood vessels of the liver. The main branches of the portal vein and the way they interdigitate with the three main hepatic veins are illustrated. Coinaud's segmental divisions are indicated in Roman numerals. ivc – inferior vena cava, lhv – left hepatic vein, lpv – left portal vein, mhv – middle hepatic vein, rhv – right hepatic vein, rpv – right portal vein.

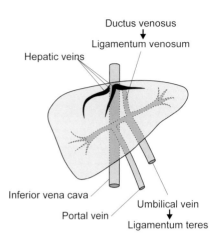

Ductus venosus
Ligamentum venosum
Hepatic veins
Inferior vena cava
Portal vein
Umbilical vein
Ligamentum teres

Fig. 9.4 Fetal circulation through the liver. The venous bypass in the fetus takes blood returning from the placenta via the umbilical vein to the left portal vein and thence directly to the left hepatic vein and on into the inferior vena cava. The temporary vessels that carry this blood (the umbilical vein and the ductus venosus) undergo vasospasm at birth and they subsequently thrombose to form the ligamentum teres and ligamentum venosum respectively. If the spasm extends into the left portal vein itself, lateral parts of the left lobe of the liver become ischaemic. This may account for the marked variability in size of this segment.

The complexity of the peritoneum of the visceral surface results from the layers that form the lesser sac of the omentum.[9] Its anterior wall consists of the lesser omentum, a double peritoneal layer that extends as a sheet from the lesser curve of the stomach to the liver and is also known as the hepatogastric ligament. It attaches in the fissure for the ligamentum venosum and from there folds back on itself to continue as the peritoneal layer covering the liver itself. At the oesophagogastric region the anterior layer continues over the diaphragm as the parietal peritoneum while the posterior layer is reflected over the posterior abdominal wall (mainly covering the body and tail regions of the pancreas) as the posterior wall of the lesser sac. On the right the two layers separate to enfold the hepatic pedicle (comprising the portal vein, the hepatic artery and the bile duct), fusing lateral to them to form a free border that stretches up from the first part of the duodenum to the lateral part of the porta hepatis where the layers again continue into the peritoneum covering the liver. Thus a foramen is formed immediately posterior to the porta hepatis where the general peritoneum communicates with the recess (the lesser sac); it is known as the 'foramen of Winslow' or the 'additus to the lesser sac' and its posterior margin overlies the inferior vena cava. The other walls of the lesser sac are formed by the posterior wall of the stomach and the peritoneum over the upper retroperitoneal structures so that part of the pancreas lies immediately posterior to it (this is why pseudocysts so commonly collect in the lesser sac). On the left it extends up to the splenic hilum. Most of the caudate lobe lies within it.

The coronary ligaments over the diaphragmatic surface of the liver divide the subphrenic peritoneal space into anterior and posterior portions which are more completely separated on the right where the ligament is more extensive. The posterior subphrenic space continues into the hepatorenal space ('Morrison's pouch'). These spaces delimit regions in which ascitic fluid and infective collections are confined.

Ultrasound appearances

In longitudinal sections through the left lobe, the liver has a triangular shape with a rounded upper surface and a sharp inferior border; its margins are clearly defined by the reflective capsule (Fig. 9.5). The parenchymal echoes are a mid-grey and consist of a uniform, sponge-like pattern interrupted by the vessels. Sections on the right show the same basic shape but the liver here is larger, especially the upper portion, while the various impressions produced by the contiguous organs are apparent (Fig. 9.6). In transverse sections the wedge shape of the liver is seen, tapering to the left (Fig. 9.7). The caudate lobe (Fig. 9.8) is seen as an extension of the right lobe in transverse sections and as an almond-shaped structure posterior to the left lobe in longitudinal views. The position of the ligamentum teres is marked by an intensely reflective focus in transverse sections (Fig. 9.9).

The appearance of the complex of vessels at the porta depends on their orientation in the slices viewed; two main projections need to be considered. When the tomogram runs along the line of the hepatic pedicle, the portal vein is cut lengthways (Fig. 9.10); tomograms slightly laterally also cut the bile duct which is seen as a smaller tubular

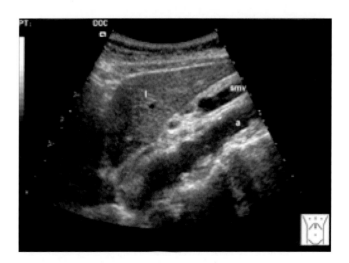

Fig. 9.5 Left lobe of liver, sagittal section. The triangular shape of the left lobe is seen in this subject in whom the liver is thinned anteroposteriorly. It overlies the aorta whose irregular walls indicate atheromatous change. a – aorta, l – liver, smv – superior mesenteric vein.

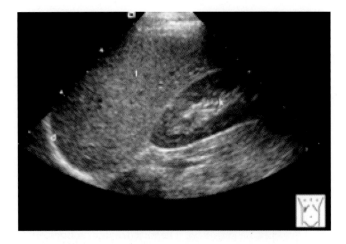

Fig. 9.6 Right lobe of liver, sagittal section. The bright bow of the diaphragm outlines the upper surface of the liver while posteriorly it overlies the right kidney. Its parenchyma is interrupted by spaces for the veins. d – diaphragm, l – liver, k – kidney.

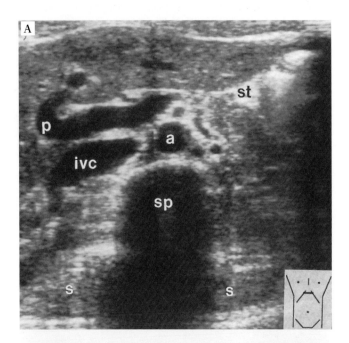

Fig. 9.7 The left and right livers. A: In transverse section the liver has a wedge shape, narrowing to the left. This means that the visceral surface is tilted to the left and also inferiorly, though this can only be appreciated on a sagittal section. This tomogram has passed through the porta hepatis. a – aorta, ivc – inferior vena cava, p – portal vein, s – sacrospinalis muscle, sp – spine, st – stomach. **B:** Transverse image showing the main inter-lobar fissure separating the left and right lobes. **C:** Longitudinal scan showing the fissure lying between the porta hepatis and the gallbladder fossa.

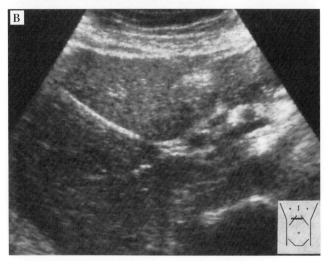

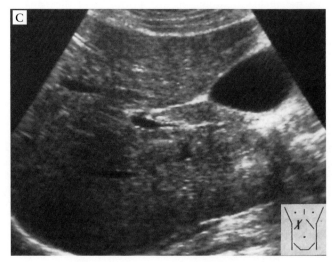

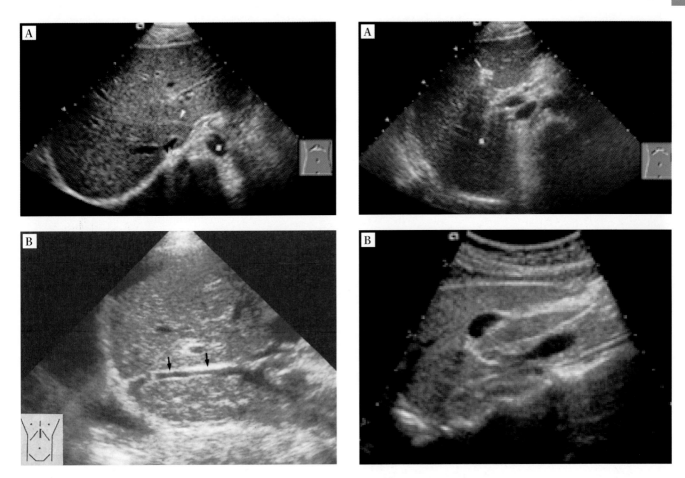

Fig. 9.8 The caudate lobe. A: In transverse section the caudate lobe is seen as an extension medially of the right lobe. It lies immediately anterior to the inferior vena cava and is separated from the overlying left lobe by a fissure (arrowhead). **B:** In longitudinal section it is seen as an oval or almond-shaped portion of liver tissue posterior to the left lobe from which it is separated by the fissure for the ligamentum venosum (arrows). In this case a trace of ascites surrounds the caudate lobe, indicating its position within the lesser sac. a – aorta, ivc – inferior vena cava, p – porta.

Fig. 9.9 The ligamentum teres. The fibrous tissue and surrounding fat give the ligamentum teres strong echoes. **A:** Cut in cross-section (arrow) it appears as a spot (arrowhead) while **B:** cut lengthways a band is seen. It often casts a marked shadow (s) which interferes with imaging of structures immediately deep to it.

structure running parallel to the portal vein and lying anterior to it. Often the duct is only apparent from the mid-position of the porta and below because further superiorly the smaller left and right ducts are cut in cross section, lying to the left and right of the portal vein respectively, and so are difficult to recognise. Sections along the hepatic pedicle and slightly medially image the hepatic artery immediately anterior to the portal vein; usually the artery divides somewhat lower than the level of junction of the hepatic ducts and so the right branch is more often imaged as a ring passing across to the right and lying between the portal vein and the bile duct (either the right hepatic or the common duct). As a normal variant the artery lies anterior to the duct but the position of both this and the bile ducts anterior to the portal vein

is practically inviolable. Seen in transverse section (Fig. 9.11) the portal vein appears as a ring with the duct and artery anterior to it in the same relative positions as in the longitudinal sections.

The portal vein branches can be traced from the porta, the right passing more or less transversely for a few centimetres before dividing into its main anterior and posterior branches (Fig. 9.12). The left portal vein curves anteriorly as well as crossing to the left (reflecting the generally more anterior position of the left lobe of the liver) before giving off superior and inferior branches to the various segments it traverses. One notable branch passes inferiorly towards the ligamentum teres; usually it thins to a fine thread as it enters the ligamentum itself, often being too small to be resolved here. It is an important vein

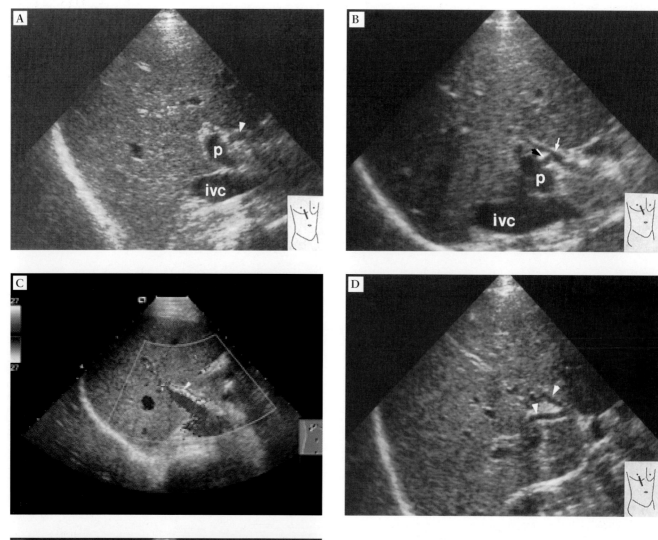

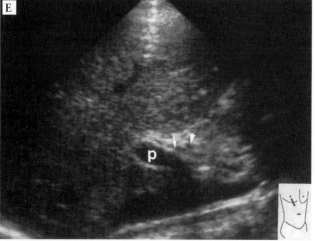

Fig. 9.10 The porta hepatis cut lengthways. Oblique cuts through the porta medially show **A:** the hepatic artery (arrowhead) lying anterior to the portal vein (p) while **B:** slightly further laterally the common bile duct (arrow) overlies the vein in a characteristic configuration with the hepatic artery (arrowhead) in between. **C:** In colour Doppler the portal vein signals are shown in red because the blood flows towards the transducer. The hepatic artery flow is in the same direction (arrowhead) but its higher velocity makes the signals prone to aliase, shown here as a mosaic of yellow and green. **D:** In this subject a cut further laterally still reveals the hepatic artery dividing into two branches (arrowheads) – presumably these represent the right and left main branches. If this is the correct interpretation, this depicts a relatively uncommon anomaly of the hepatic artery in which the main division occurs further laterally than usual. **E:** A much commoner anomaly, where the artery (arrowhead) lies anterior to the bile duct (arrow) (10% of subjects) is shown. ivc – inferior vena cava.

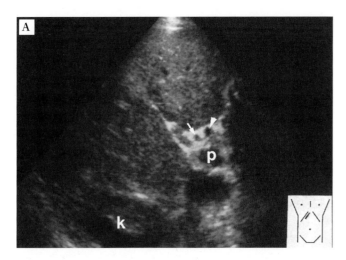

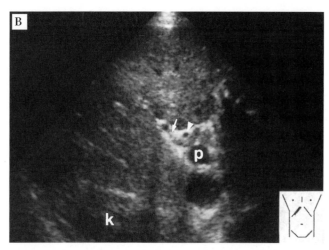

Fig. 9.11 The porta hepatis cut across. A: A cross-section through the porta (usually this will be oblique on the body, often running along the right costal margin) cuts across all three vessels of the hepatic pedicle. The hepatic artery (arrowhead) lies anteromedially while the bile duct (arrow) lies anterolaterally. **B:** A cut slightly superiorly in this subject shows the right hepatic artery crossing between the bile duct and the portal vein to curve away into the right lobe of the liver. k – kidney, p – portal vein.

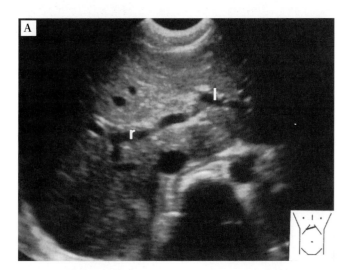

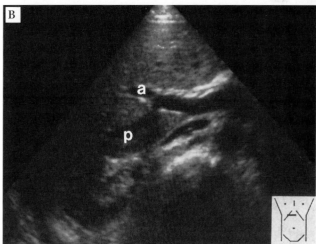

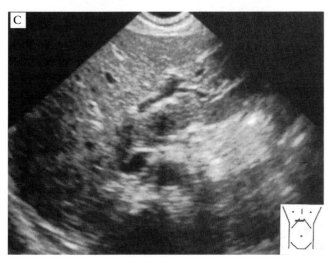

Fig. 9.12 The portal veins. The main portal vein divides into the main right and left branches within the porta. **A:** A cut just superior to this shows the main branches with the right branch (r) passing transversely and the left (l) passing anteromedially. **B:** A cut through the right branch shows its division into anterior (a) and posterior (p) segmental branches. **C:** Similarly on the left the two main segmental divisions of the portal vein are shown.

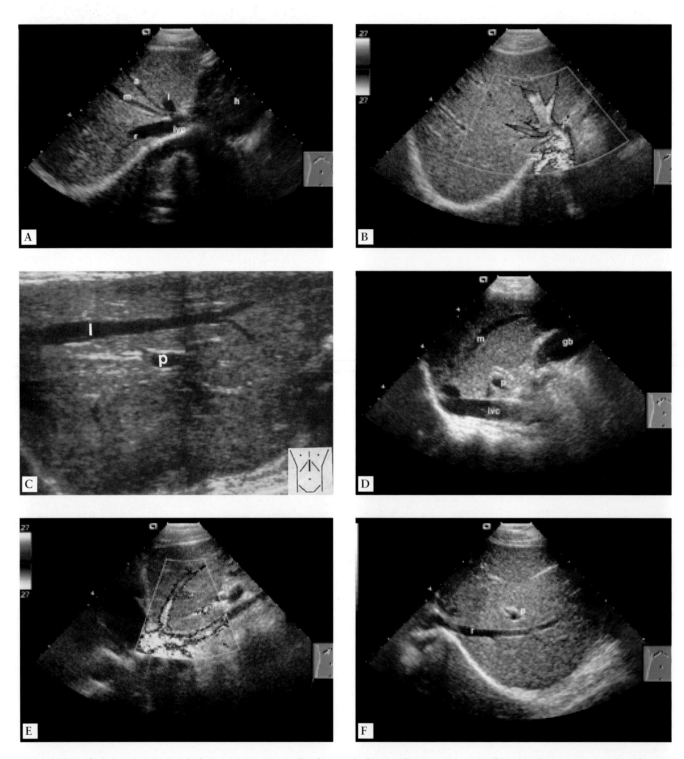

Fig. 9.13 Main hepatic veins. A: In a high transverse section inclined upwards the main hepatic veins are well-seen as they converge on the inferior vena cava. In this subject an accessory vein (a) is present. **B:** Colour Doppler shows the positions of the three main hepatic veins. **C and D:** Longitudinal sections in the sagittal plane show the path of the left and middle hepatic veins (l and m) lying approximately in the midline and in the right mid-clavicular lines respectively. **E:** Colour Doppler highlights the position of the middle hepatic vein. **F:** The right hepatic vein (r) is best demonstrated in a coronal section through the lower intercostal spaces. a – accessory hepatic vein, g – gallbladder, h – heart, ivc – inferior vena cava, l – left hepatic vein, m – middle hepatic vein, p – portal vein, r – right hepatic vein.

because, as the remnant of the left umbilical vein (Fig. 9.4), it represents one of the potential sites of portosystemic anastomoses which can open up in portal hypertension (see Ch. 13).

Sections high in the liver show the larger hepatic veins as they converge towards the upper cava (Fig. 9.13). Their relations are best shown in cross-sections: the right hepatic vein generally lies in the coronal plane and curves medially to enter the cava a centimetre or so below the diaphragm. The middle hepatic vein can be traced from the general position of the gallbladder curving superiorly and posteriorly to enter the anterior part of the cava immediately below the diaphragm. Commonly the left vein joins it so that these two empty together, the left hepatic vein having curved from left to right. Supernumerary main veins are common. The smaller inferior group of hepatic veins may sometimes be demonstrated as short vessels passing directly from the caudate lobe and the medial portion of the right lobe where the cava is in direct contact with the liver (Fig. 9.14).

The two sets of veins tend to have distinctive appearances on ultrasound, the portal veins having thicker, reflective walls while the hepatic veins appear merely as defects in the liver parenchyma. This corresponds to their anatomical structures since the hepatic veins are essentially large sinusoids whose walls are thin or absent while the portal veins have fibromuscular walls and in addition are accompanied by smaller hepatic arterial branches and by small radicals of the biliary tree. However, as always in ultrasound imaging, the actual appearances depend as much on the angle of interrogation as on the anatomy so that a portal vein cut at a more oblique angle may have inapparent walls while sometimes a hepatic vein that has been cut so that its walls lie at 90° to the ultrasound beam has strongly reflective walls. The overall anatomy also helps in their distinction and they may be traced towards the porta or the inferior vena cava where a definite designation is required. Doppler (Fig. 9.15) provides a direct means of demonstrating the flow direction[10] (though it must be remembered that flow in the portal veins may be reversed in extreme portal hypertension (see Ch. 13).

Within the liver parenchyma the normal bile ducts are too small to be demonstrated except under good imaging conditions (Fig. 9.16). However, the left and right main ducts measure a few millimetres in inner diameter and one expects to visualise them as well as the larger common hepatic and bile ducts. Only occasionally can the cystic duct be made out; the difficulty here is that it is usually extremely tortuous (Fig. 9.17). The diameter of the lumen of the bile duct increases slightly with age, as is the case also with the pancreatic duct (see Ch. 16). The conventional position to measure the bile duct lumen is within the porta at the level of the right portal vein where the duct is cut across (Fig. 9.18); at this level the hepatic artery can usually also be demonstrated, probably actually the right

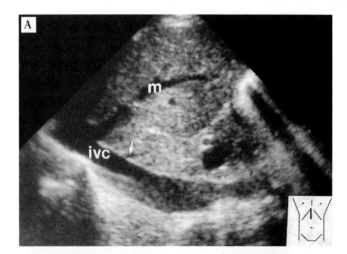

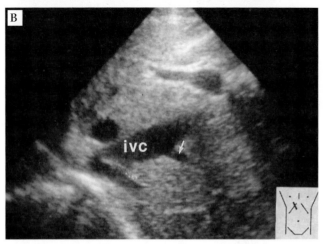

Fig. 9.14 Inferior hepatic veins. The main hepatic veins are supplemented by a small set of veins, the inferior group (arrows), which drain those parts of **A**: the caudate and **B**: right lobes that are in direct contact with the cava. ivc – inferior vena cava, m – middle hepatic vein.

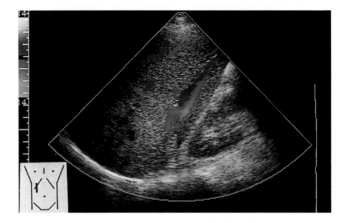

Fig. 9.15 Colour Doppler of the right lobe of the liver. The flow in the main portal vein is shown as a red colour because it runs towards the transducer; whereas the flow in the hepatic vein is coded as blue because it is away from the transducer.

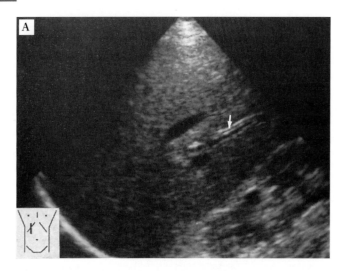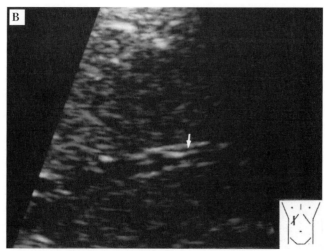

Fig. 9.16 Intrahepatic bile ducts. A: Under good imaging conditions with a high resolution scanner normal intrahepatic bile ducts (arrow) can sometimes be detected lying close to the larger portal vein branches. Provided these are less than 1 mm in calibre, they can be accepted as normal. Colour Doppler demonstrates that some of these vessels accompanying the portal veins are arterial branches; the anatomical relationship of these three vessels is more variable than at the porta hepatis. **B:** A magnification of the relevant portion of **A**.

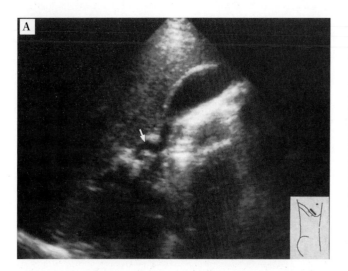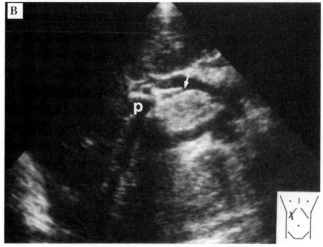

Fig. 9.17 Cystic duct. A: The cystic duct is often visualised at the point where it leaves the gallbladder (arrow) but **B:** the point of junction with the common duct (arrow) is rarely demonstrated. p – right portal vein.

hepatic artery. A convenient and easily remembered formula is 1 mm per decade of life; this allows for the smaller duct calibre in the paediatric age group and for progressive enlargement with age, while for the average adult the value of 4–5 mm corresponds with the commonly quoted measurements. The duct expands as it descends and receives the cystic duct, so if only the more inferior (extrahepatic) portions can be accessed, an additional few millimetres must be allowed.

When compared with the duct diameter measured during a cholecystogram or a cholangiogram (either percutaneous or retrograde endoscopic), the ultrasound sizes seem too small. This discrepancy caused much debate before the complex of factors that explain it was understood and the measurements could be reconciled. Ultrasound tends to underestimate the calibre of ducts in general because of infilling due to the beam width artefact that causes the reflective walls to appear thickened and to spread into the lumen. On the other hand, on X-ray the tube-film distance magnifies the image and this is added to the fact that the duct is distended either by injected contrast or by the choleresis induced by the biliary contrast agent. These factors combine to account for the discrepancy (Fig. 9.19).

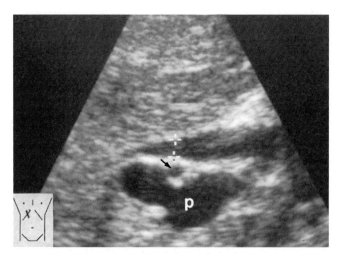

Fig. 9.18 Measurement of the common duct. The recommended position for measuring the calibre of the common duct is at the point where it crosses the hepatic artery (caliper crosses). In this patient the duct measures 4.1 mm. arrow – hepatic artery, p – portal vein.

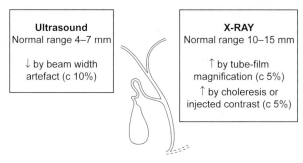

Common hepatic duct
Anatomical inner diameter 7–12 mm

Ultrasound	**X-RAY**
Normal range 4–7 mm	Normal range 10–15 mm
↓ by beam width artefact (c 10%)	↑ by tube-film magnification (c 5%)
	↑ by choleresis or injected contrast (c 5%)

Fig. 9.19 Discrepancy between X-ray and ultrasound normal ranges for the bile duct. While the ultrasound measurement of the diameter of the bile duct is underestimated because of infilling due to beam spreading, the cholangiographic measurement is exaggerated because of magnification effects. In addition the contrast-induced choleresis ensures that the duct is filled during the X-ray measurement. When the duct has an oval cross-section, the X-ray measurement is of the long axis while the ultrasound measurement is of the short axis. These factors account well for the discrepancy.

Variations

True variants of the liver may be divided into cases of failure of development of a lobe or segment and cases where abnormal development has occurred.[11] The commonest examples of failure affect the left lobe, especially its lateral segments (II and III), and are often compensated for by hypertrophy of the right and quadrate lobes. The small left lobe may result from a developmental failure (i.e. true hypoplasia) but an alternative mechanism concerning the fetal bypass system seems probable in many cases. At birth the umbilical vein and sinus venosus are occluded by vasospasm, thus

closing the placento-liver bypass; the ligamentum teres and ligamentum venosum are formed by the fibrosed remnants of these vessels (Fig. 9.4). The left portal vein branch is closely attached to these fetal blood vessels; if the spasm extends abnormally, the lateral portion of the left lobe may become ischaemic. Though difficult to establish with certainly, the frequency with which a small lateral segment of the left lobe is replaced by a fibrous band is suggestive of this aetiology. Generally this anomaly is of no clinical significance, though occasionally it is associated with defective development of the diaphragm. Absence of the right lobe is much rarer; again a diaphragmatic hernia may coexist.

Enlargement of one portion of the liver also most commonly affects the left lobe which may stretch across to the left costal margin. Here it lies superior to the spleen where it often gives a confusing appearance that is easily mistaken for a subphrenic collection. Alternatively, it may form a thin sheet of liver in the epigastrium that extends well below the costal margin. These two variants probably should be considered as changes in shape rather than as true anomalies where an additional lobe is found. Usually these more severe developmental anomalies form as sessile lobes consisting of marked enlargements of a liver segment; the Riedel's lobe, a 'linguiform prolongation of the right lobe', is very common. It may appear simply as an elongated right lobe or may have a narrowing overlying the right kidney so that it is almost pedunculated (Fig. 9.20). True pedunculated accessory lobes are rarer; the stalk may contain liver tissue or only vessels and fibrous tissue. Since they may be found in any position in the abdomen, they are particularly confusing especially when affected by pathology such as masses or torsion.

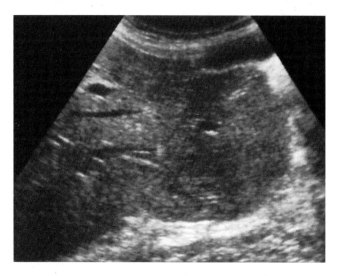

Fig. 9.20 Riedel's lobe. Riedel's lobe is an inferior extension of the right lobe which often overlies the kidney. Because it lies very superficially, it is obvious on palpation and thus raises the suspicion of hepatomegaly.

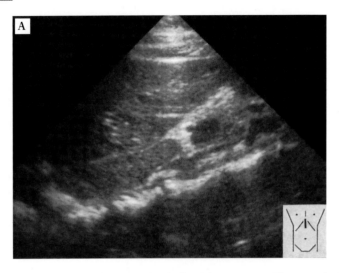
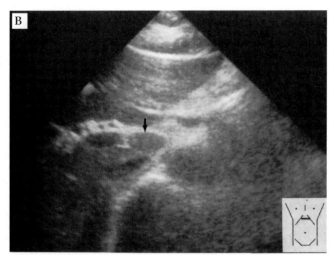

Fig. 9.21 Long caudate lobe. The caudate lobe is very variable in size. **A:** When it extends far inferiorly, as in this subject. **B:** Transverse cuts through its tip may suggest the presence of a pre-aortic mass (arrow) that is separate from the liver, such as an enlarged lymph node but cuts further superiorly demonstrate its continuity with the liver.

Marked variability of the caudate lobe has been mentioned: it may be very small or may extend inferiorly as a tongue below the level of the free border of the left lobe (Fig. 9.21). Seen in transverse section, the tip seems to be separate from the liver and at first might suggest a pancreatic mass or lymphadenopathy.

Indentations on the liver surface from adjacent structures can be quite marked and masses may impress themselves on the liver parenchyma as it is soft and yielding. The same effect often produces grooves on the diaphragmatic surface where prominent leaflets indent it, producing furrows. True accessory fissures are sometimes encountered on this surface as deep peritoneal folds in the liver substance that are fixed in position (Fig. 9.22).

Assessment of liver size

The wide normal variation in the configuration of the liver makes assessment of its size difficult, whatever means are employed. The bulk of the liver may lie mainly on the right, perhaps with a Riedel's lobe and a correspondingly small left lobe, or there may be a small right lobe with a large left lobe that extends across to lie under the left hemidiaphragm above the spleen. In the midline such a large left lobe may cover the upper epigastric organs.

Clinical evaluation is notoriously unreliable,[12,13] a Riedel's lobe, for example, easily being mistaken for hepatomegaly. Tomographic techniques are not well suited to size assessment because each image represents only one projection of the anatomy so that the full series of slices must be evaluated before the true dimensions of the liver can be appreciated. This is difficult to perform automatically and can only be approximated by eye. Because it is non-

tomographic, isotope scintigraphy is in some respects the most reliable method for size evaluation since the whole outline of the liver is demonstrated.[14] Again the problem of projections, here those of the liver surfaces rather than of slices, is difficult to overcome.

With tomographic techniques such as ultrasound, the simplest approach to the evaluation of liver size is from linear measurements in standard positions. In a series of 1000 normal subjects, anteroposterior (AP) longitudinal diameters were measured in the midline and at the mid-clavicular line with the subjects in deep inspiration.[15] The left lobe measurements were straightforward but on the right, overlying lung usually prevented access to the uppermost part of the liver, so the level of the lung was taken as the limit (Fig. 9.23). The results of the linear measurements (Table 9.1) were not improved upon by calculating areas and the longitudinal and AP measurements were closely enough correlated for most subjects so that use of the longitudinal value alone was accurate enough for routine purposes, except in very thin or very obese subjects. This is because the liver tends to be elongated in thin subjects, so that the longitudinal measurement on its own

Table 9.1 Dimensions of the normal liver[15]

	Diameter (cm) (mean ± SD)	95th percentile (cm)
Mid-clavicular		
Longitudinal	10.5 ± 1.5	12.6
AP	8.1 ± 1.9	11.3
Midline		
Longitudinal	8.3 ± 1.7	10.9
AP	5.7 ± 1.5	8.2

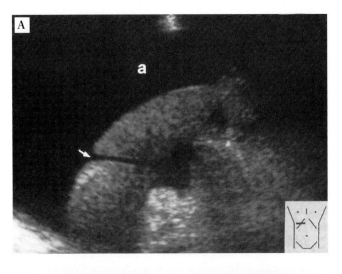

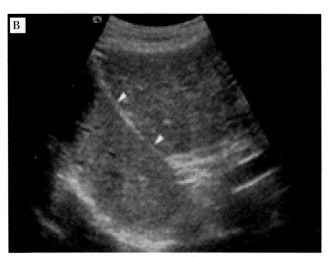

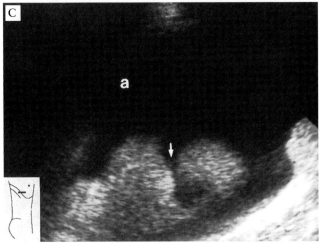

Fig. 9.22 Accessory fissure in the liver. A and B: Under normal conditions, accessory fissures are difficult to detect on ultrasound because the surfaces are apposed; in this patient ascitic fluid (a) separating the surfaces reveals the fissure (arrow) extending deep into the right lobe from its lateral surface. In another patient, **C:** a fissure is seen within the right lobe (arrowheads) in this transverse section.

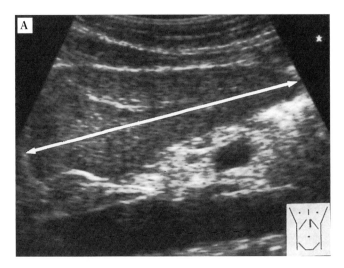

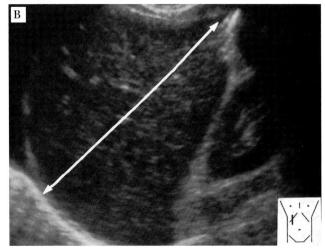

Fig. 9.23 Linear measurements of the liver. The size of the liver can be assessed by **A:** taking the span in the midline and **B:** in the mid-clavicular line; the former averages 8 cm and the latter 10 cm. Only in very thin or very heavily built patients is it necessary also to take the anteroposterior measurements to compensate for their different liver shapes.

gives an overestimation, while the reverse is true of obese subjects, whose livers tend to be short and deep.

Quite similar figures were proposed in another study[16] in which linear measurements were compared with autopsy measurements of liver size. The span (superoinferior distance) of the right lobe was measured in the scan plane halfway between the midline and the lateral extent of the right lobe (in practice this is very close to the midclavicular line). When this was correlated with autopsy measurements, 93% of those livers with a span of less than 13 cm were normal while 75% of those larger than 15 cm were abnormal. The 13–15 cm group must be considered an overlap region of uncertainty, despite which this type of linear measurement is useful for assessment of changes in liver size, for example when following the response of liver metastases to chemotherapy.

In a slight elaboration of this method, longitudinal measurements of the left lobe in the midline and of the right lobe in the mid-clavicular line have been extensively assessed and provide a surprisingly good correlation with other physical measurements such as body weight and surface area.[15] In this study of almost 1000 healthy subjects, the normal values on the left were 8.3 (±1.7), and on the right 10.5 (±1.5) cm. Only in very heavy and very light subjects was it found to be important to add AP measurements; in these somatotypes the horizontal and vertical lie of the liver respectively leads to an under- and overestimation of liver size when only longitudinal measurements are used.

A slightly more complex method, in which the height, breadth and thickness of the liver are combined, mathematically also gives good correlations.[17] The product of these three (in centimetres) divided by 27 (3^3) gives an index of liver volume which is nominally 100%. The standard deviation is between 95% and 140% (75 subjects). Since this requires the transverse span of the liver to be measured, it is not readily applied to standard scanners; possibly this is the reason for its failure to gain routine acceptance.

A more elaborate method of estimating the liver volume involves measuring the area of each of a spaced series of tomograms.[18] If all the slices are in the same plane (usually either transverse or sagittal sections) and are spaced 1 cm apart, simply summing the areas (in cm^2) gives the liver volume (in ml). A slight refinement can be incorporated to allow for the difficulty in measuring the areas of the topmost and lowermost slices whose outlines tend to be blurred because of the partial volume effect. If other sets of slices, such as radial, are chosen, more complex formulae must be used, but the same results can be obtained. Accuracies of ±5% have been obtained *in vivo* and this represents a great improvement on clinical or simple linear ultrasound measurements. However, the technique is time consuming and necessitates the use of a static scanner (the field of view of real-time systems being too small to accommodate the whole area of the central tomograms through

the liver). In addition, in many subjects, the complete set of slices cannot be obtained, gas or bone preventing access for some parts of the liver. For most departments therefore, this type of evaluation is too tedious and cumbersome for routine use; the same method is much more easily applied to CT scans.

In practice therefore, the ultrasound evaluation of liver size is a subjective affair; an experienced sonologist can gain a useful impression of liver size from tomographic views in different directions covering both lobes with due allowance for the patient's size. For example, if both left and right lobes project below the costal margin, suspicion of hepatomegaly is raised and can often be confirmed by noting that the free edge of the liver has lost its normal sharp configuration and become rounded, a non-specific feature of hepatomegaly of any cause. Though crude, this form of subjective evaluation is often useful, especially in refuting a clinical impression of hepatomegaly which is often readily explained by the presence of a Riedel's lobe (especially if it overlies a high right kidney) or perhaps by a flat right hemidiaphragm.

One lobe of the liver whose size can be assessed on a linear measurement is the caudate lobe, which is often particularly enlarged in cirrhosis and in hepatic vein occlusion (the Budd–Chiari syndrome). Again, a subjective evaluation is often sufficient, especially to exclude enlargement, but when there is doubt or when a baseline measurement is required, its transverse diameter at the level of the porta may be measured and compared with the transverse diameter of the right lobe (Fig. 9.24). The normal caudate lobe is less than two-thirds of the right lobe and there is only a small overlap with normal.[19] A simpler alternative is to compare the AP thickness of the caudate with the left lobe immediately anterior to it; the caudate should be less than half the thickness of the left lobe (Fig. 9.25).

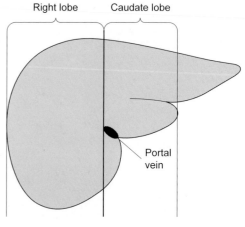

Fig. 9.24 Measurement of the caudate lobe. The position for measurement of the caudate lobe in the transverse plane is shown. The normal caudate is less than two-thirds the transverse diameter of the right lobe.

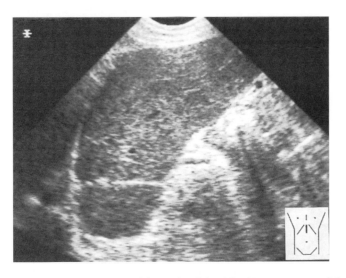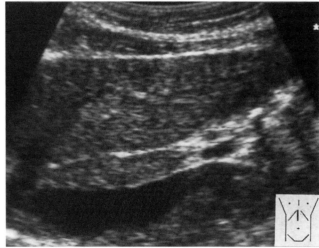

Fig. 9.25 AP measurement of the caudate lobe. The AP measurement of the caudate lobe should be no more than one-half of the AP measurement of the overlying left lobe. These two patients show that the rule applies even in wide variations of liver shape.

REFERENCES

1 Valleix D, Sautereau D, Pouget X et al. Ultrasonographic anatomy of the liver. Surg Radiol Anat 1987; 9: 123–134
2 Gelfand D W. Anatomy of the liver. Radiol Clin North Am 1980; 18: 187–194
3 Marks W M, Filly R A, Callen P W. Ultrasonic anatomy of the liver: a review with new applications. JCU 1979; 7: 137–146
4 Brown B M, Filly R A, Callen P W. Ultrasonographic anatomy of the caudate lobe. J Ultrasound Med 1982; 1: 189–192
5 Heloury Y, Leborgne J, Le Neel J C, Malvy P, Barbin J Y, Hureau J. The caudate lobe of the liver. Anatomical study. Surgical applications. J Chir (Paris) 1987; 124: 651–657
6 Couinaud C. Le Foie; études anatomique et chirurgicales. Paris: Masson, 1957
7 Mukai J K, Stack C M, Turner D A et al. Imaging of surgically relevant hepatic vascular and segmental anatomy. Part 1. Normal anatomy. AJR 1987; 149: 287–292
8 LaFortune M, Madore F, Patriquin H et al. Segmental anatomy of the liver: a sonographic approach to the Couinaud nomenclature. Radiology 1991; 181: 443
9 Balfe D M, Mauro M A, Koehler R E et al. Gastrohepatic ligament: normal and pathologic CT anatomy. Radiology 1984; 150: 485–490
10 Berland L L, Lawson T L, Foley W D. Porta hepatis: sonographic discrimination of bile ducts from arteries with pulsed Doppler with new anatomic criteria. AJR 1982; 138: 833–840
11 Champetier J, Yver R, Letoublon C, Vigneau B. A general review of anomalies of hepatic morphology and their clinical implications. Anat Clin 1985; 7: 285–299
12 Naftalis J, Leevy C M. Clinical estimation of liver size. Am J Dig Dis 1963; 8: 236–243
13 Sullivan S, Krasner N, Williams R. The clinical estimation of liver size. BMJ 1976; 2: 1042–1043
14 Peternel W W, Schaefer J W, Schiff L. Clinical evaluation of liver size and hepatic scintiscan. Am J Dig Dis 1966; 11: 346–350
15 Niederau C, Sonnenberg A, Müller J E, Erchenbrecht J F, Scholten T, Fritsch W P. Sonographic measurements of the normal liver, spleen, pancreas and portal vein. Radiology 1983; 149: 537–540
16 Gosink B B, Leymaster C F. Ultrasonic estimation of hepatomegaly. JCU 1981; 9: 37–41
17 Kardel T, Holm H H, Rasmusen S N, Mordensen T. Ultrasonic determination of liver and spleen volumes. Scand J Clin Lab Invest 1971; 27: 123–128
18 Rasmussen S N. Liver volume determination by ultrasonic scanning. Dan Med Bull 1978; 25: 1–46
19 Harbin W P, Robert N J, Ferrucci J T. Diagnosis of cirrhosis based on regional changes in hepatic morphology: a radiological and pathological analysis. Radiology 1980; 135: 273–283

Benign focal liver lesions

Keith C Dewbury

Introduction

A focal liver lesion is, by definition, a discrete abnormality arising within the liver. Clearly, to some degree the distinction between focal and diffuse abnormalities is artificial and the two merge together. Difficulty in separating an intrahepatic from an extrahepatic mass is sometimes a problem. Identification of the exact organ involved is essential in the diagnostic process as well as in treatment and prognostication. Ultrasonic features suggesting an intrahepatic origin include movement of the mass with the liver in respiration, bulging of the liver capsule, displacement and distortion of the portal and hepatic vessels and posterior displacement of the inferior vena cava. The larger the lesion, the more difficult the distinction may be. Masses of less than 10 cm in size are usually more accurately assessed. CT should be used to complement ultrasound when there are difficulties. The advantages of demonstration of all tissues including gas and bone may be invaluable. The limitless multiplanar scanning to delineate boundaries between contiguous viscera and the real-time capabilities remain important contributions for ultrasound.

Simple cysts

Ultrasound is highly accurate in the demonstration of cystic lesions in any organ and this applies particularly in the liver.[1] Fine detail is well shown and a careful evaluation of cyst wall smoothness and regularity, septa, fluid levels and internal echoes should be made in addition to the posterior acoustic accentuation. Fine internal detail may be better evaluated with ultrasound than with CT.[2]

Fine septations are not uncommonly seen and should not be cause for concern. Simple hepatic cysts may be primary or secondary. Primary liver cysts are congenital and arise from developmental defects in the formation of bile ducts.[3] They are relatively uncommon, tend to be superficial and are lined with cuboidal epithelium. They usually do not cause liver enlargement and are rarely palpable. The right lobe of the liver is affected more often than the left (Fig. 10.1). The incidence is 1 in 600 at laparotomy.[4] Occasionally simple cysts may present with pain, as a right upper quadrant mass or with symptoms secondary to haemorrhage or infection (Fig. 10.2).[5] The average cyst size is 3 cm.

Acquired cysts are usually secondary to trauma, inflammation or parasitic infection and are indistinguishable from primary cysts on ultrasound. The diagnostic accuracy of ultrasound in the diagnosis of simple liver cysts approaches 100%. The differential diagnosis includes a necrotic metastasis, hydatid cyst, hepatic cyst adenocarcinoma, haematoma or abscess (Fig. 10.3). If there is any concern about the diagnosis or the patient is symptomatic, guided percutaneous aspiration may be performed for cytological analysis.[5] In common with cysts in other organs, most simple cysts recur following aspiration.[6] Occasionally, an intrahepatic gallbladder may simulate a solitary intrahepatic cyst.[7] Biliary cystadenoma is usually quite distinctive, with multiple septations and papillary projections. The choledochal cyst, with its continuation with the extrahepatic biliary tree, is also usually quite characteristic (see Ch 15 and Vol. 2 Ch. 48).[8] Occasionally a choledochal cyst may be localised and intrahepatic in site, causing diagnostic confusion (Fig. 10.4).[8] Radioactive excretion studies with technetium-HIDA establishes the correct diagnosis in this instance.

Polycystic liver disease

Multiple cysts in the liver occasionally occur as an isolated phenomenon; however, they are most commonly seen in patients with underlying adult polycystic disease. The majority of patients with this disease have renal cysts (Fig. 10.5).[9] Polycystic renal disease is a relatively common congenital condition affecting 1 in 500. It has an autosomal dominant mode of inheritance. Approximately one-third of patients with polycystic kidney disease are found to have liver cysts.[3,4] Polycystic liver disease is more likely to be symptomatic than single cysts, the most common presentation being with hepatomegaly. As with single cysts, haemorrhage or infection in the cysts may cause pain. Multiple cysts in the liver may distort the normal liver architecture. Acoustic accentuation beyond each cyst may produce the impression of an abnormal liver texture (Fig. 10.6). A similar appearance may be seen with marked intrahepatic biliary duct dilatation and in Caroli's disease.

Biliary hamartomas (von Meyenberg complexes)

Bile duct hamartomas are small focal developmental lesions of the liver composed of groups of dilated intrahepatic bile ducts with a collageneous stroma. On ultrasound they are demonstrated as small lesions of low reflectivity or areas of high reflectivity with ring-down artefacts related to the cholesterol crystals within the dilated tubules. (Fig. 10.7) These are usually isolated and insignificant but may present with episodes of cholangitis.[10]

Echinococcal cysts (hydatid disease)

The liver is most frequently involved in hydatid disease, where more than half of the cysts are found.[12] Other sites of involvement, in decreasing order of frequency, include the lungs, the bones, the brain and the peritoneal cavity.[3] The parasite is endemic in certain areas, particularly where sheep and cattle grazing are common, such as the Middle East. The eggs of the worm *Echinococcus granulosus* are

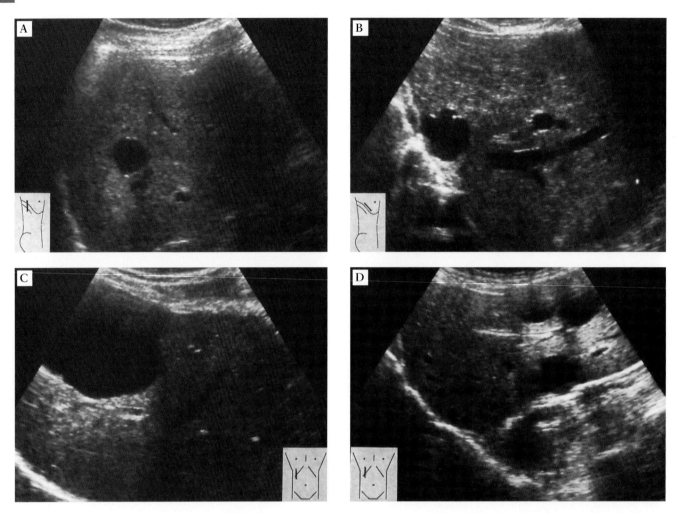

Fig. 10.1 Liver cyst. A: Small simple liver cyst in the right lobe of the liver showing a clear well-defined wall and distal acoustic enhancement. **B:** Longitudinal scan showing a simple liver cyst with partial septation anteriorly. Distal acoustic enhancement is poorly appreciated due to the lesion's location adjacent to the diaphragm. **C:** Large simple liver cyst. Note the prominence of the distal acoustic enhancement. **D:** Three simple cysts in the right lobe of the liver.

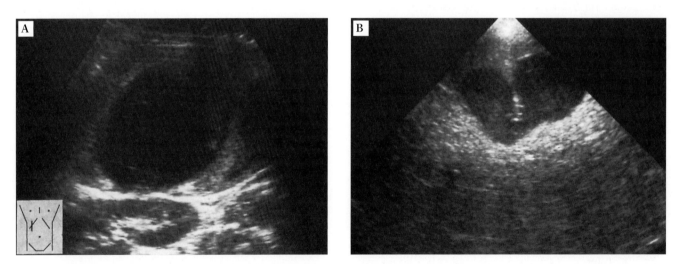

Fig. 10.2 Liver cyst. A: A large simple cyst in the right lobe of the liver showing stranding due to haemorrhage. **B:** Placement of a needle for diagnostic aspiration of a simple cyst into which haemorrhage has occurred.

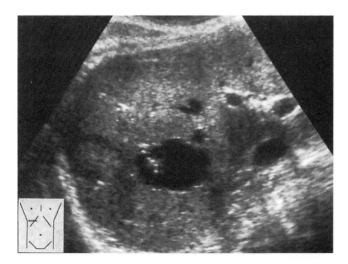

Fig. 10.3 Liver cyst and metastasis. Transverse scan of the right lobe of the liver showing a solid metastasis and adjacent to this a cystic metastasis which may be mistaken for a simple liver cyst. The irregularity of its wall should arouse suspicion.

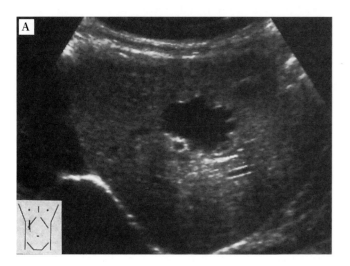

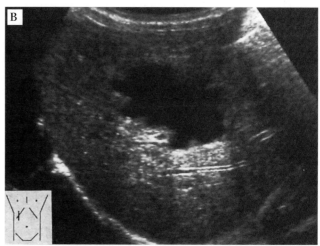

Fig. 10.4 Cyst with irregular margins. A and **B**: Longitudinal scans taken in an infant at 1 and 4 months of age. They show a unilocular cyst with a crenated margin within the right lobe of the liver. This lies centrally and has enlarged during the period of observation. The lobulated margin raises the possibility of a biliary origin.

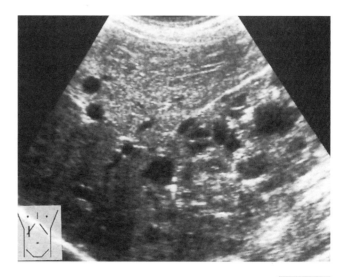

Fig. 10.5 Polycystic disease. Longitudinal scan showing the enlarged right kidney of a patient with adult polycystic renal disease with small cysts. Two or three small cysts are also noted in the liver.

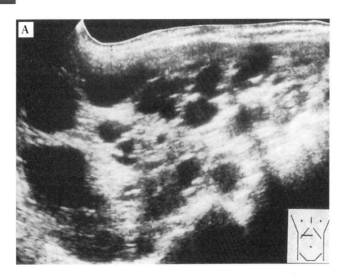
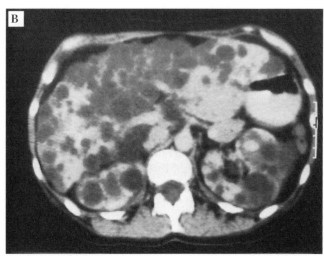

Fig. 10.6 Polycystic disease. Transverse ultrasound scan with a corresponding CT slice in a patient with marked polycystic liver disease associated with adult polycystic kidneys. Note that in the ultrasound scan the distortion of the parenchyma by the multiple cysts and the irregular distal enhancement beyond them produces a very abnormal liver textural pattern.

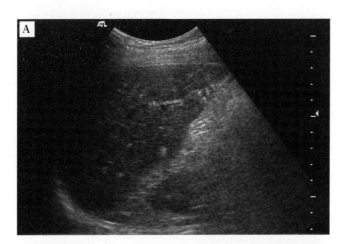
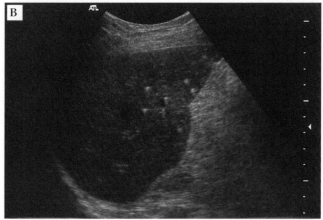

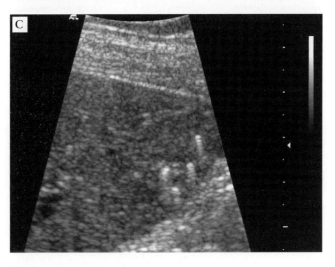

Fig. 10.7 Von Meyenberg complexes. A and **B:** Longitudinal scans. **C:** Magnified view. Note the small highly reflective foci with ring-down artefacts adjacent to portal tracts. The artefacts are probably due to cholesterol crystals.

excreted in the faeces of infected dogs. Cattle, sheep, goats and humans serve as the intermediate host. The eggs hatch in the upper intestine and the embryos permeate the intestinal mucosa to enter the bloodstream. The larvae lodge in an organ and cause an inflammatory reaction. Some larvae encyst and grow slowly, at a rate of up to 1 cm per year. Enclosing the fluid within the cyst is an inner nucleated germinal layer, which gives rise to the brood capsules, and an outer non-nucleated layer. The outer layer is quite distinctive with numerous delicate laminations like tissue paper. Outside this is an inflammatory reaction. Daughter cysts may develop from the inner germinal layer. A variety of ultrasound appearances may be demonstrated by hydatid cysts.[13]

Solitary cyst

A single cyst may vary from 1 to 20 cm in size and may be indistinguishable from a simple congenital liver cyst. In endemic regions, all liver cysts are considered to be hydatids until proven otherwise (Fig. 10.8). The distinction between simple and hydatid cysts may be aided by noting the following features:

1 Wall calcification may occur many years in hydatids after the initial infection. Simple liver cysts rarely, if ever, calcify. The presence of a complete rind of calcification suggests an inactive lesion (Fig. 10.9).[14]
2 Debris consisting of sand or scolices may be present within hydatid cysts. Visibility of this can be

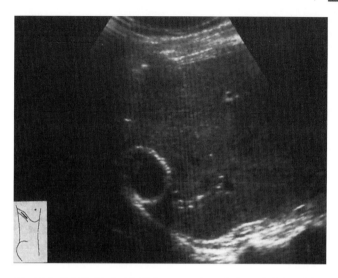

Fig. 10.9 Calcified hydatid. Oblique scan through the right lobe of the liver showing a single calcified hydatid cyst.

accentuated by moving the patient during the examination.[15]
3 It may be possible to discern the two layers of the wall of a hydatid cyst.

Separation of the membrane

Separation of the membrane producing a pathognomonic 'ultrasound waterlily sign' results from detachment and collapse of the inner germinal layer from the exocyst. The collapsed germinal layer is seen as an undulating linear collection of echoes either floating in the cyst or lying in the most dependent portion (Fig. 10.10).[16]

Daughter cysts

The development of daughter cysts from the lining germinal membrane produces a characteristic appearance of cysts enclosed within a cyst. This appearance is characteristic, producing what may be described as a cartwheel or honeycomb cyst (Fig. 10.11).[17]

Multiple cysts

With heavy or continued infestation, multiple primary parent cysts may develop within the liver, often producing hepatomegaly with normal liver tissue between the individual cysts. In the absence of membrane separation or daughter cyst formation, the diagnosis of hydatid disease may be difficult. The differential diagnosis should include necrotic hepatic metastases, chronic haematomas, abscess,

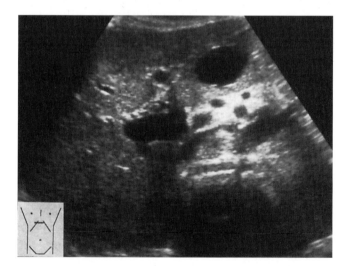

Fig. 10.8 Hydatid disease – simple type. Transverse scan through the liver showing a single simple cyst in the left lobe in a patient from the Middle East. A complement fixation test suggested the presence of hydatid disease.

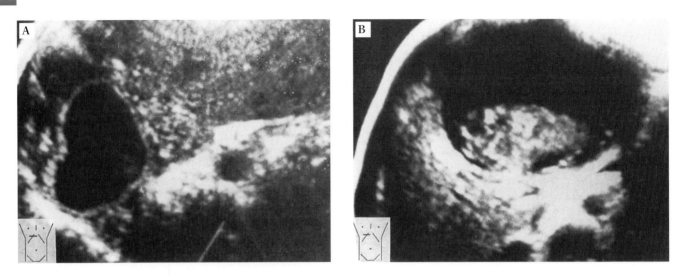

Fig. 10.10 Hydatid cysts. A: Transverse scan of the liver showing a hydatid cyst appearing as a flattened sphere. Note the early detachment of the capsule laterally. **B:** Hydatid cyst in which the membranes have become completely detached producing the 'floating membranes sign'. (Figure courtesy of Professor Sawat Hussein, Karachi.)

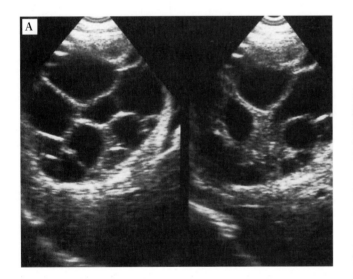

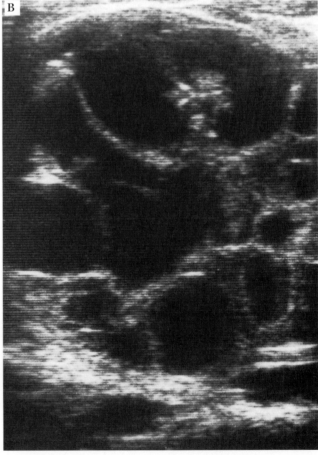

Fig. 10.11 Classical hydatid cysts. A and **B:** Examples of the pathognomonic appearance of hydatid cysts in which daughter cysts have developed from the lining germinal membrane producing the characteristic cartwheel or honeycomb pattern. (Figure courtesy of Professor Sawat Hussein, Karachi.)

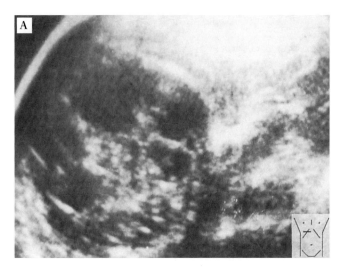
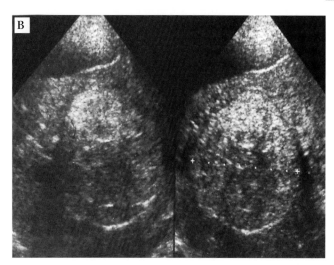

Fig. 10.12 Complicated hydatid cysts. A: Transverse scan showing an infected hydatid cyst. Many of the daughter cysts are filled with debris and the margins of the cyst have become rather indistinct. **B:** Infected hydatid cyst where the whole cyst has become more highly reflective than adjacent liver and the increased reflectivity within the cyst has almost totally obscured the margins of the daughter cysts. (Figure courtesy of Professor Sawat Hussein, Karachi.)

simple cysts, polycystic disease and bile duct cysts.[12] Uncomplicated percutaneous aspiration of hydatid cysts has been reported.[18] Anaphylaxis is a well-recorded risk of fluid leakage and skin tests or complement fixation tests should be performed if there is a suspicion of the diagnosis of hydatid disease.[5] When hydatid cysts become secondarily infected a different pattern may be seen with filling of the cyst with echoes (Fig. 10.12). The membrane may separate, producing a bizarre appearance. As cysts grow they may compress vascular structures or the biliary tree. In practice, significant biliary obstruction may mean that there is communication of the cyst with the biliary tree.[19] Cysts arising in the upper portion of the liver may communicate with the bronchi by a trans-diaphragmatic pathway.

Abscess

Pyogenic abscess

Liver abscesses most frequently arise as a complication of an intra-abdominal infection with direct portal venous spread to the liver.[20,21] Common sources of infection include the biliary tract, colonic diverticulitis and appendiceal abscess. Abscesses may also result from prior abdominal surgery, trauma, neoplasm or bacteraemia in an immunocompromised patient but often the source of infection is not found. The agent is most commonly *Escherichia coli*, but anaerobic bacteria such as *Clostridia* and *Bacteroides* are also found.[22] Rapid diagnosis and prompt appropriate treatment are important since the morbidity and mortality from untreated abscesses is high.[23,24] The clinical presentation may be variable but

fever, pain, pleurisy, nausea and vomiting are all common. There is usually a leukocytosis with abnormal liver function tests and anaemia.

Ultrasound shows a spherical, oval or slightly irregular echo-poor lesion with distal accentuation in three-quarters of cases (Fig. 10.13).[25] Great variability is common and depends upon both the age of the abscess and the causative organism. In the genesis of an abscess, inflammatory destruction of liver parenchyma is followed by pyogenic exudation within the cavity formed. The reflectivity of the contents and the definition of the margin will change in a dynamic way with time (Figs 10.14 and 10.15). A significant number of abscesses can be higher in reflectivity than adjacent normal liver. This may be caused by air or microbubbles within the fluid or to a mixture of differing content producing strong acoustic interfaces.[26,27] Larger amounts of gas within an abscess produce the typical ultrasound appearances associated with parenchymal gas.[28,29] In a chronic abscess a wall of variable thickness may be present. The differential diagnosis of an abscess includes complicated hepatic cysts and necrotic tumours. A diagnostic fine needle aspiration is invaluable and should be readily performed (Fig. 10.16 and see Ch. 7).

Amoebic abscess

Entamoeba histolytica primarily infects the colon. The disease is contracted by ingesting the cysts in contaminated food and water. The walls of the cysts dissolve in the alkaline contents of the small bowel and the trophozoites emerge to colonise and ulcerate the colon. The right half of the colon is most commonly involved.[22] Patients

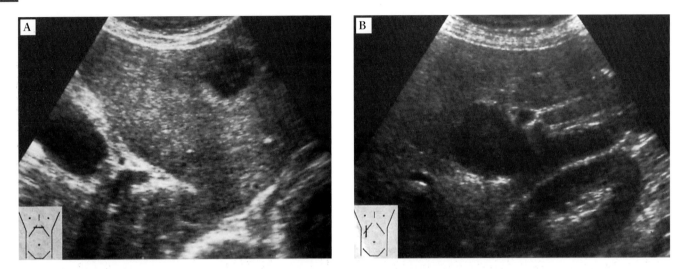

Fig. 10.13 Pyogenic abscess. A: Typical small pyogenic abscess in the left lobe of the liver. The wall is slightly thickened and irregular. A few low-level echoes are present within the abscess cavity and acoustic enhancement is noted beyond the abscess. **B:** A more clearly defined abscess in the right lobe of the liver but showing similar features with a little debris within the abscess and distal enhancement beyond. In this patient a second lesion is just visible adjacent to the hemidiaphragm. Multiplicity of pyogenic abscesses is common and should be excluded by a systematic search.

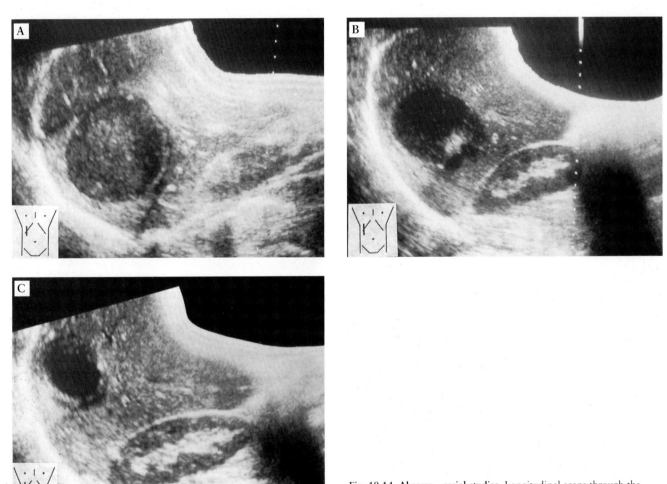

Fig. 10.14 Abscess – serial studies. Longitudinal scans through the right lobe of the liver taken at monthly intervals showing the change in size and appearance of an abscess on treatment.

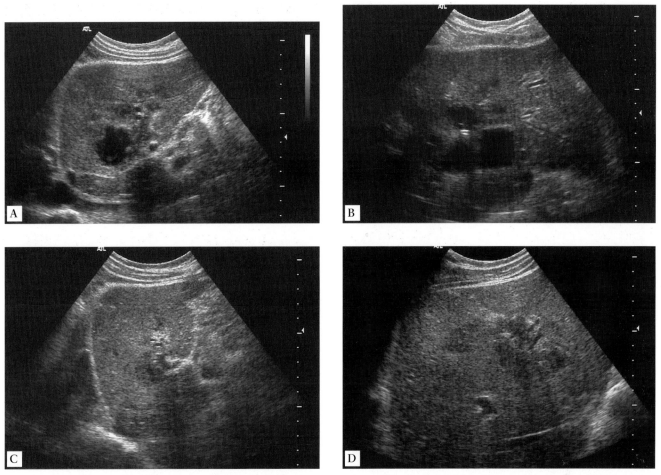

Fig. 10.15 Liver abscess with follow-up. A and **B:** Longitudinal and transverse images showing an irregular almost echo-free cavity within the centre of the liver with adjacent textural alteration. Note the highly reflective tip of the aspirating needle in the transverse image. 100 cc of pus were withdrawn at the initial scans. **C** and **D:** Corresponding longitudinal and transverse images taken 2 weeks following needle aspiration and intense antibiotic therapy. Dramatic healing of this large abscess has occurred, leaving a residual textural alteration but no cavity.

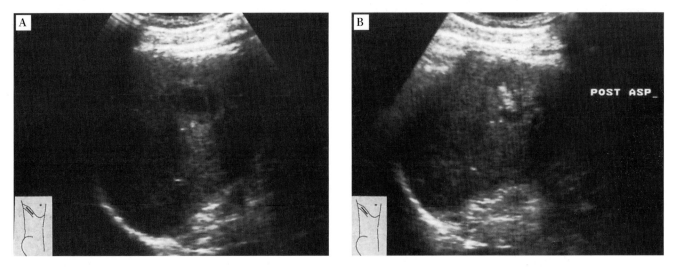

Fig. 10.16 Abscess, pre- and post-aspiration. A: Oblique scan through the right lobe of the liver showing a small echo-poor focal lesion with distal enhancement, suspicious of an abscess. **B:** Appearances after 20 ml of thick pus had been removed.

may be asymptomatic. Invasion of the colonic mucosa allows the amoebae to be carried in the portal venous system to the liver. Hepatic abscess formation occurs in 25% of infected patients and is the most common non-enteric complication.[30] An amoebic abscess may be indistinguishable from a pyogenic abscess. Characteristically there is:

1 lack of a significant wall echo so that they appear to be punched out lesions,
2 symmetric oval or round configuration,
3 lower reflectivity than liver with a homogeneous pattern of internal echoes,
4 increased sound transmission,
5 subcapsular location (Fig. 10.17).[30–34]

When the infection has been established there is liquefaction necrosis of the hepatocytes with little leukocytic response or fibrotic reaction, producing the classical 'anchovy sauce' contents. Pathologically, the walls of this abscess have a shaggy fibrin lining surrounded by scant fibrovascular response. Aspiration is rarely indicated as the diagnosis can be confirmed by haemagglutination titres and response to metronidazole therapy. Serial follow-up after therapy shows a decrease in the size of the lesion and a decrease in its reflectivity. At this stage the lesion has the characteristics of fluid on ultrasound but in fact the contents are semi-solid and cannot be aspirated easily. Complete resolution can be expected eventually, although this may take as long as 2 years.[35] Occasionally

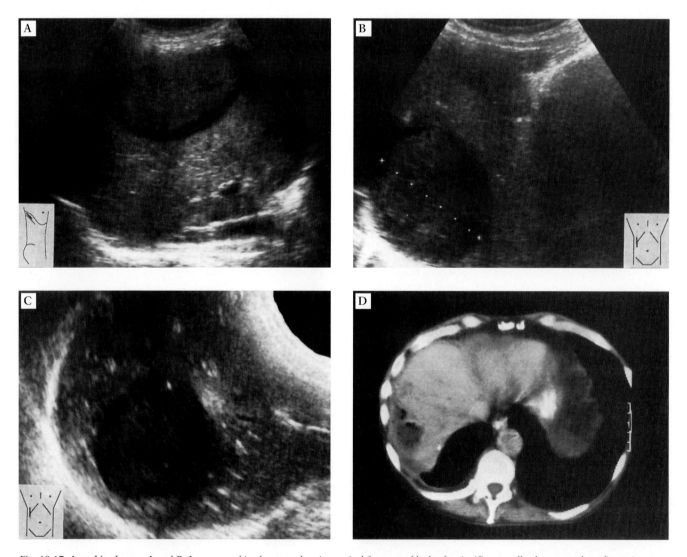

Fig. 10.17 Amoebic abscess. A and B: Large amoebic abscesses showing typical features of lack of a significant wall echo, an oval configuration, low, uniform reflectivity of internal echoes and distal acoustic enhancement. Both abscesses also show a typical peripheral location. **C:** Ultrasound and **D:** CT images of an amoebic abscess in which there is a small amount of gas present, shown by high reflectivity on ultrasound and low density on CT.

a cystic focal area may persist; it is indistinguishable from a simple liver cyst.

Candidiasis

Hepatic candidiasis is uncommon and usually follows haematogenous spread of infection to the liver in an immunologically compromised patient. The typical ultrasound appearances are of a small target lesion a few millimetres in diameter with a highly reflective centre and a poorly reflective halo. This outer halo is often a little irregular and lobular in outline (Fig. 10.18). Multiple lesions are characteristic. The outer rim is assumed to be necrotic and inflammatory debris and the central reflectivity either fungal mycelia or the collagen vascular bundle. Lymphoma and leukaemia are the important differential diagnoses, although target lesions are unusual in these conditions.[36,37] Because of their small size, a high resolution transducer such as a small parts linear array should be used. Fine needle aspiration is necessary for definitive diagnosis.

Cavernous haemangioma

Benign hepatic neoplasms are rare[38] with the exception of the cavernous haemangioma. This is the most common benign tumour of the liver and is reported in 7–20% of patients at autopsy.[39,40] The tumour is composed of a network of vascular endothelial lined spaces filled with blood. The majority of patients are asymptomatic and require no treatment.[41,42] Their importance lies in positive differentiation from lesions such as metastases that do require therapy or that may change patient management.

The spectrum of appearances on ultrasound is variable. However, the majority have a very distinctive pattern. This is of a sharply defined, highly reflective round tumour usually less than 2 cm in diameter and with a homogeneous echo pattern. Lesions may be single or multiple.[39,41,43,44] The high reflectivity is most likely due to the multiple interfaces between the vascular spaces. Lesions may occur anywhere within the liver but are more common in the right lobe. There is a tendency towards a peripheral location. Those occurring centrally usually lie close to the main hepatic veins (Fig. 10.19).[45]

Larger tumours may develop a lobular margin (Fig. 10.20). Haemangiomas larger than 2.5 cm in diameter may show posterior acoustic accentuation (Fig. 10.21).

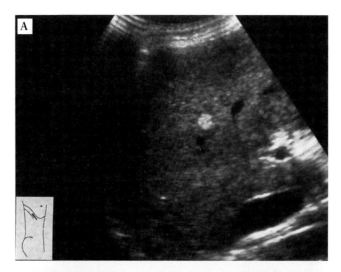

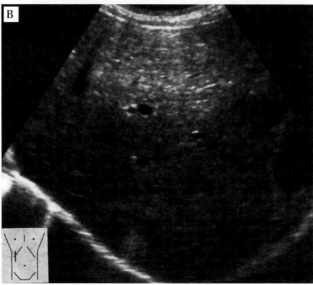

Fig. 10.19 **Haemangiomas. A:** Typical example of a tiny highly reflective cavernous haemangioma. **B:** Haemangioma of slightly lower reflectivity; detail and contrast resolution are reduced because the lesion lies beyond the focal zone.

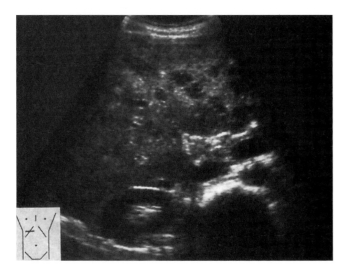

Fig. 10.18 **Fungal abscess.** Transverse scan through the liver in a patient with disseminated candidiasis. The lesions show the typical pattern of multiple slightly echo-poor lesions with a reflective nidus.

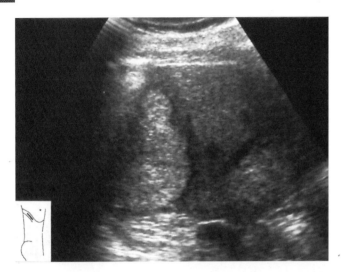

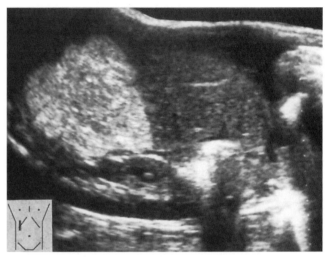

Fig. 10.20 Large haemangioma. A: Large lesion of high reflectivity with a lobular margin. **B:** Large lesions may be confusing and need either additional imaging or histology for full evaluation.

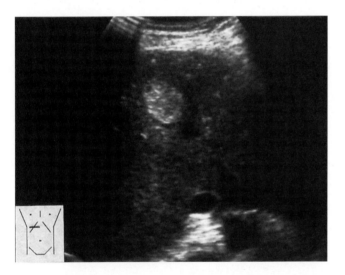

Fig. 10.21 Haemangioma with enhancement. Typical 3 cm haemangioma showing the unusual finding of slight distal accentuation.

This is an unusual feature, although not unique in highly reflective masses, and it probably relates to the vascularity.[46] As the haemangioma undergoes degeneration and fibrous replacement, the reflectivity becomes more heterogeneous. This is more frequently seen with larger lesions. Atypical appearances make distinction from other focal hepatic lesions difficult or impossible.

A further interesting variation occasionally reported is the reduction in reflectivity that can be seen within the same lesion scanned at different times and particularly over a period of time. This is difficult to explain but relates to the blood flow within the haemangioma at the time of imaging (Fig. 10.22).

In asymptomatic patients with no known history of malignancy, it is safe to consider these classical appearances as diagnostic of haemangioma. Where there is an unusual ultrasound appearance or clinical concern a dynamic CT should be done. A characteristic enhancement pattern is then typically shown (Fig. 10.23) and ultrasound contrast agents may show similar patterns (see Ch. 5). Lesions smaller than 1–1.5 cm in diameter may be difficult to evaluate accurately with dynamic CT. However, these small haemangiomas are usually extremely typical on ultrasound.[47] MRI with a dedicated protocol for evaluation for haemangioma has a better sensitivity than either ultrasound or dynamic helical CT. On T_2 weighting, haemangiomas have higher signal intensity because of their high water content and subsequent prolonged T_2 relaxation time.[48–50] If this is not available and any doubt persists, biopsy of these lesions can safely be performed with a fine needle, particularly if a long liver path is chosen (see Ch. 7).[51]

A rare but interesting group of haemangiomatous tumours is seen in the liver during infancy.[52] Again, often multiple, massive shunting can occur resulting in their occasional presentation with cardiac failure. There is hepatomegaly and there may be associated cutaneous haemangiomas. Although well defined, these generally do not have the appearance of adult haemangiomas on ultrasound but rather have a non-homogeneous, irregular appearance with mixed reflectivity (Fig. 10.24). In addition, large draining veins may be seen and there may be some enlargement of the proximal abdominal aorta due to shunting through the hepatic artery. Serial ultrasound scans are useful since the natural tendency of these lesions is to decrease in size over 6 months until they are no longer visible (Fig. 10.25).

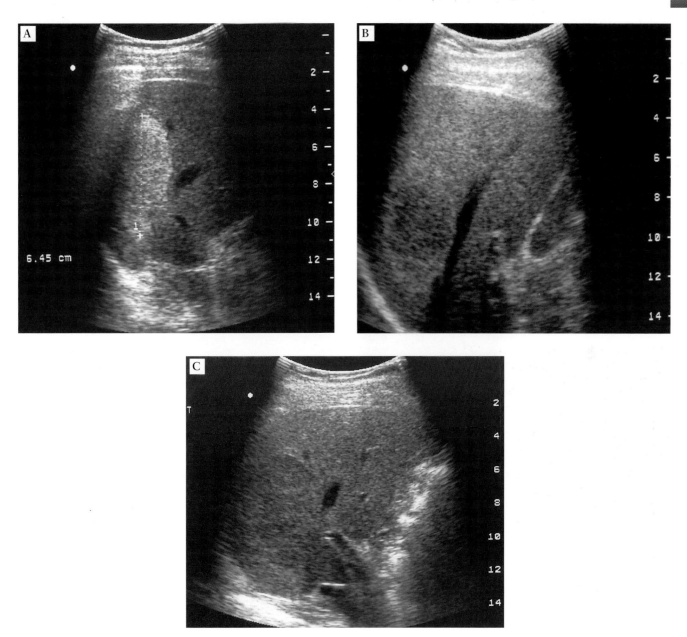

Fig. 10.22 Liver haemangioma – serial scans. A to C: A giant 6.5 cm liver haemangioma is imaged at 6-monthly intervals showing a reduction in reflectivity in the final image. The lesion has become almost invisible.

Focal nodular hyperplasia

Focal nodular hyperplasia is a rare benign tumour of the liver that is often discovered by chance. Typically it is found in women of 20–40 years of age but occurs in both sexes and in all age groups.[53] Most patients are asymptomatic but up to one-third may have pain or hepatomegaly. Focal nodular hyperplasia is generally a solid lesion in a subcapsular location. It is well circumscribed but non-encapsulated (Fig. 10.26). The mass is composed of

normal hepatocytes, Kupffer cells, bile duct elements and fibrous connective tissue. Multiple nodules are separated by bands of fibrous tissue, often radiating from a central stellate scar or a linear fibrous scar.[54] The ultrasound features are variable. The lesions are usually homogeneous with a slightly differing reflectivity from that of the normal liver, which may be higher or lower (Fig. 10.27). An echo complex corresponding to the central fibrous scar, although classical, is infrequently demonstrated.[55] Because the lesions contain Kupffer cells they may concentrate

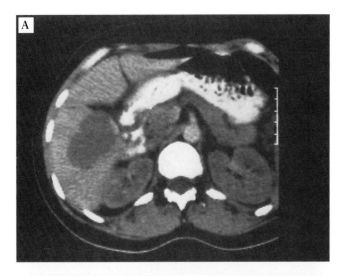

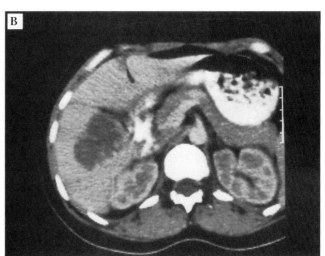

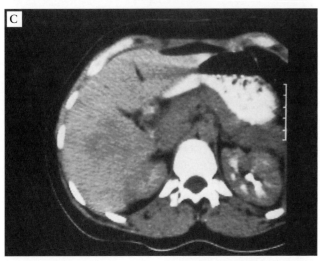

Fig. 10.23 Haemangioma – dynamic CT scan. A to **C:** Part of a dynamic CT scan following contrast, showing the typical filling-in of the lesion during the course of the examination. Delayed slices over several minutes may be required to demonstrate the infilling.

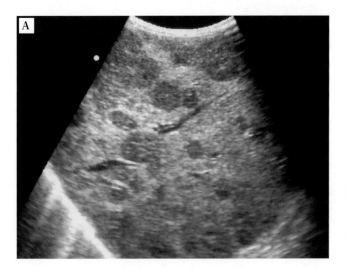

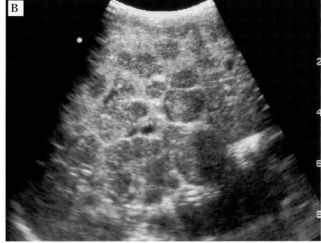

Fig. 10.24 Multiple infantile haemangiomas. A and **B:** Longitudinal and transverse scans showing the typical appearance of multiple haemangiomas in infancy. Doppler showed increased liver vascularity.

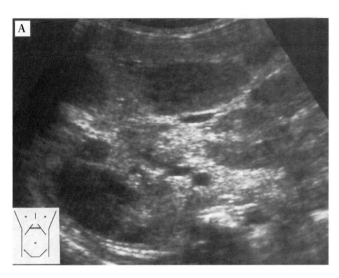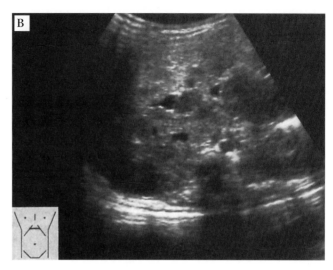

Fig. 10.25 Neonatal haemangioma. A: Transverse scan through the liver of a neonate who had a congenital cardiac anomaly and multiple visible haemangiomas on the skin. The patient was developing heart failure. The liver is full of large relatively well-defined echo-poor focal lesions. Arteriography of the liver at the time of cardiac catheterisation confirmed that these were haemangiomas. **B:** Follow-up scan 3 months later, although done at different magnification, shows a dramatic spontaneous reduction in size of the focal liver lesions; this is a typical finding in multiple haemangiomatous tumours of the liver in infancy.

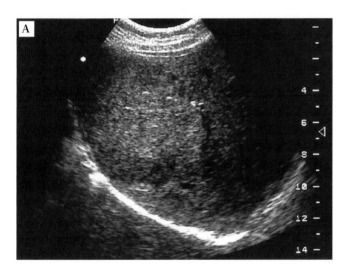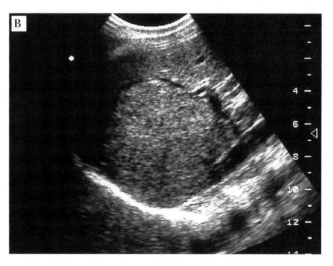

Fig. 10.26 Focal nodular hyperplasia. A and B: Longitudinal and oblique scans of the right lobe of the liver showing a large focal lesion. This is of almost the same reflectivity as adjacent liver and there is no well-defined capsule. The lesion is recognised by subtle architectural changes in the portal tracts and vessels. No central scar is demonstrated.

radiocolloids and microbubble contrast agents that show late liver-specific uptake. This combination of a lesion larger than 2 cm diameter on ultrasound (or CT) without a cold area on the isotope scan is almost diagnostic of focal nodular hyperplasia.[54,56]

The increased sensitivity of modern Doppler may be useful in diagnosis of focal nodular hyperplasia, showing a rich vascularity with both peripheral and central vessels creating the so-called spoke-wheel appearance (Fig. 10.28).[57–59]

Liver cell adenoma

Liver cell adenoma consists of normal or slightly atypical hepatocytes containing areas of bile stasis and focal haemorrhage or necrosis but, unlike focal nodular hyperplasia, not containing bile ducts or Kupffer cells.[56] They usually manifest as smooth solitary masses that are well marginated and completely or partially encapsulated. There is a close association with the use of oral contraceptives and it is much commoner in women.[22,60,61] Up to 60% of patients with hepatic

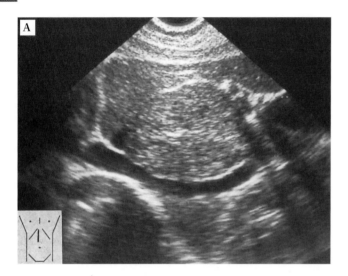

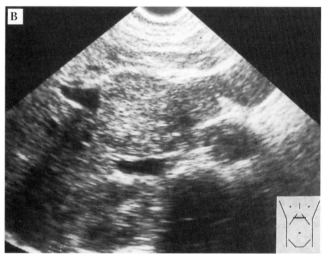

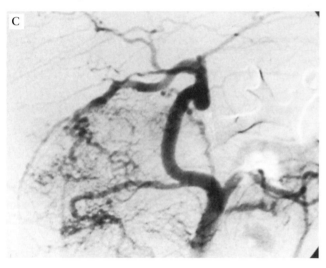

Fig. 10.27 Focal nodular hyperplasia. A: Longitudinal and **B:** transverse scans of the liver showing a well-defined focal lesion expanding the caudate lobe of the liver. Its texture is little different from adjacent liver tissue. **C:** Selective arteriogram showing a uniform vascularity of this lesion which, at biopsy, was proven to be focal nodular hyperplasia.

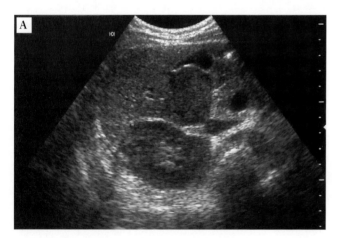

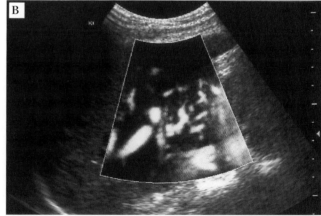

Fig. 10.28 Doppler in focal nodular hyperplasia. A and **B:** Doppler shows the typical rich vascularity of focal nodular hyperplasia with an abundance of central as well as peripheral vessels.

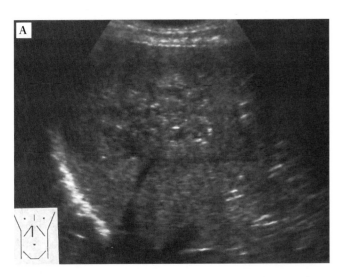
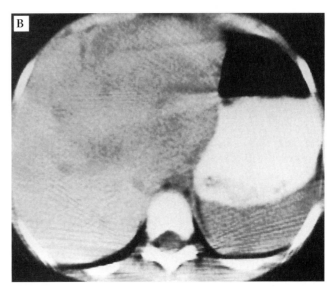

Fig. 10.29 Adenoma. A: Ultrasound and **B:** CT images showing a large rather poorly defined focal mass in the left lobe of the liver. Obvious necrotic clefts are shown on the ultrasound scan. Both ultrasound and CT suggested this was a malignant tumour but at biopsy it turned out to be a liver cell adenoma.

adenoma have areas of haemorrhage and necrosis compared with 6% with focal nodular hyperplasia (Fig. 10.29). The mass is usually symptomatic with presentations including a palpable mass, right upper quadrant pain and haemorrhage either into the tumour or from rupture into the peritoneum. There are no definitive ultrasound features that distinguish hepatic adenoma from focal nodular hyperplasia.[56] The clinical presentation should be helpful. Distinction is important as focal nodular hyperplasia may be followed conservatively while surgery is the treatment of choice for hepatic adenoma. Hepatic adenomas may regress following cessation of the contraceptive pill.

The precise ultrasound pattern is very variable depending on the amount of bleeding that has occurred and the timing of the scan in relation to the episode of bleeding.

Colour Doppler often has a non-specific appearance in adenoma. Typically, large peripheral subcapsular vessels are described. Central vessels may also be identified but they are not usually as prominent as in focal nodular hyperplasia (Fig. 10.30).

Hepatic adenomas also occur in association with glycogen storage disease, where there is an 8% incidence (see Vol. 2 Ch. 47). In type I disease the incidence is reportedly as high as 40%.[64,65] In von Geirke's disease the overall liver

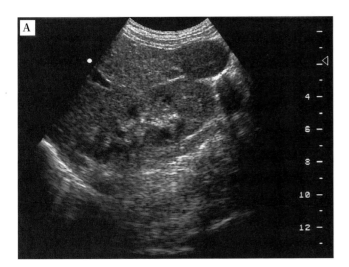
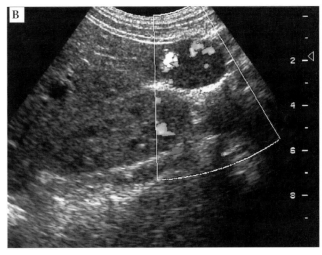

Fig. 10.30 Doppler in liver adenoma. A and **B:** A small, well-defined liver adenoma with a few central vessels but no rich central vascularity (as is more typical of FNH).

texture is abnormal with an increase in size and reflectivity due to fatty and glycogen infiltration. Against this background, adenomas stand out with a variable appearance ranging from low to high reflectivity.

Lipomas and focal fatty change

Lipomas are rare primary benign tumours arising from mesenchymal elements. They are non-encapsulated and in continuity with the normal liver parenchyma. They show the typical high reflectivity of fatty tumours (Fig. 10.31).[66]

Fatty infiltration of the liver is a common occurrence resulting from increased deposition of triglyceride in hepatocytes. This arises from a variety of nutritional disturbances or toxic insults to the liver.[67,68] These include obesity, nutritional deficiencies, diabetes mellitus, pregnancy, steroids, hepatotoxic drugs and alcoholism.[69] The development of fatty infiltration is a dynamic process and changes may be seen within a few weeks of an insult and may regress within days.[68,70] Most characteristically, the fatty involvement is uniform or geographic in distribution, but occasionally it may be nodular or multifocal, when it can be indistinguishable from other focal hepatic lesions.[71] Features suggesting the true nature of the process are sharp, angular boundaries to the lesions and no evidence of displacement or effacement of venous structures (Fig. 10.32).

Another well-recognised variant is focal sparing of small areas of normal liver in a more generalised fatty infiltration. The spared area appears as an echo-poor focal

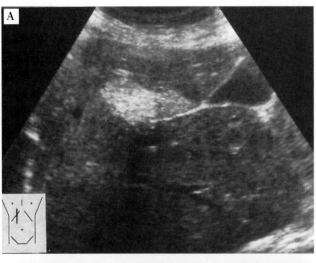
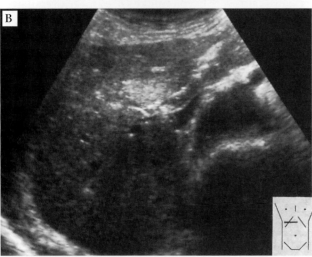
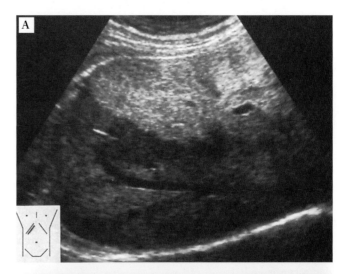
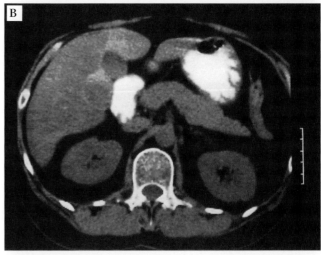

Fig. 10.31 Fatty lesion. A and **B:** A fairly well-defined reflective focal lesion lying just above the hepatic inter-lobar fissure. Guided biopsy of this lesion revealed fatty tissue; the differential diagnosis is between focal fatty change and lipoma.

Fig. 10.32 Focal fatty change. A: Transverse scan through the right lobe of the liver showing the typical geographic distribution of focal fatty infiltration, in this example most marked anteriorly with sparing posteriorly. There is no disturbance of the normal vascular architecture. **B:** CT scan in another case showing similar features.

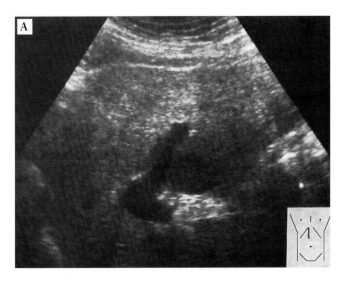

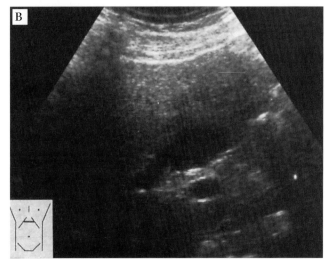

Fig. 10.33 **Focal fatty sparing. A** and **B:** The typical oval area of focal sparing from a more generalised fatty infiltration of the liver is shown.

mass. A characteristic location for the spared area is the quadrate lobe anterior to the portal vein bifurcation or related to the gallbladder bed.[70–72] The shape of the spared area or pseudomass is typically ovoid. Its location has led to the suggestion that the sparing relates to alteration of blood flow in this area (Fig. 10.33).[72]

Liver haematoma

The aetiology of a liver haematoma may be blunt abdominal trauma or rupture of a neoplasm such as a hepatic adenoma or cavernous haemangioma. In children, liver trauma due to blunt abdominal trauma is a common problem. This may be attributed to the greater flexibility of the rib cage and the lack of surrounding fat.[73–75]

There are three major categories of liver trauma:

1 rupture of the liver and its capsule. This is the most serious injury. The patient may be too ill for any imaging to be undertaken. This type of injury will usually be most fully demonstrated with CT,
2 subcapsular haematoma,
3 central haematoma.

An acute central haematoma tends to be highly reflective because of fibrin and erythrocytes forming multiple acoustic interfaces. With time, the clot undergoes liquefaction which corresponds with decreasing reflectivity and an increase in the size of the haematoma (Fig. 10.34) because of fluid absorption into the lesion as a result of increased osmotic pressure secondary to blood breakdown in the devitalised tissues. Over a period of months the haematoma may become cystic and develop internal stranding (Fig. 10.35). This eventually resolves with regen-

eration of liver tissue, but a residual fibrous scar or a small cystic space may persist.

Subcapsular haematomas, if small, go through a similar sequence of changes but if larger they may initially appear to be poorly reflective due to the larger amount of fluid blood present within them.

In addition to evaluating the liver, ultrasound is helpful in evaluating other abdominal viscera and assessing the presence of free blood. Liver rupture will often require surgical intervention but the large majority of patients with liver haematomas require minimal or no surgical intervention. Serial follow-up is of value and interest to monitor progressive resolution.

Calcification

Liver calcification is not a disease process but is seen as the end result of a number of infections and infestations including tuberculosis, syphilis and parasitic diseases.[76] Liver abscesses and haematomas may also develop dystrophic calcification in the long term. In these situations, the calcifications can be regarded as the 'tombstones' of the disease in question. As with calcification elsewhere, the appearances are typical with a focus of very high reflectivity and clear-cut distal acoustic shadowing (Figs 10.36 and 10.37).

Paediatric liver tumours

Benign tumours of the liver in children include haemangioendothelioma (Fig. 10.38), mesenchymal hamartoma, multiple haemangiomas, adenoma and cystic hepatoblastoma. These are discussed in more detail in Volume 2, Chapter 47.

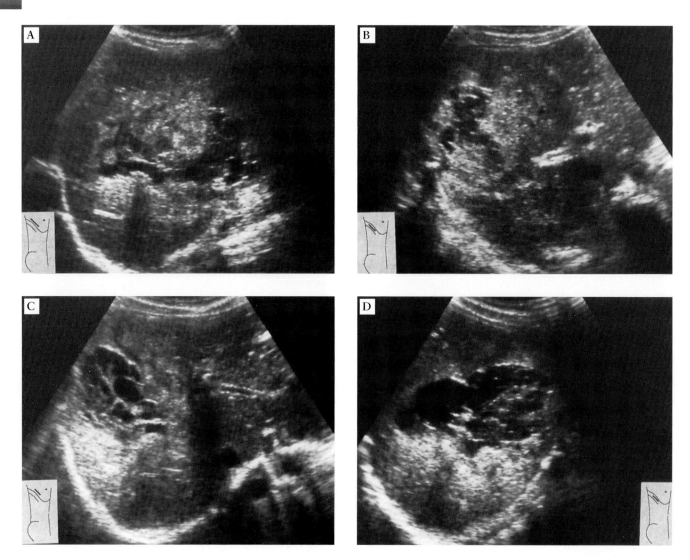

Fig. 10.34 Liver trauma. A and **B:** Oblique intercostal liver images of a child who suffered liver trauma following a fall from a horse. Note the irregular patchy high reflectivity involving much of the right lobe of the liver. **C** and **D:** Follow-up scans 4 days later showing some decrease in reflectivity corresponding to liquefaction of the clot.

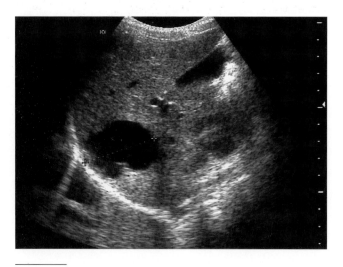

Fig. 10.35 Liver haematoma. Liver trauma in an 8-year-old boy. Scans taken 2 months following his original cycling accident show that the original haematoma has become a cystic lesion. Note the mirror artefact of the lesion above the diaphragm.

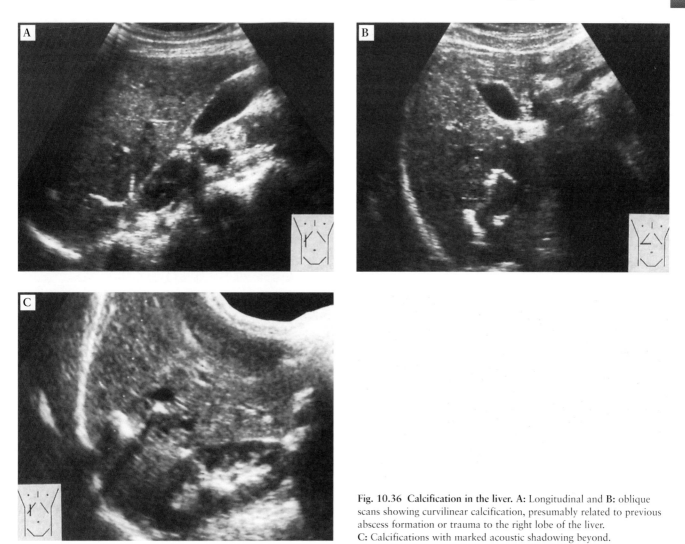

Fig. 10.36 Calcification in the liver. A: Longitudinal and **B:** oblique scans showing curvilinear calcification, presumably related to previous abscess formation or trauma to the right lobe of the liver. **C:** Calcifications with marked acoustic shadowing beyond.

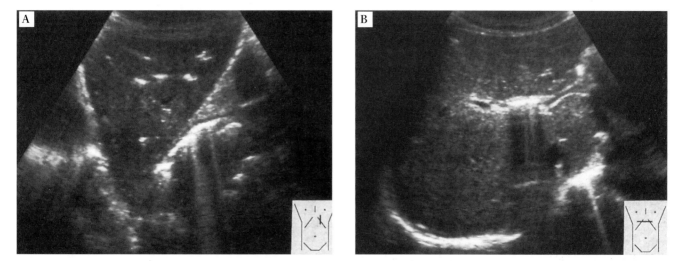

Fig. 10.37 Pneumobilia. A: Longitudinal and **B:** transverse scans showing small focal areas of high reflectivity with distal shadowing and reverberation artefacts. This is due to gas within the biliary tree and is to be compared with Figure 10.36.

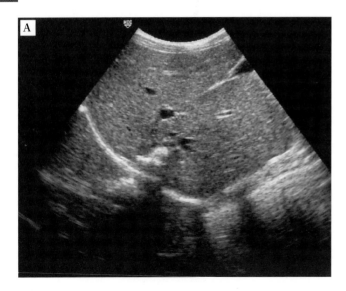
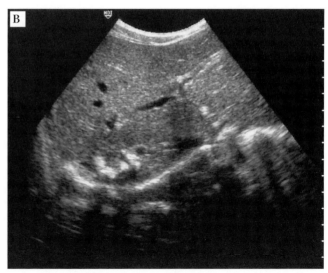

Fig. 10.38 Liver haemangioendothelioma. A: Longitudinal and **B:** transverse scans. These vascular tumours of infancy frequently calcify and may resolve or reduce in size. In this 4-year-old, little more than residual calcification is seen within the haemangioendothelioma.

REFERENCES

1 Federle M P, Filly R A, Moss A A. Cystic hepatic neoplasms: complimentary roles of CT and sonography. AJR 1981; 136: 345

2 Brick S H, Hill M C, Lande I M. The mistaken or indeterminate CT diagnosis of hepatic metastases: the value of sonography. AJR 1987; 148: 723

3 O'Brien M J, Gottlieb L S. The liver and biliary tract. In: Robins S L, Cotran R S, eds. Pathologic basis of disease. Philadelphia: Saunders, 1979: 1009

4 Taylor K J W, Viscomi G N. Ultrasound diagnosis of cystic disease of the liver. J Clin Gastroenterol 1980; 2: 197

5 Roemer C E, Ferruci J T Jnr, Mueller P R et al. Hepatic cysts: diagnosis and therapy by sonographic needle aspiration. AJR 1981; 136: 1065

6 Saini S, Mueller P R, Ferruci J T Jr et al. Percutaneous aspiration of hepatic cysts does not provide definitive therapy. AJR 1983; 141: 559

7 Spiegel R M, King D L, Green W M. Ultrasonography of primary cysts of the liver. AJR 1978; 131: 235

8 Austin R M, Sussman S, McArdle C R et al. Computed tomographic and ultrasound appearances of a solitary intrahepatic choledochal cyst. Clin Radiol 1986; 37: 149

9 Kuni C C, Johnson N L, Holmes J H. Polycystic liver disease. JCU 1978; 6: 332

10 Salo J, Shen J, Hecht A. Sonogram of multiple bile duct hamartomas. JCU 1989; 17: 667–669

11 Lev-Toaff A S, Bach A M, Wechsler R J et al. The radiologic and pathologic spectrum of biliary hamartomas. AJR 1995; 165: 309–313

12 Choliz J D, Olaverri F J L, Casas T F, Zubieta S O. Computed tomography in hepatic echinococcosis. AJR 1982; 139: 699

13 Hadidi A. Ultrasound findings in liver hydatid disease. JCU 1979; 7: 365

14 Itzchuk Y, Rubinestein Z, Shilo R. Ultrasound in tropical diseases. In Sanders R C, Hill M C, eds. Ultrasound annual. New York: Raven Press, 1983: 69

15 Lewell D B, McCorkell S J. Hepatic echinococcal cysts: sonographic appearance and classification. Radiology 1985; 155: 773

16 Niron E A, Ozer H. Ultrasound appearances of liver hydatid disease. Br J Radiol 1981; 54: 335

17 Babcock D S, Kaufman L, Cosnow I. Ultrasound diagnosis of hydatid disease (echinococcosis) in two cases. AJR 1978; 131: 895

18 Mueller P R, Dawson S L, Ferucci J T Jr, Nardi G L. Hepatic echinococcal cyst: successful percutaneous drainage. Radiology 1985; 155: 627

19 Gharbi H A, Hassine W, Brauner M W, Dupuch K. Ultrasound examination of the hydatic liver. Radiology 1981; 139: 459

20 Kuligowska E, Connors S K, Shapiro J H. Liver abscess: sonography in diagnosis and treatment. AJR 1982; 138: 253

21 Silver S, Weinstein A, Cooperman A. Changes in the pathogenesis and detection of intrahepatic abscess. Am J Surg 1979; 137: 608

22 Wright R, Milward-Sadler G H, Alberti K G M M, Karran S. The liver in infection. In: Liver and biliary disease, 2nd ed. Eastbourne: Baillière Tindall, 1985: 1077

23 Freeny P C. Acute pyogenic hepatitis: sonographic and angiographic findings. AJR 1980; 135: 388

24 Kuligowska E, Noble J. Sonography of hepatic abscess. In: Raymond H W, Zwiebel W J, eds. Seminars in ultrasound, vol 4(2). New York: Grune & Stratton, 1983: 102

25 Terrier F, Becker C D, Triller J K. Morphologic aspects of hepatic abscesses at computed tomography and ultrasound. Acta Radiol 1983; 24: 129

26 Subramanyan B R, Balthazer E J, Raghavendra B N et al. Ultrasound analysis of solid appearing abscesses. Radiology 1983; 146: 487

27 Powers T A, Jones T B, Carl J H. Echogenic hepatic abscess without radiographic evidence of gas. AJR 1981; 137: 159

28 Jones M, Kovak A, Geshner J. Acoustic shadowing by gas producing abscesses. South Med J 1981; 74: 247

29 Burt T B, Knochel J Q, Lee T G. Gas as a contrast agent and diagnostic aid in abdominal sonography. J Ultrasound Med 1982; 1: 179

30 Ralls P W, Colletti P M, Quinn M F, Halls J. Sonographic findings in hepatic amoebic abscess. Radiology 1982; 145: 123

31 Boultbee J E, Simjee A E, Rooknoodeen F, Engelbrecht H E. Experiences with grey scale ultrasonography in hepatic amoebiasis. Clin Radiol 1979; 30: 683

32 Dalrymple R B, Fataar S, Goodman A et al. Hyperechoic amoebic liver abscess: an unusual ultrasonic appearance. Clin Radiol 1982; 33: 541

33 Sukov R J, Cohen L J, Sample W F. Sonography of hepatic amoebic abscess. AJR 1980; 134: 911

34 Abul-Khair M H, Kenawi M M, Korasky E E, Arafa N M. Ultrasonography and amoebic liver abscesses. Ann Surg 1981; 193: 221

35 Ralls P W, Quinn M F, Boswell W D Jr, Colletti P M et al. Patterns of resolution in successfully treated hepatic amoebic abscess: sonographic evaluation. Radiology 1983; 149: 541

36 Ho B, Cooperberg P L, Li D K B et al. Ultrasonography and computed tomography of hepatic candidiasis in immunosuppressed patients. J Ultrasound Med 1982; 1: 157

37 Miller J H, Greenfield L D, Wald B R. Candidiasis of the liver and spleen in childhood. Radiology 1982; 142: 375

38 Mergo P J, Ros P R. Benign lesions of the liver. Radiol Clin North Am 1998; 36(2): 319–331
39 Onodera H, Ohta K, Oikawa M et al. Correlation of the real time sonographic appearance of hepatic haemangiomas with antiography. JCU 1983; 11: 421
40 Karhunen P J. Benign hepatic tumours and tumour like conditions in man. J Clin Pathol 1986; 39: 183–188
41 Wiener S N, Paruleker S G. Scintigraphy and ultrasonography of hepatic haemangioma. Radiology 1979; 132: 149
42 Park W C, Phillips R. The role of radiation therapy in the management of haemangiomas of the liver. JAMA 1970; 212: 1496
43 Mirk P, Rubaltelli L, Bazzocchi M et al. Ultrasonographic patterns in hepatic haemangiomas. JCU 1982; 10: 373
44 Freeny P C, Vimont T R, Barnett D C. Cavernous transformation of the liver: ultrasonography, arteriography and computed tomography. Radiology 1979; 132: 143
45 Bruneton J N, Drouillard J, Fenart D et al. Ultrasonography of hepatic cavernous haemangioma. Br J Radiol 1983; 56: 791
46 Taboury J, Porcel A, Tubiana J-M, Monnier J-P. Cavernous haemangiomas of the liver studied by ultrasound. Radiology 1983; 149: 781
47 Itai Y, Ohtomo K, Araki T et al. Computed tomography and sonography of cavernous haemangiomas of the liver. AJR 1983; 141: 315
48 McFarland E G, Mayo-Smith W W, Saini S et al. Hepatic hemangiomas and malignant tumors: improved differentiation with heavily T2 weighted conventional spin-echo MR imaging. Radiology 1994; 193: 43–47
49 Birnbaum B A, Weinreb J C, Megibow A J et al. Definitive diagnosis of hepatic hemangiomas: MR imaging versus Tc-99-labeled red blood cell SPECT. Radiology 1990; 176: 95–101
50 Glazer G M, Aisen A M, Francios I R et al. Hepatic cavernous haemangioma: magnetic resonance imaging. Radiology 1985; 155: 417
51 Solbiati L, Liveraghy T, De Pra L et al. Fine needle biopsy of hepatic hemangioma with sonographic guidance. AJR 1985; 144: 471
52 Stanley P, Gates G F, Eto R, Miller S W. Hepatic cavernous hemangiomas and hemangioendotheliomas in infancy. AJR 1977; 129: 317
53 Scatarige J C, Fishman E K, Sanders R C. The sonographic 'star sign' in focal nodular hyperplasia of the liver. J Ultrasound Med 1982; 1: 275
54 Rogers J V, Mack L A, Freeny P C et al. Hepatic focal nodular hyperplasia: angiography, CT, sonography and scintigraphy. AJR 1981; 137: 983
55 Welch T J, Sheedy P F, Johnson C M et al. Focal nodular hyperplasia and hepatic adenoma: comparison of angiography, CT, ultrasound and scintigraphy. Radiology 1985; 156: 593
56 Sandler M A, Petrocelli R D, Marks D S, Lopez R. Ultrasonic features and radionuclide correlation in liver cell adenoma and focal nodular hyperplasia. Radiology 1980; 135: 393
57 Shamsi K, De Schepper A, Degryse H, Deckers F. Focal nodular hyperplasia of the liver: radiologic findings. Abdom Imaging 1993; 18: 32–38
58 Shirkhoda A, Farah M C, Bernacki E et al. Hepatic focal nodular hyperplasia: CT and sonograpic spectrum. Abdom Imaging 1994; 19: 34–38
59 Buetow P C, Pantograg-Brown L, Buck J L et al. Focal nodular hyperplasia of the liver: imaging–pathologic correlation. Radiographics 1996; 16: 369–388
60 Klatstein G. Hepatic tumours: possible relationship to use of oral contraceptives. Gastroenterology 1977; 73: 386
61 Quinn S K, Hanks J, Shaffer H. Sonographic diagnosis of a liver cell adenoma. South Med J 1986; 79: 372
62 Golli M, Van Nhieu J T, Mathieu D et al. Hepatocellular adenoma: colour Doppler US and pathologic correlations. Radiology 1994; 190: 741–744
63 Rheinhold C, Hammers L, Taylor C R, Quedens-Case C L, Holland C K, Taylor K J. Characterization of focal hepatic lesions with duplex sonography: findings in 198 patients. AJR 1995; 164(5): 1131–1135
64 Bowerman R A, Samuels B I, Silver T N. Ultrasonographic features of hepatic adenomas in type I glycogen storage disease. J Ultrasound Med 1983; 2: 51
65 Brunelle F, Tammam S, Odievre M, Chaumont P. Liver adenomas in glycogen storage disease in children. Ultrasound and angiographic studies. Pediatr Radiol 1984; 14: 94
66 Kurdziel J C, Itines J, Parache R M, Chaulieu C. Adenolipoma of the liver: a unique case with ultrasound and CT pattern. Eur J Radiol 1984; 4: 45
67 Foster K J, Dewbury K, Griffith A, Wright R. The accuracy of ultrasound in the detection of fatty infiltration of the liver. Br J Radiol 1980; 53: 440
68 Quinn S F, Gosink B B. Characteristic sonographic signs of hepatic infiltration. AJR 1985; 145: 753
69 Saverymutto S H, Joseph A E A, Maxwell J D. Ultrasound scanning in the detection of hepatic fibrosis and steatosis. BMJ 1986; 292: 13
70 Bashist B, Hecht H L, Harley W D. Computed tomographic demonstration of rapid changes of fatty infiltration of the liver. Radiology 1982; 142: 691
71 Yates C K, Streight R A. Focal fatty infiltration of the liver simulating metastatic disease. Radiology 1986; 159: 83
72 Kawashima A, Suehiro S, Murayama S, Russell W J. Focal fatty infiltration of the liver mimicking a tumour: sonographic and CT features. J Comput Assist Tomogr 1986; 10: 329
73 Lam A H, Shulman L. Ultrasonography in the management of liver trauma in children. J Ultrasound Med 1984; 3: 199
74 VanSonnenberg E, Simeone J F, Mueller P R et al. Sonographic appearance of haematomas in the liver, spleen and kidney: a clinical, pathologic and animal study. Radiology 1983; 147: 507
75 Moon K L Jr, Federle M P. Computed tomography in hepatic trauma. AJR 1983; 141: 309
76 Weeks L E, McCune B R, Martin J F, O'Brien T F. Differential diagnosis of intrahepatic shadowing on ultrasound examination. JCU 1978; 6: 399

Malignant liver disease

David O Cosgrove

Introduction

Primary liver cancer comprises two major histopathological types: hepatocellular carcinoma (HCC), which is one of the commonest malignancies worldwide, and cholangiocarcinoma (see Ch. 15).[1,2] Both are rare in infancy, when hepatoblastoma predominates (see Vol. 2 Ch. 47). The liver is among the commonest sites for metastatic involvement and its assessment is an important part of the staging of patients with malignancy.

General ultrasound features

Ultrasound detects liver tumours, whether primary or secondary, by demonstrating the lesion itself as a mass of greater or less reflectivity than the surrounding liver, together with changes caused by its expanding or invasive nature. As with other applications the detection of liver lesions depends on a combination of resolution and contrast, so that smaller masses can be detected when there is a marked difference in reflectivity (and sometimes of texture) from the background, whereas low-contrast lesions must be larger to be demonstrable and those of the same reflectivity as the liver (isoechoic lesions) are only detectable by virtue of their mass effect. For low-contrast lesions the masking produced by the random speckled structure of the ultrasound image has a serious detrimental effect (see Ch. 2).

As tumours expand they distort the nearby architecture, and recognition of these features often draws attention to the abnormality. Enlargement of the liver, the most fundamental, is often difficult to detect until gross because of the wide range of normal variation (see Ch. 9), but rounding of the free edge of the liver is sometimes very obvious (Fig. 11.1): like other signs of expansion this is non-specific and can also be produced by many infective and degenerative processes (e.g. granulomata, early cirrhosis or hepatic storage diseases). Care must be taken when there is a Riedel's lobe, as these often have a bulbous shape with a rounded margin, even when normal (Fig. 11.2). Focal mass effects may be seen as local humps on the liver surface (Fig. 11.3) or as deviations of the normal straight or gently curved course of the liver veins (Fig. 11.4). As with cirrhotic nodules, malignant humps are more obvious when the liver is surrounded by ascites but, if looked for carefully, they can often be demonstrated in its absence, especially if a transducer with good near-field resolution is used. The diaphragmatic surface of the liver is often indented by prominent or hypertrophic leaflets of the diaphragmatic muscle; viewed from below these may simulate masses, but they are actually ridges of liver tissue protruding between the muscle bands (Fig. 11.5). Careful observation of their shape in two dimensions should avoid this error, and the position of the 'humps' moves as the diaphragm slides over the liver with respiration – observ-

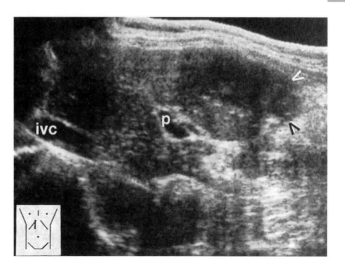

Fig. 11.1 Rounded free edge of liver. The free margin of the liver is normally sharply angled. Rounding (arrowheads) results from any disease process causing hepatomegaly and thus forms a useful but non-specific indicator of liver pathology. p – portal vein, ivc – inferior vena cava.

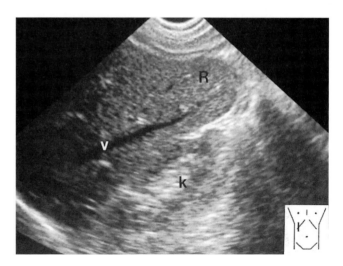

Fig. 11.2 Riedel's lobe. Although the free margin of the liver is normally sharp, in the case of a Riedel's lobe (R) it may be rounded without signifying underlying pathology. k – kidney, v – hepatic vein.

ation of the relative movements of the liver and diaphragm may provide additional important clues as to the position and nature of both real and apparent abnormalities.

Like other malignancies those in the liver provoke a neovascular supply, without which they develop ischaemic necrosis[3–5] (Fig. 11.6). These vessels characteristically penetrate the tumour from one or several sites, and are tortuous and irregular in outline. They may have abnormal branching patterns, with loops and shunts.[6] In general the neovascularity of metastases is low and often cannot be detected with current Doppler systems, though the signal boost given by microbubble contrast agents often helps

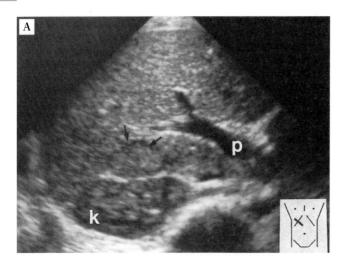

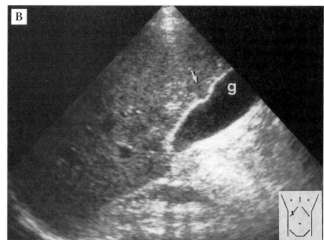

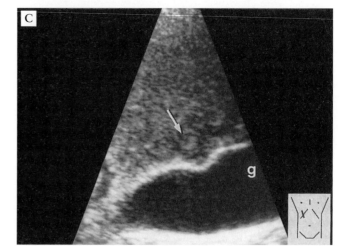

Fig. 11.3 Surface humps in liver malignancy. Subcapsular masses may cause nodularity of the liver contour. **A:** This is easier to detect when the deeper parts of the liver are affected, the indentation of the adjacent organs indicating their position. k – kidney, p – portal vein. **B** and **C:** Note that the 'hump' (arrow) may be obvious although the echo contrast is minimal ('isoechoic' lesion). Superficial 'humps' are more difficult to detect because they are obscured by reverberation and lie close to the transducer, where resolution is poor. g – gallbladder.

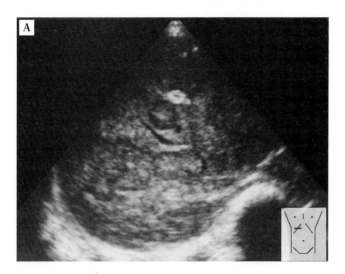

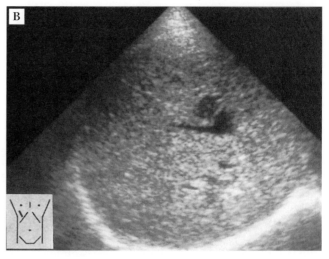

Fig. 11.4 Deviation of liver veins in malignancy. Masses may distort the normally gently curving paths of nearby blood vessels. In these examples the offending tumours (a 'target' lesion in A) are easily seen, but sometimes this feature can draw attention to an otherwise subtle lesion.

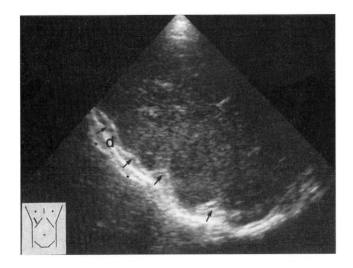

Fig. 11.5 Diaphragmatic 'humps'. Whereas the liver surface is normally smooth, because the muscle of the diaphragm may form into thickened bundles that indent the surface of the liver, 'nodularity' or 'humps' on this surface do not carry the same implications and should be ignored. This example shows marked indentations (arrowheads) of the upper surface of the liver in a patient with chronic airways obstruction. Note the mirror-image artefact (*) which gives a double outline to the hypertrophied muscular layer of the diaphragm (d) (see Ch. 4).

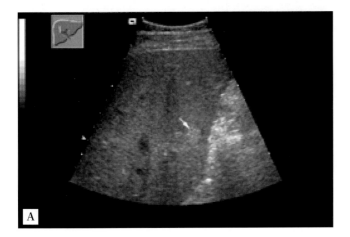

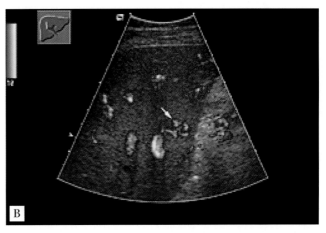

Fig. 11.6. Neovascularity in a carcinoid metastasis. A: A small reflective mass is seen in the right lobe of the liver (arrow). **B:** On power Doppler the tangle of tumour vessels is seen (arrow).

display the typical features.[7] Hepatocellular carcinomas, on the other hand, are usually well vascularised, and this is useful in distinguishing them from regenerating nodules[8] and in monitoring ablation therapy.

The invasive properties of tumours may be confirmed by the demonstration of vascular involvement (Fig. 11.7). Both the portal and the hepatic veins may be invaded, often leading to occlusion, and in the latter case extension to the cava may be observed. Intravascular tumour is usually reflective and expands the vessel, but positive differentiation from blood thrombus depends on detecting arterial Doppler signals from within the thrombus: only venous signals are found in blood thrombus as it is recanalised (Fig. 11.8). Occlusion is most directly determined with colour Doppler, which often reveals persistent marginal flow even when the thrombus is massive. Secondary signs include splenomegaly in the case of portal vein occlusion and compensatory dilatation of still-

patent hepatic veins in a partial Budd–Chiari syndrome (Figs 11.9 and 11.10). Any type of liver tumour may invade vessels, but invasion is observed more frequently with the more aggressive types and is especially common in hepatocellular carcinoma.

Bile ducts may also be invaded and occluded to produce the classic features of intrahepatic duct dilatation (see Ch. 15), with the parallel channel and double-barrel shotgun signs (Fig. 11.11). Bile duct invasion is a particular feature of cholangiocarcinoma (see Ch. 15), but may also be encountered in any other primary or secondary tumour. Obstructive jaundice does not result unless the main ducts are involved, because the liver's reserve capacity for bile excretion is able to compensate for the loss of one or even several segments. Jaundice, when it develops in liver malignancy, is more likely to be due to very extensive replacement of the liver volume by tumour, except in cholangiocarcinoma, which typically obstructs the main

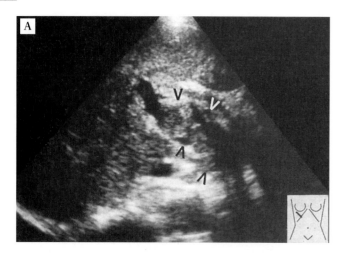

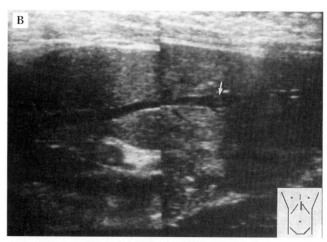

Fig. 11.7 Vascular invasion in liver malignancy. More aggressive tumours may invade the liver's blood vessels. **A:** A metastatic ovarian carcinoma has invaded the portal vein (arrowheads). **B:** A malignant melanoma has invaded the middle hepatic vein (arrow). In both cases the veins are expanded, a typical feature of tumour involvement that is not seen with simple thrombosis.

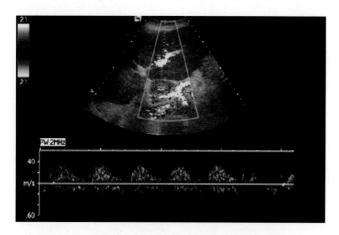

Fig. 11.8. Flow in tumour thrombus. The echogenic material filling the portal vein is shown to be tumour rather than blood thrombus by the demonstration of arterial Doppler signals from within it. This was a hepatocellular carcinoma.

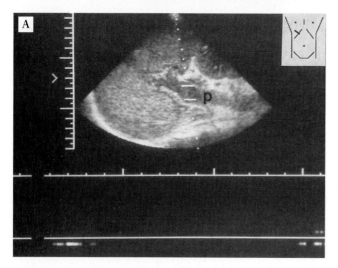

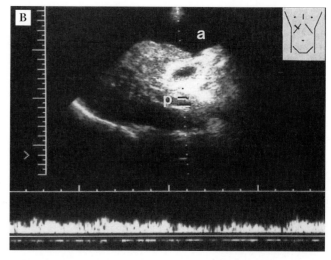

Fig. 11.9 Doppler study of portal vein invasion. A: A pulsed Doppler study of an occluded portal vein shows no signal, indicated by the flat spectral trace in the lower part of the figure. In many anatomical situations in the abdomen geometrical constraints make a negative Doppler study unreliable. **B:** The flow in a normal portal vein is so readily obtained that failure to demonstrate it is significant. The liver in **B** is heavily replaced by metastatic disease and surrounded by ascites (a). p – portal vein.

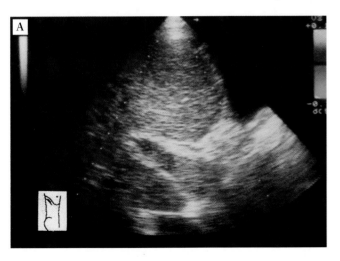 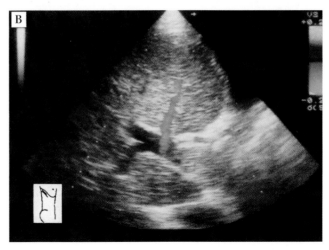

Fig. 11.10 Tumour involvement of the portal vein. A: Although solid tissue completely fills the vessel's lumen, colour flow mapping displays a little hepatopetal flow. **B:** A portal vein branch shows reversed flow.

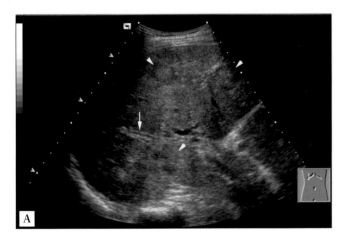 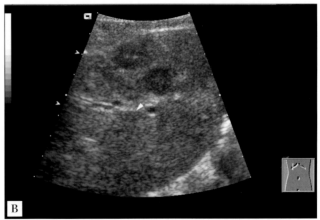

Fig. 11.11 Malignant occlusion of the biliary tree. A: When a mass lies close to the biliary tree the duct may be occluded, giving rise to the same 'parallel channel sign' (arrows) of intrahepatic biliary tree dilatation as occurs in obstruction to the main duct, but in this case confined to the affected segment. **B:** The duct dilatation is better seen in this zoomed view. The patient had a colonic carcinoma with liver metastases.

ducts at the porta. In the lymphomas the paraneoplastic syndrome of obstructive jaundice at the canalicular level should also be considered.

Segmental localisation of the position of a lesion may be important, for example, when a segmental resection is planned. The segmental numbering system described by Coinaud is used (see Ch. 9) and it is usually possible to define precisely in which segment a lesion lies by noting its position with respect to internal landmarks. The primary distinction is the main left–right division of the liver, corresponding to the lie of the middle hepatic vein, which runs from the gallbladder fossa superiorly to the IVC (inferior vena cava). The left lobe is then divided by the level of the porta hepatis into segments II (superior) and III (inferior), whereas segment IV, also in the left liver, lies between the ligamentum teres and the gallbladder fossa and is often subdivided into superior (IVA) and inferior (IVB) subsegments at the level of the porta. The right hepatic vein, usually lying in the coronal plane, demarcates the segments of the right liver that lie inferior to the porta (V and VI) from those that lie superiorly (VIII and VII), in anterior and posterior positions, respectively.

Hepatocellular carcinoma

Clinical background

Primary liver cancer is one of the major malignancies in many countries throughout the world, particularly in sub-Saharan Africa and in the Far East,[9,10] it has been increasing in incidence in many countries in recent years, but at the same time it is probably decreasing in a few others, including the USA.[11,12] A close association between hepatocellular carcinoma (HCC) and cirrhosis, particularly the post-hepatitic or macronodular variety, was demonstrated many years ago.[13] The development of hepatocellular carcinoma in cirrhotic livers is particularly frequent in the Far East and in the west, where 80% of patients with hepatocellular carcinoma have cirrhosis.[14,15] The carcinogenic properties of the hepatitis B and C viruses provides an explanation.[16–18] Chemical carcinogens, such as aflatoxin, seem to play an important role in South African hepatocellular carcinoma, where the association with hepatitis viruses is less strong (40% of cases). In alcoholic cirrhosis, which is more common in western countries, the liver has a reduced regenerative capacity compared to macronodular cirrhosis.

Grossly, hepatocellular carcinomas can be classified into four types:[19]

1   infiltrative: poorly demarcated masses with a high incidence of tumour thrombi in the portal venous system;
2   expansive: sharply demarcated nodule or nodules. Invasion of portal vein branches uncommon;
3   mixed infiltrative and expansive: when an infiltrative pattern, such as disruption of the capsule, is seen together with expansive nodules;
4   diffuse: numerous small nodules (5–10 mm diameter) scattered throughout a cirrhotic liver.

The most important serological marker of HCC is α-fetoprotein (AFP). The normal values in healthy humans are lower than 20 ng/ml, but because serum levels frequently rise in chronic liver disease, the best discriminant value for hepatocellular carcinoma is 400 ng/ml, and this high value leads to a significant false-negative rate, particularly in small hepatocellular carcinomas where its sensitivity is only about 40%.[20,21] Since the beginning of the 1980s, screening and follow-up programmes in patients with chronic liver disease have been undertaken in the Far East using a combination of ultrasonography and serum AFP measurements.[22] Ultrasonography has increased the accuracy of the diagnosis of focal lesions in the liver and significantly improved detection of early HCC, thus defining the true incidence and natural history of this disease. These studies have led to the detection of asymptomatic small hepatocellular carcinomas, opening up new therapeutic options, especially ultrasound-guided interstitial therapy, which has come to rival conventional surgery as the definitive treatment of many HCCs.[23]

Ultrasound appearances

Three forms of early disease have been described:[24–27]

a   nodular, when the contour of the tumour is regular and the boundary with the parenchyma is well defined (Figs 11.12 to 11.14); the nodules may be single or multiple,
b   massive, when the tumour is large (>5 cm) and the boundary with the liver parenchyma is difficult to recognise (Fig. 11.15),
c   diffuse, when the mass is indistinct and large portions of liver parenchyma are involved by tumour (Fig. 11.16).

The reflectivity of HCCs depends on their size (Fig. 11.17) and pathological characteristics. They may be more or less reflective than the surrounding liver, or be isoechoic (Figs 11.13 and 11.14); some have a mixed echo pattern with areas of both increased and reduced reflectivity. Small hepatocellular carcinomas (<3 cm diameter) tend to be poorly reflective (77.4% of cases) (Table 11.1).[28] Increasing reflectivity is related to the presence of necrosis and haemorrhage[29] and in larger HCCs highly reflective lesions are the commonest, being found in about half of all cases.[30,31] In a study on the natural history of small hepato-cellular carcinomas (<3 cm diameter), Ebara *et al.* correlated the ultrasound pattern of the nodules with their size,[32] and demonstrated a tendency for them to develop from generally echo-poor lesions to a pattern with an echo-poor periphery and a more reflective centre, and finally to large lesions with high-level echoes in advanced disease. The increase in reflectivity occasionally noted in small hepatocellular carcinomas is probably related to diffuse fatty change within the malignant tissue.[24,33] An echo-poor nodule may occasionally be found within a larger mass: this represents differentiation of cell lines within a pre-existing tumour – the 'tumour in tumour phenomenon' (Fig. 11.18). An echo-poor rim is frequently visualised around small nodules of hepatocellular carcinomas (Fig. 11.14). This feature helps differentiate highly reflective malignancies from haemangiomas.

Fibrolamellar HCC is a rare (2%) form of hepatocellular carcinoma which has aetiological and epidemiological differences from most HCCs. It generally arises in a previously normal liver and is usually relatively slow growing. The tumour is usually solitary and the AFP is not raised. The lesions typically present as large masses and may show a central fibrous scar, similar to the appearances seen in focal nodular hyperplasia, and sometimes have central calcification.[34]

Table 11.1 Ultrasound patterns of small hepatocellular carcinoma

Tumour size (cm)	No of tumours (%)	Reflectivity of liver		
		Low	Equal	High
1–2	15 (83.3%)	1 (5.6%)	2 (11.1%)	18 (100%)
2–3	9 (69.2%)	1 (7.7%)	3 (23.1%)	13 (100%)
Total	24 (77.4%)	2 (6.4%)	5 (16.1%)	31 (100%)

Sheu, Radiology 1984[28]

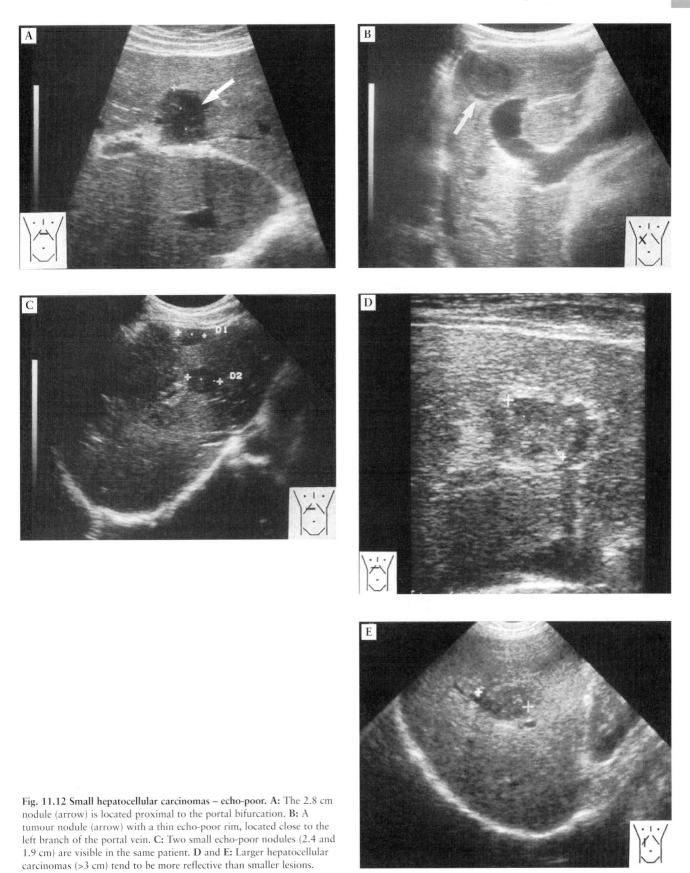

Fig. 11.12 Small hepatocellular carcinomas – echo-poor. A: The 2.8 cm nodule (arrow) is located proximal to the portal bifurcation. **B:** A tumour nodule (arrow) with a thin echo-poor rim, located close to the left branch of the portal vein. **C:** Two small echo-poor nodules (2.4 and 1.9 cm) are visible in the same patient. **D and E:** Larger hepatocellular carcinomas (>3 cm) tend to be more reflective than smaller lesions.

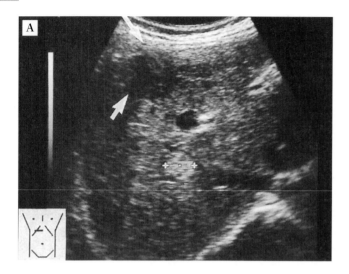

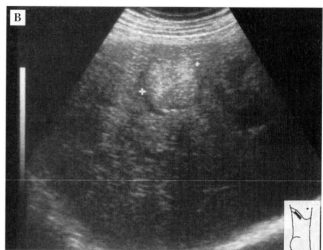

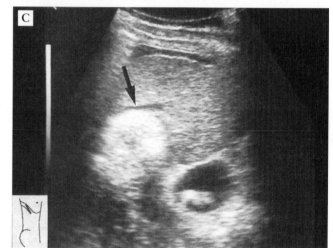

Fig. 11.13 Hepatocellular carcinomas – highly reflective. A: Small (2 cm) HCC with highly reflective pattern (between markers). A larger echo-poor nodule (arrow) is visible near to the liver surface. **B:** The nodule of HCC shows a highly reflective pattern with an echo-poor rim. **C:** HCC (4.5 cm) with intensely reflective pattern (arrow). A small quantity of ascitic fluid is visible around the liver and the gallbladder contains calculi.

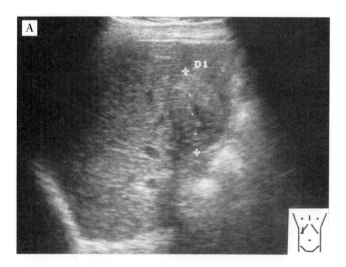

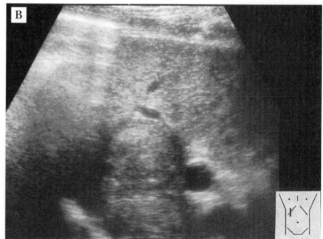

Fig. 11.14 Hepatocellular carcinoma – subtle. When the reflectivity of the tumour matches that of the surrounding liver, lesions are difficult to detect. In these examples the echo-poor halo draws attention to their presence.

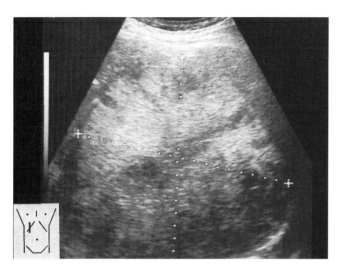

Fig. 11.15 Large hepatocellular carcinoma. Massive tumours tend to have heterogeneous internal structures.

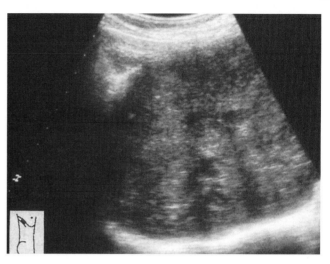

Fig. 11.16 Hepatocellular carcinoma – diffuse. A diffuse hepatocellular carcinoma involving large portions of liver parenchyma without a clear line of demarcation from the non-neoplastic tissue. The echo pattern is highly heterogeneous, with areas of both high and low reflectivity.

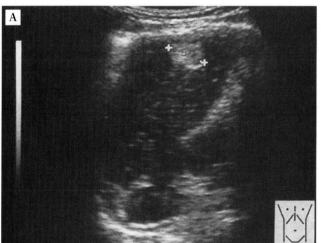

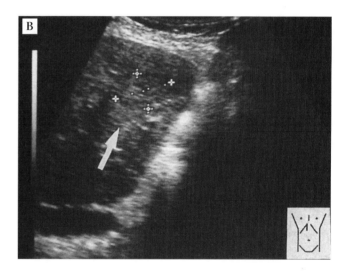

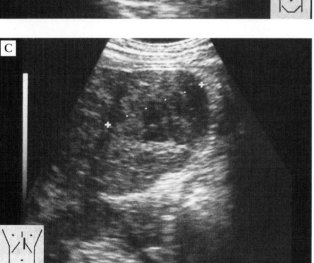

Fig. 11.17 Changing reflectivity of hepatocellular carcinomas during growth. A: At the time of the initial scan this 2 cm lesion was highly reflective. **B:** Six months later (3.4 cm) it displayed an isoechoic pattern and was difficult to visualise (arrow). **C:** After a further 3 months (4.9 cm) it displayed a poorly reflective pattern.

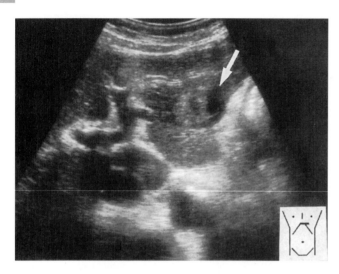

Fig. 11.18 Hepatocellular carcinoma – isoechoic. The majority of this lesion is difficult to detect because it has the same reflectivity as the surrounding liver. However, a small echo-poor nodule (arrow) is visible within the lesion ('tumour in tumour phenomenon').

Growth pattern

Some characteristics of the shape and reflectivity of hepatocellular carcinomas depend on the pattern and speed of growth of the tumour. It has been suggested that the presence of an echo-poor ring and a regular contour with sharp delimitation from the liver parenchyma represents a growth pattern of the expansive type. Partial or complete lack of these characteristics indicates an infiltrative growth pattern that produces a diffuse tumour which is difficult to recognise on ultrasound because it may be similar in appearance to the irregular texture of the liver in advanced cirrhosis. However, the ability of ultrasound to differentiate these growth patterns reliably is not fully established.

The ultrasound pattern has also been related to the growth rate of the tumour, particularly for small HCCs found in the Japanese surveys. Small echo-poor tumours tend to grow slowly, whereas those with an echo-poor rim grow faster.[32]

Vascular involvement

Hepatocellular carcinoma has a strong tendency to invade the portal venous system. The hepatic veins[35,36] and the inferior vena cava may also be involved. Vascular invasion is seen as a mass within a major portal branch or in the main portal trunk, and is readily demonstrated by ultrasound (Fig. 11.19). However, tumour spread within peripheral portal branches, which is typical of the infiltrative type of growth, is not easily visualised by ultrasound or by any other technique. Distinction from blood thrombus depends on demonstrating arterial signals from within the thrombus (see Fig. 11.8): only venous signals occur in blood thrombus as a result of recanalisation.

Doppler features

Tumour growth depends on its blood supply, and most of this neovascularisation is concentrated at the periphery of the tumour. Although these arterioles are too small to be visualised by non-invasive imaging techniques, Doppler signals may be detected from them. Arteriovenous shunts are characteristic of some hepatocellular carcinomas and they too may be detectable.[32–40] Even in small HCCs, abnormal signals, characterised by high peak Doppler shift frequencies, often over 4 kHz, are found and are

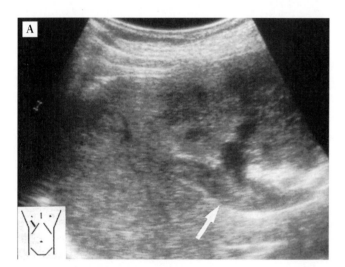 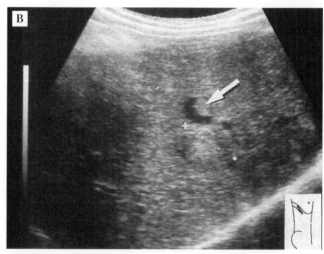

Fig. 11.19 Tumour involvement of the portal venous system. A: Echogenic material in the main and right portal veins. Material is seen within the vessel lumen (arrow). **B:** Partial occlusion of a branch of the right portal vein (arrow). The nodule of hepatocellular carcinoma (2.9 cm) is located proximal to the vessel.

attributed to the high pressure gradient in arterioportal shunting.[37,38,41] These high peak signals may be associated with broadening of the spectrum due to marked flow disturbances (Fig. 11.20). Another pulsed Doppler feature consistent with hepatocellular carcinoma is high diastolic flow, probably occurring through large intratumoural vascular lakes with low impedance (Fig. 11.21). Colour Doppler speeds the search for spectral Doppler signals and reveals the generally high vascularity that is typical of HCCs, although some cases do not show this feature.[8]

Low impedance signals are more often found in HCCs than in metastases (87% of 55 vs. 28% of 25) and are rare in haemangiomas (13% of 30).[42] In another series[39] arterial signals were found within and at the periphery of the tumour in 76% of small hepatocellular carcinomas (<3 cm in diameter) and in all those larger than 3 cm diameter. This method also proved quite sensitive (83%) in the diagnosis of HCC, but its specificity is limited by the similar signals found in some metastases, in cholangiocarcinomas, and in some benign lesions such as focal nodular hyperplasia.

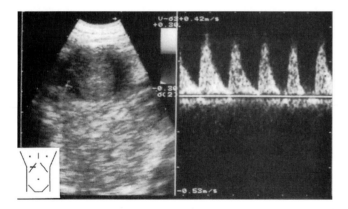

Fig. 11.20 Doppler analysis of hepatocellular carcinoma. A high peak arterial signal is detected at the periphery of the tumour.

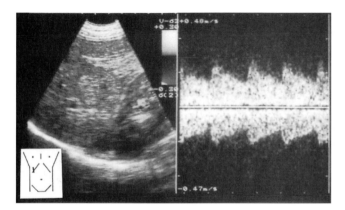

Fig. 11.21 Doppler analysis of a small highly reflective hepatocellular carcinoma. Low-impedance arterial signals within the tumour.

The vascular features of HCC are better revealed by microbubble contrast agents (see Ch. 5).[43]

Differential diagnosis

Solid focal lesions that are quite frequently detected within the liver pose a difficult diagnostic dilemma. An overall clinical assessment is fundamental to interpreting the ultrasound finding of a mass and to assessing the probability of its being malignant. In a patient with cirrhosis every solid nodule in the liver must be suspected of being a hepatocellular carcinoma until proved otherwise by guided biopsy or some other technique, such as angiography.

There are, however, some characteristic echo patterns which can help in the differential diagnosis:

a) small (1–3 cm) highly reflective nodules, single or multiple, often incidental findings in healthy subjects, are generally haemangiomas,[44]
b) an echo-poor rim or a 'target lesion' pattern suggests malignancy,
c) an anechoic area seen within a reflective lesion generally corresponds to necrosis in the centre of a metastatic deposit.

There are also other non-neoplastic lesions which sometimes require differentiation from benign and malignant tumours, for example focal fatty infiltration and hydatid cysts,[45] which sometimes display a solid pattern (see Ch. 10).

Diagnostic accuracy

Comparative studies on the sensitivity of various imaging modalities in the diagnosis of hepatocellular carcinoma in Japan indicate that real-time ultrasound has a detection rate of 94%, which is better than that of CT, angiography or scintigraphy (84%, 76% and 12%, respectively), particularly where the nodules are smaller than 2–3 cm in diameter. Ultrasound was also superior to angiography and CT in the diagnosis of neoplastic involvement of portal branches.[46]

Metastatic tumours
Clinical background

Terminal metastatic involvement of the liver is the rule in almost all but central nervous system malignancies (Table 11.2),[47] and is taken as a grave prognostic sign which underlies the importance of liver assessment in tumour staging. However, the liver may be involved early in some tumour types, particularly those arising in the splanchnic bed whose venous drainage passes directly to the liver, so that the liver may be the sole metastatic site. Colorectal carcinomas are an example in which the metastasis may be

Table 11.2 Frequency of liver metastases (adapted from[10])

Tumour type	Frequency of metastases (%)	
	At presentation	At post-mortem
Carcinomas		
Bladder	>5	30–50
Breast	1	45–60
Bronchus (oat)	10	30
Cervix	<1	15–35
Colorectal	25	70
Kidney	15	35–40
Melanoma	6	70
Nephroblastoma	3–10	40
Neuroblastoma	25	70
Ovary	<5	10–15
Pancreas	NA	50–70
Prostate	1	15
Stomach	NA	35–50
Testis	<1	s50, t80
Thyroid	4	60
Uterus	<1	15–30
Sarcomas		
Osteosarcoma	<5	<5
Rhabdomyosarcoma	10	45
Lymphoreticular		
Hodgkin's	8	60
Non-Hodgkin's	1–16	50

(s – seminoma, t – teratoma, NA – information not available)

resected if this is surgically feasible (lesions restricted to one segment or lobe). The route of tumour spread to the liver is probably haematogenous rather than lymphatic, as for the most part the liver's lymphatics are hepatofugal. An exception is the lymph drainage of the gallbladder: the early and extensive involvement of the porta hepatis region that is characteristic of this tumour, though no doubt due partly to direct contiguous invasion, may be partly lymphatic.

Whether the vascular route is arterial or via the portal venous system depends on the site of the primary.[48] Systemic lesions, such as carcinomas of the lung and breast, can only reach the liver via the arterial system (having first traversed the lung bed), whereas tumours arising in the gastrointestinal tract might spread by either route – the slight predilection for gastrointestinal tumours to involve the portion of the liver that corresponds to the distribution of the portal vein blood draining them is evidence in favour of a predominantly venous route.[49] Regardless of the vascular route, liver metastases take most of their blood supply from the hepatic artery rather than the portal vein.[50] In general they are not particularly vascular lesions, though there are exceptions – notably neuro-endocrine tumours – and the often marked vascularity of hepatocellular carcinoma has been referred to above.

Animal experiments, supported by observations in humans, show that single cells shed from a malignant tumour are not capable of growth when they embolise into the capillary bed of a potential metastatic site, and larger clumps of a few hundred cells are the smallest capable of taking root. To survive, the tumour nidus must establish its own blood supply because diffusion can only supply oxygen and nutriments to lesions smaller than about 1 mm in diameter.[51,52] Neovascularisation depends on the tumour's secreting tumour angiogenesis factors, which promote the development and ingrowth of buds from nearby capillaries. The smallest viable metastasis measures only a fraction of a millimetre in diameter: such a lesion is several orders of magnitude smaller than the smallest by any imaging technique realistically envisaged. Potentially, the lesion grows exponentially, from doubling the number of cells every week for a highly aggressive tumour such as Burkitt's lymphoma at one extreme, to doubling every 6 months for a slow-growing tumour. A tumour of 1 mm diameter, the earliest that can be detected even by the most sophisticated means under optimum circumstances, represents one that has already undergone some 20 doublings – at 40 doublings a tumour might weigh as much as 1 kg and at this size is usually lethal (Fig. 11.22).[53] Thus it is apparent that most of the growth cycle of a metastasis has already occurred by the stage at which it can be detected by imaging methods: the goal of detecting 'early' deposits is far from realised. The same depressing considerations apply to primary malignant tumours. These considerations underlie the interest in methods to detect the neovascularity of small tumours.

Liver metastases are characteristically multiple and show a range of sizes. This suggests that they have seeded on a continual basis over long periods of time, probably since the primary grew large enough to invade its vascular system. The alternative hypothesis – that seeding is a sporadic affair, tumour clumps being shed in intermittent showers – would be expected to produce size clustering of the metastases corresponding to their various ages, unless variable growth rates are assumed to occur.

Ultrasound appearances

A wide range of appearances is encountered in liver metastatic disease (Table 11.3) and their overlap with non-malignant disorders inevitably results in lack of specificity.[54,55] Focal lesions are the most common, but malignancy may also infiltrate widely. The commonest focal pattern is of echo-poor masses (Fig. 11.23), whose

Table 11.3 Ultrasonic patterns of metastases

Poorly reflective	Any type (typical of lymphomas)
Highly reflective	Typically gastrointestinal and urogenital tract 1°
Cystic	Mucin secreting 1°
Necrosis in any type	
Calcified	Typical of colorectal 1°
Confluent	Any extensive 1° or 2° tumour
Diffuse	Lymphoma and leukaemia

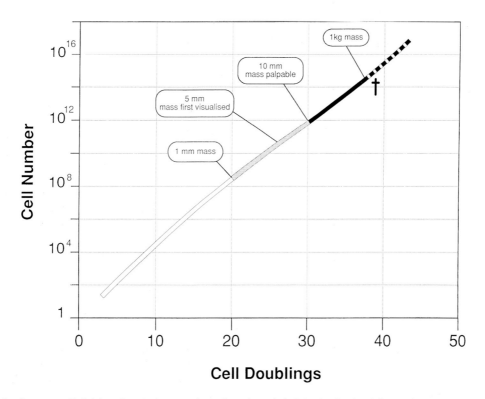

Fig. 11.22 Time scale of tumour cell division. A typical tumour has enlarged to a lethal size by the time it has undergone some 40 generations of cell division. At 20 doublings it has reached 1 mm in diameter.

texture differs little from the surrounding liver.[56] The difference in reflectivity may be such that the lesions are very obvious, and they may even be virtually echo free. This is particularly often the case for lymphomas and sarcomas, presumably because these tumours have a very uniform cellular architecture with little stromal reaction, so that few ultrasound interfaces are produced. Not uncommonly, however, the contrast in reflectivity is slight, so that the lesions are difficult to demonstrate except by recognising the mass effects and invasive features discussed above (see General ultrasound features).

Echo-poor lesions may be produced by any type of primary tumour: they are typical of many of the commonest malignancies, such as carcinoma of the breast and bronchus. Usually the attenuation in the lesion is the same as in the liver itself, so that neither distal shadowing nor increase in sound transmission is present and the surrounding liver is unremarkable. A special case occurs when metastases develop in a fatty liver: the TGC is set to be correct for the increased attenuation of the fatty liver, but this is inappropriate for the lesion itself, so that relatively increased sound transmission occurs and the resulting appearance is easily confused with simple liver cysts (Fig. 11.24). This combination of pathologies is not rare because fatty change can be produced by anorexia and by chemotherapy.

Deposits that are more reflective than the liver are easier to detect, tending to catch the eye as the beam is swept across it in the real-time search (Fig. 11.25). Again, a range of contrasts in reflectivity is found, from those that are obvious to subtle lesions that are difficult to detect, and increased through-transmission or shadowing are not generally produced. However, highly reflective lesions may be surrounded by an echo-poor band, which may be merely a fine line (known as a halo) or be obvious as a border several millimetres thick. This is known as the target or 'bull's eye' pattern (Fig. 11.26) and is more often encountered with larger lesions, perhaps representing the effects of haemorrhage or necrosis. Highly reflective and target lesions are typical of tumours originating in the gastrointestinal and urogenital tracts, being common, for example, in colorectal carcinomas and in carcinoma of the ovary, pancreas and kidney. However, it is important to note that a proportion of such tumours may also produce echo-poor deposits, and that the different types may be mixed within the same liver (Fig. 11.27).

The reasons for these different appearances on ultrasound are not clear. The low-level echoes of the common type may correspond with lesions that have a high water content: in general, high water levels are associated with low reflectivity, the clearest example being the echo-poor appearance of oedematous tissue, e.g. in acute pancreatitis.

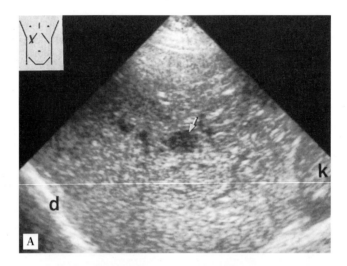

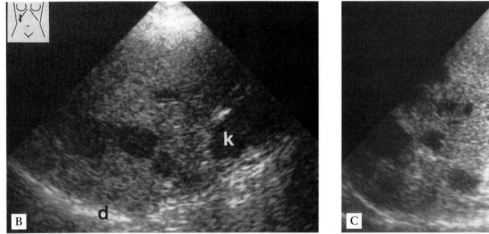

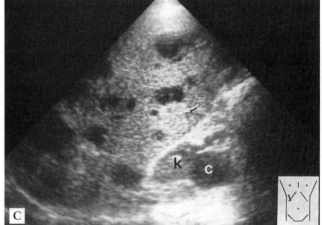

Fig. 11.23 Echo-poor metastases. Lesions with slightly lower intensity echoes than the surrounding liver are the commonest type of metastasis. **A:** The solitary deposit (arrow) was metastatic from a bronchial carcinoma. **B** and **C:** The multiple lesions were from breast and non-Hodgkin's lymphoma, respectively. The kidney in C contains a simple cyst. Note the apparent enhancement deep to some of the lesions in C (arrow): this is attributable to the relatively lower attenuation within the lesion compared to the surrounding liver (compare with Fig. 11.24). c – cyst, d – diaphragm, k – kidney.

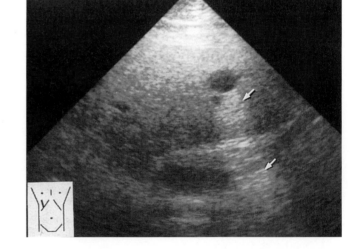

Fig. 11.24 Pseudo-enhancement of metastasis in a fatty liver. This lymphomatous lesion in the liver shows marked distal enhancement (arrows), most obviously interpreted as being due to a cystic lesion. In fact, the lesion is solid but with a lower attenuation than the fatty liver that surrounds it. As the TGC has been adjusted to compensate for the abnormally high attenuation of the fatty liver it pulls up the distal echoes, falsely suggesting that the lesion is cystic.

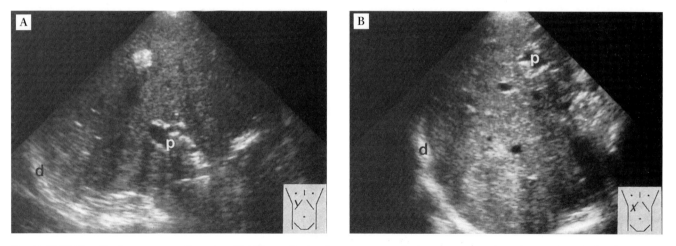

Fig. 11.25 Highly reflective metastases. Deposits with high-amplitude echoes are commonly due to metastases from the gastrointestinal and urogenital tracts. These typical solitary lesions were metastases from colonic and rectal primaries, respectively. p – portal vein, d – diaphragm.

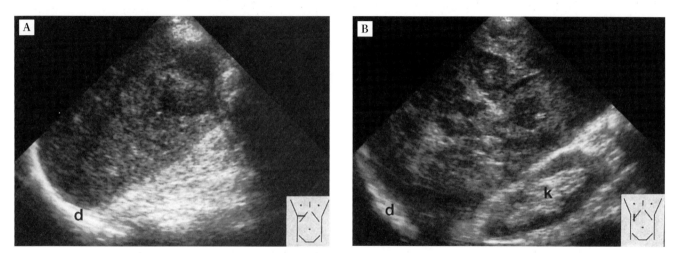

Fig. 11.26 Target lesions. A and **B:** The concentric ringed pattern of the 'target' or 'bull's eye' lesion is shown in these two cases. This pattern is more often seen with larger lesions. d – diaphragm, k – kidney.

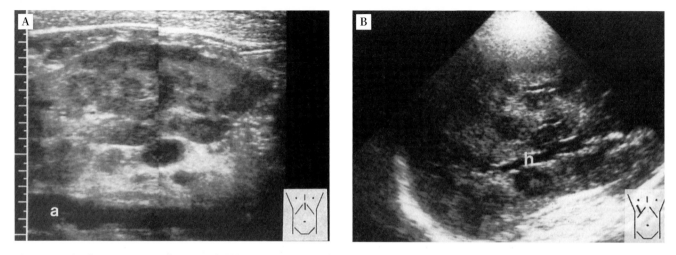

Fig. 11.27 Mixed metastases. A and **B:** Several different types of deposits often coexist in one patient: in these three examples echo-poor and target lesions are intermixed. a – aorta, h – hepatic vein.

For the highly reflective variety a correlation with vascularity has been suggested,[57] as is the case with haemangiomas,[58] but it is by no means a strong link and other factors such as stromal collagen content are equally important.[59–61] Tumour necrosis, fatty replacement[62] and calcification also play a part. The nature of the echo-poor halo surrounding highly reflective deposits remains controversial. Some authors claim that it represents an increase in fluid at the tumour margin, but others suggest that it results from pressure atrophy of the hepatocytes in response to the enlargement of the tumour, leaving the sinusoidal blood vessels as the halo.[63] However, it is by no means clear that such vessels would be echo poor, as the increased number of interfaces between the blood and the vessel walls also produces high-level echoes in other situations, such as in haemangiomas.[58]

For the less common types of liver metastasis the correspondence between pathology and ultrasonic appearance is more readily understood. Fluid-filled lesions, recognised by their increased through-transmission, are an example (Fig. 11.28): they are echo free when they contain clear fluid, such as may be produced by mucin-secreting lesions (e.g. carcinomas of the ovary, pancreas etc.), but contain debris when the fluid represents tumour necrosis.[64,65] This type tend to have a shaggy wall which may suggest an abscess, but they are not likely to be confused with simple cysts; however, the mucin-secreting types are indistinguishable except for their progressive enlargement when studied sequentially over a period of months.

Calcified lesions have very intense echoes and may produce shadowing if the foci of calcium are sufficiently large (Fig. 11.29). Calcification commonly occurs in secondaries from colorectal and gastric carcinomas, as well as in neuroblastomas.

One of the more difficult differential diagnoses is from haemangiomas, which also have a variety of appearances but are most commonly highly reflective (Fig. 11.30) (see Ch. 10).[66] Although an absolutely definite differential diagnosis is not possible, haemangiomas are typically situated in a subcapsular or perivascular position, are usually solitary, measure only a few centimetres in diameter, and have uniform, high-amplitude echoes.[44] There are no mass effects or evidence of invasion, and they lack the echo-poor halo that may be seen around highly reflective metastases. Occasionally, large haemangiomas may show increased sound transmission, a feature not described with highly reflective metastases. In children haemangiomas are echo poor and sometimes present a disorganised appearance that may suggest metastatic disease, but their marked vascularity is obvious on colour Doppler (see Vol. 2, Ch. 47). Doppler studies on adult haemangiomas are unfortunately unhelpful, generally being negative (as is usually also the case in metastases[67,68]), probably because the flow through the meshwork of tortuous vessels is too slow for detection with current equipment – in fact, apparent signals are more likely to be a form of motion artefact than true flow signals, a distinction that is readily made with spectral Doppler.[69] Microbubble enhancement techniques are promising in distinguishing haemangiomas from significant lesions (see below). Biopsy is safe, provided the lesion is approached via the surrounding liver (so that any bleeding is confined), but interpretation of a

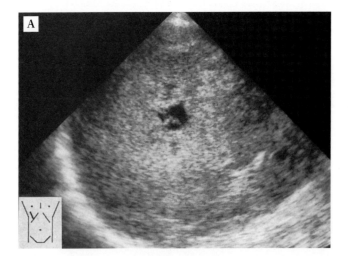 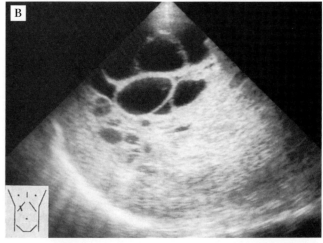

Fig. 11.28 Cystic metastases. The two varieties of cystic metastasis are illustrated. **A:** The shaggy wall of the fluid space suggests that it has resulted from necrosis in the centre of a tumour, presumably because of ischaemia. The irregularity of the surrounding tissue represents the viable portion of the metastasis. This pattern simulates an abscess cavity. **B:** When the cyst results from mucin secretion the walls of the cavity are smooth, suggesting a benign lesion; this multicystic lesion might be misdiagnosed as polycystic liver disease or as biliary cysts. If only a single cyst were present it would probably be considered to be a simple cyst. Only growth over serial observations provides the clue to their malignant nature. The commonest source of this type is the ovary, but any tissue capable of secreting mucin can be responsible: this patient had a testicular teratoma.

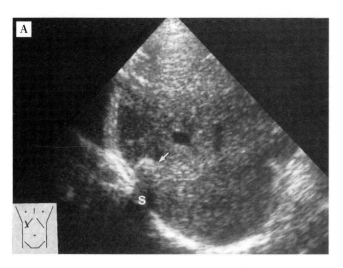
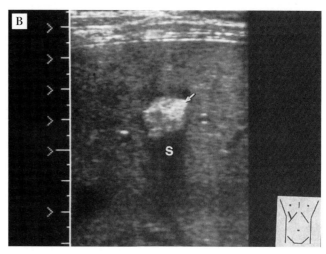

Fig. 11.29 Calcified metastases. Metastases from the gastrointestinal tract are prone to calcify. The typical ultrasound features are of a highly reflective lesion (arrows) with shadowing (s).

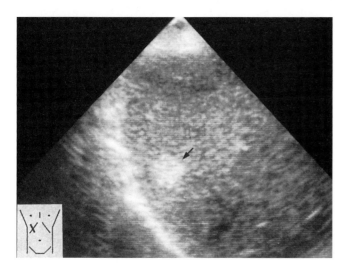

Fig. 11.30 Haemangioma. A solitary, well defined highly reflective focus (arrow) is the typical appearance of a haemangioma, but this finding in a patient undergoing a staging scan always raises doubt. The lack of any changes in the surrounding liver (halo, distortion) and the position under the capsule are helpful features suggesting a benign lesion.

cytological sample may be difficult;[70] a definitive diagnosis can usually be made on histology of a cutting needle specimen (see Ch. 7). Angiography (often performed with CT) is usually definitive,[71,72] though rare examples of metastases showing the delayed filling from the periphery that typifies haemangiomas have been reported.[73] Haemangiomas commonly show a characteristic enhancement pattern on dynamic CT and MRI after intravascular contrast, with early peripheral enhancement, often globular in distribution, followed by slow diffusion of contrast into the central vascular spaces in a centripetal pattern. In one study this pattern was seen in 67% of haemangiomas and no metastases studied.[74] Haemangiomas can also be

characterised by other features on MRI including their prolonged T_2 relaxation times, a result of their high water content, and possibly late uptake of some of the newer contrast agents, particularly the ultrasmall superparamagnetic types.[75]

Metastases (and primary hepatocellular carcinomas) may become diffuse by confluent growth of initially separate foci (Fig. 11.31). The resultant appearance is of an irregular pattern throughout the affected portion (commonly this is the entire liver), with ill-defined patchiness consisting of geographic echo-poor areas. These textural changes may be subtle and are easily missed or confused with the irregular texture of diffuse infiltrative or degenerative diseases, such as focal fatty infiltration and cirrhosis.[76] Liver enlargement, together with the absence of the typical ancillary features of cirrhosis, suggest metastatic disease or HCC. In most cases a careful search will reveal at least a few focal abnormalities that indicate the true diagnosis.

Diffuse involvement is also a feature of the lymphomas and leukaemias, though in the former there may also be focal involvement.[77] The liver is enlarged, as is the spleen, and both show reduced reflectivity identical to that produced by conditions such as acute hepatitis and acute cardiac failure (Fig. 11.32) (see Ch. 12). However, in lymphoma and leukaemia the liver is commonly affected by a reactive cellular infiltration (round-cell inflammatory changes) that produces the same ultrasonic appearance, therefore this finding is of little diagnostic value.

In general the differential diagnostic considerations for focal liver lesions include all the benign focal processes, but often the clinical picture will make some so unlikely (or probable) as to shorten the list of possible causes considerably. A pyogenic or amoebic abscess, for example, can simulate a metastasis but the liver is usually locally

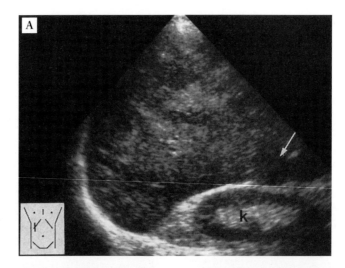

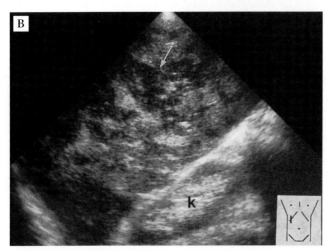

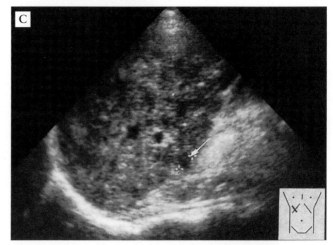

Fig. 11.31 Diffuse metastases. When metastatic disease becomes extensive the individual lesions may coalesce, so that their margins are lost. The resulting pattern is of a grossly distorted texture whose malignant origin may not be obvious. Usually, as in these examples (arrows), some definable masses can be detected among the overall texture disturbance. k – kidney.

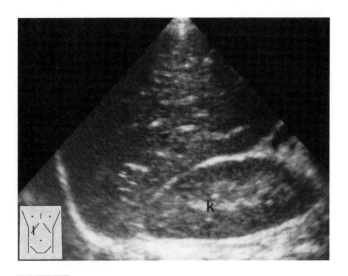

Fig. 11.32 Dark liver – lymphoma. The liver's echoes are normally higher than those of the renal cortex (evaluated at the same depth in the scan). Some acute diffuse processes cause a reduction in the liver's echo intensity (the so-called 'dark liver'): these include lymphomatous and leukaemic infiltration. Because identical changes are sometimes produced by reactive infiltration in the same patients, the findings are non-specific and biopsy confirmation is required. In this patient diffuse lymphoma was found. k – kidney.

tender and the history of fever is suggestive. Likewise, trauma will usually be suspected from the history. Hepatic (oestrogen) adenomas and focal nodular hyperplasia (FNH) pose diagnostic problems but the history of oestrogen administration suggests the former diagnosis. Both are typically vascular lesions and this can be demonstrated on colour Doppler, which often shows the central artery of FNH together with the smaller vessels radiating from it that is recognised on angiography. The Kupffer cells usually present in FNH take up colloids, producing a normal isotope scan or a hot spot, and the same effect can be exploited using non-linear techniques with micro-bubbles (see below).[78,79]

Focal fatty change can also be a difficult diagnostic problem (see Ch. 10), the fatty tissue appearing as regions of increased reflectivity which can be misdiagnosed as reflective masses.[80] Features that should be looked for are the typical pattern of focal fatty change as triangular or polygonal regions that project onto one of the liver surfaces (perhaps a fissure or the porta), and the uniform echoes with no disturbance of the adjacent liver architecture (no halo, no mass or invasive effects). In addition, the foci may progress or regress rapidly, so that a study a week or so later may reveal complete clearing or wide extension. The counterpart, focal fatty sparing, where all but a small portion of the liver has become infiltrated with fat, leaving an apparently dark segment, is even more difficult to distinguish from a deposit.[81] Again, the process develops on a segmental basis so that the spared region is seen as a wedge projecting onto a liver surface; this is especially common close to the gallbladder. As with focal fatty change there are no mass or invasive effects. Confirmation can be obtained with a liver scintigram (using S-colloid) or a delayed-phase microbubble study which show no loss of uptake in the affected region. CT is sometimes helpful, showing a low density in the fatty segments without any mass effect, but ultrasound seems to be more sensitive than CT, which may be negative when the changes are obvious on ultrasound. MRI can also be helpful by showing characteristic features of fat, such as chemical shift alterations that result from differences in proton precessional frequency between lipids and water. T_2-weighted imaging with fat saturation may also be helpful: fatty lesions show a signal drop whereas tumours show high signal intensity. If focal fatty change (or sparing) is considered before a biopsy, then it is prudent to take samples both from the apparent abnormality and from the surrounding liver: the seemingly normal liver may actually turn out to be the abnormality! The predilection for the portions of the liver near the gallbladder (especially segment IV) is interesting because this region may have an unusual arterial and portal blood supply.[82] In some subjects it is supplied by portal veins passing directly from the gallbladder; in others the cystic veins first empty into one of the main portal vein branches before passing into the

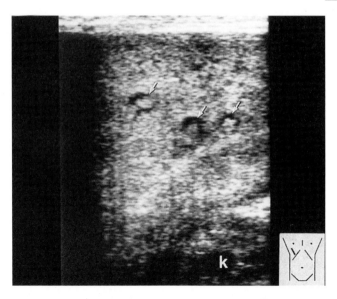

Fig. 11.33 *Candida* micro-abscess. Multiple small lesions of a target pattern (arrows) are seen in patients with fungal septicaemia and liver (or spleen) involvement. The central punctum may represent the arteriole in which the septic embolus lodged. This patient, who was recovering from a bone marrow transplant, developed monilial infection of the upper gastrointestinal tract and subsequently a fever. Typical lesions were seen on the scan and confirmed by the demonstration of hyphae on fine needle biopsy. k – kidney.

liver sinusoids. Possibly the cystic blood does not contain the toxic substance that causes fatty change in the main part of the liver, accounting for the focal sparing (or *vice versa*, toxins being present in the cystic veins in the case of focal fatty change occurring here).

Patients who are severely immunocompromised may develop widespread multifocal fungal abscesses which, if present in the liver, may be difficult to distinguish from malignancy (Fig. 11.33) (see Ch. 10).[83]

Accuracy of ultrasound in liver malignancy

Overall, transabdominal ultrasound is probably of moderate to good sensitivity in the detection of metastatic disease (Table 11.4). Although figures vary widely, most studies suggest a range of sensitivity of between 50 and 80%.[84,85] Developments in CT, especially improvements in helical scan technology, with dual-phase imaging and computer-automated scan triggering, have improved its sensitivity and this can be improved further by CT aorto-portography to give a sensitivity of up to 90%, although the latter is an invasive method. The sensitivity of MRI has also been greatly improved by the development of fast abdominal imaging, which allows the whole liver to be scanned during a single breath hold, and of liver-specific contrast agents.[86] Both CT and MRI suffer from a lack of specificity, however, as some benign lesions such as hepatic

Table 11.4 Table of reported accuracy of ultrasound in liver metastases

1° Tumour	Type	Sens	Spec	Acc	Cases	Reference
mixed	54	92	–	137	59	
lymphoma	85	72	–	51	59	
GI tract	84	90	–	100	prospective laparoscopy	72
mixed	73	94	84	108	retrospective	67
colon & breast	82	85	–	122	prospective	72
GI tract	–	–	88	50	prospective, op correlation	79
mainly GI tract	61	94	80	80	prospective, op correlation	74

cysts can mimic more aggressive pathologies. In the current climate of resource limitation ultrasound compares favourably in cost-effectiveness, portability, patient acceptability and radiation dosage.

Special techniques

Intra-operative ultrasound

Using small, high-frequency linear array transducers applied directly to the liver surface after laparotomy produces very high-resolution images which allow the detection of metastases missed on conventional studies.[87–90] Any abnormality demonstrated can be biopsied under ultrasound guidance. More accurate staging, for example in colorectal carcinoma, allows more appropriate surgical management: a segmental resection can be added when a solitary lesion is found, or a planned radical procedure limited to simple resection of the primary if multiple metastases are demonstrated[91,92] (see Ch. 8).

Interventional guidance

Using ultrasound to guide the placement of fine or cutting biopsy needles improves tissue sampling and so reduces false-negative and indeterminate results.[93,94] It also reduces risk because vulnerable structures such as the gallbladder can be avoided. Ultrasound guidance should be used for any focal lesion unless it is massive and obviously palpable (see Ch. 7).

Ultrasound is increasingly important as a means to guide interstitial therapy of liver lesions using sclerosants such as percutaneous ethanol injection (PEI) or heating with lasers or microwaves.[95] It is under investigation as a means of directing high-power interstitial focused ultrasound (HIFU) therapy, also a means of heat coagulation. In all of these the detection of residual viable tumour at the end of the planned session is also important and Doppler, with microbubble enhancement if necessary, is emerging as a fast and reliable means of demonstrating this. It has the major advantage that it can be used at the end of the treatment session, so that further treatment can

be applied if needed; contrast CT is equally effective but the patient must be moved and so it is less easily integrated into the treatment session.[96]

Doppler perfusion index

The arterialisation of the blood supply to malignant liver lesions has been exploited as a means of detecting even occult tumours (i.e. lesions too small to image or detect at surgery).[97] If the flow to the liver via the hepatic artery and via the portal vein is measured, the fraction supplied by the artery – the Doppler perfusion index (DPI) – can be calculated as the arterial component divided by the total flow. The artery supplies less than 25% in the normal liver (DPI <0.25), but when there is arterialisation the fraction increases. In studies of the liver in patients with colorectal and gastric carcinomas, a high correlation between a raised DPI and the detectable metastases was noted and, in an important group with no obvious metastases at pre-operative staging, the prognosis and disease-free survival were much lower in those with a high DPI, the difference being accounted for by local recurrent tumour in a few cases but in most by liver metastases that became overt in the 6- and 12-month follow-up scans. Thus, not only does this index detect overt metastases, it also predicts those patients at increased risk of developing metastases at follow-up, presumably because they had occult micro-metastases at presentation. However, other groups have found it difficult to reproduce these results,[98] probably because of the errors in measuring volume flow in vessels as small as the hepatic artery (see Ch. 6), and a more robust method using a microbubble agent injected as a bolus is under investigation.

Ultrasound contrast enhancement
(see Ch. 5)

The liver has emerged as a particularly promising application of the microbubble contrast agents for ultrasound because not only can Doppler and grey-scale techniques be used to demonstrate the vascular phases much more effectively than with non-enhanced Doppler, but also the liver-specific late phase of some microbubbles depicts normally functioning liver with great precision.[99,100] The vascular phases are analogous to a three-phase contrast CT scan, with arterial and portal venous components at 20 seconds and around 1 minute after an intravenous bolus, followed by an extra later 'tissue' phase. The first two phases can be demonstrated with colour Doppler, but the third phase requires a non-linear technique because the microbubbles are too slow-moving to give detectable Doppler shifts. In practice phase inversion, with its excellent spatial resolution and lack of artefacts, seems to be the most useful all-round method. Many malignancies show a rapid and spectacular uptake of contrast in the arterial phase and the chaotic pattern of the vessels is readily distinguished from the spoke-wheel pattern of FNH. The adult type of haemangioma shows minimal or no microbubble signals in this phase, but scans after a minute or two often show marked peripheral clumping of contrast which slowly percolates through the lesion in a centripetal fashion, exactly as is seen on delayed contrast CT scanning.[101]

When one of the agents that has a liver-specific phase is used, scanning late in the post-vascular phase (i.e. after 3–5 minutes) shows the distribution of normally functioning liver in a very spectacular way.[100] Again, the spatial resolution of the phase inversion mode has advantages in the detection of small lesions, and metastases down to 3 mm diameter have been convincingly demonstrated – sometimes smaller than can be detected with contrast-enhanced CT or MRI. The alternative non-linear method, stimulated acoustic emission (SAE) with colour Doppler, has poorer spatial resolution but seems to allow even a few microbubble events to be detected and so has higher sensitivity (Fig. 11.34). This is useful in characterising lesions because it has been found that whereas metastases and HCC have no or only very scanty signals, haemangiomas show some or moderate signals. Lesions that contain functioning liver tissue have the same SAE signal intensity as normal liver: this applies to regenerating nodules, focal fatty change and sparing, and to FNH (which may actually show higher signals than the surrounding liver). The combination of the vascular and the later liver-specific phases promises to expand the role of ultrasound in the liver.

The properties of microbubbles can also be exploited in entirely new ways to reveal the way they flow through the liver and its lesions, thereby providing functional haemodynamic information. Although this may prove useful for studying focal lesions themselves (and the interval imaging approach described is an approximation to this),[102] one timing method seems to be approaching acceptance as a clinical tool for studying arteriovenous shunting in the liver.[103] AV shunts are found in malignancy and in cirrhosis and in a few benign masses, notably FNH and oestrogen adenomas, but importantly, not in haemangiomas of the adult type. If a microbubble bolus is given via a peripheral vein, it arrives in the hepatic veins draining the liver earlier than normal when shunts are present. This can be timed simply by noting the delay from the injection time until the signal increase in a spectral Doppler gate placed on a hepatic vein. Early arrival seems to be very sensitive to the presence of liver malignancy, though the limits have not yet been defined, particularly the critical question of whether malignancies too small to be imaged can be detected, although the pathophysiology of malignant neovascularisation suggests that this may prove to be the case. Obviously cirrhosis will be a source of false positives, as will the other benign conditions known to have such shunts, but haemangiomas, at least of the adult type, seem to have a normal transit time. This method relies on

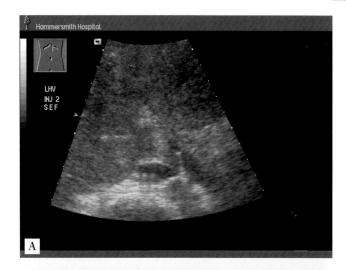

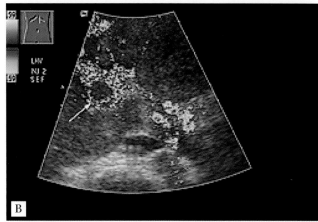

Fig. 11.34 Stimulated acoustic emission reveals liver metastases.
A: Although the liver is heterogeneous in texture, no discrete lesion could be identified in this patient being staged for liver metastases.
B: In the late phase after administration of Levovist, a clear-cut defect could be identified (arrow) because it did not take up the microbubbles in the same way as the surrounding liver.

a similar haemodynamic change to the Doppler perfusion index, and the relative advantages of the two approaches remain to be evaluated.[16,104–106]

REFERENCES

1 Okuda K, Kubo Y, Okazaki N et al. Clinical aspects of intrahepatic bile duct carcinoma including hilar carcinoma. A study of 57 autopsy-proven cases. Cancer 1977; 39: 232–246

2 Ishiguchi T, Shimamoto K, Fukatsu H, Yamakawa K, Ishigaki T. Radiologic diagnosis of hepatocellular carcinoma. Semin Surg Oncol 1996; 12: 164–169

3 Hirai T, Ohishi H, Yamada R et al. Three-dimensional power Doppler sonography of tumor vascularity. Radiat Med 1998; 16: 353–357

4 Jakab F, Rath Z, Schmal F, Nagy P, Faller J. Changes in hepatic hemodynamics due to primary liver tumours. HPB Surg 1996; 9: 245–248

5 Kamalov I R, Sandrikov V A, Gautier S V, Tsirulnikova O M, Skipenko O G. The significance of colour velocity and spectral Doppler ultrasound in the differentiation of liver tumours. Eur J Ultrasound 1998; 7: 101–108

6 Ho S, Lau W Y, Leung W T, Chan M, Chan K W, Johnson P J, Li A K. Arteriovenous shunts in patients with hepatic tumors. J Nucl Med 1997; 38: 1201–1205

7 Ernst H, Hahn E G, Balzer T, Schlief R, Heyder N. Color Doppler ultrasound of liver lesions: signal enhancement after intravenous injection of the ultrasound contrast agent Levovist. JCU 1996; 24: 31–35

8 Koito K, Namieno T, Morita K. Differential diagnosis of small hepatocellular carcinoma and adenomatous hyperplasia with power Doppler sonography. AJR 1998; 170: 157–161

9 Kew M C, Geddes E W. Hepatocellular carcinoma in rural Southern African blacks. Medicine 1982; 61: 98–108

10 Yu S Z. Epidemiology of primary liver cancer. In: Tang Z Y, ed. Subclinical hepatocellular carcinoma. Beijing, China: China Academic Publishers, 1985: 189–211

11 Saracci R, Repetto F. Time trends of primary liver cancer: Indication of increased incidence in selected cancer registry populations. J Natl Cancer Inst 1980; 65: 241–247

12 Curciarello J O, Diaz Velez L, Bosia J D et al. Hepatocellular carcinoma: clinical and epidemiological characteristics. Acta Gastroenterol Latinoamericana 1998; 28: 243–247

13 Edmondson H A, Steiner P E. Primary carcinoma of the liver. A study of 100 cases among 48 900 necropsies. Cancer 1954; 7: 462–503

14 Shikata T. Primary liver carcinoma and liver cirrhosis. In: Okuda K, Peters R L, eds. Hepatocellular carcinoma. New York: Wiley, 1976: 53–72

15 Peters R L. Pathology of hepatocellular carcinoma. In: Okuda K, Peters R L, eds. Hepatocellular carcinoma. New York: Wiley, 1976: 53–72

16 Parker K J, Tuthill T A, Lerner R M, Violante M R. A particulate contrast agent with potential for ultrasound imaging of liver. Ultrasound Med Biol 1987; 13: 555–566

17 Bruno S, Silini E, Crosignani A et al. Hepatitis C virus genotypes and risk of hepatocellular carcinoma in cirrhosis: a prospective study [see comments]. Hepatology 1997; 25: 754–758

18 Tsai J F, Jeng J E, Ho M S et al. Effect of hepatitis C and B virus infection on risk of hepatocellular carcinoma: a prospective study. Br J Cancer 1997; 76: 968–974

19 Kojiro M, Nakashima T. Pathology of hepatocellular carcinoma. In: Okuda-Ishak, ed. Neoplasms of the liver. Tokyo: Springer Verlag, 1987: 81–104

20 Chen D S, Sung J L, Sheu J C et al. Serum alpha feto protein in the early stage of human hepatocellular carcinoma. Gastroenterology 1984; 86: 1404–1409

21 Bolondi L, Benzi G, Santi V et al. Relationship between alphafeto protein serum levels, tumor volume and growth rate of hepatocellular carcinoma in a European series. Ital J Gastroenterol 1990; 22: 190–194

22 Shinagawa T, Ohto M, Kimura K et al. Diagnosis and clinical features of small hepatocellular carcinoma with emphasis on the utility of real time ultrasonography. A study in 51 patients. Gastroenterology 1984; 86: 495–502

23 Goldberg S, Livraghi T, Solbiati L, Gazelle G. In situ ablation of focal hepatic neoplasms. In: Hepatobiliary and pancreatic radiology. New York: Thieme, 1998;

24 Ohto M, Ebara M, Okuda K. Ultrasonography in the diagnosis of hepatic tumor. In: Okuda-Ishak, ed. Neoplasms of the liver. Tokyo: Springer Verlag, 1987: 251–258

25 Larcos G, Sorokopud H, Berry G, Farrell G C. Sonographic screening for hepatocellular carcinoma in patients with chronic hepatitis or cirrhosis: an evaluation. AJR 1998; 171: 433–435

26 Sarasin F P, Giostra E, Hadengue A. Cost-effectiveness of screening for detection of small hepatocellular carcinoma in western patients with Child–Pugh class A cirrhosis. Am J Med 1996; 101: 422–434

27 Bottelli R, Tibballs J, Hochhauser D, Watkinson A, Dick R, Burroughs A K. Ultrasound screening for hepatocellular carcinoma (HCC) in cirrhosis: the evidence for an established clinical practice. Clin Radiol 1998; 53: 713–716

28 Sheu J C, Sung J L, Chen D S et al. Ultrasonography of small hepatic tumors using high-resolution linear-array real time instruments. Radiology 1984; 150: 797–802

29 Itoh K, Yasuda Y, Ueno E, Kasahara K, Zhao L. Studies on the relationships between acoustic patterns produced by liver carcinoma in ultrasonography and in scanning acoustic microscopy. Asian Med J 1983; 26: 585–597

30 Cottone M, Marcenò M P, Maringhini A et al. Ultrasound in the diagnosis of hepatocellular carcinoma associated with cirrhosis. Radiology 1983; 147: 517–519

31 Zhi-zhang Xu. Real time B-mode ultrasonography in localization of subclinical carcinoma. In: Tang Zhao-you, ed. Subclinical hepatocellular carcinoma. Berlin: Springer Verlag, 1985: 36–53

32 Ebara M, Ohto M, Shinagawa T et al. Natural history of minute hepatocellular carcinoma smaller than three centimeters complicating cirrhosis. A study in 22 patients. Gastroenterology 1986; 90: 289–298

33 Yoshikawa J, Matsui O, Takashima T. Fatty metamorphosis in hepatocellular carcinoma: radiological features in 10 cases. AJR 1988; 151: 717–720

34 Brandt D J, Johnson C D, Stephens D H, Weiland L H. Imaging of fibrolamellar hepatocellular carcinoma. AJR 1988; 151: 295–299

35 Mathieu D, Guinet C, Bouklia-Hassane A, Vasile N. Hepatic vein involvement in hepatocellular carcinoma. Gastrointest Radiol 1988; 13: 55–60

36 Sugiura N, Ohto M, Kimura K, Ebara M, Okuda K. Imaging diagnosis of portal vein tumour thrombosis and its pathophysiology in hepatocellular carcinoma. Jpn J Gastroenterol 1986; 83: 2151–2160

37 Taylor K J W, Ramos I, Morse S S, Fortune K L, Hammers L, Taylor C R. Focal liver masses: differential diagnosis with pulsed Doppler US. Radiology 1987; 164: 643–647

38 Bolondi L, Gaiani S, Li Bassi S et al. Colour Doppler and duplex investigation of vascular signals arising from hepatocellular carcinoma (HCC). Gastroenterol Int 1989; 2: 30–32

39 Ohnishi K, Nomura F. Ultrasonic Doppler studies of hepatocellular carcinoma and comparison with other hepatic focal lesions. Gastroenterology 1989; 97: 1489–1497

40 Taylor K J W, Ramos I, Carter D, Morse S S, Snower D, Fortune K L. Correlation of Doppler US tumor signals with neovascular morphologic features. Radiology 1988; 166: 57–62

41 Taylor C R, Taylor K J W. Diagnostic imaging of hepatocellular carcinoma: progress in non invasive tissue characterization. J Clin Gastroenterol 1988; 10: 452–457

42 Yasuhara K, Kimura K, Ohto M et al. Pulsed Doppler in the diagnosis of small liver tumors. Br J Radiol 1988; 61: 898–902

43 Choi B, Kim T, Han J, Kim A, Seong C, Park S. Vascularity of hepatocellular carcinoma: assessment with contrast-enhanced second-harmonic versus conventional power Doppler US. Radiology 2000; 214: 381–386

44 Leifer D, Middleton W, Teefey S, Menias C, Leahy J. Follow-up of patients at low risk for hepatic malignancy with a characteristic hemangioma at US. Radiology 2000; 214: 167–172

45 Lewall D B, McCorkell S J. Hepatic echinococcal cyst: sonographic appearance and classification. Radiology 1985; 155: 773–775

46 Igawa S, Sakai K, Kinoshite H, Hirohashi K. Intraoperative sonography: clinical usefulness in liver surgery. Radiology 1985; 156: 473–478

47 Gilbert H A, Kagan A R. Liver metastases. In: Weiss L, ed. Fundamental aspects of metastases. Amsterdam: Elsevier, 1976: Ch. 26

48 Wilson M A. Metastatic disease of the liver. In: Wilson M A, Ruzicka F F, eds. Modern imaging of the liver. New York: Marcel Dekker, 1989: Ch. 17

49 Desai A G, Bennet R, Sheriff S. Streaming in the portal vein: its effect on the spread of metastases to the liver. Clin Nucl Med 1985; 10: 556–559

50 Ackerman N B. The blood supply of experimental liver metastases. Surgery 1974; 75: 589–596

51 Schor A M, Schor S L. Tumour angiogenesis. J Pathol 1983; 141: 385–413

52 Folkman J, Merler E, Abernathy C, Williams G. Isolation of a tumor factor responsible for angiogenesis. J Exp Med 1971; 33: 275

53 DeVita V. Single agent vs combination chemotherapy. CA Cancer J Clin 1975; 25: 152

54 Green B, Bree R L, Goldstein H M, Stanley C. Gray scale evaluation of hepatic neoplasms: patterns and correlations. Radiology 1977; 124: 203–208

55 Scheible W, Gosink B B, Leopold G R. Gray scale echographic patterns of hepatic metastatic disease. AJR 1977; 129: 983–987

56 Koischwitz D. Sonomorphologie primäre and secondäre leberneoplasmen. Fortschr Rontgenstr 1980; 133: 372–378

57 Rubaltelli L, Del Maschio A, Candiani F. The role of vascularisation in the formation of echographic patterns of hepatic metastases. Br J Radiol 1980; 53: 1166–1168

58 Marchal G, Baert A L, Favery J. Ultrasonography of liver haemangioma. Fortschr Rontgenstr 1983; 138: 201–207

59 Marchal G, Tshibwabwa-Tumba E, Verbeken E, Baert A, Lauweryns J. Influence of tumoral and peritumoral vascularization on the sonographic appearance of liver metastases. In: Ferrucci J T, Mathieu D G, eds. Advances in hepatic radiology. St Louis: Mosby, 1990: 109–128

60 Marchal G J, Pylyser K, Tshibwabwa-Tumba E A et al. Anechoic halo in solid liver tumors: sonographic, microangiographic, and histologic correlation. Radiology 1985; 156: 479–483

61 Marchal G, Tshibwabwa-Tumba E, Oyen R, Pylyser K, Goddeeris R. Correlation of sonographic patterns with histology and microangiography. Invest Radiol 1985; 20: 79–84

62 Tanaka S, Kitamura T, Imaoka S. Hepatocellular carcinoma: sonographic and histological correlation. AJR 1983; 140: 701–707

63 Schonland M M, Milward-Sadler G H, Wright D H, Wright R. Hepatic tumours. In: Wright R, Alberti K G, Karran S, Milward-Sadler G H, eds. Liver and biliary diseases. London: W B Saunders, 1979: 919

64 Federle M P, Filly R A, Moss A A. Cystic hepatic neoplasms: complementary roles of CT and ultrasonography. AJR 1981; 136: 345–348

65 Schlauri H, Hacki W H, von Schulthess G K, Stamm B. Liver apudoma simulating cystic liver. Dtsch Med Wochenschr 1987; 112: 1986–1989

66 Reading N G, Forbes A, Nunnerley H B, Williams R. Hepatic haemangioma: a critical review of diagnosis and management. Q J Med 1988; 67: 431–445

67 Yasuhara K, Kimura K, Ohto M et al. Pulsed Doppler in the diagnosis of small liver tumours. Br J Radiol 1988; 61: 898–902

68 Taylor K J, Ramos I, Morse S S, Fortune K L, Hammers L, Taylor C R. Focal liver masses: differential diagnosis with pulsed Doppler US. Radiology 1987; 164: 643–647

69 Kim T K, Han J K, Kim A Y, Park S J, Choi B I. Signal from hepatic hemangiomas on power Doppler US: real or artefactual? Ultrasound Med Biol 1999; 25: 1055–1061

70 Brambs H J, Spamer C, Volk B, Wimmer B, Koch H. Histological diagnosis of liver hemangiomas using ultrasound-guided fine needle biopsy. Hepatogastroenterology 1985; 32: 284–287

71 Freeny P C, Marks W M. Patterns of contrast enhancement of benign and malignant hepatic neoplasms during bolus dynamic and delayed CT. Radiology 1986; 160: 613–618

72 Suramo I, Lahde S. Computed tomography of small asymptomatic haemangiomas of the liver. Acta Radiol Diagn 1982; 23: 577–583

73 Brick S H, Hill M C, Lande I M. The mistaken or indeterminate CT diagnosis of hepatic metastases: the value of sonography. AJR 1987; 148: 723–726

74 Leslie D F, Johnson C D, MacCarty R L, Ward E M, Ilstrup D M, Harmsen W S. Single-pass CT of hepatic tumors: value of globular enhancement in distinguishing hemangiomas from hypervascular metastases. AJR 1995; 165: 1403–1406

75 Mergo P, Ros P. Benign lesions of the liver. Radiol Clin North Am 1998; 36: 319–331

76 Chafetz N, Taylor A, Alazraki N P, Gosink B B. The heterogeneous liver scan: ultrasound correlation. Radiology 1979; 130: 201–213

77 Scholmerich J, Volk B A, Gerok W. Value and limitations of abdominal ultrasound in tumour staging – liver metastases and lymphoma. Eur J Radiol 1987; 7: 243–245

78 Sandler M A, Petrocelli R D, Marks D S, Lopez R U. Ultrasonic features and radionuclide correlation in liver cell adenoma and focal nodular hyperplasia. Radiology 1980; 135: 393–397

79 Kerlin P, Davis G L, McGill D B, Weil L H, Adson M A, Sheedy P F. Hepatic adenoma and focal nodular hyperplasia: clinical, pathologic, and radiologic features. Gastroenterology 1983; 84: 994–1002

80 Kawashima A, Suehiro S, Murayama S, Russell W J. Focal fatty infiltration of the liver mimicking a tumor: sonographic and CT features. J Comput Assist Tomogr 1986; 10: 329–331

81 Kissin C M, Bellamy E A, Cosgrove D O, Slack N, Husband J E. Focal sparing in fatty infiltration of the liver. Br J Radiol 1986; 59: 25–28

82 Gabata T, Matsui O, Kadoya M J et al. Aberrant gastric venous drainage in a focal spared area of segment IV in fatty liver: demonstration with color Doppler sonography. Radiology 1997; 203: 461–463

83 Maxwell A J, Mamtora H. Fungal liver abscesses in acute leukaemia – a report of two cases. Clin Radiol 1988; 39: 197–201

84 Ohlsson B, Tranberg K, Lundstedt C et al. Detection of hepatic metastases in colorectal cancer: a prospective study of laboratory and imaging methods. Eur J Surg 1993; 159: 275–281

85 Carter R, Poon F, Hemingway D et al. A prospective study of six methods for detection of hepatic colorectal metastases. Ann Roy Coll Surg 1996; 78: 27–30

86 Paley M, Ros P. Hepatic metastases. Radiol Clin North Am 1998; 36: 319–331

87 Gozzetti G, Mazziotti A, Bolondi L et al. Intraoperative ultrasonography in surgery for liver tumors. Surgery 1986; 99: 523–530

88 Simeone J T. Intraoperative ultrasonography of liver tumours. In: Ferrucci J T, Mathieu D G, eds. Advances in hepatobiliary radiology. New York: Mosby, 1990: 229–238

89 Machi J, Sigel B. Operative ultrasound in general surgery. Am J Surg 1996; 172: 15–20

90 Bezzi M, Silecchia G, De Leo A, Carbone I, Pepino D, Rossi P. Laparoscopic and intraoperative ultrasound. Eur J Radiol 1998; 27: S207–214

91 Castaing D, Garden O J, Bismuth H. Segmental liver resection using ultrasound-guided selective portal venous occlusion. Ann Surg 1989; 210: 20–23

92 Machi J, Isomoto H, Kurohiji T et al. Detection of unrecognized liver metastases from colorectal cancers by routine use of operative ultrasonography. Dis Colon Rectum 1986; 29: 405–409

93 Huber K, Heuhold N. Rapid diagnosis of liver cancer by ultrasound-guided fine-needle aspiration biopsy. Cancer Detect Prev 1987; 10: 383–387

94 Limberg B, Hopker W W, Kommerell B. Histological differential diagnosis of focal liver lesions by ultrasonically guided fine needle biopsy. Gut 1987; 28: 237–241

95 Livraghi T. Percutaneous ethanol injection of hepatocellular carcinoma: survival after 3 years in 70 patients. Ital J Gastroenterol 1992; 24: 72–74

96 Solbiati L, Goldberg S N, Ierace T et al. Hepatic metastases: percutaneous radio-frequency ablation with cooled-tip electrodes. Radiology 1997; 205: 367–373

97 Leen E, Angerson W G, Cooke T G, McArdle C S. Prognostic power of Doppler perfusion index in colorectal cancer. Correlation with survival. Ann Surg 1996; 223: 199–203

98 Oppo K, Leen E, Angerson W J, Cooke T G, McArdle C S. Doppler perfusion index: an interobserver and intraobserver reproducibility study. Radiology 1998; 208: 453–457

99 Cosgrove D. Ultrasound contrast enhancement of tumours. Clin Radiol 1996; 51(Suppl 1): 44–49

100 Blomley M, Albrecht T, Cosgrove D et al. Improved imaging of liver metastases using stimulated acoustic emission in the late enhancement phase of the ultrasound contrast agent Levovist. Radiology 1999; 210: 409–416

101 Choi B I, Lim J H, Han M C et al. Biliary cystadenoma and cystadenocarcinoma: CT and sonographic findings. Radiology 1989; 171: 57–61

102 Eckersley R, Cosgrove D, Blomley M, Hashimoto H. Functional imaging of tissue response to bolus injection of ultrasound contrast agent. Proc IEEE Ultrasonics Symposium 1998; 2: 1779–1782

103 Blomley M J, Albrecht T, Cosgrove D O et al. Liver vascular transit time analyzed with dynamic hepatic venography with bolus injections of an US contrast agent: early experience in seven patients with metastases. Radiology 1998; 209: 862–866

104 Mattrey R F, Strich G, Shelton R E et al. Perfluorochemicals as US contrast agents for tumor imaging and hepatosplenography: preliminary clinical results. Radiology 1987; 163: 339–343

105 Matsuda Y, Yabuuchi I. Hepatic tumors: ultrasound contrast enhancement with CO_2 microbubbles. Radiology 1986; 161: 701–705

106 Hilpert P L, Mattrey R F, Mitten R M, Peterson T A D. IV injection of air-filled human albumin microspheres to enhance arterial Doppler signals: a preliminary study in rabbits. AJR 1989; 153: 613–616

Diffuse liver disease

Hylton B Meire and Henry C Irving

Introduction

The assessment of the echoes from the liver parenchyma forms part of virtually every upper abdominal ultrasound examination, and yet the information derived from these ultrasound reflections is one of the least well utilised facets of ultrasound scanning.

The normal liver parenchyma returns a homogeneous background of low-level echoes within which the normal hepatic and portal venous structures can be identified. Various pathological processes may result in either an increase or a decrease in echo amplitude, disturbances in echo pattern and alterations in the size and shape of the liver. All these features need to be evaluated whenever the liver is examined. Unfortunately, the ultrasound appearance of the liver is to a considerable degree determined not only by the nature of the liver but also by the technical characteristics of the ultrasound system in use. It is therefore important for the user to be familiar with the normal appearances of the liver on each of the makes of scanner in his or her department. Confirmation of a normal appearance of the liver may be a valuable diagnostic tool in a variety of circumstances, such as the exclusion of evidence of chronic liver disease in patients with cholestasis of pregnancy.[1] Similarly, the user must be aware of all of the indicators for both acute and chronic liver disease when examining patients with acute hepatic failure in whom the treatment and prognosis will be greatly influenced by whether or not there is underlying long-standing liver disease.

Echo amplitude

The echo amplitude of the liver parenchyma can be assessed by comparing it with the reflectivity of the right renal parenchyma and the portal vein walls.

The amplitude of the parenchymal liver echoes is slightly higher than those returned from the renal cortex at the same depth in the image (Fig. 12.1A). It is important that the comparison is between echoes at similar depths, in order to avoid errors introduced by the application of swept gain (time–gain compensation). Obviously, the comparison is only valid if the renal parenchyma is itself normal: many intrinsic renal diseases affect the reflectivity of the renal parenchyma and may lead to false diagnoses of liver disease if this is not recognised (Fig. 12.1B).

The echoes from the walls of the portal venous radicles should be higher in amplitude than the adjacent liver parenchyma, so that these vessel walls can be resolved as clear white lines (Fig. 12.2A). Loss of this clarity of the portal vein wall echoes is a reliable indicator of increased reflectivity of the liver parenchyma (Fig. 12.2B).[2] Conversely, the portal vein wall echoes may become unduly prominent, signifying reduced reflectivity of the liver parenchyma – the so-called 'dark liver'.

Attenuation

Loss in amplitude with depth is known as attenuation, and attempts to measure attenuation are a logical extension of the visual assessment of liver parenchymal reflectivity described above. Normal liver parenchyma attenuates the ultrasound beam at around 0.5 dB/MHz/cm of path length (or 1 dB/MHz/cm of depth), and it has been shown that abnormal liver parenchyma does show either increased or decreased attenuation.[3] Attenuation may be measured using the reflected signal amplitude, or alternatively by using frequency shift (based on the principle that higher frequencies are attenuated more rapidly than lower, resulting in a shift in spectral content towards the lower frequencies). Many studies have been performed to evaluate

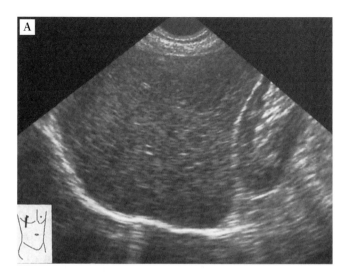
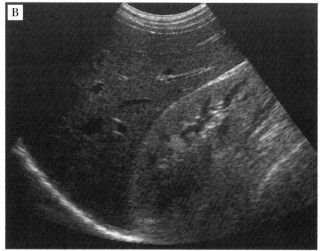

Fig. 12.1 Relationship between renal and hepatic echoes. A: Scan to show relationship between echo amplitude of normal liver and normal renal parenchyma. **B:** Scan to show abnormal kidney with increased parenchymal echoes giving a false diagnosis of 'dark' liver.

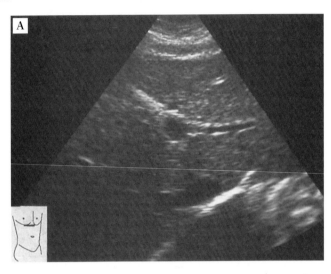
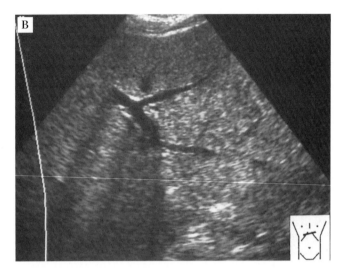

Fig. 12.2 Periportal echoes. A: Scan to show normal portal vein wall echoes standing out from adjacent liver parenchyma. **B:** Loss of portal vein wall echo, indicating 'bright' liver.

the different methods of measuring liver attenuation and to correlate the changes in attenuation with pathological processes,[3–7] and although some encouraging results have been published, the techniques have not been adopted for general clinical use.

Echo pattern

The other component of echo texture that can be assessed visually is echo pattern. Normal liver parenchyma consists of interleaving linear echoes that are uniform in size and shape, forming a homogeneous network. These echoes may become finer and more closely packed (Fig. 12.3A),

coarser and more loosely arranged (Fig. 12.3B), or irregular and non-uniform in size, shape and pattern, according to the nature of the pathology. However, it must be realised that the apparent 'texture' of the liver is at least as dependent on technical factors in the ultrasound scanner as on liver architecture. There is not a one-to-one correlation between small-scale liver anatomy and the ultrasound echo pattern.

Liver size

Estimation of liver size has long been one of the key components of a general physical examination and ultrasound

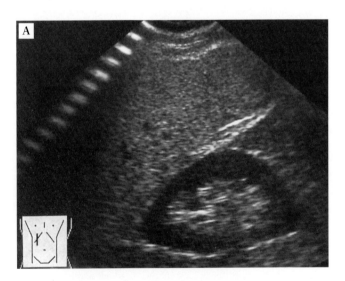
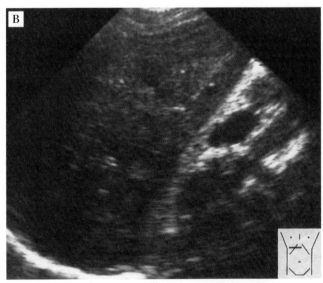

Fig. 12.3 Abnormal echo patterns in 'bright' liver. A: Fine, closely packed echoes. **B:** Coarse, loosely arranged echoes.

imaging offers a scientific approach to this (Ch. 9). Because of the complex shape of the liver, accurate estimation of its volume is tedious and time-consuming,[8,9] and some investigators have suggested that unidimensional longitudinal measurements[10,11] or bidimensional longitudinal and transverse measurements[12] can quantify hepatomegaly reasonably accurately. A useful single measurement is the longitudinal mid-clavicular diameter, which is less than 13 cm in over 95% of normals.[11] However, most ultrasonographers find that a subjective assessment of liver size, using reference organs such as the kidneys and observations of shape and surface contours, is sufficiently accurate for clinical purposes, and measurements tend to be reserved for therapeutic trials when serial estimations of liver size are required.

Accuracy

Using the ultrasound criteria described above, questions arise as to the reliability of ultrasound in predicting the presence of diffuse parenchymal liver disease, its accuracy in suggesting the correct histological diagnosis, and the possibility of replacing the invasive liver biopsy. Although many workers agree that ultrasound is a sensitive technique for distinguishing normal from abnormal liver,[11,13–21] there has been much less confidence about the ability of ultrasound to specify individual pathological processes such as steatosis and fibrosis,[14,15,18–23] and the consensus is that liver biopsy for histological diagnosis remains the gold standard, although ultrasound has much to offer in detecting and monitoring liver disease and its complications.

Fatty infiltration

The accumulation of fatty droplets within hepatocytes occurs in response to a variety of injuries to the liver that interfere with normal metabolism, deficiency of lipotropic factors, or the transportation of abnormally large amounts of fat to the liver cells. The more important causes encompass a long list, including alcohol, diabetes mellitus, obesity, pregnancy, drugs (especially corticosteroids) and toxic substances, malnutrition due to dietary deficiency or wasting disease, parenteral hyperalimentation and inborn errors of metabolism.[24,25] Fatty infiltration is a dynamic process: its severity may alter rapidly, over weeks or even days,[26,27] and is usually completely reversible.[17,28]

Ultrasound appearances

Fat causes increased reflectivity,[29] presumably owing to the interfaces produced by the multiple fat droplets producing increased echo amplitude of the liver parenchyma, giving the typical appearances of a 'bright liver'.[15,20,22,24] The pattern is usually that of fine, closely packed echoes (Fig. 12.4),[23,24] and there is often hepatomegaly (75% of

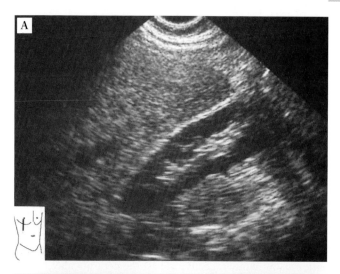

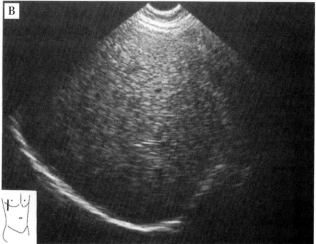

Fig. 12.4 Fatty liver. A and **B:** Longitudinal sections to show the increased reflectivity of the 'bright' liver. Note that the liver is enlarged with increased attenuation, so that the deeper parts are not imaged.

cases[23]), which is a helpful distinguishing feature from cirrhosis when the liver is normal in size or shrunken.[30]

It is the fat which is predominantly responsible for the increased attenuation of the ultrasound beam that is seen in some 'bright livers', and this feature may also be used to distinguish fatty infiltration from other causes of this ultrasound appearance.[3,7,19,31] It is important that as high a frequency transducer as possible (e.g. 5 MHz) be used in order to optimise the detection of increased attenuation if mild degrees of fatty infiltration are not to be missed.[21,23]

However, although ultrasound is highly sensitive for the detection of fatty infiltration (sensitivity 86% for mild and almost 100% for moderate and severe degrees[23]), the specificity is lower, probably owing to the fact that fatty infiltration may develop concurrently with other pathological changes, such as fibrosis, in many of the conditions listed above.

Focal fatty infiltration

Fatty infiltration is commonly a generalised process, affecting the entire liver volume in a uniform fashion and causing a diffuse abnormality. However, this is not always the case: fatty infiltration may be patchy, i.e. lobar, segmental or subsegmental in distribution, when it is known as focal fatty infiltration (or focal steatosis).[32,33]

In these situations regions of increased reflectivity form adjacent to regions of normal liver echo texture. The boundaries are often angulated or geometric in shape, or there may be characteristic interdigitating margins.[34] Regions of fatty infiltration have no mass effect and normal vessels can be seen to pass through the affected portions of liver without displacement.[35] These features usually allow a confident ultrasonographic diagnosis to be made, but the differentiation from highly reflective metastatic deposits may be difficult when the fatty infiltration results in single or multiple discrete areas of increased reflectivity (Fig. 12.5).[28,36–38]

Fatty infiltration with focal areas of sparing

Similar diagnostic dilemmas may be encountered when the fatty infiltration is almost totally uniform but there are single or multiple islands of liver that are spared. These regions of normal liver echo texture appear reduced in echo amplitude compared to the surrounding 'bright liver', and may be misinterpreted as echo-poor lesions (Fig. 12.6).[39]

Typical sites of focal fatty sparing are the quadrate lobe anterior to the portal vein bifurcation (segment 4), areas adjacent to the gallbladder fossa, and subsegmental subcap-

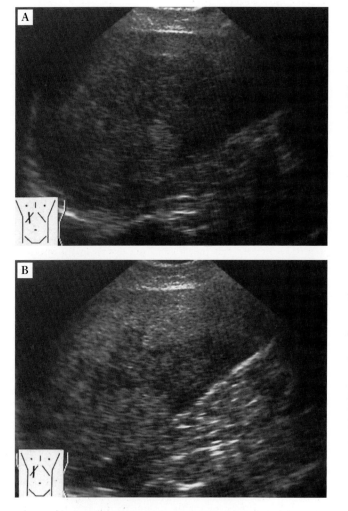

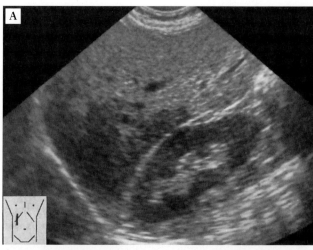

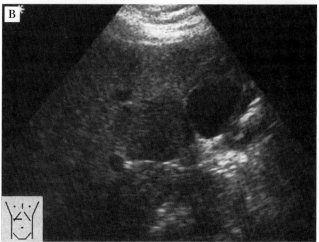

Fig. 12.5 Focal fatty infiltration. A and **B:** Two longitudinal sections showing the geographic areas of increased reflectivity typical of irregular fatty infiltration.

Fig. 12.6 Focal fatty sparing. A: Geographic echo-poor area in the posterior portion of the right lobe. **B:** Similar region in a typical position close to the gallbladder. Both are due to focal sparing in extensive but incomplete fatty change.

sular regions.[40–42] The location of these spared areas has led to speculation that there is a vascular factor associated with the aetiology of this phenomenon,[43] such as the presence of portosystemic venous collaterals permitting shunting which may act as protection from the fatty infiltration.[40]

Metabolic liver diseases

An overwhelming number of different metabolic liver abnormalities have now been identified, and a minority of these may give rise to abnormalities detectable on ultrasound. Wilson's disease without cirrhosis and Gilbert's syndrome are not associated with any abnormality on ultrasound imaging.

One of the most common groups are the glycogen storage diseases (GSD). These are a heterogeneous range of disorders of glycogen metabolism, 14 of which have been fully described to date: type 0, type IA to ID and types II to X. In all types there is excessive storage of glycogen within the liver, giving rise to a combination of hepatomegaly and an increase in parenchymal reflectivity. The appearances are similar, if not identical, to the changes seen in fatty liver disease, and ultrasound cannot reliably differentiate these two conditions. Although hepatomegaly is almost invariable only a minority of patients have splenomegaly, the cause for which is not entirely clear. A well recognised complication is the development of hepatic adenomas, which probably occur in over 25% of GSD patients. It has also been reported that approximately 25% of these adenomas may become malignant. Ultrasound is therefore valuable for serial monitoring of GSD patients to identify the adenomas and to try to detect any sudden changes in lesion characteristics which may suggest malignant change. The adenomas may be either highly or poorly reflective, and malignant change cannot be excluded on the basis of ultrasound imaging alone.[44,45]

Amyloid

Familial amyloid affects the liver and many other tissues, including the myocardium and nervous system. The diffuse deposition of amyloid within the liver does not cause any alteration in liver echo pattern and can therefore be neither diagnosed nor excluded on ultrasound imaging.

Haemochromatosis

Primary haemochromatosis gives rise to excessive iron deposition in many tissues, including the liver. The condition usually gives rise to a progressive hepatic cirrhosis, and these patients are at particular risk for the development of primary hepatocellular carcinoma. Although ultrasound can identify the cirrhotic changes the underlying haemochromatotic change cannot be diagnosed or excluded by ultrasound.

Cirrhosis

The pathological features of cirrhosis of the liver are parenchymal destruction with nodular regeneration and fibrosis resulting in architectural distortion. It is an end result of a wide variety of causes, which may be classified on either an aetiological or a morphological basis, or using a combination of both systems.

Ultrasound appearances

The ultrasound appearances are not specific for any particular type of cirrhosis, and although some cirrhotic livers may appear normal on ultrasound, abnormalities can be recognised in approximately two-thirds of cases.[13,22] The essential ultrasonographic features are increased reflectivity of the fibrous tissue and a concomitant loss of definition of portal vein walls[17,19,20,22] but no significant increase in attenuation,[3,6,7] disturbance of echo pattern, which is usually coarse and irregular,[16] although the echoes can be fine and even,[13] and a generalised heterogeneity of texture partly corresponding to the disorganisation of structure seen pathologically (Fig. 12.7).[17]

The lack of attenuation of the ultrasound beam by fibrosis is useful in distinguishing fibrosis from fatty infiltration[3,6,7] but, especially in alcoholic disease, the two pathologies often coexist, causing confusion.[17] However, some workers have been able to identify the coarse echo pattern of fibrosis in the background of the fine echo pattern of fatty infiltration, and have suggested that the mixed pattern of pathologies is recognisable on ultrasound.[23]

Regenerative nodules may give a generalised granularity to the liver echo texture in forms of micronodular cirrhosis, and the larger nodules of macronodular disease may give an ultrasonically recognisable surface nodularity. Surface nodularity is most easily detected in the presence of ascites; otherwise it can be identified by careful examination of the inferior surface of the liver, especially in relation to the gallbladder and right kidney (Fig. 12.8). Larger nodules may mimic tumour masses[46] – an awkward differential diagnosis, as cirrhosis is a risk factor for hepatoma and ultrasound is used to screen for this complication (Fig. 12.9) (Ch. 11).[47] As most hepatomas are vascular whereas regenerating nodules are not, Doppler studies are helpful in this problem (Ch. 11).

The morphology of the liver may assist in the ultrasound diagnosis of cirrhosis. Although a cirrhotic liver may be normal in size, it tends to shrink as the disease progresses. Furthermore, the right lobe may shrink, so that the caudate lobe occupies a relatively larger proportion of the liver volume.[48] A ratio of caudate lobe to right lobe can be derived from a transverse scan of the liver immediately below the portal vein bifurcation: this is less than 0.6 in normals (Ch. 9) and greater than 0.65 in cirrhosis, with 100% specificity but sensitivities of 84% and 43% in two

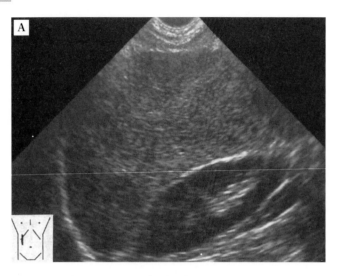 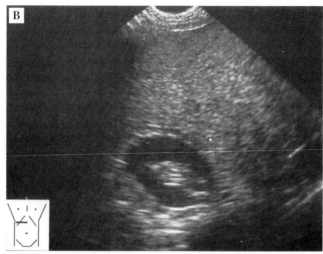

Fig. 12.7 Cirrhosis. A: Longitudinal and **B:** transverse scans to show the increased echo amplitude and irregular echo pattern without increase in attenuation typical of cirrhosis without additional fatty change.

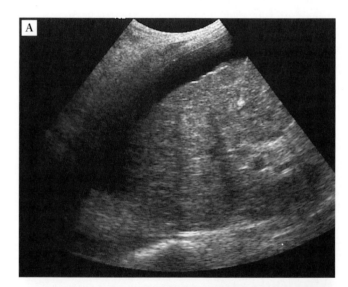

Fig. 12.8 Nodular liver surface. A: Nodularity of the liver surface is most easily seen when there is ascites. **B:** In the absence of ascites the nodularity may be apparent on the inferior liver surface. Note the right pleural effusion. **C:** A distended gallbladder facilitates assessment of the inferior surface of the liver, revealing mild nodularity in this case.

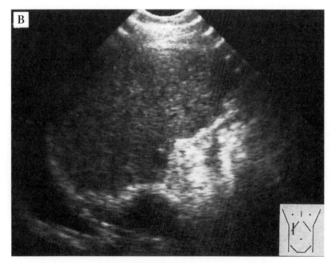 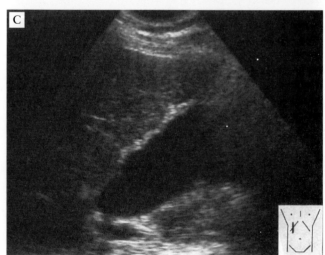

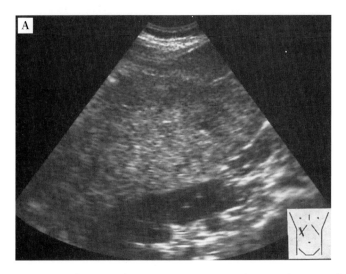

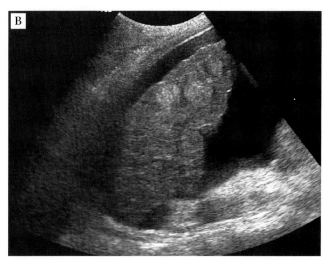

Fig. 12.9 Cirrhosis. A: The nodular echo pattern is shown in this case with advanced cirrhosis. **B:** The masses of increased reflectivity represent hepatoma formation.

different series.[48,49] Similar results have been obtained for right lobe to left lobe longitudinal diameter ratios,[30] and the two later studies found that the sensitivity rates were higher in post-necrotic (post-hepatitic) cirrhosis than in the alcohol-related disease.

Shrinkage of the right lobe with sparing or hypertrophy of the caudate and/or left lobes is thought to be related to the vascular anatomy – probably the arrangement of venous drainage, which leads to more extensive fibrosis and relatively less compensatory hypertrophy and regeneration in the right lobe than elsewhere in the liver.

Other ultrasound findings in cirrhosis are related to the complications associated with hepatocellular failure and portal hypertension: these include ascites, splenomegaly, the development of collateral venous channels and other abnormalities of the portal venous system, all of which are discussed in detail in Chapter 13.

Hepatitis

Acute viral hepatitis

The main value of ultrasound in acute viral hepatitis is in excluding an obstructive (surgical) cause of jaundice (Ch. 15), but once bile duct dilatation has been excluded the ultrasonographer may be able to suggest hepatitis as the underlying aetiology of the hepatocellular (medical) jaundice.

The so-called 'dark liver' of ultrasound refers to an appearance in which the portal vein walls appear of higher echo amplitude than usual compared to the surrounding liver parenchyma, which appears less reflective than normal (Fig. 12.10). This appearance has also been termed the 'centrilobular pattern'[20,50] and is thought to be caused by the cellular swelling and oedema in the centrilobular

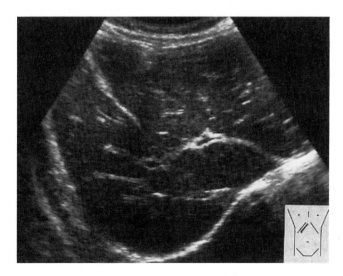

Fig. 12.10 'Dark' liver (centrilobular) pattern.

portion of the liver lobules with sparing of the portal tracts. However, although in the original description the centrilobular pattern was seen in 13 of 16 patients with acute hepatitis,[50] a later study which included 791 patients with acute hepatitis failed to show a significant increase in the incidence of this pattern in the hepatitis patients over a control group (32% and 31%, respectively).[51]

Another often striking feature of acute hepatitis is marked thickening of the gallbladder wall (Ch. 15). This may also be seen to a lesser extent in patients with a wide variety of chronic liver diseases.

The 'dark liver' appearance has also been observed in leukaemic infiltration,[50] toxic shock syndrome,[52] congestive cardiac failure, AIDS[53] and radiation injury,[54] as well as in normals,[43] so caution must be advised in the clinical application of this ultrasound sign.

Many patients with acute viral hepatitis, especially hepatitis C, have periportal adenopathy.[55,56] This finding is particularly prevalent in patients with active viraemia, but is not specific for hepatitis C and may be seen in other viral infections as well as primary biliary cirrhosis. Periportal lymphadenopathy has also been noted in systemic mastocytosis.[57]

Acute alcoholic hepatitis

Acute alcoholic hepatitis can vary from a mild anicteric illness to fulminant hepatic failure. It may be completely reversible, but may progress to frank cirrhosis. The liver is almost always enlarged and there is increased reflectivity and attenuation.[17,58]

These appearances of an enlarged 'bright' liver are indistinguishable from other causes of fatty infiltration, and the ultrasound appearances must be correlated with the clinical history.

Chronic hepatitis

The classification of chronic hepatitis is complex, but the underlying pathological changes that give rise to abnormal ultrasound findings are diffuse inflammation with varying degrees and distributions of necrosis, fatty change and fibrosis.

The ultrasound findings are of increased parenchymal reflectivity and altered echo patterns. Increased attenuation is not a marked feature of chronic hepatitis but sometimes occurs, depending upon the amount of fatty infiltration and necrosis compared to fibrosis.[14,50]

Granulomatous hepatitis

Some chronic inflammatory diseases characteristically form granulomata. In these, epithelioid macrophages and tissue histiocytes aggregate and become surrounded by small lymphocytes, and multinucleated giant cells may be formed by the coalescence of epithelioid cells. In tuberculosis the granulomata often undergo central necrosis (caseation) and subsequent fibrosis and calcification.

Granulomatous liver diseases may produce a 'bright liver' indistinguishable from other causes,[53,59] but it has been reported that the granulomata can be recognised as small, moderately reflective lesions 3–5 mm in diameter surrounded by an echo-poor halo (Fig. 12.11).[59] These granulomata have been seen in tuberculosis, sarcoidosis, toxoplasmosis and brucellosis. The echo-poor nodules in tuberculous hepatitis have been confused with metastatic disease.[60,61] Occasionally the granulomata of tuberculosis may be small in number and large in size – the so-called macronodular tuberculoma. Although the majority of these are seen as echo-poor nodules on ultrasound,[62] highly reflective masses have also been reported.[63] Both of

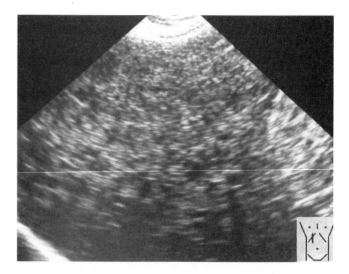

Fig. 12.11 Granulomatous hepatitis – 'target lesion' representing a granuloma. (Figure courtesy of Dr A Joseph.)

these appearances can easily be confused with infiltrative tumour, and there are no specific ultrasound features that facilitate a correct differential diagnosis. Large tuberculomas may undergo necrosis and caseation and, rarely, a frank tuberculous abscess may be present.[64] Once again there are no ultrasound features specific to this form of liver abscess. Tuberculous liver disease is more common in immunocompromised patients, especially HIV-positive subjects. In these patients multiple granulomas measuring up to 1.5 cm in diameter may be present within the liver and spleen: although usually echo-poor, these may also occasionally be highly reflective.[65]

The majority of patients with brucellosis show only non-specific hepatosplenomegaly, the typical granulomatous appearance being seen in the minority. Rarely the granulomata associated with brucellosis may undergo caseation, with the formation of a brucelloma. If these are large enough and sufficient central necrosis takes place a frank liver abscess may be formed. This is indistinguishable from other forms of suppurative liver abscess, although the relatively chronic nature of many cases of brucellosis may give rise to an appearance similar to that seen in amoebic liver abscess.[66,67]

Infestations

Infestations of the liver are well described as causes of focal lesions on ultrasound (Ch. 10). However, on a worldwide basis the single most common infestation of the liver is by the blood fluke *Schistosoma mansoni*, which causes a form of cirrhosis that eventually results in portal hypertension.

Marked fibrosis occurs around the portal tracts throughout the liver in response to a granulomatous reaction caused by the parasite implanting along portal vein branches. This is referred to pathologically as 'pipe-stem fibrosis', and is seen on ultrasound as increased reflectivity and thickening of portal vein walls. This ultrasound pattern of periportal fibrosis is typical of schistosomiasis.[68-70] Although splenomegaly usually coexists, in endemic areas the ultrasound appearance of the liver may be the only clue to the diagnosis of hepatosplenic schistosomiasis,[68,71] and ultrasound has been used to assess the success of a large-scale chemotherapy programme.[72]

Toxoplasma gondii is being identified within the liver with increasing frequency, usually in immunocompromised patients with HIV infection or post liver transplantation. The majority of cases show only hepatomegaly on imaging but occasionally the granulomatous reactions around the parasites may be detectable as 3–4 mm echopoor nodules. There are no specific ultrasound features of this condition.

Cystic fibrosis

Liver disease in cystic fibrosis becomes commoner with increasing age, and is therefore seen more frequently as patients survive the respiratory complications of the disease and live longer. Fatty infiltration may occur, especially in patients on hyperalimentation, giving the typical ultrasound features, but is of little clinical consequence. Of more importance is a distinctive type of focal biliary cirrhosis with eosinophilic concretions: in approximately 5% of cases this progresses to a multilobular biliary cirrhosis, eventually giving rise to portal hypertension.

The clinical diagnosis of liver involvement is difficult because overinflation of the lungs makes assessment of liver and spleen size unreliable.

Ultrasound of the liver may show diffuse or patchy increase in reflectivity[73] and accentuation of the periportal echoes has also been described,[74,75] as has an irregularity of the liver edge[76] – presumably indicating surface nodularity (Fig. 12.12). In established cases a fairly characteristic very coarse nodularity is seen, the nodules being between 2 and 3 cm in diameter.

The sensitivity of ultrasound for the detection of liver disease related to cystic fibrosis remains unproven, but it has been shown that hepatobiliary scintigraphy (DISIDA) can reveal early evidence of nodular change although the ultrasound findings remain normal.[77]

Biliary cirrhosis

Biliary cirrhosis is divided into primary and secondary, depending on the aetiology.

Primary biliary cirrhosis

The aetiology of primary biliary cirrhosis (PBC) remains obscure, but autoimmune factors are implicated; the

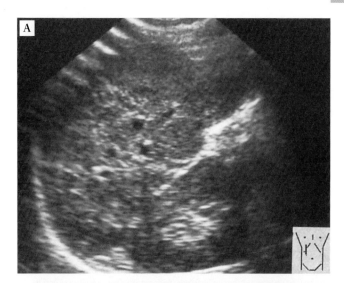
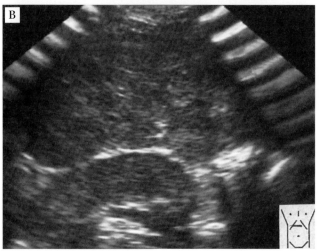

Fig. 12.12 Cystic fibrosis. A: Longitudinal and B: transverse scans to show diffuse changes and patchy (periportal) changes.

disease is far more common in females. It typically presents with pruritis in middle-aged women and progresses slowly, giving rise to jaundice after an interval of several years. Ultrasound imaging is disappointing, the size and appearances of the liver often being normal during the first few years of the disease.[14] There is, however, usually evidence of portal hypertension and splenomegaly is invariably present. In advanced cases texture changes, consisting of coarse nodularity and accentuation of the portal tracts develop (Fig. 12.13). Very rarely the liver may be small in size with a nodular surface. There is a significant increase in the incidence of gallstones in primary biliary cirrhosis, many patients having required cholecystectomy prior to diagnosis. Perihepatic lymphadenopathy is now well described in PBC, being present in almost all patients.[78] The size and number of lymph nodes correlate well with the histological stage of the disease but shows poor

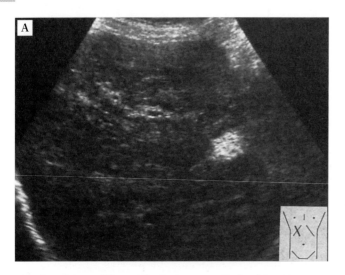 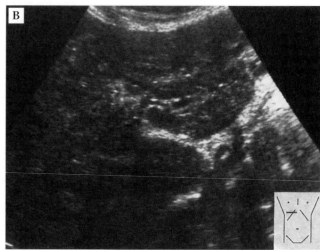

Fig. 12.13 Primary biliary cirrhosis. A: Longitudinal and **B:** transverse scans. Note the prominent periportal reflectivity and the coarse, slightly irregular texture of the liver.

correlation with clinical and biochemical variables. This lymphadenopathy is, however, not specific for PBC and has also been shown in hepatitis C,[55,56] especially in patients with active viraemia. Periportal lymphadenopathy has also been noted in systemic mastocytosis.[57]

Secondary biliary cirrhosis

Secondary biliary cirrhosis arises as a result of long-standing bile duct obstruction. The dilated ducts may be apparent but often are remarkably minor. There are no characteristic ultrasound findings apart from those relating to the initiating cause (e.g. Caroli's disease, choledochal cyst, bile duct stricture).

Secondary biliary cirrhosis may also occur as part of the disease complex of sclerosing cholangitis. Many patients with this disorder show no abnormality on ultrasound scanning, but occasionally irregular segmental duct dilatations may be seen and in advanced cases there is a marked increase in periportal reflectivity. The cirrhotic change may be identified by nodularity of the liver with increased attenuation, and by splenomegaly. The appearances are similar to those seen in schistosomiasis.

Budd–Chiari syndrome

This is caused by partial or complete obstruction of the hepatic venous outflow. The obstruction may be central or peripheral and is occasionally a result of an inferior vena caval web, but is more frequently associated with hypercoagulable states. If the venous obstruction is complete and of rapid onset, patients usually die of acute liver failure. Those who present for imaging investigations usually have a disease of slow onset and sparing of one or more of the major hepatic veins.

The ultrasound features in the acute phase are of hepatomegaly and ascites and relatively normal spleen size. Thrombus may be seen within the major hepatic veins (Fig. 12.14A) and there is often reverse flow in the portal vein (Fig. 12.14B). As the disease progresses there is compensatory hypertrophy of the caudate lobe (Fig. 12.14C), often with the detection of dilated serpiginous veins (Fig. 12.14D) and there is progressive splenomegaly. In long-standing Budd–Chiari syndrome the liver texture is abnormal, often with small focal areas of high attenuation giving rise to acoustic shadowing (Fig. 12.14E).

Some experience has now been obtained with the use of percutaneous trans-hepatic stenting in Budd–Chiari syndrome. Two groups have reported satisfactory results, even if only to improve the patient's condition while awaiting a donor liver.[79,80] Chunqing *et al.*[79] successfully used ultrasound to guide their stents in 25 patients with Budd–Chiari syndrome.

Veno-occlusive disease

Although this term can be applied to Budd–Chiari syndrome it is generally reserved for the range of conditions in which the small hepatic veins or venules become occluded, usually with sparing of the larger trunks. This condition may occur *de novo* but is usually secondary to chemotherapy for malignant disease or the consumption of a range of herbal teas.

The obstructed vessels are too small to be identified by ultrasound, but their occlusion leads to a reduction or abolition in hepatic vein flow and Doppler studies reveal bidirectional oscillating flow in the patent portions of the hepatic veins. In the acute phase there may also be reversal of portal vein flow, ascites, and a rapidly increasing spleen size. The liver sometimes shows an apparent generalised

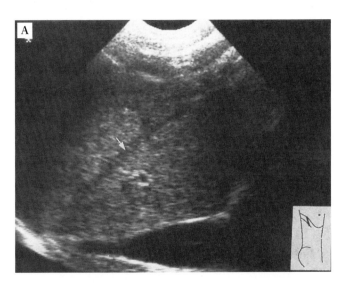

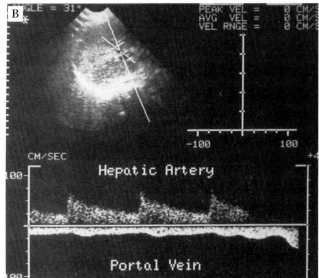

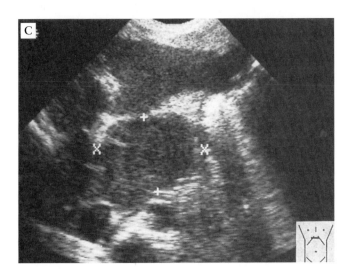

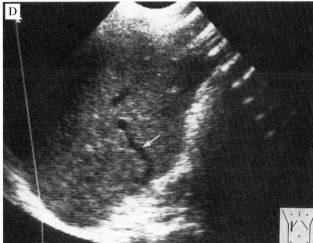

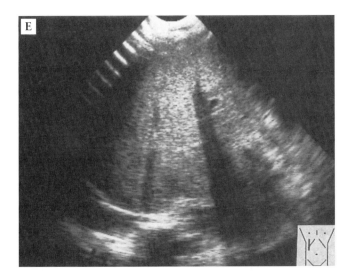

Fig. 12.14 Budd–Chiari syndrome. A: Thrombus (arrow) within a major hepatic vein. **B:** Reverse flow in the portal vein, with a compensatory increase in hepatic arterial flow. **C:** In this well established case the caudate lobe (+X) shows marked enlargement. **D:** Serpiginous dilated peripheral segment of an hepatic vein (arrow). **E:** Focal areas of attenuation with acoustic shadowing.

increase in parenchymal reflectivity which is not seen in acute large vessel disease. If the patient improves the portal flow may ultimately return to normal, but the hepatic vein waveform usually remains flattened, probably as a result of hepatic fibrosis or frank cirrhosis.

Conclusions

Ultrasound can provide a great deal of useful information about the nature and extent of diffuse liver disease, although the differential diagnosis usually remains wide (Tables 12.1 and 12.2), and liver biopsy for histological diagnosis remains the final arbiter.[81] Even in this context ultrasound has a role to play in guiding biopsy needles to maximise diagnostic accuracy and safety. It should also be noted that ultrasound can be used for guiding 'plugged' biopsies, thereby enabling tissue cores to be obtained from patients in whom the liver disease has rendered conventional biopsy unsafe owing to impaired blood coagulation.[82,83]

Table 12.1 Causes of the 'bright' liver

Fatty infiltration[15,22]
Cirrhosis[13,14]
Chronic hepatitis[14,50]
Alcoholic hepatitis[17,58]
Granulomatous hepatitis[59]
Chronic congestive cardiac failure[14]
Portal fibrosis[14]
Schistosomiasis[68,70]
Cystic fibrosis[73,74]
Glycogen storage (Gaucher's) disease[7]
Niemann–Pick disease[7]

Table 12.2 Causes of the 'dark' liver

Acute viral hepatitis[50,51]
Congestive cardiac failure
Leukaemic infiltration[50]
Toxic shock syndrome[52]
AIDS[53]
Radiation injury[54]
Normal[51]

REFERENCES

1 McDonald J A. Cholestasis of pregnancy. J Gastroenterol Hepatol 1999; 14: 515–518
2 Kurtz A B, Dubbins P A, Rubin C S. Echogenicity: analysis, significance, and masking. AJR 1981; 137: 471
3 Taylor K J W, Riely C A, Flax S, Weltin G, Kuc R, Barwick K W. Quantitative US attenuation in normal liver and in patients with diffuse liver disease: importance of fat. Radiology 1986; 160: 65–71
4 Ralls P W, Johnson M B, Kanel G et al. FM sonography in diffuse liver disease: prospective assessment and blinded analysis. Radiology 1986; 161: 451–454
5 Aufrichtig D, Lottenberg S, Hoefs J et al. Frequency-demodulated US: evaluation in the liver. Radiology 1986; 160: 59–64
6 Kuni C C, Johnson T K, Crass J R, Snover D C. Correlation of Fourier spectral shift-determined hepatic acoustic attenuation coefficients with liver biopsy findings. J Ultrasound Med 1989; 8: 631–634
7 Garra B S, Insana M F, Shawker T H, Russell M A. Quantitative estimation of liver attenuation and echogenicity: normal state versus diffuse liver disease. Radiology 1987; 162: 61–67
8 Rasmussen S N. Liver volume determination by ultrasonic scanning. Br J Radiol 1972; 45: 579–585
9 Van Thiel D H, Hagler N G, Scade R R et al. In vivo hepatic volume determination using sonography and computed tomography. Gastroenterology 1985; 88: 1812
10 Gosink B B, Laymaster C E. Ultrasonic determination of hepatomegaly. JCU 1981; 9: 37
11 Niederau C, Sonnenberg A. Liver size evaluated by ultrasound: ROC curves for hepatitis and alcoholism. Radiology 1984; 153: 503
12 Niederau C, Sonnenberg A, Muller J E, Erckenbrecht J F, Scholten T, Fritsch W P. Sonographic measurements of the normal liver, spleen, pancreas, and portal vein. Radiology 1983; 149: 537–540
13 Dewbury K C, Clark B. The accuracy of ultrasound in the detection of cirrhosis of the liver. Br J Radiol 1979; 52: 945–948
14 Joseph A E, Dewbury K C, McGuire P G. Ultrasound in the detection of chronic liver disease (the 'bright' liver). Br J Radiol 1979; 52: 184–188
15 Foster K J, Dewbury K C, Griffith A H, Wright R. The accuracy of ultrasound in the detection of fatty infiltration of the liver. Br J Radiol 1980; 53: 440–442
16 Debongie J C, Pauls C, Fievez M, Wibin E. Prospective evaluation of the diagnostic accuracy of liver ultrasonography. Gut 1981; 22: 130
17 Taylor K J W, Gorelick F S, Rosenfield A T, Riely C A. Ultrasonography of alcoholic liver disease with histological correlation. Radiology 1981; 141: 157–161
18 Meek D R, Mills P R, Gray H W, Duncan J G, Russel R I, McKillop J H. A comparison of computed tomography, ultrasound and scintigraphy in the diagnosis of alcoholic liver disease. Br J Radiol 1984; 57: 23–27
19 Sanford N L, Walsh P, Matis C, Baddeley H, Powell L W. Is ultrasonography useful in the assessment of diffuse parenchymal liver disease? Gastroenterology 1985; 89: 186–191
20 Needleman L, Kurtz A B, Rifkin M D, Cooper H S, Pasto M E, Goldberg B B. Sonography of diffuse benign liver disease: accuracy of pattern recognition and grading. AJR 1986; 146: 1011–1015
21 Saverymuttu S H, Joseph A E, Maxwell J D. Ultrasound scanning in the detection of hepatic fibrosis and steatosis. BMJ 1986; 292: 13–15
22 Gosink B B, Lemon S K, Scheible W, Leopold G R. Accuracy of ultrasonography in diagnosis of hepatocellular disease. AJR 1979; 133: 19–23
23 Joseph A E A, Saverymuttu S H, Al-Sam S, Cook M G, Maxwell J D. Comparison of liver histology with ultrasonography in assessing diffuse parenchymal liver disease. Clin Radiol 1991; 43: 26–31
24 Scatarige J C, Scott W W, Donovan P J, Seigelman S S, Sanders R C. Fatty infiltration of the liver: ultrasonographic and computed tomographic correlation. J Ultrasound Med 1984; 3: 9–14
25 Campillo B, Bernuau J, Witz M O et al. Ultrasonography in acute fatty liver of pregnancy. Ann Intern Med 1986; 105: 383–384
26 Bashist B, Hecht H L, Harley W D. Computed tomographic demonstration of rapid changes in fatty infiltration of the liver. Radiology 1982; 142: 691
27 Clain J E, Stephens D H, Charboneau J W. Ultrasonography and computed tomography in focal fatty liver. Report of two cases with special emphasis on changing appearances over time. Gastroenterology 1984; 87: 948
28 Swobodnik W, Wechsler J G, Manne W, Ditschuneit H. Multiple regular circumscript fatty infiltrations of the liver. JCU 1985; 13: 577–580
29 Behan M, Kazam E. The echographic characteristics of fatty tissues and tumours. Radiology 1978; 129: 143–151
30 Goyal A K, Pokharna D S, Sharma S K. Ultrasonic diagnosis of cirrhosis: reference to quantitative measurements of hepatic dimensions. Gastrointest Radiol 1990; 15: 32–34
31 Lin T, Ophir J, Potter G. Correlation of ultrasonic attenuation with pathologic fat and fibrosis in liver disease. Ultrasound Med Biol 1988; 14: 729–734
32 Scott W W Jnr, Sanders R C, Siegelman S S. Irregular fatty infiltration of the liver: diagnostic dilemmas. AJR 1980; 135: 67–71

33 Mulhern C B, Arger P H, Coleman B G, Stein G N. Nonuniform attenuation in computed tomography study of the cirrhotic liver. Radiology 1979; 132: 399

34 Quinn S F, Gosink B B. Characteristic sonographic signs of hepatic fatty infiltration. AJR 1985; 145: 753–755

35 Halvorsen R A, Korobkin M, Ram P C, Thompson W M. CT appearances of focal fatty infiltration of the liver. AJR 1982; 139: 277–281

36 Middleton W D. Sonography case of the day: focal hepatic fatty infiltration adjacent to falciform ligament. AJR 1989; 152: 1326–1327

37 Yoshikawa J, Matsui O, Takashima T et al. Focal fatty change of the liver adjacent to the falciform ligament: CT and sonographic findings in five surgically confirmed cases. AJR 1987; 149: 491–494

38 Kawashima A, Suehiro S, Murayama S, Russell W J. Case report: focal fatty infiltration of the liver mimicking a tumour: sonographic and CT findings. J Comput Assist Tomogr 1986; 182: 239

39 Kissin C M, Bellamy E A, Cosgrove D O, Slack N, Husband J E. Focal sparing in fatty infiltration of the liver. Br J Radiol 1986; 59: 25–28

40 Marchal G, Tshibwabwa-Tumba E, Verbeken E et al. 'Skip areas' in hepatic steatosis: a sonographic-angiographic correlation. Gastrointest Radiol 1986; 11: 151–157

41 Sauerbrei E E, Lopez M. Pseudotumor of the quadrate lobe in hepatic sonography: a sign of generalised fatty infiltration. AJR 1986; 147: 923–927

42 White E M, Simeone J F, Mueller P R, Grant E G, Choyke P L, Zeman R K. Focal periportal sparing in hepatic fatty infiltration: a cause of hepatic pseudomass on US. Radiology 1987; 162: 57–59

43 Arai K, Matsui O, Takashima T, Ida M, Nishida Y. Focal spared areas in fatty liver caused by regional decreased portal flow. AJR 1988; 151: 300–302

44 Mieli-Vergani G, Mowat A P. Paediatric liver disease: medical aspects. In: Millward-Sadler G H, Wright R, Arthur M J P, eds. Wright's liver and biliary disease, 3rd edn. London: W B Saunders, 1992: 1189–1207

45 Mowat A P. Inborn errors of metabolism associated with disordered liver function or hepatomegaly. In: Liver disorders in childhood, 3rd edn. Oxford: Butterworth–Heinemann, 1994: 244–302

46 Okazaki N, Yoshida T, Yoshino M, Matue H. Screening of patients with chronic liver disease for hepatocellular carcinoma by ultrasonography. Clin Oncol 1984; 10: 241

47 Cottone M, Marceno M P, Maringhini A et al. Ultrasound in the diagnosis of hepatocellular carcinoma associated with cirrhosis. Radiology 1983; 147: 517–519

48 Harbin W P, Rabert N J, Ferrucci J T Jr. Diagnosis of cirrhosis based on regional changes in hepatic morphology. A radiological and pathological analysis. Radiology 1980; 135: 273

49 Giorgio A, Amoroso P, Lettieri G et al. Cirrhosis: value of caudate to right lobe ratio in diagnosis with US. Radiology 1986; 161: 443

50 Kurtz A B, Rubin C S, Cooper H S et al. Ultrasound findings in hepatitis. Radiology 1980; 136: 717–723

51 Giorgio A, Amoroso P, Fico P et al. Ultrasound evaluation of uncomplicated and complicated acute viral hepatitis. JCU 1986; 14: 675–679

52 Lieberman J M, Bryan P J, Cohen A M. Toxic shock syndrome: sonographic appearances of the liver. AJR 1981; 137: 606

53 Grumbach K, Coleman B G, Gal A A et al. Hepatic and biliary tract abnormalities in patients with AIDS. Sonographic-pathologic correlation. J Ultrasound Med 1989; 8: 247–254

54 Garra B S, Shawker T H, Chang R, Kaplan K, White R D. The ultrasound appearance of radiation-induced hepatic injury. Correlation with computed tomography and magnetic resonance imaging. J Ultrasound Med 1988; 7: 605–609

55 Dietrich C F, Zeuzem S. Sonographic detection of perihepatic lymph nodes: technique and clinical value [German]. Zeitschr Gastroenterol 1999; 37: 141–151

56 Cassani F, Valentini P, Cataleta M et al. Ultrasound detected abdominal lymphadenopathy in chronic hepatitis C: high frequency and relationship with viremia. J Hepatol 1997; 26: 479–483

57 Avila N A, Ling A, Worobec A S, Mican J M, Metcalfe D D. Systemic mastocytosis: CT and US features of abdominal manifestations. Radiology 1997; 202: 367–372

58 Shepherd D F C, Dewbury K C. Sequential imaging of the process of acute alcoholic hepatitis with ultrasound and isotopes. Br J Radiol 1980; 53: 163–165

59 Mills P, Saverymuttu S, Fallowfield D, Nussey S, Joseph A E. Ultrasound in the diagnosis of granulomatous liver disease. Clin Radiol 1990; 41: 113–115

60 Blangy S, Cornud F, Sibert A, Vissuzaine C, Saraux J L, Benacerraf R. Hepatitis tuberculosis presenting as tumoral disease on ultrasonography. Gastrointest Radiol 1988; 13: 52–54

61 Ferandes J D, Nebesar R A, Wall S G, Minihan P T. Report of tuberculous hepatitis presenting as metastatic disease. Clin Nucl Med 1984; 9: 245–247

62 Amaris J, Kardache M, Soyer P et al. Radiological aspects of hepatic tuberculoma. 3 cases. [French] Gastroentérol Clin Biol 1997; 21: 888–892

63 Tan T C, Cheung A Y, Wan W Y, Chen T C. Tuberculoma of the liver presenting as a hyperechoic mass on ultrasound. Br J Radiol 1997; 70: 1293–1295

64 Jain R, Sawhney S, Gupta R G, Acharya S K. Sonographic appearances and percutaneous management of primary tuberculous liver abscess. JCU 1999; 27: 159–163

65 Monill-Serra J M, Martinez-Noguera A, Montserrat E, Maideu J, Sabate J M. Abdominal ultrasound findings of disseminated tuberculosis in AIDS. JCU 1997; 25: 1–6

66 Halimi C, Bringard N, Boyer N et al. Hepatic brucelloma: 2 cases and a review of the literature. [French] Gastroentérol Clin Biol 1999; 23: 513–517

67 Vallejo J G, Stevens A M, Dutton R V, Kaplan S L. Hepatosplenic abscesses due to *Brucella melitensis*: report of a case involving a child and review of the literature. Clin Infect Dis 1996; 22: 485–489

68 Hussain S, Hawass N D, Zaidi A J. Ultrasonographic diagnosis of schistosomal periportal fibrosis. J Ultrasound Med 1984; 3: 449–452

69 Abdel-Wahab M F, Esmat G, Milad M, Abdel-Razek S, Strickland G T. Characteristic sonographic pattern of schistosomal hepatic fibrosis. Am J Trop Med Hyg 1989; 40: 72–76

70 Cerri G G, Alves V A F, Magalhaes A. Hepatosplenic schistosomiasis mansoni: ultrasound manifestations. Radiology 1984; 153: 777

71 Homeida M, Ahmed S, Dafalla A et al. Morbidity associated with *Schistosoma mansoni* infection as determined by ultrasound: a study in Gezira, Sudan. Am J Trop Med Hyg 1988; 39: 196–201

72 Homeida M A, Fenwick A, DeFalla A A et al. Effect of antischistosomal chemotherapy on prevalence of Symmers' periportal fibrosis in Sudanese villages. Lancet 1988; ii: 437–440

73 Wilson-Sharpe R C, Irving H C, Brown R C, Chalmers D M, Littlewood J M. Ultrasonography of the pancreas, liver and biliary system in cystic fibrosis. Arch Dis Child 1984; 59: 923–926

74 Willi U V, Reddish J M, Littlewood Teele R. Cystic fibrosis: its characteristic appearance on abdominal ultrasonography. AJR 1980; 134: 1005–1010

75 Graham N, Manhire A R, Stead R J, Lees W R, Hodson M E, Batten J C. Cystic fibrosis; ultrasonographic findings in the pancreas and hepatobiliary system correlated with clinical data and pathology. Clin Radiol 1985; 36: 199–203

76 McHugo J M, McKeown C, Brown M T, Weller P, Shah K J. Ultrasound findings in children with cystic fibrosis. Br J Radiol 1987; 60: 137–141

77 O'Connor P J, Southern K W, Bowler I M, Irving H C, Robinson P J, Littlewood J M. The role of hepatobiliary scintigraphy in cystic fibrosis. Hepatology 1996; 23: 281–287

78 Dietrich C F, Leuschner M S, Zeuzem S et al. Perihepatic lymphadenopathy in primary biliary cirrhosis reflects progression of the disease. Eur J Gastroenterol Hepatol 1999; 11: 747–753

79 Chunqing Z, Lina F, Guoquan Z et al. Ultrasonically guided percutaneous transhepatic hepatic vein stent placement for Budd–Chiari syndrome. J Vasc Intervent Radiol 1999; 10: 933–940

80 Ganger D R, Klapman J B, McDonald V et al. Transjugular intrahepatic portosystemic shunt (TIPS) for Budd–Chiari syndrome or portal vein thrombosis: review of indications and problems. Am J Gastroenterol 1999; 94: 603–608

81 Celle G, Savarino V, Picciotto A, Magnolia M R, Scalabrini P, Dodero M. Is hepatic ultrasonography a valid alternative tool to liver biopsy? Report on 507 cases studied with both techniques. Dig Dis Sci 1988; 33: 467–471

82 Riley S A, Ellis W R, Irving H C, Lintott D J, Axon A T R, Losowsky M S. Percutaneous liver biopsy with plugging of the needle track: a safe method for use in patients with impaired coagulation. Lancet 1984; ii: 436

83 Irving H C. Sheath needle for liver biopsy. Radiology 1988; 168: 879

The portal venous system

Luigi Bolondi, Stefano Gaiani,
Fabio Piscaglia and Carla Serra

Portal hypertension

Portal hypertension develops when increased resistance to portal flow ('backward flow theory') and/or increased portal blood flow ('forward flow theory') occur; recent evidence suggests that both mechanisms are involved in the maintenance of chronic portal hypertension.[1–3] They result in enlargement of the extrahepatic portal vessels, the development of spontaneous portosystemic collaterals and slow portal vein flow. Sonographic examination of the abdomen can usually display all of these abnormalities, providing fundamental diagnostic information, and it has become generally accepted as a basic step in the management of all patients with suspected portal hypertension and other alterations of the portal circulation.[4]

Sonographic findings in portal hypertension

Changes in portal vein calibre

The portal vessels have been measured both in normal subjects and in patients with portal hypertension[5–16] and wide variations in the normal limits of the diameter of the portal vein have been reported (Table 13.1).[6,10–16] It is known that many factors, such as respiration,[15] posture changes[17] and post-prandial state[18,19] influence its calibre. Measurements should therefore be taken in basal conditions (quiet respiration, supine and fasting). In patients with advanced cirrhosis and portal hypertension a threshold of 13 mm can be used: this provides almost 100% specificity but is less sensitive.[5,13] Dilatation of the portal vein to over 13 mm occurred in 56% of 129 cirrhotic patients with established portal hypertension (Fig. 13.1).[5,13] A value of 12 mm may be useful to differentiate chronic hepatitis from compensated cirrhosis.[20] In attempts to identify patients with a high risk for variceal bleeding, some authors[11,14] have demonstrated that the presence of oesophageal varices is correlated with dilatation of the portal vein: a calibre over 17 mm is 100% predictive for large varices.[11] Some discrepancies may be explained by the populations studied, since patients with advanced disease tend to have larger calibre veins. A normal calibre

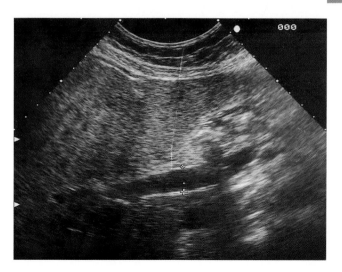

Fig. 13.1 **Dilated portal vein** (over 14 mm) in a patient with liver cirrhosis and portal hypertension.

of the portal vein does not, however, exclude portal hypertension: in some patients with alcoholic cirrhosis we found 11–12 mm portal veins even in the presence of large varices.

The main intrahepatic portal branches are usually also dilated in portal hypertension, whereas the peripheral intrahepatic branches appear narrowed and tortuous, presumably due to the parenchymal fibrosis and nodular regeneration.

Varying degrees of dilatation of the splenic and superior mesenteric veins also occur in portal hypertension. The upper limit of the normal splenic and superior mesenteric veins ranges from 10 to 12 mm.[5,13,15,16] Weill reported that a calibre of the splenic vein of 20 mm or greater should be considered a specific sign of portal hypertension[21] while splenic veins over 12 mm diameter should be regarded as suspicious. Splenomegaly of all types is usually associated with dilatation of the splenic vein, possibly because of the increased splenic blood flow (Fig. 13.2) and it may be difficult to establish whether this indicates portal hypertension or is simply a physiological consequence of the splenomegaly. Other signs of portal hypertension, such as dilatation of the superior mesenteric vein, which does not depend on spleen size, may be helpful. Splenomegaly is also accompanied by a dilatation of the splenic artery, which is required to supply a more extensive capillary bed. Dilatation of the splenic artery was found to occur more frequently in cirrhosis caused by a chronic viral hepatitis than in alcohol abuse.[22] A ratio between the diameter of the hepatic and splenic arteries above 0.9, measured at 1.5–3 cm from their origins, suggests an alcoholic cause for the cirrhosis, with a specificity of 88%, whereas a lower ratio is indicative of an infectious cause.[22] In measurements of the splenic artery, the possibility of a splenic artery aneurysm should be borne in mind; though rare

Table 13.1 Calibre of the normal portal vein (in mm)

Webb et al[6]	10
Weinreb et al[10]	15
Cottone et al[11]	17
Niederau et al[12]	14
Bolondi et al[13]	13
Zoli et al[14]	14
Kurol & Forsberg[15]	16
Goyal et al[16]	16

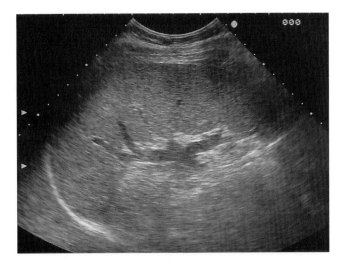

Fig. 13.2 **Splenomegaly.** Severe splenomegaly with a dilated splenic vein at the hilum.

in the general population (0.04%), it is more frequent in patients with portal hypertension (prevalence 8.8–13%).[23–25] The pathogenesis is probably excessive flow in the vessel resulting from both the hyperdynamic splanchnic circulation and the splenomegaly. A splenic aneurysm can be misdiagnosed as a collateral vessel on B-mode ultrasound alone; hence Doppler confirmation of the arterial or venous nature of the flow in any echo-free structure located along the course of the splenic artery should be performed, especially in patients who are potential candidates for liver transplantation, because splenectomy is recommended at the time of surgery in patients with an aneurysm (Fig. 13.3).

Another important sign of portal hypertension is the lack of variation in calibre with respiration in the splenic and superior mesenteric veins (Fig. 13.4).[5] In normal subjects there is a dilatation of the portal vessels during sus-

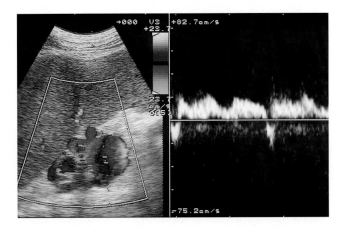

Fig. 13.3 **Splenic artery aneurysm.** A dilated rounded vascular structure is visible at the hilum of the spleen. Colour Doppler and spectral analysis show biphasic turbulent flow.

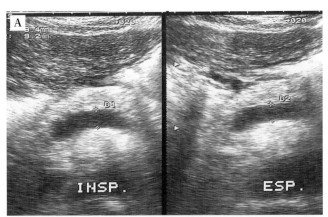

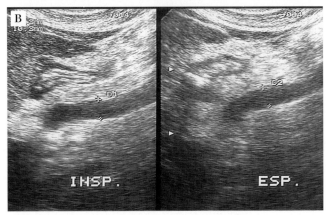

Fig. 13.4 **Dilated splanchnic vessels. A:** Dilatation of the splenic vein and **B:** the superior mesenteric vein. During respiration there was no variation in the calibre of the vessels.

pended inspiration because of the reduced venous outflow from the liver.[26] In patients with portal hypertension the intrahepatic resistance is increased and this minimises further dilatation of the portal vessels during a Valsalva manoeuvre. This lack of respiratory calibre variation has good sensitivity (80%) and is specific.[5]

Detection of spontaneous portosystemic collaterals

Opening up of vessels between the high-pressure portal venous system and the low-pressure systemic circulation is usually seen in patients with portal hypertension.

An important example is the umbilical vein, which runs within the ligamentum teres in the left lobe of the liver and when recanalised is easily visible as a channel greater than 3 mm in diameter (Fig. 13.5).[7,27] Recanalisation of the umbilical vein is a highly specific sign of portal hypertension. Colour Doppler facilitates its identification, particularly when it is small; hepatofugal flow in this vein is pathognomonic of portal hypertension. In a series of 184 cirrhotic patients, the umbilical vein was patent in 33.7%,

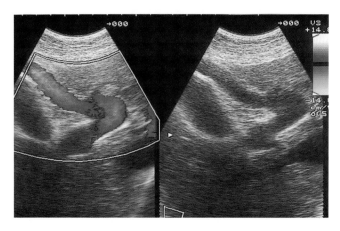

Fig. 13.5 **The umbilical vein** may be dilated in portal hypertension. In this case the umbilical vein is seen in the ligamentum teres. Colour flow signals are shown inside the vein.

but the prevalence was even higher (56.8%) in patients with more severe (Child C) cirrhosis.[28] Para-umbilical collaterals may be located within the liver parenchyma close to the falciform ligament and, in some cases two (or, rarely, more) umbilical veins are detectable. The umbilical vein may also be visible distally, where it can be followed along the abdominal wall towards the umbilical region (Fig. 13.6). Once outside the liver it lies relatively superficially and care should be taken not to exert too much pressure with the transducer to avoid compressing the vein and thus hindering correct evaluation.

Other collaterals, such as the left gastric vein and retroperitoneal veins around the pancreas, may be difficult to detect because of intestinal gas. The left gastric vein can be visualised at its origin (from the splenic vein or from its confluence with the portal vein). In a series of 187 consecutive patients, this vein could be visualised in 46% of cases and had a mean diameter of 2.4 mm. It terminated in the

portal vein in 30% of cases, at the splenoportal junction in 33% and in the splenic vein in 37%.[29] In cirrhotic patients, visualisation is likely to be easier due to its enlargement in portal hypertension (Fig. 13.7).[30] Dilatation of the left gastric vein suggests the presence of large oesophageal varices.[7]

The short gastric veins may be detectable between the upper pole of the spleen and the wall of the stomach and their visualisation suggests the presence of gastric (and oesophageal) varices. They appear as anechoic tubes with venous flow towards the oesophagus on spectral Doppler (Fig. 13.8).

Large splenorenal shunts, connecting splenic varices with the left renal vein, may relieve the portal hypertension and lead to flow reversal in the splenic and even in the portal veins.[31] They appear as tortuous vessels near the lower pole of the spleen (Fig. 13.9). This spontaneous shunt is usually massive so that flow in gastric varices is

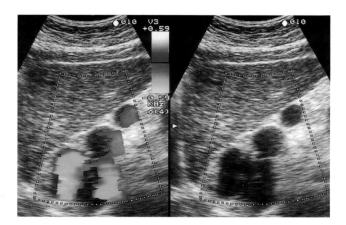

Fig. 13.7 **Left gastric vein.** Marked dilatation of the left gastric vein seen as tortuous channels located behind the left lobe of the liver. Colour mapping confirms its vascular nature.

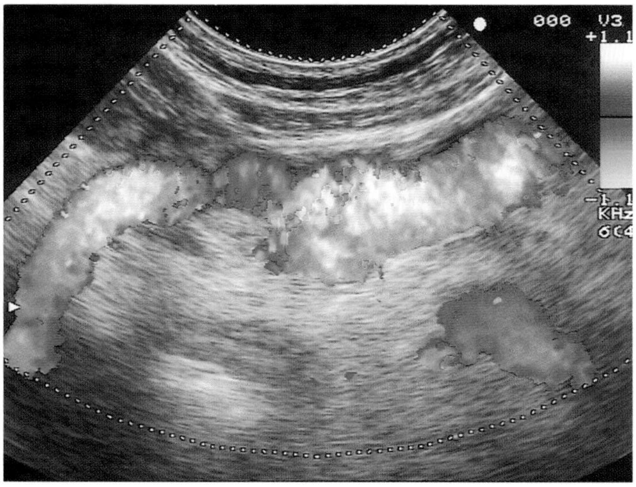

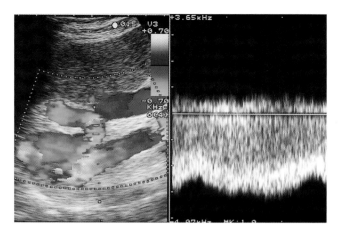

Fig. 13.8 **Short gastric veins** appear as dilated, winding vessels near the upper pole of the spleen. The Doppler trace demonstrates venous flow towards the diaphragm.

Fig. 13.6 **Dilated umbilical vein** followed along the abdominal wall.

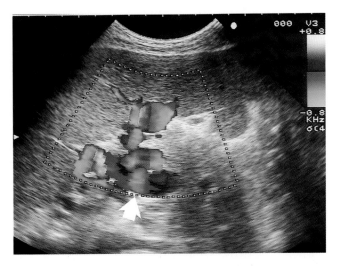

Fig. 13.9 Splenorenal collaterals. Dilation of the venous radicle at the hilum of the spleen connected with the left renal vein (arrow).

low and consequently gastro-oesophageal bleeding is reduced.[32] When there is suspicion of a spontaneous splenorenal shunt, the main left renal vein should also be examined: typically it is dilated.

Occasionally collaterals may be seen within the gallbladder wall (Fig. 13.10).[33] They connect the extrahepatic portal venous system with the intrahepatic portal branches, and may be prominent in portal vein thrombosis.[34]

Direct visualisation of oesophageal varices is often difficult or impossible, though their presence may be inferred by demonstrating thickening of the oesophageal wall, irregularity of the lumen and, particularly, variation of oesophageal wall thickness with respiration. In one report these features detected all cases of moderate or large varices confirmed at endoscopy, but their adequate evalu-

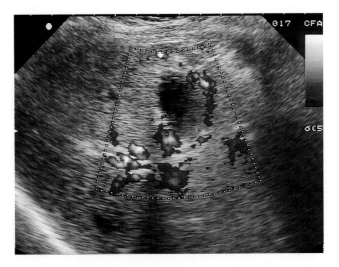

Fig. 13.10 Pericholecystic collaterals. They are detected on power Doppler as vessels with low velocity flow in the wall of the gallbladder in a case of portal vein thrombosis with cavernous transformation.

ation is time consuming, operator dependent and feasible only in a minority of patients; therefore, it cannot be recommended as routine clinical practice.[35]

Other portosystemic collaterals that may be detected, for example omphalo-iliocaval, spleno-retroperitoneal and splenoportal anastomoses, have been described in patients with uncomplicated portal hypertension.[36] In these cases the large spontaneous shunts tend to prevent the development of ascites and gastrointestinal bleeding.[37]

Portal vein thrombosis

In adults, portal vein thrombosis may be caused by haematological or clotting disorders, acute inflammatory diseases of the digestive tract (e.g. necrotising enteritis, intestinal infarction, acute cholecystitis, pancreatitis), pancreatic or gastric tumours, or it may occur as a surgical complication; overall, cirrhosis remains the most common cause. Its incidence is debated, around 10% being reported in an old autopsy series[38] whereas a more recent angiographic study has indicated an incidence of about 1%.[39] Because it is invasive, angiography cannot be performed as a screening examination and might therefore underestimate the true prevalence.

Ultrasonography is routinely used in suspected portal thrombosis, because it is simple, non-invasive and accurate.[13,40] Partial thrombosis typically appears as a reflective band adhering to the wall of the vessel. Recent thrombosis may be undetectable on grey scale imaging, since early thrombus is echo-poor and indistinguishable from blood. In these cases Doppler ultrasound (especially colour or power Doppler) is essential for confirming the absence of portal flow (Fig. 13.11). As the thrombus organises its reflectivity increases and can then be visualised as reflective material within the lumen (Fig. 13.12). In chronic thrombosis reflective fibrous tissue replaces the portal vein.[13] Complete occlusion may be followed by cavernous transformation of the portal vein, in which collateral vessels develop around the thrombosed portal vein, which appears as a solid elongated structure at the porta hepatis, surrounded by numerous tortuous channels (Fig. 13.13).

Portal vein occlusion occurs frequently (up to 25%) in patients with hepatocellular carcinoma, while it is seen in less than 1% in patients with metastases. Tumour invasion of the portal vein may have an echo pattern similar to that of the surrounding (neoplastic) liver parenchyma and there is often a marked dilatation of the vessel, probably related to growth of the tumour within the lumen itself (Fig. 13.14).

Doppler ultrasound findings in portal hypertension

The clinical applications of Doppler studies of the splanchnic vessels include the assessment of the presence, direction and characteristics of blood flow. Doppler not only

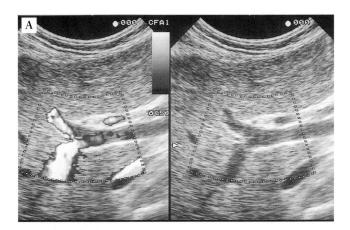

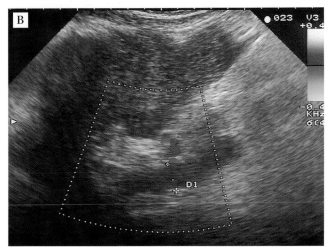

Fig. 13.11 Recent thrombosis. A: Partial thrombosis of the bifurcation of the right portal trunk. The thrombus is echo-poor and cannot be identified by grey scale imaging alone, though it is well defined by power Doppler flow mapping. **B:** Complete recent thrombosis of the portal trunk. No flow signals are seen on colour Doppler.

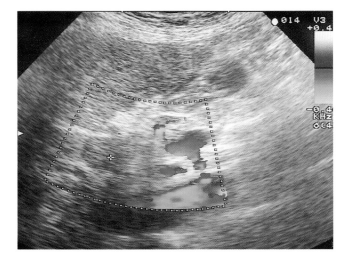

Fig. 13.12 Complete thrombosis of the portal vein. The portal trunk (+) is filled with echogenic material.

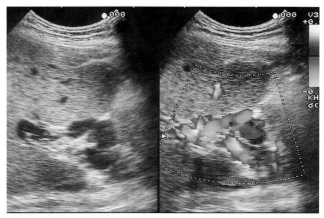

Fig. 13.13 Cavernous transformation of the portal vein. The portal vein is replaced by a series of tortuous irregular vessels. Colour Doppler demonstrated turbulent flow.

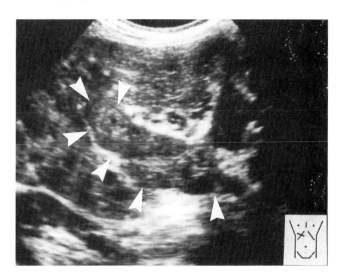

Fig. 13.14 Thrombosed and dilated portal vein. Tumour thrombus of the portal vein (arrowheads) in a case of diffuse hepatocellular carcinoma. The vessel is markedly dilated.

clarifies doubtful real-time images but also provides new insights in many clinical conditions. Quantification of the volume of blood flow in some of the major abdominal arteries and veins has also been attempted as it might provide important clinical information. However, its reliability is still not accepted unanimously.

Detection of blood flow

Establishing the presence of blood flow within the portal vein is the simplest Doppler finding and is usually easy to perform. Colour and power Doppler facilitate the task by directly visualising flow within vessels (Fig. 13.15).

In chronic portal vein thrombosis, when the portal vein is small and highly reflective, Doppler of the porta hepatis

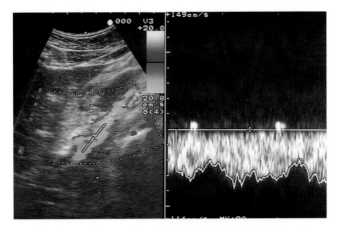

Fig. 13.15 Doppler of the normal portal vein. Colour Doppler facilitates identification of the vessel and positioning of the sample volume. Spectral analysis shows a phasic high-velocity profile.

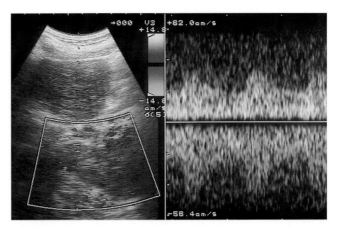

Fig. 13.16 Tumour portal thrombosis in hepatocellular carcinoma. The portal trunk is enlarged and filled by echogenic material. Doppler shows arterial signals with a high-velocity, turbulent flow profile.

reveals no evidence of blood flow. When cavernous transformation has occurred, continuous low-velocity flow can be demonstrated within the small tortuous vessels, best depicted with colour Doppler (Fig. 13.13). Partial thrombosis appears as an absence of colour signal and this can equally be identified when the thrombus is anechoic (Fig. 13.11A). Appropriate scanner settings and technique are required to avoid false-positive findings.

Given its reliability, sensitivity and non-invasiveness, Doppler is considered as the most suitable technique to assess the prevalence of portal thrombosis in cirrhosis. In a series of 228 consecutive cirrhotic patients (without hepatocellular carcinoma) the prevalence of partial and complete vein thromboses were 1.8% and 4.4%.[41] The sensitivity of Doppler ultrasound in diagnosing portal vein thrombosis is similar to that of dynamic computed tomography,[42] but it may be less accurate in partial or branch vein thrombosis, although the high sensitivity of modern scanners may improve on this.[43] In some instances Doppler ultrasound is more accurate than arterioportography, which can erroneously suggest portal thrombosis when there is reverse flow in a patent portal vein.[44] Doppler ultrasound may therefore be considered as sensitive in the diagnosis of portal thrombosis and it is the first imaging technique to be chosen when there is a clinical suspicion.[45] Neovascularisation within the thrombus, a pathognomonic sign of tumour thrombus, may be identified as arterial signals within the thrombus (Fig. 13.16).[46]

Direction of blood flow

Flow direction is another unequivocal qualitative finding provided by Doppler ultrasound (Fig. 13.15); its importance in the investigation of hepatic haemodynamics is obvious. L'Herminè *et al*[47] reported reversed intrahepatic portal flow (demonstrated by arterioportography) in about 5% of their cases, one-third of whom had complete hepato-

fugal flow. However, the rate of reversed flow detected by arterioportography may not accurately reflect its prevalence in a non-selected population of cirrhotics, because only patients with complicated portal hypertension or who are surgical candidates are subjected to this invasive procedure. Kawasaki *et al*[48] reported a prevalence of spontaneous hepatofugal flow of 6.1% in cirrhotic patients and of 5.3% in patients with hepatocellular carcinoma. The overall prevalence of hepatofugal flow in liver cirrhosis (without hepatocellular carcinoma) was 8.3% of 228 patients.[41] Reversed portal flow was associated with a significantly reduced calibre of the portal vein but it is not clear if this finding carries a poor prognosis. Hepatofugal portal flow is associated with a decreased risk of variceal bleeding, while it does not predict survival.[41] In addition, hepatofugal flow in the splenic vein (Fig. 13.17) has proved to be closely correlated with hepatic encephalopathy,[49] probably due to the drainage of large amounts of blood into large splenorenal collaterals.

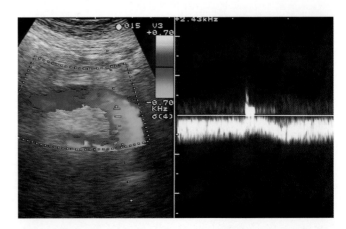

Fig. 13.17 Reversed flow in the splenic vein. The blue colour and the spectral trace below the baseline indicate flow directed towards the spleen.

Characteristics of blood flow and its disturbances

The pattern of the Doppler signals (whether presented as an audio signal or a spectral tracing), can be used to identify a vessel, even when the grey scale image is equivocal, because vessels tend to have a Doppler 'signature'.[50]

The impedance changes in the splanchnic vessels have been studied in the three main arterial beds: the superior mesenteric, splenic and hepatic. The superior mesenteric artery supplies a large part of the intestine and subsequently the portal system. Elevated sinusoidal pressure triggers a reduction of mesenteric arterial resistance, resulting in a hyperdynamic splanchnic circulation.[1] Thus the portal vein flow is increased and this contributes to the maintenance of portal hypertension.[1,51] This dilatation of the intestinal arterioles decreases the impedance indices in the superior mesenteric artery (Fig. 13.18).[52–56] In this vessel the use of the pulsatility index (PI) is more suitable than that of the resistance index (RI), due to the high downstream impedance in fasting normal subjects.[53] A decrease in the PI has been reported to accompany worsening liver function[53] and the development of oesophageal varices.[53,54] Iwao and co-workers have shown that dilatation of this vascular bed plays an important role in the reduction of total peripheral vascular resistance.[55] The reliability of these indices has been debated, especially concerning intra- and inter-observer variability. Recent studies, however, have demonstrated that skilled operators can reduce the variability to insignificant levels by a preliminary training period.[57,58]

Doppler impedance indices, measured in the intraparenchymal branches of the splenic artery, were found to be increased in patients with cirrhosis (Fig. 13.19)[59,60] irrespective of spleen size, and they correlate closely with splenoportal vascular resistance.[59] After liver transplantation, a rapid drop to normal values has been observed, while this seems to be abolished or reversed in patients

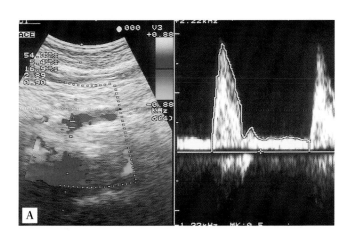 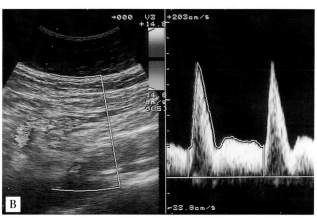

Fig. 13.18 Superior mesenteric artery. A: Doppler study of the superior mesenteric artery in a normal fasting subject shows a low diastolic flow. **B:** In a patient with portal hypertension, there is a marked increase of diastolic flow because of the decreased resistance of the splanchnic vascular bed.

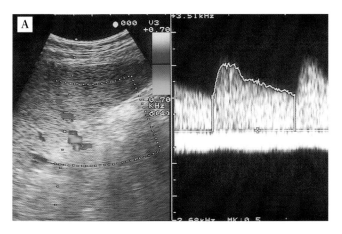 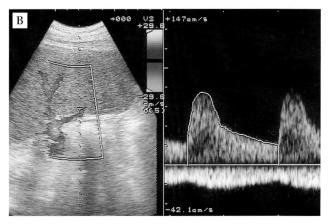

Fig. 13.19 Splenic artery. A: Doppler trace shows a normal flow profile with high diastolic phase in a normal subject with an RI of 0.5. **B:** In patients with portal hypertension there is a decrease in diastolic flow with an RI of 0.7.

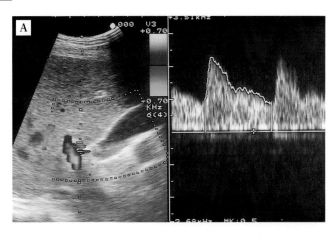
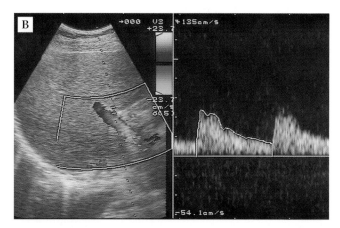

Fig. 13.20 Hepatic artery. A: Doppler trace shows a normal flow profile with high diastolic phase in a normal subject with an RI of 0.61. **B:** In patients with portal hypertension there is decreased diastolic flow with an RI of 0.71.

suffering from complications that increased portal resistance.[61]

In patients with liver cirrhosis, hepatic arterial impedance indexes are increased compared both to controls (Fig. 13.20)[62] and to patients with chronic hepatitis.[63] This increase, which seems to correlate with the increase of sinusoidal resistance,[62] becomes even more pronounced if portal vein thrombosis occurs.[62]

Doppler examination of the hepatic veins may also provide useful data. Normally they display a triphasic waveform determined by the cardiac cycle, particularly the fluctuating right atrial pressure. These phasic variations of flow are completely lost in some 25% of cases of liver cirrhosis with portal hypertension (Fig. 13.21) and greatly reduced in a further 25%.[64] The pathophysiology of this alteration is still unclear but is presumably attributable to an increase in liver stiffness. The identification of these abnormalities has diagnostic and prognostic meaning: loss of triphasicity suggests the presence of large varices[65] and

a completely flat waveform was associated with an unfavourable prognosis in a multivariate analysis that also incorporated clinical indices.[66]

Hepatic vein pulsatility is also altered in patients with portal hypertension due to cardiac failure.[67] In this case, however, while the antegrade flow components decrease, the retrograde components become more pronounced (Fig. 13.22). The portal vein pulsatility may also be increased, occasionally with transient reversal of flow in each cardiac cycle (Fig. 13.23),[68] a finding that is suggestive of high right atrial pressure.[68-71]

Quantitative measurement of blood flow

A complete haemodynamic evaluation of the portal venous system in portal hypertension should include measurement of: (a) the volume of portal venous flow (Qpv); (b) the portal perfusion pressure (pressure gradient between the portal vein and the hepatic veins; Ppv – Phv);

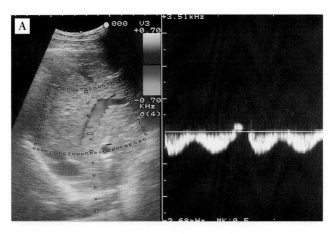
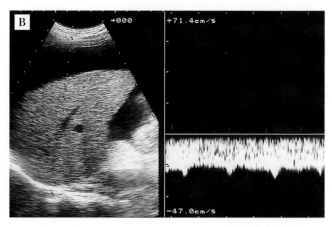

Fig. 13.21 Hepatic vein Doppler. A: Doppler flow profile in a normal hepatic vein is characterised by a phasic waveform. **B:** In some patients with cirrhosis the flow profile may be continuous.

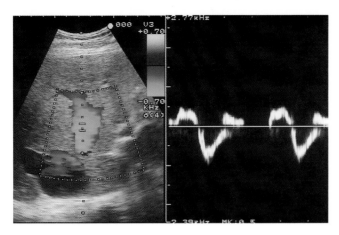

Fig. 13.22 Hepatic vein Doppler in cardiac failure. The hepatic veins are dilated and the Doppler trace shows an increase of the retrograde phase.

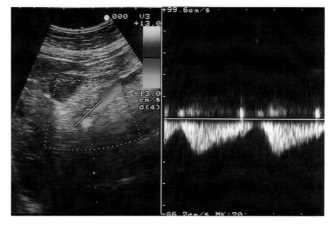

Fig. 13.23 Portal flow in cardiac failure is characterised by a pulsatile waveform.

and (c) the portal vascular resistance (Pvr), which is calculated as:[72]

$$Pvr = Ppv - Phv/Qpv$$

from the volume and gradient.

While several invasive methods have been developed to measure portal and hepatic venous pressures,[73,74] measurement of flow volume has always proved much more difficult, so non-invasive measurements using Doppler ultrasound have attracted attention. The measurement presupposes uniform insonation in which the entire volume of blood in a cross-section of the vessel is exposed to a uniform ultrasonic beam. The time-averaged mean velocity (V), calculated from the mean Doppler shift, is multiplied by the cross-sectional area (A) of the vessel, to give the volume flow (Q):

$$Q = VA$$

Important sources of error include the non-uniform insonation, which cannot be controlled by the operator, measurement of the cross-sectional area of the vessel and the assessment of the beam/vessel angle (necessary to convert the frequency shifts of the Doppler signal into velocity); the angle errors increase rapidly with increasing obliquities of approach (see Ch. 6).[75] Measurement of the cross-sectional area of the vessel presents even greater problems not only because of the small size of most of the vessels of interest but also because they are often not circular, especially the veins,[12] while their calibre varies through the cardiac and respiratory cycles. For these reasons, flow velocity and volume calculations taken at angles over 60° or in small and tortuous vessels, have poor reproducibility and are unacceptable in clinical practice. Another critical point is the calculation of the mean velocity. Both direct calculation by the software of the instrument and its estimation as a fixed fraction of the maximal velocity may be inaccurate: estimated mean velocity is greatly influenced by Doppler spectral gain while differences of flow profile from patient to patient can produce major errors. On the other hand, estimates of the average peak velocity have been found to be reasonably reproducible, particularly after a preliminary training programme to standardise methodology (Table 13.2).[76]

Although ultrasound cannot directly measure portal pressure, an indirect assessment can be made using the 'congestion index' which correlates with portal pressure[76] or, more strictly, with portal resistance.[61] The congestion index is the ratio between the cross-sectional area and the mean flow velocity of the portal trunk. It takes into account the fact that in portal hypertension the portal vein tends to dilate and the blood velocity to decrease, so that higher values are found in patients with more severe portal resistance[61] and pressure[77] and larger varices.[78] The addition of this index to the endoscopic feature of oesophageal varices improves the prediction of early bleeding in patients with cirrhosis.[79]

For the portal vein, its straight course over 3–4 cm, its relatively large calibre and its oblique position with

Table 13.2 Guidelines for Doppler measurements of the portal vein (from Sabbà et al 1995[76])

1 Measure in suspended normal respiration
2 Longitudinal scan of the portal vein
3 Sample volume in the centre of the vessel, at the level of the hepatic artery, covering 50% of the vessel diameter
4 Doppler angle of 55° or less
5 Pulse repetition frequency (PRF) = 4 kHz; wall filter = 100 Hz
6 Doppler and B-mode tracings recorded simultaneously
7 Average maximum velocity obtained by manual tracing of the envelope of the Doppler waveform
8 Doppler waveform calculation obtained by covering two cardiac cycles between three arterial wall artefacts
9 Portal vein diameter measured from the inner anterior to the inner posterior wall
10 Values result from the mean of three consistent measurements

respect to the abdominal wall are favourable factors for Doppler investigations. Measurements of flow velocity should be made according to the reported guidelines (Table 13.2). Errors in measuring the cross-sectional area do affect the calculation of flow volume in the portal vein but repeated measurements of the diameter reduce the error of flow calculations to within 10%[80] and they correlate well with the results of lipiodol droplet cine-angiography[81] and electromagnetic flowmetry,[82] though the coefficient of variation in the Doppler measurements was higher than for electromagnetic measurements (10.9% versus 5.9%). In humans the total hepatic flow volume measured by Doppler flowmetry as the sum of portal and hepatic artery flow volumes correlates well with the functional hepatic flow volume measured by the clearance of D-sorbitol in healthy subjects ($r = 0.83$).[83] In patients with cirrhosis this correlation breaks down because intrahepatic portosystemic shunting precludes measuring functional flow. Even portal flow alone correlates well with the total hepatic flow measured by the indocyanine green constant infusion clearance method ($r = 0.80$).[84]

Based on these findings, it is reasonable to affirm that the Doppler spectrum can be used as a measure of portal vein flow, even though the absolute values expressed in ml/min may not correspond to the actual flow volumes. Changes of flow velocity and volume assessed by Doppler flowmetry in the same subject under different conditions are more reliable, since possible sources of errors in measuring the absolute values would be expected to affect different measurements in the same way. The method seems to be suitable for *in vivo* monitoring of acute haemodynamic changes in the portal vein such as those induced by feeding, hormones and drugs.[52,56,85,86]

Despite these limitations, many papers dealing with quantitative measurements of flow in the portal vein have been published in recent years and they agree that velocity is reduced, to a greater or lesser degree, in cirrhotic patients (Figs 13.15 and 13.24). Mean portal flow velocity in healthy subjects is usually 12–20 cm/s, whereas a series of cirrhotic patients showed mean values in the range of 8–13 cm/s.[19,62,72,81,83–85,87–90] The variation of reported values for portal vein flow velocity is partly dependent on the methodology (see Ch. 6) and partly on the variation of the haemodynamic patterns with the stage and aetiology of the cirrhosis. It is recommended that the threshold for defining a reduction of portal flow velocity is established in each ultrasound unit, depending on the equipment and the methodology used. For instance, in our experience a threshold of 15 cm/s for the mean portal flow velocity has a sensitivity of 88% and a specificity of 96% in identifying patients with cirrhosis.[89] Even more interestingly, portal flow velocity proved to be the best ultrasound feature, together with the liver biochemical profile, to differentiate compensated cirrhosis from chronic hepatitis: in our scoring system a mean velocity between 16 and 12 cm/s

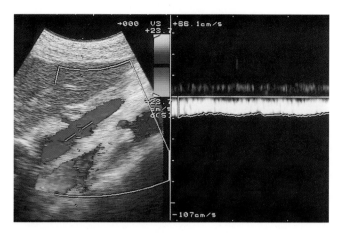

Fig. 13.24 Doppler of the portal vein. Decrease of flow velocity in a patient with cirrhosis: the peak velocity is 16 cm/s and the mean velocity is less than 10 cm/s.

had a moderate weight for the diagnosis of cirrhosis and a velocity below 12 cm/s was highly suggestive.[20]

Influence of collateral pathways on portal flow

Data about portal flow volumes in cirrhosis are even more variable because of the influences of collateral pathways, whose extent varies from case to case. Several studies indicate that mean values of portal flow are comparable to those of normal subjects, as can be observed from the baseline values of patients undergoing beta-blocker treatment compared to the average values in normal subjects that are 700–900 ml/min. To understand this some pathophysiological features of cirrhosis need to be considered. First, the total flow measured in the portal trunk is affected by the location of any portosystemic shunts. Total portal inflow, calculated as the sum of the flow volumes in the superior mesenteric and splenic arteries, is significantly greater in patients with large oesophageal or gastric varices than in controls or in patients with no or small varices.[55] A patent umbilical vein (Figs 13.5 and 13.6) may also explain high portal velocity and flow volume, while large splenorenal collaterals may reduce portal flow[81] and eventually produce flow reversal.[49] In the former therefore, the evaluation of velocity and flow may underestimate the degree of portal hypertension, so that the congestion index seems to be a more reliable index.[28] Portal flow volume is significantly higher in patients with a patent umbilical vein than in those without, but effective liver portal perfusion is lower, as calculated from flow volume in the portal trunk minus portal flow volume in the umbilical vein.[28,91] These discrepancies are particularly evident in patients with more advanced liver functional impairment, whereas they are not seen with the congestion index.[28]

Patients with portal hypertension lack the normal post-prandial increase in portal flow;[19] this is probably related to the hypertensive state of the splanchnic venous bed and to diversion of blood flow through portosystemic collaterals. The decreased post-prandial impedance in the superior mesenteric artery is the same in cirrhotics as in healthy subjects:[52,92] since splenic arterial flow does not decrease after a meal, the lack of portal flow increase in cirrhotics seems to be determined by flow through collateral pathways rather than by reduced portal inflow.[92]

Measurements of flow in the winding and irregular collateral vessels that develop in portal hypertension is difficult, with the exception of the recanalised umbilical vein.[28,91] Only the presence and direction of flow can be assessed in the splenorenal collaterals, though flow in the coronary vein (left gastric vein) can be estimated in some patients.[93]

Diagnosis of Budd–Chiari syndrome

The Budd–Chiari syndrome is a rare disorder in which the hepatic veins are obstructed. The most important sonographic findings are hepatomegaly, with particular enlargement of the caudate lobe (because the inferior hepatic veins are usually spared), non-visualisation or dilatation and irregularity of the main hepatic veins and non-visualisation of the confluence of the hepatic veins with the inferior vena cava (IVC; Fig. 13.25), which may also be narrowed or obstructed (Fig. 13.26).[94–97] Since the IVC is often also involved in the Budd–Chiari syndrome, confirmation may be obtained by demonstrating steady reversed flow in the lower portion of the IVC. In other cases flow in the IVC is in the normal direction but loses its phasic oscillation, suggesting partial obstruction. Changes in the Doppler waveform of the hepatic veins is

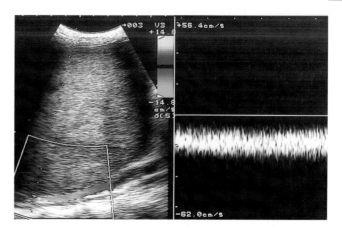

Fig. 13.26 Budd–Chiari syndrome. Narrowing of the IVC with continuous turbulent high velocity flow profile.

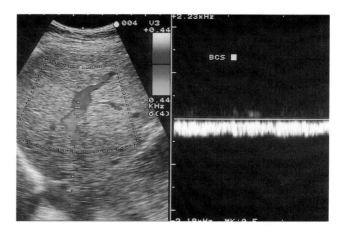

Fig. 13.27 Budd–Chiari syndrome. Doppler ultrasound of the hepatic vein shows a flat waveform indicating continuous flow.

useful in the diagnosis of Budd–Chiari syndrome.[98] Absence of phasic variation resulting in steady forward flow suggests obstruction of the upper portion of the IVC or of the hepatic vein outlet, preventing retrograde transmission of the pressure variations of the right atrium (Fig. 13.27). This has been proposed as a major Doppler sign of Budd–Chiari syndrome[97] but a similar pattern is found in advanced cirrhosis,[64] so that its specificity is poor. Reversed flow in one or more of the hepatic veins is pathognomonic,[98] though seldom found, while reversed flow in the portal vein is more commonly seen, though this is also non-specific. A comparison with magnetic resonance angiography showed that similar diagnostic information is provided by the two techniques so that MR should be a second-choice diagnostic tool when sonography fails to confirm the diagnosis.[99] Venography remains the gold standard, but can be restricted to cases where ultrasound and MR were inconclusive.

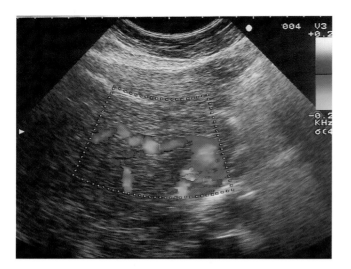

Fig. 13.25 Budd–Chiari syndrome. Tortuous and irregular hepatic vein in the enlarged caudate lobe.

Evaluation of portosystemic surgical shunts

Ultrasonography is a useful method in the follow-up of patients after portosystemic shunt surgery, allowing assessment of patency in 75% of cases.[13] The shunt is deemed patent when a direct confluence between the portal vein and the IVC, or between the splenic and left renal vein, is demonstrated.

When the shunt itself is not displayed, indirect signs of patency may be used: in portocaval shunts a decrease in calibre of the portal vein, compared with the pre-operative value, is a useful sign of patency, as is widening of the IVC above the level of the anastomosis (Fig. 13.28).[100] Similarly, dilatation of the left renal vein is consistent with a patent distal splenorenal shunt, while reversed flow in the superior mesenteric vein indicates a patent mesocaval shunt (Fig. 13.29). All the above observations are only valid if adequate pre-operative measurements of the same parameters have been obtained for comparison.

Doppler has proved useful in pre-operative evaluation of patients as well as postoperative follow-up. Pre-operatively, it can guide the choice of surgery: thrombosis or flow reversal in the portal vein suggests that shunts may be technically impossible or unhelpful. In the postoperative period Doppler is the investigation of choice to assess shunt patency and the haemodynamic consequences of the procedure. Provided pre-operative baseline studies have been performed, it is possible within certain limits to assess flow through the shunt and to gauge changes in portal perfusion.

With regard to the direct assessment of flow through the anastomosis, the series published in the literature show wide variations in sensitivity, ranging from 55% to 87%.[101–103] Turbulent high-speed flow towards the

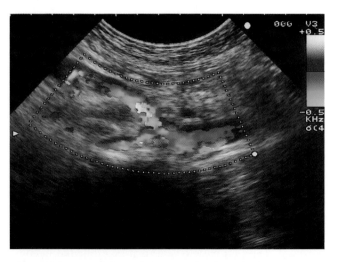

Fig. 13.29 Mesocaval shunt. Colour Doppler shows the direct communication between the superior mesenteric vein and the IVC with reversed flow in the superior mesenteric vein.

systemic circulation can be detected within the shunt itself (Fig. 13.28). In some cases this flow may show a phasic profile in response to variations in caval pressure.

Indirect signs of patency can be found in practically all patients by examining the direction of flow in the portal vein or the characteristics of flow towards the shunt. When a side-to-side portocaval shunt cannot be visualised on conventional ultrasound, the presence of hepatofugal flow in the intrahepatic portal branches is a reliable indicator of patency of the shunt.[102] However, it must be remembered that the haemodynamics change gradually and, in the immediate postoperative period, slow hepatopetal portal flow may still be detected despite a patent shunt. Conversely, hepatopetal portal flow detected in a late postoperative study raises the suspicion of thrombosis of the shunt, especially if flow was hepatofugal at a previous examination.

In end-to-side portocaval shunts, portal flow is usually absent or hepatofugal in the intrahepatic branches, despite the literature reports of the appearance of hepatopetal flow in an intrahepatic branch due to anomalous pathways, such as arterioportal fistulae.[102] Demonstration of reversal of flow in the splenic, and sometimes also the portal, veins is proof of patency of a conventional splenorenal shunt.

Visualisation of distal splenorenal shunts is not always feasible on real-time ultrasound (53.5% in our group of patients; Fig. 13.30)[104] but useful information can usually be obtained from the pattern in the splenic vein which displays phasic flow synchronous with caval pulsatility if the shunt is patent. The goal of this kind of shunt is to decompress gastro-oesophageal varices while maintaining hepatopetal flow in the mesoportal venous bed (in order to reduce the incidence of hepatic encephalopathy). Doppler studies showed low-velocity hepatopetal flow at 12

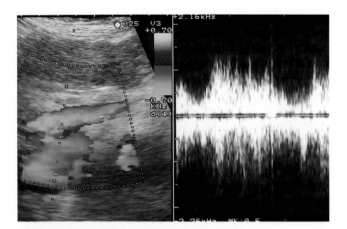

Fig. 13.28 Side-to-side portocaval shunt. A direct communication between the portal vein and the enlarged IVC is seen on colour Doppler. The spectral trace is turbulent and phasic in response to caval pressure variation.

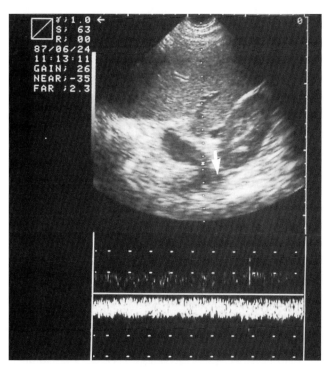

Fig. 13.30 **Distal splenorenal shunt (Warren).** Doppler study shows continuous flow directed from the splenic to the left renal vein (arrow).

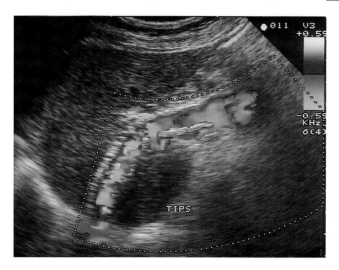

Fig. 13.31 **TIPS.** The intrahepatic stent is visualised in the right lobe of the liver on colour flow mapping.

months after surgery in 77% of cases,[104] with a low incidence of late reversal of flow.[105] Sequential measurements of the impedance indices in the intrasplenic arteries before and after surgery have been proposed as an indicator of shunt patency.[59] They are increased in cirrhosis but fall after successful surgical shunting.

Trans-jugular intrahepatic portosystemic shunt (TIPS)

A minimally invasive option for complications of portal hypertension, including variceal bleeding and refractory ascites, has been developed: positioning a metallic stent between a hepatic vein and an intrahepatic portal vein branch (usually the right) by a percutaneous trans-jugular approach. This avoids open surgery and is safe for patients with severe liver failure. Results are comparable to sclerotherapy in the prevention of variceal rebleeding.[106] A major problem of TIPS is stenosis or occlusion of the shunt: malfunction occurs in about 50% of cases at 1 year and carries the risk of rebleeding. While occlusion is irreversible, early diagnosis of stent stenosis allows angioplasty. Follow-up by repeated venography is the most reliable approach but it is an expensive and invasive procedure. Routine follow-up is therefore by repeated sequential Doppler examinations (Fig. 13.31).

Several haemodynamic changes occur immediately after TIPS placement; both portal vein diameter and mean

velocity have been reported to increase, resulting in a marked increase in portal vein flow volume (Fig. 13.32).[107] Blood flow in the main portal vein is hepatopetal but flows towards the shunt in the intrahepatic segments in 55% of patients with well-functioning TIPS.[108] Conversely, flow in other collaterals, such as the left gastric and the para-umbilical veins, may decrease, cease or reverse.[107] Shortly after TIPS placement, mean flow velocity in the shunt is high, ranging normally from 100 to over 200 cm/s (Fig. 13.33).[108–112]

Duplex Doppler is accepted as a reliable technique in the long-term surveillance for complications such as stent thrombosis or stenosis and hepatic vein stenosis.[108,109,111,113,114] The absence of detectable flow within a stent by Doppler sonography has proved to be sensitive (100%) and specific (96%) for occlusion.[109] On the other hand, numerous criteria have been proposed for the diagnosis of stenosis, but the overall accuracy is still debated.

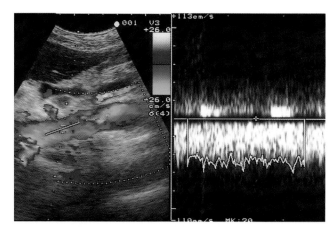

Fig. 13.32 **Portal flow after TIPS.** The portal vein is dilated with high-velocity hepatopetal flow (mean velocity 47 cm/s).

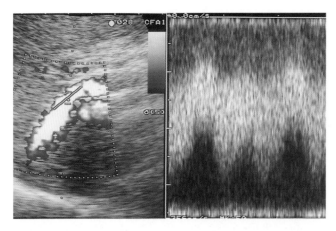

Fig. 13.33 TIPS. Power Doppler clearly depicts the stent. Spectral analysis shows phasic high-velocity flow (200–250 cm/s).

Stenosis of the distal end of the shunt or of the hepatic vein outflow is associated with a decrease of flow velocity through the stent.[108,109,115] A stent velocity less than 50 cm/s achieved a sensitivity of 100% and a specificity of 93% in the diagnosis of hepatic vein stenosis[109] while others suggest the use of two diagnostic criteria such as progressive reduction of peak velocity in the stent and a stent velocity less than 60 cm/s.[108] Reversed flow in the proximal portion of the hepatic vein has also been reported in cases of hepatic vein stenosis.[111]

Localised acceleration of flow suggests stent stenosis[108,109] while high flow velocity throughout the stent can simply represent high-volume flow without pathological significance.[107] Other signs, such as a marked decrease of portal flow velocity over time and a change from hepatofugal to hepatopetal flow in the intrahepatic branches, help confirm the diagnosis of stent stenosis. Contrast-enhanced power Doppler sonography has been reported to improve sensitivity and specificity in the diagnosis of stent dysfunction.[116,117]

Evaluation of medical treatment in portal hypertension

Doppler flowmetry is a reliable method for evaluating haemodynamic changes following the administration of vasoactive drugs such as vasopressin and terlipressin and the somatostatin-analogue octreotide used in the treatment of acute variceal bleeding.[118–122] Several studies have used Doppler to investigate their prophylactic use, to monitor the individual response to the drugs and to clarify their mechanisms of action. Beta-blockers are used for chronic prevention of variceal bleeding in portal hypertension. Their effect has been attributed to a direct reduction of heart rate and cardiac output, mediated by beta-1 receptor blockade, as well as to probable vasoconstriction of the splanchnic bed, mediated by beta-2 receptor blockade.

These two effects lead to a reduction of the splanchnic inflow. The administration of beta-blockers markedly decreases portal flow velocity and volume both in acute[32,123–128] and chronic settings,[125,127] whereas their effects on the splanchnic arterial impedance are still debated. The mean response is a decrease of flow volume of 13–30%, but the individual responses vary greatly.[125,127] Propranolol also reduces blood flow in the left gastric vein.[32]

Nitrates are also used in the long-term prevention of variceal bleeding, either when beta-blockers are contraindicated or as an addition to them to potentiate the portal effects. They act by producing peripheral vasodilatation, thus decreasing cardiac preload and output, resulting in reduction of portal inflow and reflex arterial vasoconstriction. A decrease in portal resistance is a second mechanism of action. Some of these effects are easily detectable by duplex Doppler as a decrease of portal flow, whose extent is similar to that produced by beta-blockers,[123,124,128,129] and an increase in the PI in the superior mesenteric artery.[124,129] Both oral propranolol and trans-cutaneous nitroglycerin maintain reduced portal flow over 24 hours.[126,129,130] Preliminary reports suggest a correlation between hepatic venous pressure and Doppler portal flow measurements in the assessment of response to beta-blockers.[131–133] If these are confirmed, Doppler could be used to optimise the individual treatment for prevention of bleeding.

REFERENCES

1 Vorobioff J, Bredfeldt J E, Groszmann R J. Increased blood flow through the portal system in cirrhotic rats. Gastroenterology 1984; 87: 1120–1126

2 Benoit J N, Womack W A, Hernandez L, Granger D N. 'Forward' and 'backward' flow mechanisms of portal hypertension. Relative contribution in the rat model of portal vein stenosis. Gastroenterology 1985; 89: 1092–1096

3 Sikuler E, Groszmann R J. Interaction of flow and resistance in maintainance of portal hypertension in a rat model. Am J Physiol 1986; 250: 205–212

4 Bolondi L, Piscaglia F, Siringo S, Gaiani S, Zironi G. Imaging techniques and haemodynamic measurements in portal hypertension. In: DeFranchis R, ed. Portal hypertension II. London: Blackwell Science, 1996: 56–66

5 Bolondi L, Gandolfi L, Arienti V et al. Ultrasonography in the diagnosis of portal hypertension: diminished response of portal vessels to respiration. Radiology 1982; 142: 167–172

6 Webb L J, Berger L A, Sherlock S. Gray-scale ultrasonography of portal vein. Lancet 1977; ii: 675–677

7 Lafortune M, Marleau D, Breton G et al. Portal venous measurements in portal hypertension. Radiology 1984; 151: 27–30

8 Juttner H U, Jenney J M, Ralls P W, Goldstein L I, Reynolds T B. Ultrasound demonstration of portosystemic collaterals in cirrhosis and portal hypertension. Radiology 1982; 142: 459–463

9 Dach J L, Hill M C, Pelaez J C et al. Sonography of hypertensive portal venous system: correlation with arterial portography. AJR 1981; 137: 511–517

10 Weinreb J, Kumari S, Phillip G et al. Portal vein measurements by real time sonography. AJR 1982; 139: 497–499

11 Cottone M, Sciarrino E, Marceno M P et al. Ultrasound in the screening of patients with cirrhosis with large varices. BMJ 1983; 533: 287

12 Niederau C, Sonnen A, Muller J E et al. Sonographic measurements of the normal liver, spleen, pancreas and portal vein. Radiology 1983; 149: 537–540

13 Bolondi L, Mazziotti A, Arienti V et al. Ultrasonographic study of portal venous system in portal hypertension and other portosystemic shunt operation. Surgery 1984; 95: 261–269

14 Zoli M, Dondi C, Marchesini G et al. Splanchnic vein measurements in patients with liver cirrhosis: a case-control study. J Ultrasound Med 1985; 4: 641–646

15 Kurol M, Forsberg L. Ultrasonographic investigation of respiratory influence on diameters of portal vessels in normal subjects. Acta Radiol Diagn 1986; 27: 675–680

16 Goyal A K, Pokharna D S, Sharma S K. Ultrasonic measurements of portal vasculature in diagnosis of portal hypertension. J Ultrasound Med 1990; 9: 45–48

17 Rahim N, Adam E J. Ultrasound demonstration of variation in normal portal vein diameter with posture. Br J Radiol 1985; 58: 313–314

18 Bellamy E A, Bossi M C, Cosgrove D O. Ultrasound demonstration of changes in the normal portal venous system following a meal. Br J Radiol 1984; 57: 147–149

19 Gaiani S, Bolondi L, Li Bassi S, Santi V, Zironi G, Barbara L. Effect of meal on portal hemodynamics in healthy humans and in patients with chronic liver disease. Hepatology 1989; 9: 815–819

20 Gaiani S, Gramantieri L, Venturoli N et al. What is the criterion standard for differentiating chronic hepatitis from compensated cirrhosis? A prospective study comparing ultrasonography and percutaneous liver biopsy. J Hepatol 1997; 27: 979–985

21 Weill F S. Cirrhosis and portal hypertension. In: Weill F S, ed. Ultrasound diagnosis of digestive diseases. Berlin: Springer Verlag, 1990

22 Bolondi L, Zironi G, Gaiani S, Li Bassi S, Benzi G, Barbara L. Caliber of splenic and hepatic arteries and spleen size in cirrhosis of different etiology. Liver 1991; 11: 198–205

23 Puttini M, Aseni P, Brambilla G, Belli L. Splenic artery aneurysms in portal hypertension. J Cardiovasc Surg 1982; 23: 490–493

24 Ayalon A, Wiesner R H, Perkins J D, Tominaga S, Hayes D H, Krom R A. Splenic artery aneurysms in liver transplant patients. Transplantation 1988; 45: 386–389

25 Kobori L, van der Kolk M J, de Jong K P et al. Splenic artery aneurysms in liver transplant patients. Liver Transplant Group. J Hepatol 1997; 27: 890–893

26 Moreno A H, Burchell A R, Van der Woude R, Burke J H. Respiratory regulation of splanchnic and systemic venous return. Am J Physiol 1967; 213: 455–465

27 Glazer G M, Laing F C, Brown T W, Gooding G A W. Sonographic demonstration of portal hypertension: the patent umbilical vein. Radiology 1980; 136: 161–163

28 Sacerdoti D, Bolognesi M, Bombonato G, Gatta A. Paraumbilical vein patency in cirrhosis: effects on hepatic hemodynamics evaluated by Doppler sonography. Hepatology 1995; 22: 1689–1694

29 Roi D J. Ultrasound anatomy of the left gastric vein. Clin Radiol 1993; 47: 396–398

30 Matsutani S, Furuse J, Ishii H, Mizumoto H, Kimura K, Ohto M. Hemodynamics of the left gastric vein in portal hypertension. Gastroenterology 1993; 105: 513–518

31 Takayasu K, Moriyama N, Shima J et al. Sonographic detection of large spontaneous splenorenal shunt, and its clinical significance. Br J Radiol 1984; 57: 565–570

32 Gaiani S, Bolondi L, Fenyves D, Zironi G, Rigamonti A, Barbara L. Effect of propranolol on portosystemic collateral circulation in patients with cirrhosis. Hepatology 1991; 14: 824–829

33 Marchal G F J, Van Holsbeeck M, Tshibwabwa-Ntumba E et al. Dilatation of cystic veins in portal hypertension: sonographic demonstration. Radiology 1985; 154: 187–189

34 Gaiani S, Bolondi L, Barbara L. Duplex Doppler evaluation of cystic veins in prehepatic portal hypertension. Ital J Gastroenterol 1988; 20: 19

35 Saverymuttu S H, Wright J, Maxwell J D, Joseph A E A. Ultrasound detection of oesophageal varices – comparison with endoscopy. Clin Radiol 1988; 39: 513–515

36 Di Candio G, Campatelli A, Mosca F, Santi V, Casanova P, Bolondi L. Ultrasound detection of unusual spontaneous portosystemic shunts associated with uncomplicated portal hypertension. J Ultrasound Med 1985; 4: 297–305

37 Wexler M J, MacLean L D. Massive spontaneous portal-systemic shunting without varices. Arch Surg 1975; 110: 995–1003

38 Hunt A H, Whittard B R. Thrombosis of the portal vein in cirrhosis hepatis. Lancet 1954; i: 281

39 Okuda K, Ohnishi K, Kimura K et al. Incidence of portal vein thrombosis in liver cirrhosis. An angiographic study in 708 patients. Gastroenterology 1985; 89: 279–286

40 Merrit C R. Ultrasonographic demonstration of portal vein thrombosis. Radiology 1979; 133: 425

41 Gaiani S, Bolondi L, Li Bassi S, Zironi G, Barbara L. Prevalence of spontaneous hepatofugal portal flow in liver cirrhosis. Clinical and endoscopic correlation in 228 patients. Gastroenterology 1991; 100: 160–167

42 Miller V E, Berland L L. Pulsed Doppler duplex sonography and CT of portal vein thrombosis. AJR 1985; 145: 73–76

43 Alpern M B, Rubin J M, Williams D M, Cape K P. Porta hepatis: duplex Doppler ultrasound with angiographic correlation. Radiology 1987; 162: 53–56

44 Raby N, Meire H B. Duplex Doppler ultrasound in the diagnosis of cavernous transformation of the portal vein. Br J Radiol 1988; 61: 586–588

45 Scoutt L M, Zawin M L, Taylor K J W. Doppler ultrasound. Part II. Clinical applications. Radiology 1990; 174: 309–319

46 Lencioni R, Caramella D, Sanguinetti F, Ballotta L, Falaschi F, Bartolozzi C. Portal vein thrombosis after percutaneous ethanol injection for hepatocellular carcinoma: value of color Doppler sonography in distinguishing chemical and tumor thrombi. AJR 1995; 164: 1125–1130

47 L'Herminè C. Radiology of liver circulation. Dordrecht: Martinus Nijhoff, 1985

48 Kawasaki T, Moriyasu F, Nishida O et al. Analysis of hepatofugal flow in portal venous system using ultrasonic Doppler duplex system. Am J Gastroenterol 1989; 84: 937–941

49 Ohnishi K, Saito M, Sato S et al. Direction of splenic venous flow assessed by pulsed Doppler flowmetry in patients with a large splenorenal shunt. Relation to spontaneous hepatic encephalopathy. Gastroenterology 1985; 89: 180–185

50 Taylor K J W, Burns P N, Woodcock J P et al. Blood flow in deep abdominal and pelvic vessels: ultrasonic pulsed Doppler analysis. Radiology 1985; 154: 487–493

51 Schrier R W, Arroyo V, Bernardi M, Epstein M, Henriksen J H, Rodés J. Peripheral vasodilation hypothesis: a proposal for the initiation of renal sodium and water retention in cirrhosis. Hepatology 1988; 8: 1151–1157

52 Sabbà C, Ferraioli G, Genecin P et al. Evaluation of postprandial hyperemia in superior mesenteric artery and portal vein in healthy and cirrhotic humans in an operator-blind echo-Doppler study. Hepatology 1991; 13: 714–718

53 Piscaglia F, Gaiani S, Gramantieri L, Zironi G, Siringo S, Bolondi L. Superior mesenteric artery impedance in chronic liver diseases: relationship with disease severity and portal circulation. Am J Gastroenterol 1998; 93(10): 1798–1799

54 Nakano R, Iwao T, Oho K, Toyonaga A, Tanikawa K. Splanchnic hemodynamic pattern and liver function in patients with cirrhosis and esophageal or gastric varices. Am J Gastroenterol 1997; 92: 2085–2089

55 Iwao T, Oho K, Sakai T et al. Splanchnic and extrasplanchnic arterial hemodynamics in patients with cirrhosis. J Hepatol 1997; 27: 817–823

56 Ray-Chaudhuri K R, Ryder S A, Thomaides T, Mathis C H, Phil D. The relationship between blood flow and pulsatility index in the superior mesenteric artery at rest and during constrictor stimuli in normal subjects. JCU 1994; 22: 149–160

57 Zoli M, Merkel C, Sabbà C, Sacerdoti D, Gaiani S, Ferraioli G, Bolondi L. Interobserver and inter-equipment variability of echo-Doppler sonographic evaluation of the superior mesenteric artery. J Ultrasound Med 1996; 15: 99–106

58 Sacerdoti D, Gaiani S, Buonamico P, Merkel C, Zoli M, Bolondi L, Sabba C. Interobserver and interequipment variability of hepatic, splenic, and renal arterial Doppler resistance indices in normal subjects and patients with cirrhosis. J Hepatol 1997; 27: 986–992

59 Bolognesi M, Sacerdoti D, Merkel C et al. Splenic Doppler impedance indices: influence of different portal hemodynamic conditions. Hepatology 1996; 23: 1035–1040

60 Piscaglia F, Gramantieri L, Gaiani S, Cavalli G C, Bolondi L. Possible mechanisms for changes of intrasplenic arterial impedance indices in portal hypertension. Hepatology 1997; 26: 513–514

61 Bolognesi M, Sacerdoti D, Bombonato G et al. Splenic impedance indices: a useful method to monitor patients after liver transplantation? Hepatology 1998; 27: 674–678

62 Sacerdoti D, Merkel C, Bolognesi M, Amodio P, Angeli P, Gatta A. Hepatic arterial resistance indexes in cirrhosis without and with portal vein thrombosis: relationships with portal hemodynamics. Gastroenterology 1995; 108: 1152–1158

63 Piscaglia F, Gaiani S, Zironi G et al. Intra- and extra-hepatic arterial resistance in chronic hepatitis and liver cirrhosis. Ultrasound Med Biol 1997; 23: 675–682

64 Bolondi L, Li Bassi S, Gaiani S, Benzi G, Santi V, Barbara L. Changes in the hepatic vein waveform detected by Doppler ultrasound in liver cirrhosis. Radiology 1991; 178: 513–516

65 Gorka W, Al Mulla A, Al Sebayel M, Altraif I, Gorka T S. Qualitative hepatic venous Doppler sonography versus portal flowmetry in predicting the severity of esophageal varices in hepatitis C cirrhosis. AJR 1997; 169: 511–515

66 Ohta M, Hashizume M, Kawanaka H et al. Prognostic significance of hepatic vein waveform by Doppler ultrasonography in cirrhotic patients with portal hypertension. Am J Gastroenterol 1995; 90: 1853–1857

67 Hosoki T, Arisawa J, Marukawa T et al. Portal blood flow in congestive heart failure: pulsed duplex sonographic findings. Radiology 1990; 17: 733–736

68 Alvarez G, Sanchez la Fuente J, Lopez J, Gomez A. Flow changes in hepatic veins in congestive cardiac insufficiency. A study using pulsed Doppler US. Eur J Radiol 1989; 9: 163–166

69 Wachsberg R H, Needleman L, Wilson D J. Portal vein pulsatility in normal and cirrhotic adults without cardiac disease. JCU 1995; 23: 3–15

70 Duerinckx A J, Grant E G, Perrella R R, Szeto A, Tessler F N. The pulsatile portal vein in cases of congestive heart failure: correlation of duplex Doppler findings with right atrial pressures. Radiology 1990; 176: 655–658

71 Catalano D, Caruso G, DiFazzio S, Carpinteri G, Scalisi N, Trovato G M. Portal vein pulsatility ratio and heart failure. JCU 1998; 26: 27–31

72 Moriyasu F, Nishida O, Ban N et al. Measurement of portal vascular resistance in patients with portal hypertension. Gastroenterology 1986; 90: 710–716

73 Paton A, Reynolds T B, Sherlock S. Assessment of portal venous hypertension by catheterisation of hepatic vein. Lancet 1953; i: 918

74 Groszmann R J, Glickmann M, Blei A et al. Wedged and free hepatic venous pressure measured with a balloon catheter. Gastroenterology 1978; 76: 253–258

75 Burns P N. Interpretation and analysis of Doppler signals. In: Taylor K J W, Burns P N, Wells P N T, eds. Clinical applications of Doppler ultrasound. New York: Raven, 1988

76 Sabbà C, Merkel C, Zoli M et al. Interobserver and interequipment variability of echo Doppler examination of the portal vein: effect of a cooperative training program. Hepatology 1995; 21: 428–433

77 Moriyasu F, Ban N, Nishida O et al. 'Congestion index' of the portal vein. AJR 1985; 146: 735–739

78 Siringo S, Bolondi L, Gaiani S et al. The relationship of endoscopy, portal Doppler ultrasound flowmetry, and clinical and biochemical tests in cirrhosis. J Hepatol 1994; 20: 11–18

79 Siringo S, Bolondi L, Gaiani S et al. Timing of the first variceal hemorrhage in cirrhotic patients: prospective evaluation of Doppler flowmetry, endoscopy and clinical parameters. Hepatology 1994; 20: 66–73

80 Eik-Nes S H, Marsal K, Kristoffersen K. Methodology and basic problems related to blood flow studies in the human fetus. Ultrasound Med Biol 1984; 10: 329–337

81 Ohnishi K, Saito M, Nakayama T et al. Portal venous hemodynamics in chronic liver disease: effects of posture change and exercise. Radiology 1985; 155: 757–761

82 Dauzat M, Pomier Layrargues G. Portal vein blood flow measurements using pulsed Doppler and electromagnetic flowmetry in dogs: a comparative study. Gastroenterology 1989; 96: 913–919

83 Zoli M, Magalotti D, Bianchi G et al. Functional hepatic flow and Doppler-assessed total hepatic flow in control subjects and in patients with cirrhosis. J Hepatol 1995; 23: 129–134

84 Bolognesi M, Sacerdoti D, Merkel C, Gatta A. Relationship between portal blood flow measured by image-directed Doppler ultrasonography and hepatic blood flow measured by indocyanine green constant infusion in patients with cirrhosis. JCU 1995; 23: 297–303

85 Brown H S, Halliwell M, Qamar M, Read A E, Evans J M, Wells P N T. Measurement of normal portal venous blood flow by Doppler ultrasound. Gut 1989; 30: 503–509

86 The value of Doppler ultrasound in the study of hepatic hemodynamics. Consensus conference. Bologna, Italy, 12 September 1989. Chairman: L. Barbara. J Hepatol 1990; 10: 310

87 Zoli M, Marchesini G, Cordiani M R et al. Echo-Doppler measurement of splanchnic blood flow in control and in cirrhotic subjects. JCU 1986; 14: 429–435

88 Pugliese D, Ohnishi K, Tsunoda T, Sabbà C, Albano O. Portal hemodynamics after meal in normal subjects and in patients with chronic liver disease studied by echo-Doppler flowmeter. Am J Gastroenterol 1987; 10: 1052–1056

89 Zironi G, Gaiani S, Fenyves D, Rigamonti A, Bolondi L, Barbara L. Value of measurement of mean portal flow velocity by Doppler flowmetry in the diagnosis of portal hypertension. J Hepatol 1992; 16: 298–303

90 Piscaglia F, Zironi G, Gaiani S et al. Relationship between splanchnic, peripheral and cardiac hemodynamics in liver cirrhosis of different degree of severity. Eur J Gastroenterol Hepatol 1997; 9: 799–804

91 Mostbeck G H, Wittich G R, Herold C et al. Hemodynamic significance of the paraumbilical vein in portal hypertension: assessment with duplex ultrasound. Radiology 1989; 170: 339–342

92 Iwao T, Toyonaga A, Oho K et al. Postprandial splanchnic hemodynamic response in patients with cirrhosis of the liver: evaluation with 'triple-vessel' duplex US. Radiology 1996; 201: 711–715

93 Gaiani S, Bolondi L, Fenyves D, Zironi G, Rigamonti A, Barbara L. Effect of propanolol on portosystemic colateral circulation in patients with cirrhosis. Hepatology 1991; 14: 824–829

94 Weill F S, Le Mouel A, Bihr E, Rohmer P, Zeltner F, Perrisney G. Ultrasonic patterns of acquired Budd–Chiari's syndromes. Eur J Radiol 1981; 1: 236–237

95 Baert A L, Fevery J, Marchal G et al. Early diagnosis of Budd–Chiari syndrome by computed tomography and ultrasonography: report of five cases. Gastroenterology 1983; 84: 587–595

96 Makuuchi M, Hasegawa H, Yamazaki S et al. Primary Budd–Chiari syndrome: ultrasonic demonstration. Radiology 1984; 152: 775–779

97 Hosoki T, Kuroda C, Tokunaga K et al. Hepatic venous outflow obstruction: evaluation with pulsed Doppler sonography. Radiology 1989; 170: 733–737

98 Bolondi L, Gaiani S, Li Bassi S, Zironi G et al. Diagnosis of Budd–Chiari syndrome by pulsed Doppler ultrasound. Gastroenterology 1991; 100: 1324–1331

99 Kane R, Eustace S. Diagnosis of Budd–Chiari syndrome: comparison between sonography and MR angiography. Radiology 1995; 195: 117–121

100 Holmin T, Alwmark A, Forsberg L. The ultrasonic demonstration of portacaval and interposition mesocaval shunt. Br J Surg 1982; 69: 673–675

101 Ackroyd N, Gill R, Griffiths K, Kossoff G, Reeve T. Duplex scanning of the portal vein and portosystemic shunts. Surgery 1986; 99: 591–597

102 Lafortune M, Patriquin H, Pomier G et al. Hemodynamic changes in portal circulation after portosystemic shunts: use of Duplex sonography in 43 patients. AJR 1987; 149: 701–706

103 Moriyasu F, Nishida O, Ban N et al. Ultrasonic Doppler duplex study of hemodynamic changes from portosystemic shunt operation. Ann Surg 1987; 205: 151–156

104 Bolondi L, Gaiani S, Mazziotti A et al. Morphological and hemodynamic changes in the portal venous system after distal spleno-renal shunt: an ultrasound and pulsed Doppler study. Hepatology 1988; 8: 652–657

105 Tylen U, Simert G, Vang J. Hemodynamic changes after distal spleno-renal shunt studied by sequential angiography. Radiology 1986; 121: 585–589

106 Shiffman M L, Jeffers L, Hoofnagle J H, Tralka T S. The role of transjugular intrahepatic portosystemic shunt for treatment of portal

hypertension and its complications: a conference sponsored by the National Digestive Diseases Advisory. Hepatology 1995; 22: 1591–1597

107 Lafortune M, Martinet J P, Denys A et al. Short- and long-term hemodynamic effects of transjugular intrahepatic portosystemic shunts: a Doppler/manometric correlative study. AJR 1995; 164: 997–1002

108 Foshager M C, Ferral H, Nazarian G K, Castaneda-Zuniga W R, Letourneau J G. Duplex sonography after transjugular intrahepatic portosystemic shunts (TIPS): normal hemodynamic findings and efficacy in predicting shunt patency and stenosis. AJR 1995; 165: 1–7

109 Chong W K, Malisch T A, Mazer M J, Lind C D, Worrell J A, Richards W O. Transjugular intrahepatic portosystemic shunt: US assessment with maximum flow velocity. Radiology 1993; 189: 789–793

110 Kimura M, Sato M, Kawai N et al. Efficacy of Doppler ultrasonography for assessment of transjugular intrahepatic portosystemic shunt patency. Cardiovasc Intervent Radiol 1996; 19: 397–400

111 Feldstein V A, Patel M D, LaBerge J M. Transjugular intrahepatic portosystemic shunts: accuracy of Doppler US in determination of patency and detection of stenoses. Radiology 1996; 200: 141–147

112 Dodd G D 3rd, Zajko A B, Orons P D, Martin M S, Eichner L S, Santaguida L A. Detection of transjugular intrahepatic portosystemic shunt dysfunction: value of duplex Doppler sonography. AJR 1995; 164: 1119–1124

113 Surratt R S, Middleton W D, Darcy M D et al. Morphologic and hemodynamic findings at sonography before and after creation of a tranjugular intrahepatic portosystemic shunt. AJR 1993; 160: 627–630

114 Longo J M, Bilbao J I, Rousseau H P et al. Transjugular intrahepatic portosystemic shunt: evaluation with Doppler sonography. Radiology 1993; 186: 529–534

115 Haskal Z J, Pentecost M J, Shlanky-Golderg R D et al. Tranjugular intrahepatic portosystemic shunt stenosis and revision: early and midterm results. AJR 1994; 163: 439–444

116 Uggowitzer M M, Kugler C, Machan L et al. Value of echo-enhanced Doppler sonography in evaluation of transjugular intrahepatic portosystemic shunts. AJR 1998; 170: 1041–1046

117 Furst G, Malms J, Heyer T et al. Tranjugular intrahepatic portosystemic shunts: improved evaluation with echo-enhanced color Doppler sonography, power Doppler sonography, and spectral duplex sonography. AJR 1998; 170: 1047–1054

118 Iwao T, Toyonaga A, Oho K et al. Effect of vasopressin on esophageal varices blood flow in patients with cirrhosis: a comparison with the effects on portal vein and superior mesenteric artery blood flow. J Hepatol 1996; 25: 491–497

119 Iwao T, Toyonaga A, Shigemori H et al. Hepatic artery hemodynamic responsiveness to altered portal blood flow in normal and cirrhotic livers. Radiology 1996; 200: 793–798

120 Matsutani S, Mizumoto H, Fukuzawa T, Ohto M, Okuda K. Response of blood flow to vasopressin in the collateral left gastric vein in patients with portal hypertension. J Hepatol 1995; 23: 557–562

121 Zironi G, Rossi C, Siringo S et al. Short- and long-term hemodynamic response to octreotide in portal hypertensive patients: a double-blind, controlled study. Liver 1996; 16: 225–234

122 Buonamico P, Sabbà C, Garcia-Tsao G et al. Octreotide blunts postprandial splanchnic hyperemia in cirrhotic patients: a double-blind randomized echo-Doppler study. Hepatology 1995; 21: 134–139

123 Zoli M, Marchesini G, Brunori A, Cordiani M R, Pisi E. Portal venous flow in response to acute betablocker and vasodilatatory treatment in patients with liver cirrhosis. Hepatology 1986; 6: 1248–1255

124 Bolognesi M, Sacerdoti D, Merkel C, Gatta A. Duplex Doppler sonographic evaluation of splanchnic and renal effects of single agent and combined therapy with nadolol and isosorbide-5-mononitrate in cirrhotic patients. J Ultrasound Med 1994; 13: 945–952

125 Bolognesi M, Sacerdoti D, Merkel C, Bombonato G, Enza E, Gatta A. Effects of chronic therapy with nadolol on portal hemodynamics and on splanchnic impedance indices using Doppler sonography: comparison between acute and chronic effects. J Hepatol 1997; 26: 305–311

126 Alvarez D, de las Heras M, Abecasis R et al. Daily variation in portal blood flow and the effect of propranolol administration in a randomized study of patients with cirrhosis. Hepatology 1997; 25: 548–550

127 Piscaglia F, Gaiani S, Siringo S, Gramantieri L, Serra C, Bolondi L. Duplex Doppler evaluation of the effects of propranolol and isosorbide-5-mononitrate on portal flow and spanchonic arterial circulation in cirrhosis. Aliment Pharmacol Therap 1998; 12(5): 475–481

128 Tincani E, Cioni G, Cristani A et al. Duplex Doppler ultrasonographic comparison of the effects of propranolol and isosorbide-5-mononitrate on portal hemodynamics. J Ultrasound Med 1993; 12: 525–529

129 Zoli M, Magalotti D, Ghigi G, Marchesini G, Pisi G. Transdermal nitroglycerin in cirrhosis. A 24-hour echo-Doppler study of splanchnic hemodynamic. J Hepatol 1996; 25: 498–403

130 Garcia-Pagan J C, Navasa M, Bosch J, Bru C, Pizcueta P, Rodes J. Enhancement of portal pressure reduction by the association of isosorbide-5-mononitrate to propranolol administration in patients with cirrhosis. Hepatology 1990; 11: 230–238

131 Albillos A, Paramo M P, Cacho G et al. Accuracy of the noninvasive measurement of portal (PBF) and forearm blood flow (FBF) in the assessment of the portal pressure response to propranolol. Hepatology 1996; 24 (suppl): 206A

132 Merkel C, Sacerdoti D, Bolognesi M, Enzo E, Marin R, Gatta A. Failure of acute challenge with nadolol to predict long-term portal hemodynamic effect in patients with cirrhosis: an assessment using invasive and non-invasive techniques. Ital J Gastroenterol 1994; 26: 208

133 Viudez P, Castano G, Carlevaro O et al. Comparative study between duplex-Doppler US and invasive hemodynamic measurements: response to i.v. propranolol in cirrhotic patients with portal hypertension. Hepatology 1996; 24 (suppl): 205A

Liver transplants

Hylton B Meire and Pat Farrant

Introduction

Liver transplantation is now an acceptable option for patients with end-stage chronic liver disease[1] or fulminant hepatic failure[2], and may also offer prolonged survival for certain patients with hepatic malignances. Transplantation of only part of the liver is now used for the treatment of some otherwise uncorrectable metabolic disorders and enzyme defects, such as Crigler–Najjar syndrome, urea cycle defects and proprionic acidaemia. In this group of disorders the patient's liver is intrinsically normal, with the exception of a single metabolic abnormality. The abnormality can often be corrected entirely by transplanting only a small fraction of the liver volume – usually the left lobe, although rarely a right lobe may be used – in a procedure termed auxiliary liver transplantation. The same procedure can be used in patients with acute or fulminant hepatic failure in whom it is considered that there may be some chance of recovery of the native liver but temporary support is necessary to enable the patient to survive until such recovery takes place.

The progressive improvement in survival from liver transplantation over the past few years has been due to a combination of factors, including better patient selection, improved organ preservation, developments in surgical technique, modern immunosuppressive agents and improved postoperative management. Medical imaging, especially ultrasound, plays an important role in patient selection and management, being used in the pre-operative, operative and postoperative periods,[3,4] depending upon factors such as the surgical technique and the patient's original diagnosis.

Pre-operative patient assessment

The initial role for ultrasound in the pre-operative assessment of patients considered for liver transplantation is in confirming the diagnosis. For patients with fulminant hepatic failure or end-stage liver disease the changes associated with the disease can be identified, although the cause of the disease cannot, of course, be determined by ultrasound. An exception to this rule is the Budd–Chiari syndrome, where ultrasound imaging and Doppler studies can confirm occlusion of the hepatic veins and usually also show enlargement of the caudate lobe, together with any other lobe or segment in which the major vein has been spared.

If transplantation is being considered as a treatment for suspected malignant hepatic tumours it is essential that the malignant nature of the lesion is confirmed histologically. Patients referred for liver transplantation with liver tumours have, on occasion, proved to have complex hydatid cysts, amoebic abscesses or haemangiomas. In addition, the true histological nature of some tumours may be difficult to identify, particularly for pathologists not used to evaluating the rarer types. Both focal nodular hyperplasia and hepatic adenoma can be indistinguishable from hepatocellular carcinoma on ultrasound imaging, and these diagnoses should therefore always be borne in mind and, if necessary, ultrasound-guided biopsy, angiography and dynamic CT undertaken. On rare occasions transplantation may be offered to patients with benign tumours, such as giant haemangiomas, in whom surgical resection is not possible.

In addition to confirming the diagnosis, ultrasound imaging should be directed towards assessing the complications of the disease. In patients with chronic liver disease this includes confirmation of portal vein patency and assessment of paraportal collaterals. If the liver failure is secondary to biliary atresia, associated anatomical abnormalities should be sought and, for those with malignant disease, the size and extent of the tumour and the presence of extrahepatic spread should be assessed. The exact role of ultrasound in the pretransplant patient therefore varies somewhat according to the diagnosis, and each of the main diagnoses is considered separately below. However, perhaps the most important role for ultrasound is that of confirming portal vein patency, as portal vein occlusion may be a contraindication to surgery.

Portal vein patency

Successful liver transplantation depends upon several factors, but among the most important are successful vascular anastomoses. Portal vein occlusion is a recognised sequel of long-standing liver disease and causes rapid hepatic decompensation; it is therefore important for the status of the portal vein to be assessed pre-operatively. Patency of the portal vein used to be an essential prerequisite for liver transplantation. Some transplant surgeons now attempt portal thrombectomy or construct portal conduits,[5] but if either of these procedures is to be undertaken it is important that accurate pre-operative information is available. In many patients this can all be obtained from an ultrasound examination, but angiography is still often required in difficult cases.

The extrahepatic components of the portal venous system can normally be assessed via subcostal scans, and the combination of imaging and colour flow Doppler usually rapidly confirms their patency (Fig. 14.1). In patients with gaseous distension and very small livers, imaging of the extrahepatic portal vein may be difficult or impossible and angiography remains necessary in a minority.

Both imaging and Doppler studies of the intrahepatic portal venous system are best achieved via right lateral intercostal scans, which allow visualisation of the main and right portal veins even in the smallest of livers (Fig. 14.2). It is important to be aware that flow within the intrahepatic portal vein does not necessarily imply patency of the extrahepatic venous system: low-velocity forward intrahepatic flow can occur in patients in whom splenic and

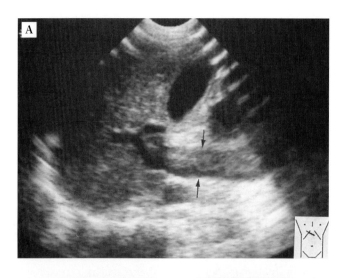

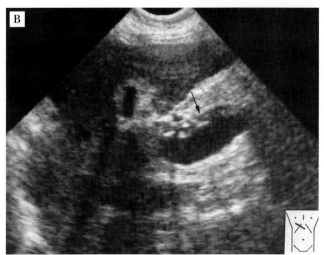

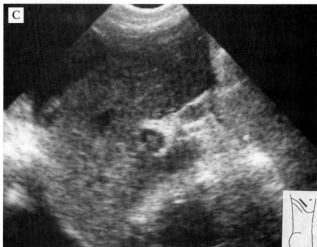

Fig. 14.1 Assessment of portal vein patency. A: Oblique subcostal scan of extrahepatic portal vein. The main portal vein (arrows) is dilated and there is thrombus adherent to its anterior wall. **B:** There is old partially calcified thrombus adherent to the anterior portal vein wall (arrow). **C:** Same patient as in B. There is fresh thrombus within the intrahepatic portal vein.

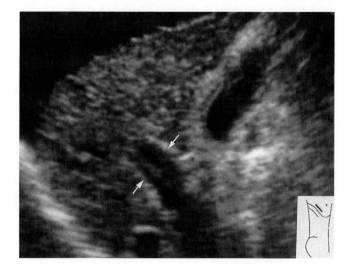

Fig. 14.2 Lateral intercostal scan of the portal vein. In this patient with a small cirrhotic liver and ascites, this approach shows partial thrombosis of the intrahepatic portal vein. Arrows – portal vein walls.

superior mesenteric venous occlusion have been proven. Both components of the portal system must be examined.

If colour flow and power Doppler studies fail to detect flow within the portal vein the equipment control settings must be optimised to detect low-velocity flow. In particular the high-pass filter (wall thump filter), often invaluable for arterial studies, should be set at the lowest possible value consistent with excluding flash artefact from the image. In addition, the Doppler shift frequency must be optimised by minimising the beam/vessel angle, particularly by using lateral intercostal scans. Even if all these measures fail to detect portal flow, portal occlusion cannot be considered proven as flow velocities below 2 or 3 cm/s are below the threshold of some scanners. If no flow is found the examination should be repeated after an interval or after a meal, particularly if the patient's clinical condition improves. If doubt persists after a second or subsequent examination, the use of ultrasound contrast agents may be helpful by increasing the signal intensity from any blood within the portal vein.[6] However, care must be exercised as contrast agents may give a positive signal owing to slow flow within paraportal collaterals or small recanalised channels within the portal vein. Contrast agents usually cause the colour image to flare, thereby greatly reducing the spatial resolution and causing the signal from multiple small vessels to appear to be a good signal from a single large vessel.

If all the above techniques fail to confirm patency with confidence, angiography or dynamic CT is required.

The direction and absolute velocity of portal flow are unimportant in this context (Fig. 14.3) and, in patients with severe decompensated liver disease, rapid changes in both velocity and direction of flow may be observed as their condition varies. The presence of a patent extra-hepatic iatrogenic portosystemic shunt usually gives rise to continuous reversed flow in the portal vein, although reverse flow may, of course also be present in the absence of an artificial shunt. The presence of a patent shunt is important, as this will need to be closed during the transplant operation to ensure adequate portal perfusion of the new liver.[7]

If little or no flow is detected in the intrahepatic portal veins, and if there is imaging evidence of either fresh or old thrombus in the intrahepatic portal system, the superior mesenteric vein must be assessed. If the superior mesenteric vein remains patent at the level of the splenic vein confluence the surgeon may be able to use this as a source of portal supply to the grafted liver.

In patients in whom low-velocity flow is detected within the portal vein the examination should be repeated if transplantation is not undertaken within 1–2 weeks (Fig. 14.4). Similarly, even if flow is normal or high the examination should be repeated if transplantation is not undertaken within 4–6 weeks. All patients with chronic liver disease are at increased risk for spontaneous portal vein thrombosis, and this is particularly likely if the flow velocity is low (Fig. 14.5). A false impression of low portal flow may be obtained, particularly when using the right lateral intercostal approach, if Doppler signals are obtained only from the right branch of the portal vein. In patients in whom there has been recanalisation of the umbilical vein most or all of the portal inflow may be diverted into the umbilical vein. In this situation there may be little or no flow, or even reverse flow, in the right branch of the portal vein in the presence of relatively normal forward flow velocity in the main portal vein. It is therefore important to be confident that the main portal vein has been examined.

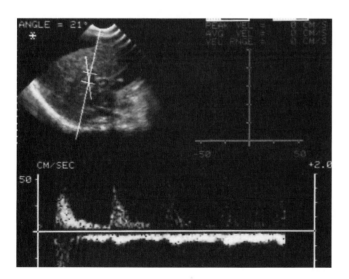

Fig. 14.3 Portal vein Doppler. There is low-velocity reversed flow in the portal vein. The simultaneous acquisition of an arterial signal confirms that the venous signal is portal in origin.

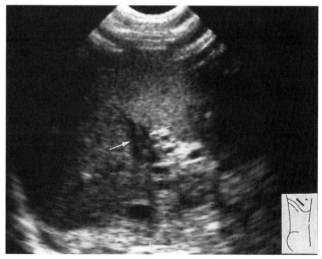

Fig. 14.4 Acute portal thrombosis. The portal vein (arrows) contains fresh thrombus 4 weeks after an initial pretransplant study confirmed portal vein patency.

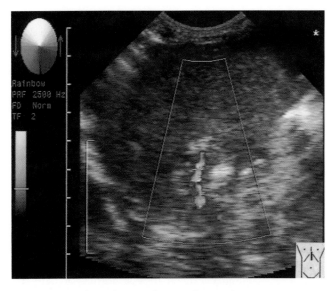

Fig. 14.5 Arterial signal in portal vein occlusion. There is a strong forward flow signal in the region of the porta hepatis. This is due to continuous high-velocity flow in the hepatic artery in the absence of portal vein flow.

A further source of error in the diagnosis of portal vein occlusion is cavernous transformation of the portal vein, which develops as a long-term sequel to portal vein thrombosis. Imaging alone may suggest the diagnosis by detecting numerous serpiginous channels replacing the portal vein at the porta hepatis. However, in a minority of patients with this condition a single large collateral channel may be present and may be mistaken for the main portal vein (Fig. 14.6). In the majority of patients with cavernous transformation the intrahepatic portal vein branches are either abnormally small or absent, and therefore the assessment should include both the intra- and extrahepatic components of the portal vein.

In patients in whom transplantation is being considered for malignant liver disease it is important to determine whether or not there is vascular invasion by the tumour, particularly in primary hepatocellular carcinoma (Fig. 14.7). Up to 25% have been reported to invade the intrahepatic portal venous system, and tumour thrombus may occupy the whole of the intrahepatic system and extend into the extrahepatic portal vein (Fig. 14.8).

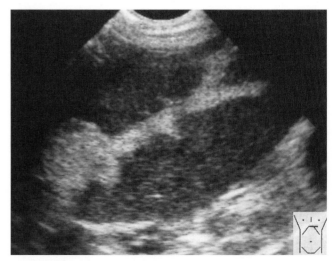

Fig. 14.7 Portal invasion by hepatocellular carcinoma. Transverse scan of the left lobe of the liver showing a highly reflective primary hepatocellular carcinoma which has extended into the left intrahepatic portal system.

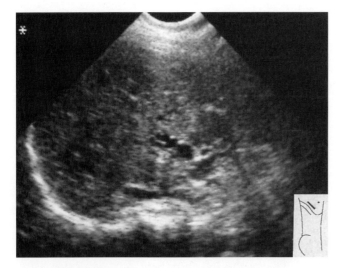

Fig. 14.6 Cavernous transformation of the portal vein. In this patient with long-standing portal vein thrombosis there has been cavernous transformation with the production of a dominant collateral anteriorly within the porta; this can easily be mistaken for the main portal vein.

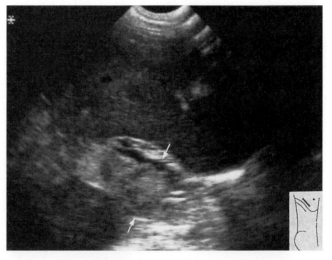

Fig. 14.8 Tumour thrombus in main portal vein. In this patient with hepatocellular carcinoma the main portal vein (arrows) is greatly expanded and is filled with tumour thrombus.

The final component of portal assessment is the detection of paraportal collaterals, particularly those in the right side of the abdomen, which may give rise to surgical problems during hepatectomy. Foreknowledge of the presence of major subhepatic collaterals helps the surgeon to plan the operative approach.

It is customary to measure the maximum diameter of the spleen when assessing patients with liver disease, and this should always be recorded prior to liver transplantation. Although the presence and degree of splenomegaly are of no importance at this stage in the patient's management, progressive splenic enlargement in the postoperative period may be the first indication of portal vein stenosis or occlusion, recurrent liver disease or rejection. A preoperative baseline measurement is therefore important, and in many patients with successful transplantation the spleen may be found to decrease in size postoperatively as successful transplantation immediately reduces the portal pressure to normal.

Hepatocellular carcinoma

Patients with chronic liver disease, especially that due to the hepatitis B and C viruses, have a greatly increased incidence of hepatocellular carcinoma (HCC) (Fig. 14.9). The most important factor in the selection of HCC patients for liver transplantation is the total tumour volume; the number of tumours is also important. Survival beyond 1 year is uncommon in patients with multiple tumours or those with a single lesion greater than 3 cm in diameter. If the HCC is of the fibrolamellar variety the prognosis may be significantly better, even when the primary tumour is very large. It is therefore important to obtain a very skilled

pre-operative histological diagnosis in patients with large tumours, especially in the younger age group, in whom the lesion may be fibrolamellar in type.

Pre-operative assessment of the HCC patient for transplantation is therefore aimed at confirmation of the number and size of tumours (Fig. 14.10). If the total tumour bulk is greater than 15 ml the chances of 1-year survival are less than 5%, and liver transplantation is therefore contraindicated.

HCC is particularly prone to invade the portal vein and may also extend into the hepatic veins. The ultrasound examination should therefore be directed towards the exclusion of vascular invasion.

In those patients with HCC superimposed on a relatively normal or only moderately compromised liver, the

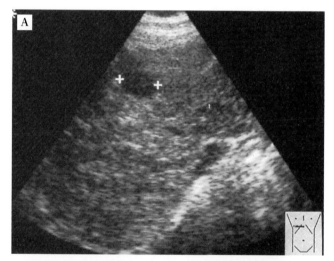
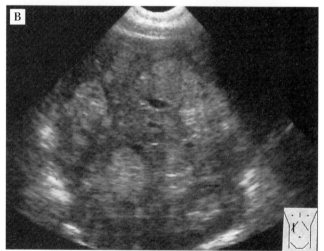

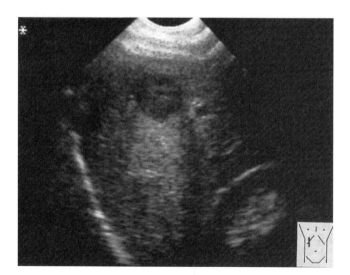

Fig. 14.9 Hepatocellular carcinoma in chronic liver disease. In this routine pretransplant examination a 2.5 cm diameter poorly reflective and poorly attenuating mass has developed and was proved to be a hepatocellular carcinoma.

Fig. 14.10 Assessment of hepatocellular carcinoma. A: In this child with tyrosinaemia a solitary 15 mm diameter nodule has arisen; its presence expedited transplantation. B: In this adult patient multifocal hepatoma has developed and excludes the possibility of curative transplantation.

question of resectability should always be considered. The patient is likely to have a longer survival with a curative resection. If the tumour is relatively small and can be shown to be confined to a single segment or lobe of the liver with no vascular invasion, a partial hepatectomy may be the most appropriate course of treatment.

HCC most often metastasises to the lungs and bones, which are best investigated by CT and nuclear medicine studies. Occasionally lymphatic spread gives rise to adenopathy in the porta hepatis or upper abdomen, and ultrasound examination can confirm the presence of lymph node enlargement.

Other tumours

Liver transplantation may occasionally be offered to patients with other forms of hepatic malignancy which are not amenable to resection. Tumours in this group include cholangiocarcinoma, other very rare primary hepatic tumours, and metastases from carcinoid (Fig. 14.11), provided the tumour is confined to the liver. Liver transplantation is seldom curative in this group of patients, but may extend the period of good-quality survival and palliate the severe endocrine manifestations of the neuroendocrine tumours. In these patients ultrasound is aimed at confirmation of the original diagnosis, assessment of the resectability and possible spread of the disease, and confirmation of portal vein patency.

Budd–Chiari syndrome

Budd–Chiari syndrome (BCS) may present as acute hepatic venous congestion, fulminant hepatic failure

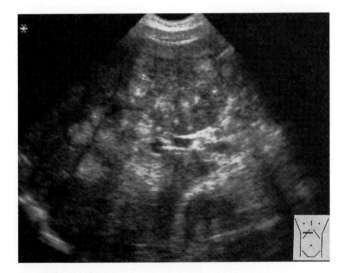

Fig. 14.11 Metastatic carcinoid of the liver. The symptoms associated with carcinoid are related to the tumour volume within the liver. Carcinoid deposits are almost always clearly defined and highly reflective.

(FHF) or established cirrhosis. Patients in the first category may achieve almost complete recovery if an early porto-systemic shunt is created; those with FHF or late decompensated cirrhosis may require transplantation.

The role of ultrasound in BCS is firstly to confirm the original diagnosis.[8] Imaging and Doppler studies, especially colour flow imaging, should be directed towards confirming occlusion of all the major hepatic veins. In patients with long-standing BCS numerous serpiginous intrahepatic collaterals are usually detected, and retrograde flow may occasionally be seen in patent central segments of the major hepatic veins (see Ch. 12). Rarely the hepatic vein occlusion may be secondary to an inferior vena caval abnormality, particularly a web, and attempts should be made to assess the IVC. However, this is often difficult in the presence of a swollen liver, and biplane contrast vena cavography or spiral CT with contrast are more accurate than ultrasound in assessment of the IVC.

Many patients with BCS also suffer thrombotic occlusion of the portal venous system, either in the acute phase or later in the disease process. In acute complete BCS flow within the portal vein is almost always reversed, but as hepatic venous collaterals develop flow within the portal vein may reduce, thereby increasing the risk of spontaneous thrombosis, particularly if the original vascular occlusions were secondary to an underlying abnormality of thrombogenesis.

Fulminant hepatic failure

The clinical management of fulminant hepatic failure has changed rapidly in recent years, with a marked improvement in survival. However, there remains a group of patients in whom liver recovery can be predicted to be very unlikely, and these patients may be offered emergency liver transplantation. Their clinical diagnoses vary widely and include paracetamol and other drug overdoses, Wilson's disease and acute viral hepatitis (Fig. 14.12), but are often uncertain until after transplantation. The main role of preoperative ultrasound in these patients is to exclude extensive hepatic malignancy as the cause of the failure and to confirm portal vein patency. It is possible that Doppler studies of hepatic artery resistance index (HARI) may be helpful in determining the prognosis in fulminant hepatic failure. Our own experience in 18 adult cases showed a highly significant increase in the HARI in those patients who ultimately required transplantation. These changes were not seen in patients who subsequently recovered without transplantation.[9]

Chronic liver disease

Patients with a variety of chronic liver disorders comprise the largest group considered for liver transplantation. Preoperative ultrasound imaging is directed to confirming the

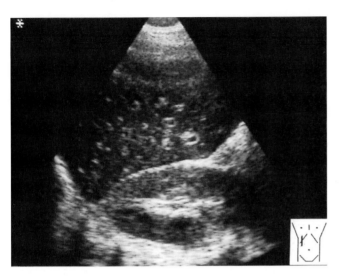

Fig. 14.12 Acute viral hepatitis. This child presented with fulminant hepatic failure. The ultrasound reveals uniform decrease in parenchymal reflectivity, the portal vein branches standing out against the poorly reflective parenchymal background.

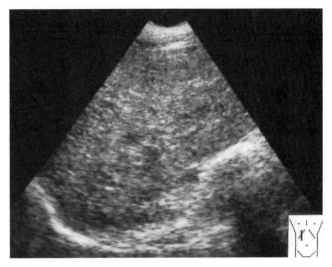

Fig. 14.13 Heterogeneous liver of secondary biliary cirrhosis. In this child with a failed Kasai procedure the liver has become extremely heterogeneous and the main portal vein and portal tracts can no longer be identified by ultrasound imaging.

presence of severe liver disease, if necessary with the use of ultrasound-guided liver biopsy in those with very small livers.

These patients are at increased risk for the development of primary HCC, and it is therefore essential that the whole volume of the liver is examined carefully to detect any focal lesion. If focal lesions or suspicious areas are detected on ultrasound imaging, further investigations are indicated, including ultrasound-guided biopsy, angiography and CT scanning after lipiodol injection into the hepatic artery. If imaging procedures confirm the presence of a small HCC this finding will generally expedite transplantation, but if larger volumes of tumour are present transplantation is unlikely to be appropriate.

Confirmation of the patency of the intra- and extrahepatic portal vein is important, and any patient with low-velocity flow or in whom there is a significant delay before transplantation should be re-examined in the pre-operative period to exclude subsequent thrombosis of the portal vein.

Biliary atresia

Patients with severe progressive liver failure secondary to a failed Kasai procedure or undiagnosed biliary atresia constitute an important group in whom liver transplantation offers the only hope of prolonged survival. These are almost always children, varying in age from a few months to a few years. In this group ultrasound assessment is technically difficult as a result of several factors, including previous surgery, associated congenital anomalies, ascites, heterogeneous and highly reflective livers (Fig. 14.13), and a lack of patient cooperation.

Previous surgical intervention, particularly the Kasai procedure, usually gives rise to adhesions in the upper abdomen, with gas-filled bowel in the subhepatic space extending up to the porta hepatis. This may make visualisation of the extrahepatic portal venous system difficult or impossible, and may necessitate recourse to angiography if doubt about their patency persists.

Patients with biliary atresia have an increased incidence of congenital anomalies, including situs inversus abdominis, situs ambiguous, malrotation of the gut, abnormalities of the hepatic artery, portal vein and inferior vena cava and polysplenia or asplenia. It is important that as many of these as possible are identified or excluded on the pre-operative investigations, so that the surgeon can be warned of their existence.[10] In particular, the hepatic artery anatomy is frequently abnormal, with multiple arteries and/or an anomalous extrahepatic course. Very rarely the portal vein may drain directly into the vena cava, or may lie in a preduodenal position. The IVC may be absent, left-sided, or subject to a number of other anomalies, the commonest of which is caval interruption with azygos continuation.

The heterogeneous and highly reflective liver in end-stage secondary biliary cirrhosis may render imaging of the intrahepatic portal venous system difficult, and indeed the portal vein radicals may be compressed by the abnormal liver. In this situation colour flow imaging usually permits confirmation of portal vein patency. However, care should be exercised when interpreting colour flow images as these patients often have a particularly rapid flow in relatively large hepatic arteries (Fig. 14.5). Any high-velocity forward-flowing colour signal within the liver must also be subjected to spectrum analysis to determine whether it is arterial or venous in origin. Recent research has shown that unexpected death from ischaemic hepatitis in these patients may be predicted by serial measurements of the hepatic artery resistance index (HARI).[11] It is therefore important to monitor the HARI at regular intervals in children with well established cirrhosis. If the end-diastolic flow becomes absent or reversed, the frequency of monitoring should be increased and transplantation expedited if at all possible.

Pre-operative donor assessment

The continuing lack of donors for paediatric recipients has led to the development of living related-donor transplantation. With this procedure a relative, usually mother, father, uncle or aunt, is used as the donor. Generally the donor's segments II and III are removed and used for the transplant procedure. Prior to removal of these segments it is important to exclude the presence of liver disease in the donor and to assess the presence of any vascular anomalies.[12] Ultrasound is essential for both of these purposes, although some centres still insist on angiography to assess the arterial anatomy, as certain variations in the arterial supply to the liver may make it difficult or impossible to remove segments II and III with a suitable arterial supply.

Peroperative scanning

Intra-operative ultrasound is now an accepted technique (see Ch. 8) and may fulfil a number of roles in the transplant patient.

Prehepatectomy intra-operative ultrasound may be helpful to confirm the number and extent of neoplasms and to assess vascular invasion. Absence of the intervening abdominal wall permits better-quality images to be obtained on intra-operative scans than is possible pre-operatively, and thus makes the technique worthwhile even when pre-operative imaging has been reassuring.

If the donor liver is too large for the recipient it may be necessary to reduce its size, usually using segments II, III and IV.[13,14] Scanning of the donor liver to identify the major intrahepatic vessels may be helpful in speeding reduction operations. A further variation on this theme is the division of a donor liver into separate right and left lobe units to be transplanted into two recipients. This so-called 'split liver' procedure usually requires bisection of the liver through the plane of the middle hepatic vein, and on-the-table intra-operative ultrasound is essential.

Similarly, harvesting of the donor segments from a living related donor requires accurate mapping of the hepatic venous, portal venous and arterial anatomy, and this is greatly aided by intra-operative ultrasound examination.[15,16]

After successful transplantation intra-operative Doppler studies are invaluable in confirming good flow through the vascular anastomoses,[17] especially if conduits have been used or if the anatomy is abnormal, for example if a donor liver reduction procedure has been performed. The portal vein anatomy will certainly be abnormal in patients who have received a left lobe graft, either a cutdown liver, a split liver or a living related-donor procedure. In all these instances there is usually insufficient portal vein length with the donor segments to attach to the recipient, and a variety of non-anatomical vascular connections may be achieved. Flow in these is almost always disturbed and frequently frankly turbulent, particularly if there is a mismatch between the size of the donor and the recipient vessels. Doppler studies are important to confirm adequate total flow in the portal system prior to abdominal closure.

In auxiliary transplantation there is often difficulty in ensuring adequate portal flow into the transplanted segments. To overcome this problem it is frequently necessary to apply a surgical band around the branch of the portal vein supplying the native lobe, in order to restrict flow into this lobe and encourage flow into the donor liver. The degree to which the band is tightened should be judged with intra-operative Doppler studies, to try to confirm roughly even flow between donor and recipient lobes.

Postoperative scanning

The role of ultrasound in the postoperative period varies according to the time elapsed since the operation. There are cogent arguments in favour of performing routine imaging and Doppler examinations during the early postoperative period,[18–21] although the need for and the frequency of these examinations remains controversial. If circumstances permit, it is probably ideal to perform routine examinations on days 1, 3, 5 and 7, and weekly thereafter, unless otherwise indicated by clinical or biochemical findings. Indeed, it has even been suggested that routine postoperative scans should be undertaken three times per day so as to detect unsuspected vascular complications.[22]

Before undertaking postoperative examinations it is important for the equipment operator to be fully conversant with the surgical details. In particular it is important to know whether or not a cutdown procedure has been used (Fig. 14.14) and to have detailed information concerning the hepatic artery, portal vein, IVC and biliary anastomoses. Many different variants of these anastomoses may be used, according to the preference of the surgeon, the nature of the underlying disease process or the anatomy of the donor and recipient vessels. For example, patients with biliary atresia, sclerosing cholangitis and other bile duct abnormalities are likely to have a Roux loop for the biliary conduit. Patients with abnormal arterial anatomy or who are being retransplanted for arterial occlusions may have an arterial conduit, often arising anteriorly from the distal abdominal aorta.

The operator should follow a predetermined protocol to ensure that all aspects of the transplant anatomy are

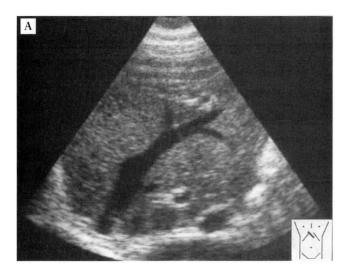
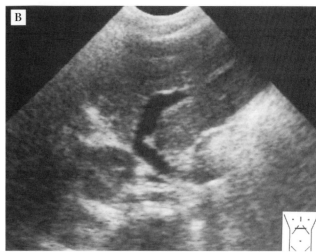

Fig. 14.14 Cutdown liver. A: Oblique subcostal scan and **B:** transverse subcostal scan. The unusual hepatic vein anatomy (A) and portal vein anatomy (B) result from transplantation of segments II, III and IV only from the donor liver.

carefully assessed and that all possible sites for fluid collections are evaluated.

Hepatic artery

Problems related to the hepatic artery anastomosis are the most common vascular complications after liver transplantation.[23] Most patients suffer a minor degree of postoperative haemorrhage, giving rise to haematomas of 3–5 cm diameter at the porta hepatis (Fig. 14.15). In adults early arterial occlusion occurs in 1–3% of patients but is more common in the paediatric age group, especially in patients under 1 year of age. Early arterial occlusion is almost always a catastrophic event, with rapid and irre-

versible liver cell death. The resultant hepatic necrosis can usually be diagnosed on ultrasound scanning by the detection of areas of liquefaction (Fig. 14.16).[24] Rarely surgical revascularisation procedures may be successful,[25] but in general, if the patient is to be saved urgent retransplantation is necessary.

Postoperative occlusion of the hepatic artery most commonly occurs at the site of the vascular anastomosis, but may occur elsewhere in the main vessel (possibly as a result of clamp injury) and intrahepatic obstructions of individual major branches have also been documented.

Impending or complete occlusion of the hepatic artery is often indicated by generalised non-specific deterioration of the liver function tests, with a characteristic rise in the

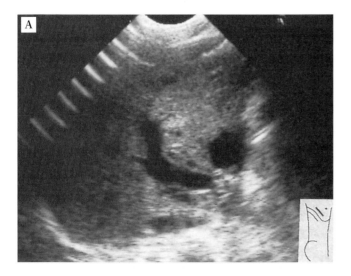
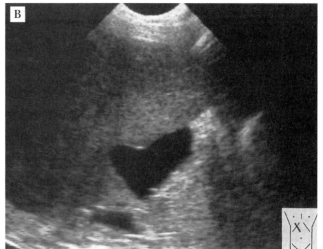

Fig. 14.15 Porta hepatis fluid collections. These small periportal fluid collections are almost invariable in the early post-transplant phase and are usually of no clinical significance.

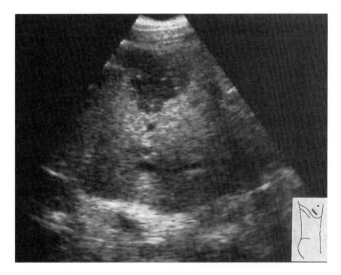

Fig. 14.16 Hepatic infarction. Segmental infarction due to occlusion of a branch artery gives rise to an irregular area of reduced reflectivity, which may be the first indicator of arterial occlusion.

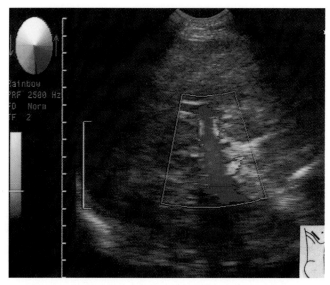

Fig. 14.17 Colour Doppler detection of the hepatic artery. The colour map velocity coding has been adjusted to highlight the higher systolic velocities in the artery as orange against the slower red portal vein flow.

AST, or with a bile leak. Platt *et al.*[26] have suggested that regular Doppler surveillance with measurement of the HARI and systolic acceleration time may help to identify cases of hepatic artery stenosis.

Ideally all segments of the arterial system should be studied, including the extrahepatic and intrahepatic main hepatic artery and the right and left intrahepatic branches. In practice, the extrahepatic artery is often difficult to identify owing to upper abdominal bowel gas. The intrahepatic portion of the main hepatic artery and the right hepatic arterial branch can normally be identified via the right lateral intercostal approach, and the left branch can be visualised on transverse subcostal scans using the left portal vein branch as a landmark. The anatomical location of the artery and its branches is somewhat variable, and colour flow imaging (CFI) may be helpful in its detection (Figs 14.17 and 14.18). Both the portal vein and the hepatic artery have flow in the same direction, and if there is high-velocity or disturbed flow within the portal vein it may partially or completely mask the small adjacent hepatic artery. A spectral Doppler trace should therefore be obtained from the hepatic artery before its patency can be confirmed with certainty (Fig. 14.19).[27] The velocity of flow within the artery is very variable in the early post-operative phase, and both colour flow and spectral scans may show the artery to have flow either higher or lower in velocity than that in the adjacent accompanying portal vein (Fig. 14.18). Where the flow velocity is low and CFI is not available, duplex scanning alone may fail to detect the artery.[28,29]

The flow–velocity waveform obtained from the hepatic artery in the acute post-transplant phase is variable and, as with velocity values, the significance of the various waveforms is uncertain. However, if the velocity is found to be

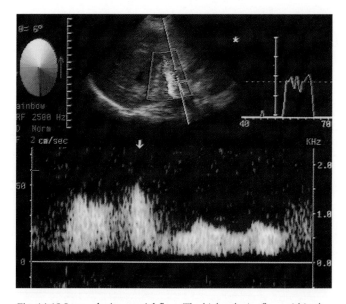

Fig. 14.18 Low-velocity arterial flow. The high-velocity flow within the portal vein prevented identification of the artery on the colour flow image. Spectral Doppler studies reveal the presence of a low-velocity arterial signal adjacent to the high-velocity venous signal.

extremely low or the waveform very damped (Fig. 14.20) this strongly raises the suspicion of a significant anastomotic stenosis. Similar appearances may result from hepatocellular problems due either to poor preservation of the donor organ or to early acute rejection. Occasionally waveforms are found in which there is no evidence of diastolic flow (Fig. 14.21). Although this was initially thought to indicate the presence of acute rejection, this waveform

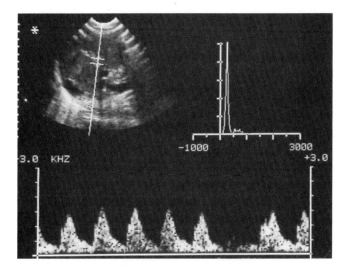
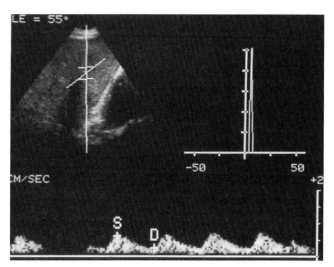

Fig. 14.19 Hepatic artery Doppler. Patency of the main and right hepatic artery is confirmed by this lateral intercostal duplex Doppler study.

Fig. 14.20 Damped arterial flow. This low-amplitude intrahepatic arterial signal raises the suspicion of significant anastomotic stenosis.

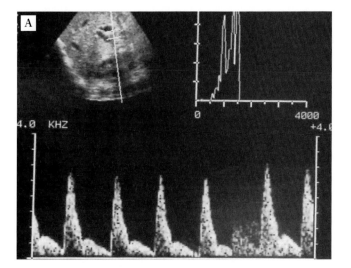
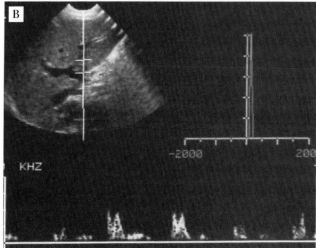

Fig. 14.21 Absence of hepatic artery diastolic flow. A: There is good systolic and early diastolic perfusion with very little end-diastolic flow. This was a transient finding of uncertain origin. **B:** There is a low-velocity biphasic systolic pulse and no diastolic flow. This trace indicates poor arterial perfusion, possibly as a result of severe parenchymal damage.

is now known to be non-specific[30,31] and may indicate liver parenchymal problems, kinking of the hepatic artery, the existence of a long and compliant arterial conduit, or be of no significance at all. Usually the arterial waveform is unremarkable, and therefore any patient in whom the waveform is felt to be abnormal should receive frequent follow-up examinations to confirm continuing vascular patency. If the Doppler studies show a progressive reduction in arterial velocity or a fall-off in diastolic flow in the absence of obvious parenchymal abnormality, the possibility of a progressive arterial obstructive lesion should be considered and angiography must be advised. Operative relief of a stenosis or inadequate anastomosis is much

more satisfactory than an urgent retransplantation.[32] Percutaneous hepatic artery angioplasty probably has no role in the immediate post-transplant phase, a period of about 2 weeks being necessary for the anastomosis to heal to a point where it can withstand balloon dilatation.[33]

When the liver is transplanted all possible collateral arterial routes are interrupted. After transplantation potential collaterals readily develop, particularly in children, and may be capable of maintaining adequate arterial perfusion by the third postoperative week.[34] In adults they develop more slowly, though are probably both quicker and more efficient if a Roux loop has been used in place of the recipient's common duct.

Doppler studies of the intrahepatic arterial tree become more difficult to interpret with increasing time after the operation. If good collateral supply has been established an entirely normal intrahepatic arterial waveform may be detected, even in the presence of total occlusion of the main hepatic artery. More commonly, however, there is some damping of the intrahepatic systolic arterial wave with maintenance of the diastolic flow (Fig. 14.22).[29] Conversely, the technical limitations of colour and duplex Doppler systems may prevent the operator from obtaining a Doppler signal even in the presence of a patent hepatic artery. Doppler studies of the hepatic artery are important, but in any patient in whom the Doppler findings do not concur with the clinical context angiography must be performed, particularly if there is likely to be a therapeutic implication.

If the hepatic artery remains patent but the portal vein becomes occluded there is almost always a marked increase in arterial flow, with an increase in systolic velocity and a reduction in the resistance index (Fig. 14.23).

Very rarely liver biopsy may lead to an arterioportal shunt and this may also give rise to high arterial flows, but the true nature of the lesion can generally be established by detecting alteration in the portal flow, usually manifested by flow reversal in the portal vein branch draining the affected segment. Such arterioportal shunts are of little clinical significance and almost always resolve spontaneously.

Although some patients with late-onset arterial obstruction may show little clinical evidence of this, the majority suffer one or more complications. In the first few weeks after transplantation the most likely consequence is breakdown of the biliary anastomosis. Bile leaks should therefore be searched for in any patient thought to have a compromised artery, and the artery should be studied in

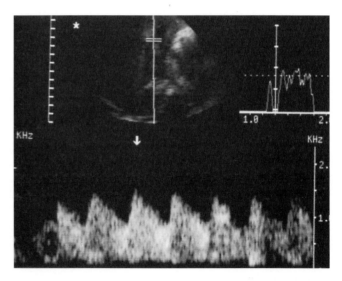

Fig. 14.23 Hepatic arterial waveform in portal occlusion. In this patient late portal occlusion had occurred but liver perfusion was maintained by a compensatory increase in arterial flow.

any patient thought to have a biliary leak (Fig. 14.24). If the biliary anastomosis survives the arterial deprivation a biliary stricture may develop, either at the site of anastomosis or, more commonly, at the junction of the left and right hepatic ducts.[35,36] A consequence of this may be segmental or asymmetrical intrahepatic duct dilatation and, once again, it is important to study both ducts and artery.

A further complication of hepatic artery occlusion is the increased risk of intrahepatic abscess formation. Even if Doppler studies reveal an adequate collateral supply, the risk remains and is further enhanced if there is associated biliary stenosis, with intrahepatic bile duct dilatation and

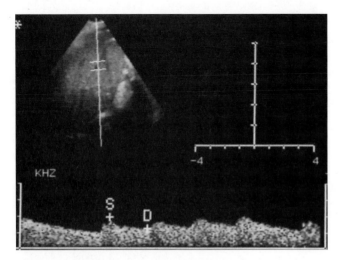

Fig. 14.22 Hepatic artery perfusion via collaterals. There was total occlusion of the hepatic artery developing several weeks after transplantation. The intrahepatic branches remain perfused via collaterals with a very damped waveform.

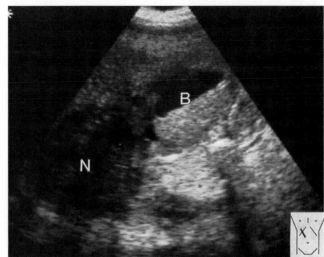

Fig. 14.24 Consequences of arterial occlusion. This patient with complete arterial occlusion has developed an area of necrosis in the right lobe (N) and a biliary leak with subhepatic biloma (B) in which the bile is sedimenting out.

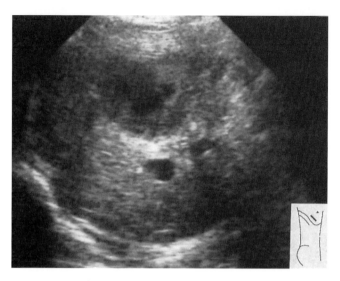

Fig. 14.25 Hepatic abscess secondary to ischaemia. The area of necrosis shown in Figure 14.16 has progressed to frank abscess formation.

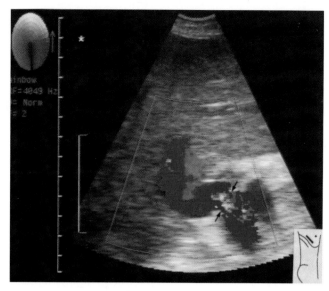

Fig. 14.26 Post-transplant portal vein study. There is a mild narrowing at the anastomosis (arrows) with a moderately high-velocity jet through the anastomosis (coded yellow). Within the intrahepatic portal vein there is a coarse vortex; the reverse flow component is coded purple.

stasis increasing the chance of cholangitis. Therefore, the whole volume of the liver must be scanned in any patient with known or suspected arterial occlusion or biliary stenosis, with a view to detecting abscess formation as early as possible (Fig. 14.25). If a suspected abscess is identified this should be confirmed by CT scan, and its communication with the biliary tree can be demonstrated by cholangiography. Ultrasound may be helpful for both diagnostic and therapeutic drainage of liver abscesses and, with aggressive treatment, these may resolve despite continuing arterial occlusion.

If the arterial stenosis is treated by trans-luminal angioplasty serial Doppler studies are invaluable for confirming improvement in the arterial flow and for monitoring the patient's subsequent progress. It is not yet clear what percentage of arterial stenoses can be treated by angioplasty alone and how many ultimately require reoperation.

Although the majority of arterial occlusions occur relatively soon after transplantation those patients with an arterial conduit are at particular risk of very late occlusion, sometimes several years postoperatively. These occlusions are caused by intimal or pseudo-intimal hyperplasia and are thus slow in onset. They are usually accompanied by good collateral formation and may have little adverse effect on liver function. However, this is not invariably the case, and we have seen one case of acute conduit occlusion 1 year post-transplant which gave rise to hepatic necrosis.

Portal vein

Early postoperative occlusion of the portal vein is rare in adults and uncommon in children. However, early occlusion may have catastrophic consequences, with early graft dysfunction or variceal bleeding; confirmation of portal

patency is therefore very important. Colour flow imaging alone is almost always sufficient for confirmation of patency (Fig. 14.26), problems being experienced only when the anatomy is abnormal after liver reduction procedures. Patients with BCS, abnormal portal vein anatomy, including those with a cutdown liver or living related donor, a portal vein conduit, or who have had an operative thrombectomy are all at increased risk of portal vein thrombosis and deserve special attention.

The flow characteristics within the transplanted portal vein are often abnormal owing to a degree of infolding at the portal anastomosis (Fig. 14.27). There may be severe flow disturbance beyond the anastomosis (Fig. 14.28) and a relatively high-velocity jet may be found at the anastomosis. For this reason, velocity measurements distal to the anastomosis are difficult or impossible. However, spectral Doppler studies should be attempted using colour flow imaging to detect the highest velocity, and a peak velocity estimate should be performed. If this is more than 100 cm/s the anastomosis is likely to be unacceptably tight (Fig. 14.29) and the patient must be carefully monitored for the development of portal stenosis and evidence of extrahepatic portal hypertension. In patients with significant subhepatic fluid collections the portal vein can be compressed or displaced, and this may give rise to stenosis or kinking. Aspiration of the collection may prevent subsequent portal vein thrombosis.

Delayed portal vein compression, kinking or thrombosis may be caused by hypertrophy of the grafted liver. This is particularly likely to occur where a cutdown graft is inappropriately small for the size of the recipient. We have seen a few cases in which portal vein reconstruction has

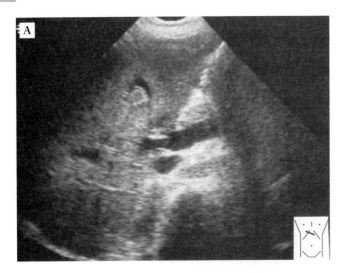

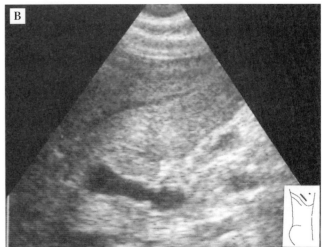

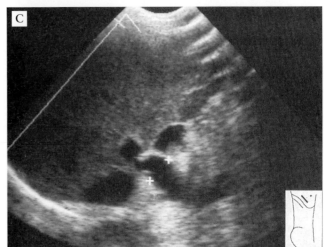

Fig. 14.27 Portal vein anastomoses. The portal vein anastomosis is frequently visible and may appear as **A**: a sudden change in calibre, **B**: a circumferential flap or **C**: an eccentric flap.

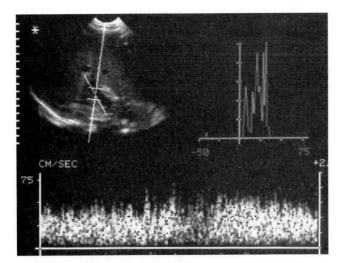

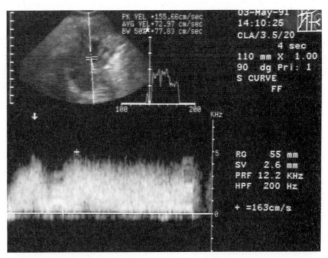

Fig. 14.28 Normal post-transplant portal vein Doppler. The irregularity at the portal anastomosis almost invariably gives rise to disturbed flow distal to the anastomosis.

Fig. 14.29 Portal vein stenosis. In this early post-transplant patient the lumen at the portal vein anastomosis is very small and the peak velocity through the anastomosis is 163 cm/s.

been necessary to overcome kinking or compression several weeks or months after a segmental graft. It is possible that the appropriate choice of surgical technique for the anastomosis may reduce or prevent the incidence of this problem.[37]

Transient highly reflective foci within the portal vein lumen indicate gas bubbles. These may be an incidental finding[38] but can also indicate grave intra-abdominal pathology, such as bowel infarction. We have seen only two examples of intraportal gas bubbles in many thousands of examinations (Fig. 14.30): one patient died within 48 hours because of overwhelming gas gangrene, and one survived after vigorous antibiotic therapy. Jantsch *et al.*[39] identified three cases in 120 liver transplantation patients. All were found to be

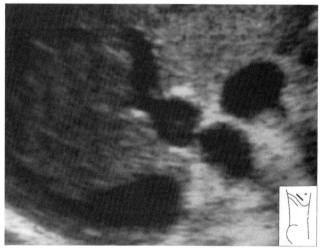

Fig. 14.31 **Late-onset portal vein stenosis.** There is a very tight stenosis with a residual lumen of only 2 mm and both pre- and post-stenotic dilatation.

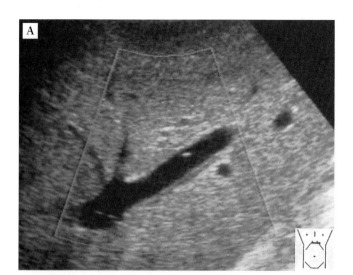

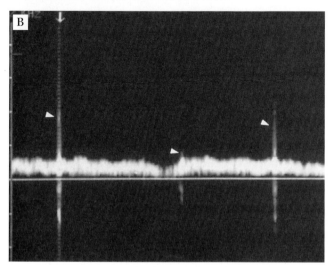

Fig. 14.30 **Intraportal gas. A:** Rapidly moving highly reflective foci were seen within the lumen of the portal vein; three are captured in this still frame. **B:** The passage of gas bubbles through the Doppler range gate gives rise to high-amplitude transient signals (arrowheads) superimposed on the portal venous signal.

due to septicaemia by gas-forming organisms. Conversely, King *et al.*[40] identified two cases, both of which were apparently associated with benign pneumatosis intestinalis.

As with pre-operative investigations, assessment of the portal system includes measurement of spleen size. Many post-transplant patients show a small reduction in spleen size; a significant enlargement suggests unresolved portal hypertension.

Late stenosis of the portal vein is an uncommon but serious complication[41] and can usually be predicted by detecting a narrow anastomosis on the early postoperative scans (Fig. 14.31). In these patients serial measurements of the jet velocity[42] permit the detection of a progressive stenosis, and the spleen is seen to enlarge if the lesion becomes haemodynamically significant.

Many cases can be successfully treated by angioplasty, and Doppler ultrasound is essential to monitor the success of this therapy.[43,44]

Portal vein stenosis may rarely occur as a very late complication, even several years after successful transplantation. The diagnosis may be made incidentally by detection of intrahepatic post-stenotic dilatation of the portal vein (Fig. 14.32) with an associated high-velocity jet and increasing splenomegaly. These patients may also present with ascites or haematemesis.

Late and sudden portal vein occlusion is rare and usually presents with a sudden deterioration in liver function tests, the onset of resistant ascites and rapidly increasing splenomegaly. Occasionally the only symptom is acute gastrointestinal haemorrhage, indicating the recurrence of portal hypertension. Any patient with one or more of these signs or symptoms should receive immediate and thorough ultrasound examination of the liver and spleen, with full Doppler assessment.

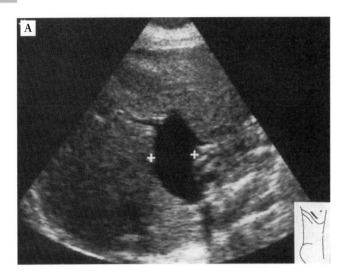
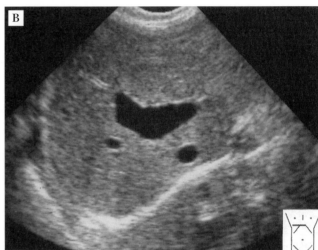

Fig. 14.32 **Portal vein stenosis with post-stenotic dilatation. A:** Lateral intercostal scan and **B:** transverse scan. There is marked dilatation of the intrahepatic portal vein associated with a high-velocity vortex secondary to anastomotic stenosis.

Hepatic veins and IVC

In the majority of liver transplant patients examination of the hepatic veins need be only fairly cursory. Hepatic vein dilatation due to upper IVC anastomotic stenosis is rare and early hepatic vein thrombosis is almost unheard of, except in patients who have been transplanted for BCS. In these cases the major hepatic veins and IVC must be scanned carefully to confirm flow and to exclude the presence of thrombi.

A non-specific correlation has been shown between the pulsatility of the hepatic vein waveform and the presence and severity of a range of hepatic parenchymal abnormalities. The clinical relevance of hepatic vein Doppler studies in liver transplantation remains uncertain. After some initial enthusiasm our own results have been disappointing, showing no correlation between hepatic vein waveform and the presence of liver abnormality and duration of patient survival. More encouraging shorter-term results have been reported in which deterioration of pulsatility of the hepatic vein waveforms was 100% correlated with deterioration in the patient's liver status (Fig. 14.33).[45,46] Our own experience suggests that there is a large number of extraneous factors affecting hepatic vein pulsatility, including the presence and severity of ascites, pleural effusions and other collections, patient obesity and the degree to which the transplanted liver matches the size of the recipient abdomen. Similarly disappointing results have been reported by Kok *et al.*[21] For the moment it seems prudent to study the hepatic vein waveform and to be aware that significant progressive reductions in pulsatility may be a non-specific indicator of the presence of one of many clinical complications.

Stenosis of the IVC is extremely rare and generally presents with ascites and increasing lower limb oedema.

The diagnosis can be established with ultrasound by the demonstration of a dilated and pulseless cava below the level of the stenosis (Fig. 14.34),[47] but contrast cavography is the definitive diagnostic test.

Fluid collections

Upper abdominal fluid collections are common in the early postoperative period and are seldom of any clinical significance.[3] The commonest causes are unresolved ascites, small periportal haematoma (Fig. 14.35) and sub-capsular intrahepatic haematomas (Fig. 14.36), which usually occur on the superior aspect of the left lobe or the inferior lateral aspect of the right lobe. In a minority of patients the collections are found to be of bile. These may arise either by leakage from the bile duct anastomosis, from the cystic duct remnant after the routine cholecystectomy normally undertaken on the transplanted liver, or from segmental ducts in a cutdown liver. The majority of bile collections are non-progressive and slowly resolve without intervention. Of these, the periportal collections are the only ones likely to become of significance, as they may compress or displace the portal vein or bile duct. Fine linear echoes are frequently detected within haematomas, thereby differentiating them from bile collections, which may contain amorphous and unstructured reflective material which may precipitate with time (Fig. 14.37). During the first week or two of postoperative management the majority of haematomas are comprised of clotted blood (Fig. 14.38) and aspiration is seldom either necessary or possible.

An early scan to identify and measure fluid collections is an important component of postoperative care, the majority of collections stabilising in size in the first few days. Any collections that arise *de novo* several days after

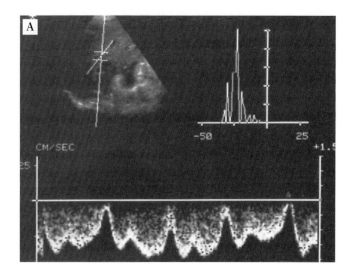

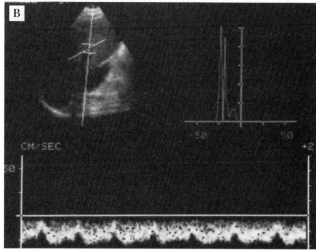

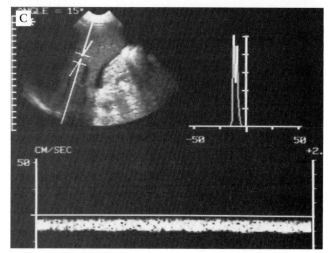

Fig. 14.33 Doppler studies of the hepatic veins. A: Normal hepatic vein tracing. **B:** The tracing is moderately damped and **C:** severely damped, indicating increased liver stiffness.

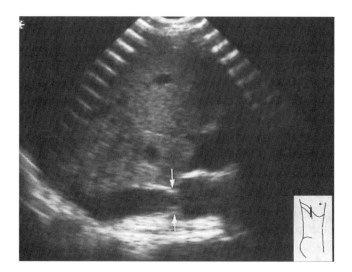

Fig. 14.34 Stenosis of the IVC. The inferior IVC anastomosis (arrows) is rather tight, with dilatation of the IVC inferior to the anastomosis

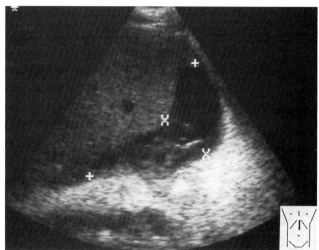

Fig. 14.35 Periportal haematoma. This subhepatic periportal haematoma shows retraction of the blood clot inferiorly, with clear serous fluid superiorly.

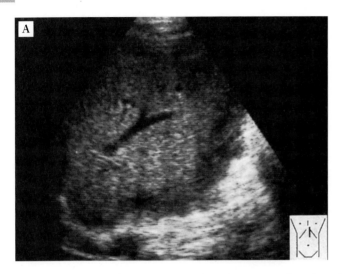

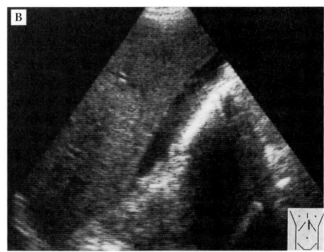

Fig. 14.36 Subcapsular haematoma. A: In the early post-transplant phase the inferior subcapsular haematoma is only just detectable as an irregular area of reduced reflectivity. B: As the haematoma matures it acquires the more typical 'lens' shape, with indentation of the liver margin.

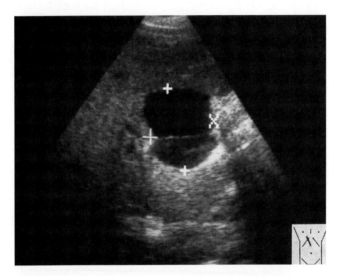

Fig. 14.37 Subhepatic bile collection. Bile salts have precipitated out to give a fluid/fluid level. This is suggestive but not definitely diagnostic of a biloma.

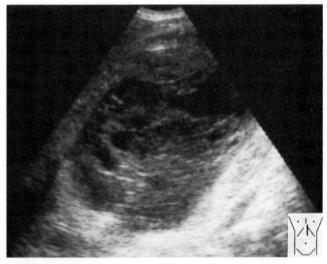

Fig. 14.38 Subhepatic haematoma. In this fresh haematoma the true fluid nature is indicated by the marked distal accentuation, and the linear echoes of freshly clotted blood are well seen within the haematoma.

a transplant, or any that progressively increase in size, may compress adjacent structures and warrant further investigation.

In our experience infection of fluid collections during the early postoperative phase is rare. However, if the patient's clinical condition suggests the presence of infection the fluid collections should be examined in detail to determine whether the nature of the fluid within any of them has altered, especially with the development of gas bubbles (Fig. 14.39). Any collection with features suspicious of infection warrants ultrasound-guided diagnostic aspiration.

Large right-sided (Fig. 14.40) and small left-sided pleural effusions are very common and are almost never of any clinical consequence.

The fluid collections occurring in the early postoperative period may be slow to clear, haematomas frequently persisting for 6–12 weeks or more. However, the development of new collections in the late postoperative period is of serious significance and raises the possibility of a bile leak (possibly indicating hepatic artery occlusion) or ascites, raising questions about the patency of the portal vein and IVC.

Fluid collections which have been confidently demonstrated to be persistent and unchanged in size can usually

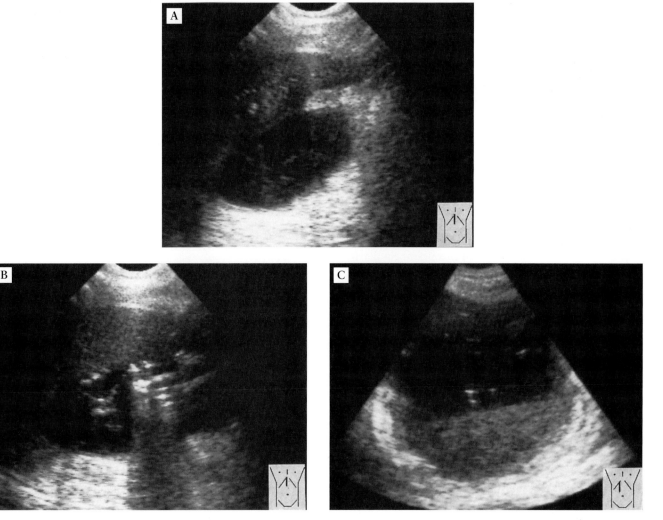

Fig. 14.39 Infected haematoma. A: In the early postoperative phase an uncomplicated haematoma is noted. **B:** Several days later the patient developed a pyrexia and gas bubbles have arisen within the haematoma, indicating a pyogenic infection. **C:** This subhepatic bile collection had been known to be present for several days. Repeat examination when the patient developed a pyrexia revealed small gas bubbles rising slowly to the surface within the fluid collection.

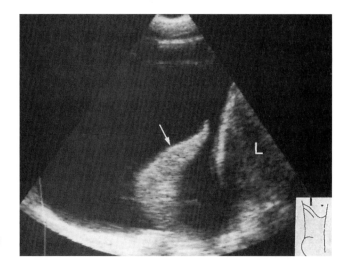

Fig. 14.40 Large right pleural effusion. There is a large right pleural effusion with a compressed and airless right lower lobe of the lung (arrow) above the diaphragm. L – liver.

be successfully drained by ultrasound-guided catheter placement in the late postoperative phase.[3] By this stage the majority consist of only thin fluid, usually liquefied blood or bile-stained ascites. In patients with proven bile leaks catheter placement and subsequent continuous drainage of the collection may promote healing of the biliary leak and prevent the need for more radical reconstructive surgery.

The bile ducts

Many surgical variations of bile duct anastomosis have been used, but current practice favours an end-to-end anastomosis where the recipient bile duct can be used. However, if the recipient has an underlying biliary abnormality, such as biliary atresia or sclerosing cholangitis, it will be necessary to employ a Roux loop. Similarly, in patients receiving a cutdown graft there is insufficient bile duct present to permit a direct biliary anastomosis and a Roux loop is again likely to be used.

Bile duct dilatation in the early postoperative period is unusual. Rarely inspissated bile may occlude the common duct, with consequent obstruction (Fig. 14.41). It is, however, important to identify and measure the common, left and right hepatic ducts to confirm their normality and to establish baseline values for comparison with subsequent examinations (Fig. 14.42).

Patients who have received a cutdown liver may be at increased risk of biliary anastomotic complications, and the altered anatomy makes imaging of these livers more taxing. This group of patients deserves particularly careful monitoring of the intrahepatic duct diameters. It must be remembered that in paediatric patients receiving a left lobe

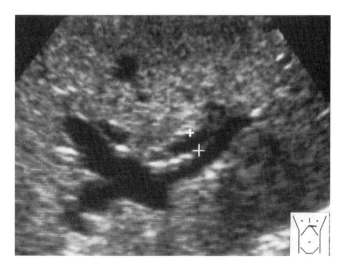

Fig. 14.42 Measurement of bile duct diameter. The proximal left hepatic duct diameter has been measured for monitoring in this patient receiving balloon dilatation of a late biliary stricture.

graft from an adult donor the diameter of the bile duct will be appropriate for an adult and may be unusually large for a child. It is therefore important to record the size of the bile duct in such cases during the early postoperative phase, and to monitor for any subsequent dilatation. Failure to do this may give rise to an erroneous diagnosis of biliary dilatation in this group of patients.

The bile ducts within transplanted livers seem less compliant than normal and may fail to return to a normal calibre after early and successfully treated bile duct dilatation (Fig. 14.43). This persistent dilatation is generally of little clinical significance, though it is important to

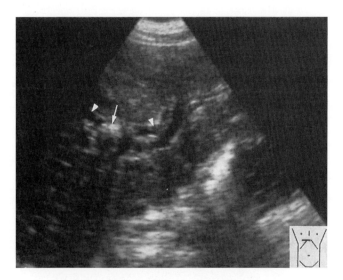

Fig. 14.41 Inspissated bile. Inspissated bile (arrow) has become adherent to the upper limb of the T-tube, with subsequent obstruction and intrahepatic duct dilatation (arrowheads).

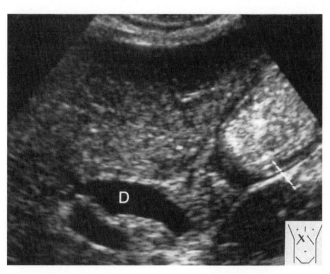

Fig. 14.43 Persistent duct dilatation after relief of obstruction. This patient received surgical correction for a biliary stenosis but the dilatation of the common hepatic duct (D) never resolved, despite good bile drainage.

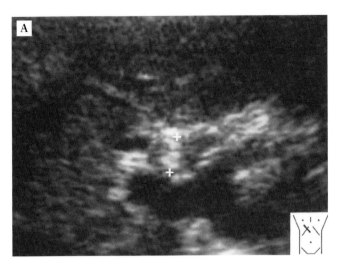
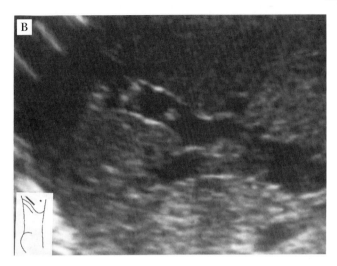

Fig. 14.44 Biliary concretions and cholangitis. A: Biliary concretions are seen within a non-dilated common duct (between calipers) and **B:** within a dilated system. Cholangitis cannot be diagnosed by ultrasound unless frank abscess formation is detected.

monitor the patient's serum bilirubin carefully. Ascending cholangitis and biliary sludge formation with concretions are more likely to develop in these patients (Fig. 14.44).[3]

The late onset of biliary strictures is not uncommon after liver transplantation and may occur either at the anastomotic site or higher within the biliary tree (Fig. 14.45), possibly at a vascular watershed. The former are probably complications of surgical technique and generally respond satisfactorily to percutaneous trans-hepatic dilatation. Non-anastomotic stenoses are likely to be ischaemic in origin, and in these patients the hepatic arterial tree must be studied. There is a small subgroup of patients with post-operative biliary obstruction in whom extensive epithelial

casts form within the biliary tree. These patients usually have a patent hepatic artery with good flow, and the lesions are almost certainly therefore not vascular in origin. It is possible that this is a late manifestation of preservation injury to the harvested liver, leading to late onset of epithelial sloughing within the biliary tree. The treatment of this condition is extremely unsatisfactory and most patients ultimately require retransplantation.

Late-onset biliary leaks are extremely uncommon.

Gas within the intrahepatic bile ducts may be noted on routine examination (Fig. 14.46). If the patient is afebrile and asymptomatic this is of no significance and is almost certainly a consequence of a previous sphincterotomy or the

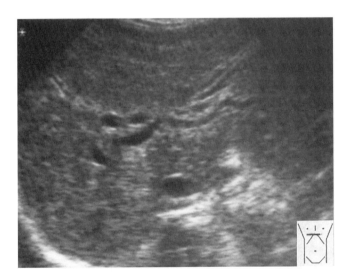
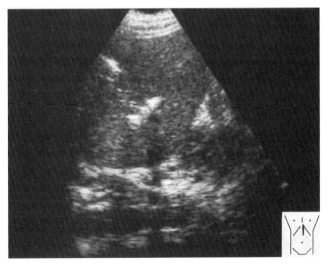

Fig. 14.45 Ischaemic biliary stricture. This patient became jaundiced several weeks post transplant. There is mild dilatation of the left and right duct systems but the common hepatic duct was collapsed. This pattern of bile duct dilatation suggests an ischaemic cause.

Fig. 14.46 Gas within the biliary tree. The highly reflective foci with shadowing are caused by gas within the left duct system. The diameters cannot be assessed.

use of a Roux loop as a biliary conduit. There may be an increased incidence of ascending cholangitis in these patients and careful monitoring for early hepatic abscesses is therefore indicated, though large quantities of intra-hepatic gas may prevent a complete evaluation with ultrasound.

Parenchymal changes

Subjective assessment of the parenchymal echo pattern and reflectivity seldom reveals any significant change in the majority of liver transplant patients. A minority show a variable degree of progressive increase in reflectivity (Fig. 14.47), possibly indicating fat deposition, which is of no clinical significance.

In patients who are acutely unwell a generalised reduction in reflectivity may occasionally be detected and should raise the possibility of viral hepatitis, particularly in the first few months after transplantation.

There are no identifiable parenchymal changes in patients with either acute or progressive chronic rejection.

If the original transplantation was undertaken for malignancy, both the liver and the upper abdominal cavity must be checked for any evidence of tumour recurrence. Once the acute postoperative phase has been successfully overcome, the commonest cause of death in these patients is recurrent tumour, usually in the transplanted liver.

There is also a significantly increased risk in all liver transplant patients from new primary malignancies, especially lymphoma, as a consequence of prolonged immuno-suppression.[48]

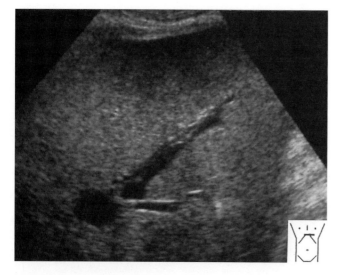

Fig. 14.47 Post-transplant fatty change. The uniform increase in parenchymal reflectivity in this transplanted liver was associated with normal liver function and is probably due to moderate fatty change. Note: the non-dilated left hepatic duct is outlined anterior to the left portal vein branch.

Diaphragmatic function

Diaphragmatic paralysis with consequent respiratory compromise has been identified in a minority of young children following liver transplantation.[49] Ultrasound is valuable in these patients to establish the diagnosis by observing the diaphragm movement during spontaneous respiration. The condition is probably caused by damage to the phrenic nerve during clamping of the suprahepatic vena cava. In our own series of four cases ultrasound was useful in establishing the diagnosis and confirming the return of normal diaphragmatic function after plication of the diaphragm.

Ultrasound-guided procedures

Although the majority of postoperative fluid collections do not require diagnostic or therapeutic aspiration, ultrasound remains a useful technique for guiding needle or catheter placement where collections of bile, blood or ascites are slow to resolve or are thought to have become infected. Similarly, intrahepatic abscesses can be diagnosed and treated by ultrasound-guided catheter placement, and chronic drainage of bile collections may permit spontaneous healing of bile duct leaks.

Ultrasound-guided biopsy is often necessary for patients with a left lobe graft and may be helpful in those where blind biopsy has failed to produce an adequate specimen, or where the ultrasound examination has shown suspicion of a focal lesion in patients at risk for malignant disease.

In patients with biliary or portal stenoses in whom percutaneous trans-hepatic balloon dilatation is considered, ultrasound imaging may be invaluable in guiding the initial needle and catheter into the appropriate vessel. Once the dilatation has been successfully accomplished, imaging and, where relevant, Doppler studies, are important for monitoring subsequent progress and assessing the need for further intervention.

REFERENCES

1 Bismuth H, Castaing D, Ericzon B G et al. Hepatic transplantation in Europe. First report of the European liver transplant registry. Lancet 1987; ii: 674–676
2 Bismuth H, Samuel D, Gugenheim J. Emergency liver transplantation for fulminant hepatitis. Ann Intern Med 1987; 10: 337–341
3 Raby N, Meire H B, Forbes A, Williams R. The role of ultrasound screening in management after liver transplantation. Clin Radiol 1988; 39: 507–510
4 Lengley D G, Skolnick M L, Zajko A B, Bron K M. Duplex Doppler sonography in the evaluation of adult patients before and after liver transplantation. AJR 1988; 151: 687–696
5 Tzakis A G, Todo S, Steiber A, Starzl T E. Venous jump grafts for liver transplantation in patients with portal vein thrombosis. Transplantation 1989; 48: 530–531
6 Teefey S A, Middleton W D, Crowe T M, Peters M G. Doppler sonographic evaluation of the portal vein: effects of intravenous dodecafluoropentane. J Ultrasound Med 1997; 16: 641–645

7 Margarit C, Lazaro J L, Charco R, Hidalgo E, Revhaug A, Murio E. Liver transplantation in patients with splenorenal shunts: intraoperative flow measurements to indicate shunt occlusion. Liver Transplantation Surg 1999; 5: 35–39

8 Powell-Jackson P R, Karani J, Ede R J et al. Ultrasound and ^{99m}Tc sulphur colloid scintigraphy in diagnosis of Budd–Chiari syndrome. Gut 1986; 27: 1502–1506

9 Deasy N P, Wendon J, Meire H B, Sidhu P S. The value of serial Doppler ultrasound as a predictor of clinical outcome and the need for transplantation in fulminant and severe acute liver failure. Br J Radiol 1999; 72: 134–143

10 Bisset G S III, Strife J, Balistrevi W F. Evaluation of children for liver transplantation: value of MR imaging and sonography. AJR 1990; 155: 351–356

11 Broide E, Farrant P, Reid F et al. Hepatic artery resistance index can predict early death in children with biliary atresia. Liver Transplantation Surg 1997; 3: 604–610

12 Seu P, Imagawa D K, Olthoff K M et al. A prospective study on the reliability and cost effectiveness of preoperative ultrasound screening of the 'marginal' liver donor [published erratum in Transplantation 1996; 62: 704]. Transplantation 1996; 62: 129–130

13 De Hamptinne B, de Goyet J de V, Kestens P J, Otte J B. Volume reduction the liver graft before orthotopic transplantation. Transplantation Proc 1987; 19: 3317–3322

14 Broelsch C E, Emond J C, Whitington P F, Thistlethwaite J R, Baker A L, Lichtor J L. Application of reduced-size liver transplants as split grafts, auxillary orthotopic grafts and living related segmental transplants. Ann Surg 1990; 212: 368–377

15 Cheng Y F, Chen C L, Huang T L et al. Magnetic resonance of the hepatic veins with angular reconstruction: application in living-related liver transplantation. Transplantation 1999; 68: 267–271

16 Kawasaki S, Makuuchi M, Miyagawa S et al. Extended lateral segmentectomy using intraoperative ultrasound to obtain a partial liver graft. Am J Surg 1996; 171: 286–288

17 Waldman D L, Lee D E, Bronsther O, Orloff M S. Use of intraoperative ultrasonography during hepatic transplantation. [Published erratum in J Ultrasound Med 1998; 17: 415]. J Ultrasound Med 1998; 17: 1–6

18 Kubota K, Billing H, Ericzon B G, Kelter U, Groth C G. Duplex Doppler ultrasonography for monitoring liver transplants. Acta Radiol 1990; 31: 279–283

19 Kok T, Sloof M J, Thijn C J et al. Routine Doppler ultrasound for the detection of clinically unsuspected vascular complications in the early postoperative phase after orthotopic liver transplantation. Transplant Int 1998; 11: 272–276

20 Pinna A D, Smith C V, Furukawa H, Starzl T E, Fung J J. Urgent revascularisation of liver allografts after early hepatic artery thrombosis. Transplantation 1996; 62: 1584–1587

21 Kok T, Haagsma E B, Klompmaker I J et al. Doppler ultrasound of the hepatic artery and vein performed daily in the first two weeks after orthotopic liver transplantation. Useful for the diagnosis of acute rejection? Invest Radiol 1996; 31: 173–179

22 Hellinger A, Roll C, Stracke A, Erhard J, Eigler F W. Impact of colour Doppler sonography on detection of thrombosis of the hepatic artery and the portal vein after liver transplantation. Langenbecks Arch Chir 1996; 381: 182–185

23 Wozeney P, Zajko A B, Bron K M. Vascular complications after liver transplantation: a five year experience. AJR 1986; 147: 657–663

24 Cook G J, Crofton M E. Hepatic artery thrombosis and infarction: evolution of the ultrasound appearances in liver transplant recipients. Br J Radiol 1997; 70: 248–251

25 Klintmalm B G, Olson L M, Nery J R, Husberg B S, Paulsen A W. Treatment of hepatic artery thrombosis after liver transplantation with immediate vascular reconstruction: a report of three cases. Transplant Proc 1988; 20 (Suppl. 1): 610–612

26 Platt J F, Yutzy G G, Bude R O, Ellis J H, Rubin J M. Use of Doppler sonography for revealing hepatic artery stenosis in liver transplant recipients. AJR 1997; 168: 473–476

27 Flint E W, Sumkin J H, Zajko A B. Duplex sonography of hepatic artery thrombosis after liver transplantation. AJR 1988; 151: 481–483

28 McDiarmid S V, Hall T R, Grant E G et al. Failure of duplex sonography to diagnose hepatic artery thrombosis in a high risk group of pediatric liver transplant recipients. J Pediatr Surg 1991; 26: 710–713

29 Hall T R, McDiarmid S V, Grant E G, Boechat M I, Busultil R W. False negative duplex Doppler studies in children with hepatic artery thrombosis after liver transplantation. AJR 1990; 154: 573–575

30 Longley D G, Skolnick M L, Sheahan D G. Acute allograft rejection in liver transplant recipients: lack of correlation with loss of hepatic artery diastolic flow. Radiology 1988; 169: 417–420

31 Propeck P A, Scanlan K A. Reversed or absent hepatic arterial diastolic flow in liver transplants shown by duplex sonography: a poor predictor of subsequent hepatic artery thrombosis. AJR 1992; 159: 1199–1201

32 Marujo W C, Langnas A N, Wood R P, Stratta R J, Li S, Shaw B W Jr. Vascular complications following orthotopic liver transplantation: outcome and the role of urgent revascularisation. Transplant Proc 1991; 23: 1484–1486

33 Mondragon R S, Karani J B, Heaton N D. The use of percutaneous transluminal angioplasty in hepatic artery stenosis after transplantation. Transplantation 1994; 57: 228–231

34 Pariente D, Riou J Y, Schmit P, Verlhac S, Bernard O, Devictor D. Variability of clinical presentation of hepatic artery thrombosis in paediatric liver transplantation: role of imaging modalities. Pediatr Radiol 1990; 20: 253–257

35 Zajko A B, Campbell W L, Logsdon G A et al. Cholangiographic findings in hepatic artery occlusion after liver transplantation. AJR 1987; 149: 485–489

36 Evans R A, Raby N D, O'Grady J G et al. Biliary complications following orthotopic liver transplantation. Clin Radiol 1990; 41: 190–194

37 Saad S, Tanaka K, Inomata Y. Portal vein reconstruction in pediatric liver transplantation from living donors. Ann Surg 1998; 227: 275–281

38 Chezmar J L, Nelson R C, Bernardino M E. Portal venous gas after hepatic transplantation: sonographic detection and clinical significance. AJR 1989; 153: 1203–1205

39 Jantsch H, Barton P, Fugger R *et al*. Sonographic demonstration of septicaemia with gas-forming organisms after liver transplantation. Clin Radiol 1991; 43: 397–399

40 King S, Shuckett B. Sonographic diagnosis of portal venous gas in two pediatric liver transplant patients with benign pneumatosis intestinalis. Case reports and literature review. Pediatr Radiol 1992; 22: 577–578

41 Malassagne B, Soubrane O, Dousset B, Legmann P, Houssin D. Extrahepatic portal hypertension following liver transplantation: a rare but challenging problem. HPB Surg 1998; 10: 357–363

42 Lee J, Ben-Ami T, Yousefzadeh D et al. Extrahepatic portal vein stenosis in recipients of living-donor allografts: Doppler sonography. AJR 1996; 167: 85–90

43 Funaki B, Rosenblum J D, Leef J A et al. Portal vein stenosis in children with segmental liver transplants: treatment with percutaneous transhepatic venoplasty. AJR 1995; 165: 161–165

44 Funaki B, Rosenblum J D, Leef J A, Hackworth C A, Szymski G X, Alonso E M. Angioplasty treatment of portal vein stenosis in children with segmental liver transplants: midterm results. AJR 1997; 169: 551–554

45 Coulden R A, Britton P D, Farman P, Noble-Jamieson G, Wight D G D. Preliminary report: hepatic vein Doppler in the early diagnosis of acute liver transplant rejection. Lancet 1990; 336: 273–274

46 Britton P D, Lomas D J, Coulden R A, Farman P, Revell S. The role of hepatic vein Doppler in diagnosing acute rejection following paediatric liver transplantation. Clin Radiol 1992; 45: 228–232

47 Brouwers M A, de Jong K P, Peeters P M, Bijleveld C M, Klompmaker I J, Slooff M J. Inferior vena cava obstruction after orthotopic liver transplantation. Clin Transplantation 1994; 8: 19–22

48 Nalesnik M A, Makowka L, Starzl T E. The diagnosis and treatment of post-transplant lymphoproliferative disorders. Curr Probl Surg 1988; 25: 367–472

49 Smyrniotis V, Andreani P, Muiesan P, Mieli-Vergani G, Rela M, Heaton N D. Diaphragmatic nerve palsy in young children following liver transplantation. Successful treatment by plication of the diaphragm. Transplant Int 1998; 11: 281–283

15

Gallbladder and biliary tree

Jane Bates and Henry C Irving

Normal anatomy of the biliary tree

The intrahepatic bile ducts run in the portal tracts alongside the portal vein radicles and hepatic artery branches. At the porta hepatis the right and left hepatic ducts join to form the common hepatic duct, which passes inferiorly for approximately 3 cm before being joined by the cystic duct to form the common bile duct. The common bile duct continues caudally for approximately 7 cm, lying anterior to the right margin of the portal vein and lateral to the hepatic artery (Figs 15.1 and 15.2). It runs parallel with both vessels for a short distance before passing behind the first part of the duodenum. Distally, the common duct lies in a deep groove on the posterior aspect of the head of the pancreas and may be completely surrounded by pancreatic tissue. Within the posterolateral part of the pancreatic head the distal end of the common bile duct passes laterally, accompanying the pancreatic duct into the second part of the duodenum.

Gallbladder

The gallbladder lies in a fossa on the undersurface of the right lobe of the liver. It has a thin smooth wall, up to 2 mm in thickness (Fig. 15.3),[1] composed of an outer serosal layer, a middle fibromuscular layer and an inner mucosa. The bulbous distal portion of the gallbladder, the fundus, is generally in the most caudal and anterior position, often projecting below the inferior margin of the liver. The fundus tapers into the body and finally into the neck, which curves posterocaudally before becoming continuous with the cystic duct (Fig. 15.4).

The gallbladder serves as a reservoir for bile secreted by the liver; its size therefore varies according to digestive requirements throughout the day. The wall of the gallbladder is at its thickest in the region of the neck – normally up to 3 mm (Fig. 15.5). A small expansion of the gallbladder neck – Hartman's pouch – often becomes more marked in gallbladder dilatation.

Cystic duct

The cystic duct, 3–4 cm in length, is lined by mucosal folds which project into the lumen in a spiral arrangement – hence the term 'spiral valve'. It is not in fact a true valve and bile can flow in both directions, determined by differences in pressure between the gallbladder and the common bile duct. Its importance to the sonographer is that there may be an acoustic shadow beyond the valve, falsely suggesting the presence of a stone in the cystic duct (Fig. 15.6).[2]

Normal anatomical variants

Ducts

Normal variations in the anatomy of the ducts are common. The point at which the cystic duct joins the common hepatic duct is particularly variable: usually they unite just inferior to the porta hepatis, but the cystic duct may join the right hepatic duct or the junction may be much lower – occasionally within the head of the pancreas itself. The cystic duct may pass medially either posterior or anterior to the common hepatic duct, and then curve laterally to join its medial border. On ultrasound scans it is not usually possible to recognise the exact point of union of the cystic and common hepatic ducts, and it has therefore become accepted convention to refer to the extrahepatic bile duct as 'the common duct'.[3]

Gallbladder

The shape, size and position of the gallbladder are highly variable. In some cases the gallbladder fossa lies deep within the liver and the gallbladder appears to be surrounded by hepatic tissue – the so-called 'intrahepatic gallbladder' – which may mimic an intrahepatic cyst (Fig. 15.7). At the other end of the spectrum the gallbladder may be attached to the liver by a long mesentery, forming a very mobile structure which may be found in the right iliac fossa or very rarely even in the pelvic region, depending upon patient position. The neck of the gallbladder can, however, still be found at the porta.

In some subjects the fundus of the gallbladder is folded over – the 'Phrygian cap' – which can make examination of the lumen difficult.[4] Often, rotating the patient into the left lateral decubitus position unfolds the gallbladder, making it more accessible to full ultrasound interrogation (Fig. 15.8). Failing this, a more prolonged fast may dilate the gallbladder sufficiently for a successful study to be performed.

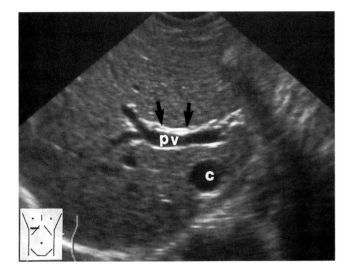

Fig. 15.1 Right hepatic duct. Transverse scan through liver showing a normal-calibre right hepatic duct (arrows), anterior to the right branch of the portal vein (pv). (c – inferior vena cava).

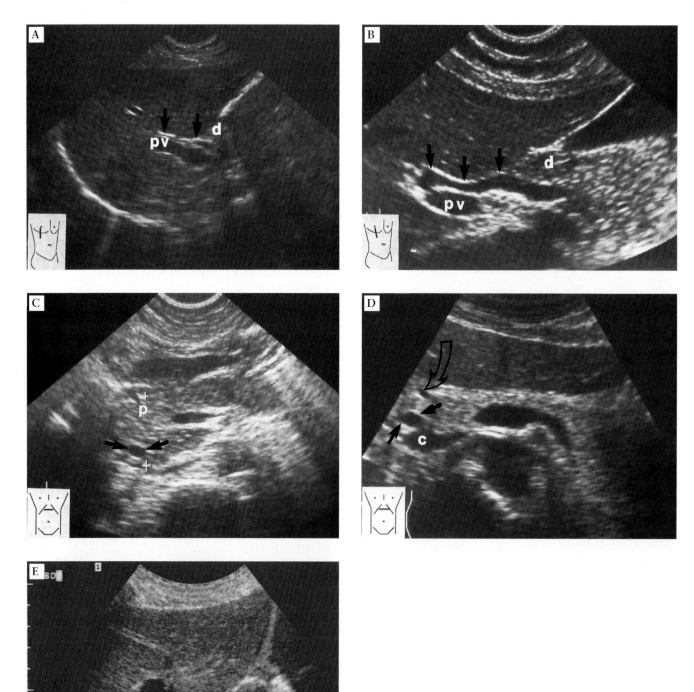

Fig. 15.2 Normal common duct. A: Longitudinal scan showing duct (arrows) anterior to portal vein (pv), and passing posterior to gas-filled duodenum (d). **B:** Longitudinal scan showing duct passing posterior to fluid-filled duodenum (d). **C:** Transverse scan showing duct (arrows) within head of pancreas (p). **D:** Transverse scan showing duct (arrows) about to enter duodenal papilla (open arrow – gastroduodenal artery, c – inferior vena cava). **E:** Longitudinal scan showing cystic duct (arrow) joining common duct just proximal to the first part of the duodenum.

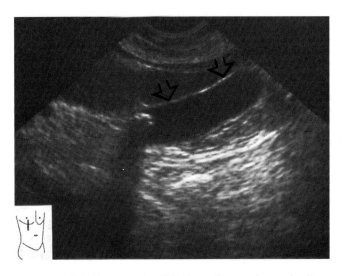

Fig. 15.3 Gallbladder. Normal gallbladder wall seen only as a thin line (arrows) when the gallbladder is filled (cf. Fig. 15.14). Note the stone in the neck of the gallbladder.

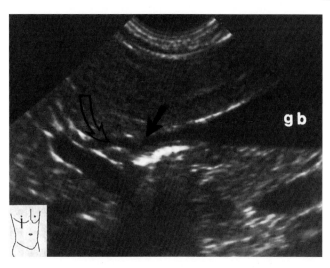

Fig. 15.4 Neck of gallbladder. Body of gallbladder tapers down to the neck (arrow), which becomes continuous with the cystic duct (open arrow).

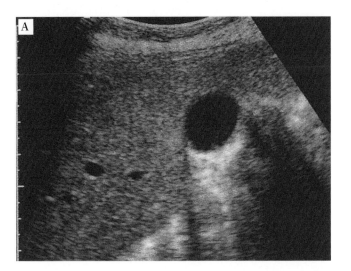

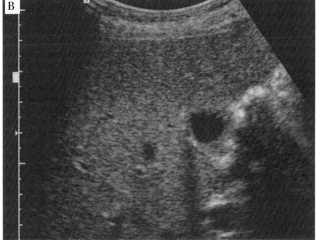

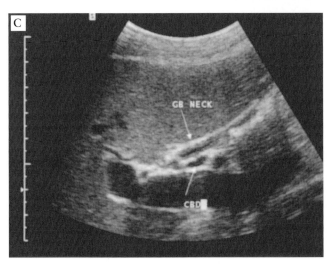

Fig. 15.5 Neck of gallbladder. Transverse scans through gallbladder showing how the wall becomes thicker in the neck. **A:** Fundus. **B:** Neck. **C:** Longitudinal scan through gallbladder neck.

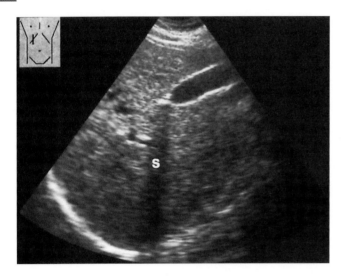

Fig. 15.6 Shadow from neck of gallbladder. Acoustic shadow (s) from normal neck of gallbladder.

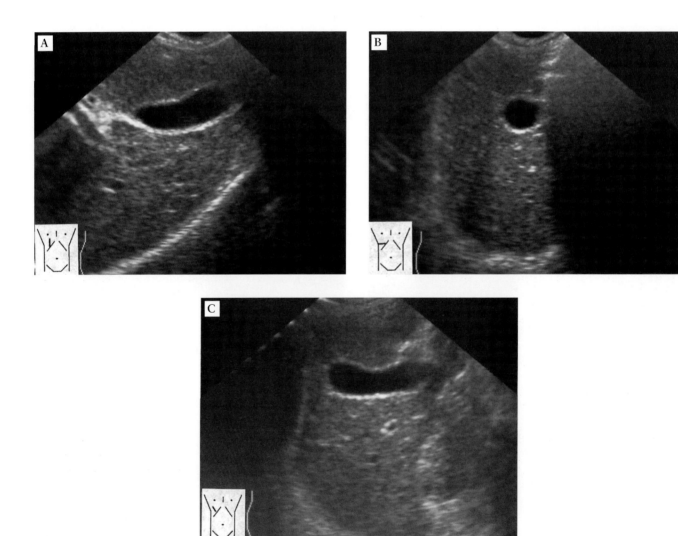

Fig. 15.7 Intrahepatic gallbladder. A: Longitudinal scan. **B:** Transverse scan. **C:** Oblique scan.

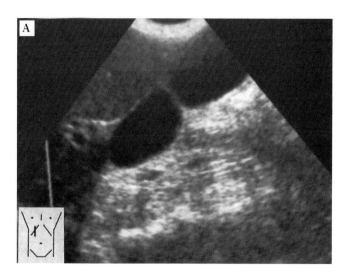 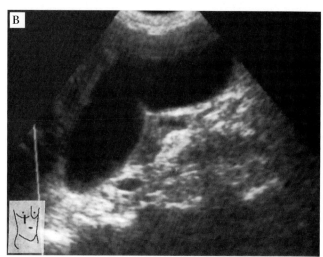

Fig. 15.8 Phrygian cap. A: Patient supine. **B:** Patient in right anterior oblique position.

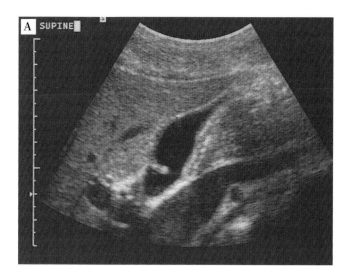 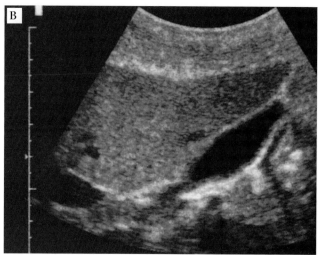

Fig. 15.9 Folded gallbladder. A: Patient supine. **B:** Patient in right anterior oblique position.

Folding of the gallbladder is a common variation which may mimic septation. The protuberance of the mucosa at the apex of the fold has led to false diagnoses of stones, but scanning in both longitudinal and transverse axes should help avoid this pitfall (Fig. 15.9).[5] True septa are uncommon and not usually of clinical significance. They can be distinguished from folding of the gallbladder by scanning in both longitudinal and transverse planes with the patient supine and in the left decubitus position. Septa can lead to errors in diagnosis when the sonographer reports one portion of the gallbladder as free of stones and misses a stone in the distal portion (Fig. 15.10).[6] The septum can also be mistaken for a small polyp.

The gallbladder may be totally absent, or there may be double or even triple gallbladders with either a single cystic duct or with multiple separate cystic ducts – these anomalies are extremely rare.

Hepatic artery

Usually the hepatic artery arises from the coeliac axis and runs for a short distance to the right before turning superiorly. At this point the artery lies anterior to the portal vein with the common duct to its right. Just proximal to the porta hepatis the artery branches and the right hepatic artery crosses to the right, posterior to the common hepatic duct, before entering the substance of the liver (Fig. 15.11).

In about 15% of subjects the right hepatic artery passes anterior to the common hepatic duct, and in a smaller proportion (approximately 5%) it originates from the

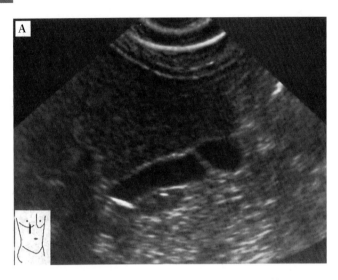 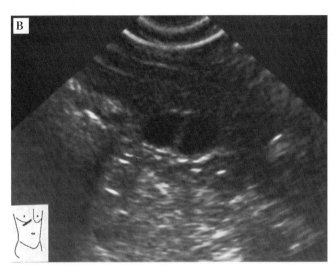

Fig. 15.10 Septated gallbladder. A: Longitudinal scan. **B:** Oblique scan.

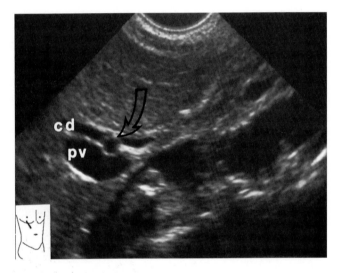 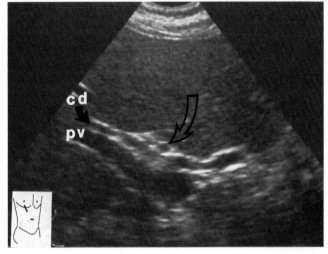

Fig. 15.11 Normal hepatic artery (arrow) crossing between common duct (cd) and portal vein (pv).

Fig. 15.12 Anomalous hepatic artery (open arrow) crossing anterior to common duct (cd).

superior mesenteric artery – the replaced right hepatic artery – and passes posterior to the superior mesenteric vein before turning anterior to the portal vein.[7] Colour Doppler ultrasound is useful in sorting out the anatomy in these cases,[8] although it is usually possible to identify the vessels by tracing them back to their point of origin (Fig. 15.12).

Technique and ultrasound appearances

The biliary system should be examined after the patient has fasted: not only does this distend the gallbladder with bile to allow investigation of its lumen, it also helps to

reduce the contents of the stomach and duodenum, which sometimes obscure the common duct and pancreas.

In some patients the posterior wall of the gallbladder is closely adjacent to the duodenum and distal acoustic shadowing from the latter may simulate gallbladder pathology (Fig. 15.13). In such cases, giving the patient a drink of water usually helps to outline the duodenum and display the gallbladder wall more clearly.

The normal gallbladder in the non-fasted state is contracted and thick walled (Fig. 15.14). This is generally indistinguishable from pathological contraction, and care should always be taken to ensure that the patient has adhered to the correct preparation if the gallbladder is small or not visualised on ultrasound.[9]

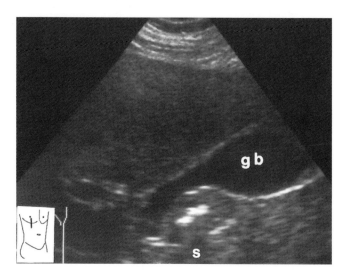

Fig. 15.13 **Bowel indenting posterior wall of gallbladder** (gb) with intraluminal gas casting an acoustic shadow (s).

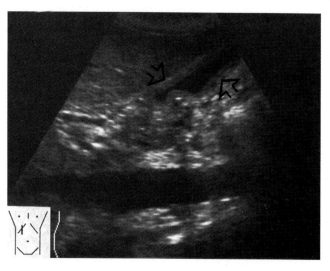

Fig. 15.14 **Normal contracted gallbladder.** Normal wall thickness of physiologically contracted gallbladder (open arrows).

The equipment of choice for examination of the gallbladder and biliary tree is a curved-array transducer which allows good acoustic access both subcostally and intercostally, with an adequate near field to accommodate superficial gallbladders. A frequency of 5 MHz with a focal zone at the appropriate depth generally provides sufficiently good resolution to detect even small stones within the gallbladder. The penetration at this frequency may not, however, be adequate in large or obese patients, in whom a 3.5 MHz transducer is necessary. With the lower frequency the width of the beam is greater and small stones may not be recognised as they lack acoustic shadowing (see Fig. 15.25).[10] Similarly, if the stone is outside the focal zone of the transducer, in the near or far fields, acoustic shadowing from a stone may be lost because the beam is wider than the stone.[11] With electronic focusing the position of the focal zone is under user control and should be at an appropriate depth.

A comprehensive examination of the biliary system naturally includes imaging of both the liver and the pancreas. The normal intrahepatic bile ducts are rarely visualised during routine scans, but it is not uncommon to display the main right and left hepatic ducts as thin tubular structures running parallel to the main branches of the portal vein (see Fig. 15.1).[12]

An initial survey of the gallbladder with the patient supine is usual. It is helpful to align the transducer along the long axis of the gallbladder and then angle it both laterally and medially, so that the entire volume of the gallbladder is interrogated by the ultrasound beam. A subcostal approach in deep inspiration brings the liver down, so that the right lobe provides an acoustic window for the gallbladder. However, an intercostal approach is the most successful technique in the majority of patients, allowing the gallbladder to be imaged through the right lobe of the liver in quiet respiration, with minimum artefact from adjacent bowel.

The normal gallbladder has an echo-free lumen and is surrounded by a smooth, moderately reflective wall. Because there is little attenuation of the ultrasound beam, the time–gain compensation used appropriately for the adjacent liver results in acoustic accentuation behind the gallbladder. However, this may not be apparent if gas-filled bowel lies immediately posteriorly (Fig. 15.15). In transverse scans the gallbladder appears circular,

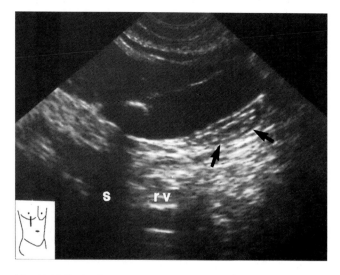

Fig. 15.15 **Shadowing – stone versus gas.** Posterior to the gallbladder there is shadowing (s) beyond a stone, reverberation (rv) beyond gas-containing bowel, and transmission of sound beyond empty bowel (arrows).

increasing in diameter towards the fundus. If possible the transducer should be maintained at right angles to the long axis of the gallbladder, as an oblique section may give a spurious impression of wall thickening (Fig. 15.16).[13]

The gallbladder must be examined with the patient in at least two different positions if small mobile stones or non-mobile polyps are to be correctly diagnosed. Following initial scans in the supine position the patient is turned into the left decubitus position. This allows the liver and gallbladder to fall away medially from the ribs, unfolding the gallbladder, and may also be useful in moving overlying bowel from the region of interest. Other patient posi-

tions may sometimes be necessary, for example erect scans with the patient either sitting or standing.

The right anterior oblique or left decubitus positions are indispensable for examining the common duct, which can then be traced distally running from the porta hepatis to the head of the pancreas as an immediate anterior relation of the portal vein (Fig. 15.17).[14] The lower end of the duct is best demonstrated on transverse scans through the head of the pancreas (Fig. 15.18) and, although a supine position is usually adequate, a semi-erect position with the left side raised is recommended by some.[15] A water load may be helpful in allowing visualisation of the lower end of the

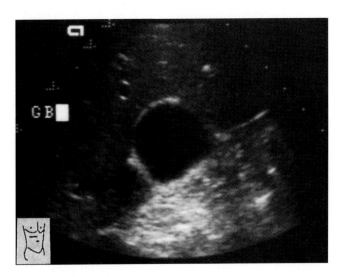

Fig. 15.16 Spurious gallbladder wall thickening (arrow) due to angulation of the beam.

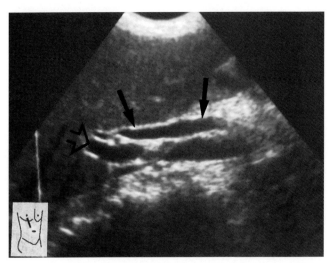

Fig. 15.17 Normal common duct (arrow) anterior to portal vein (open arrow). Note how the duct widens as it travels in the free edge of the lesser omentum.

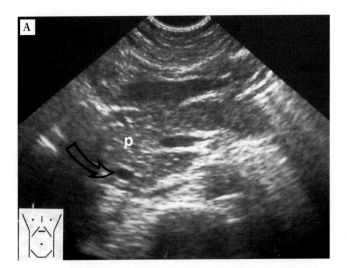

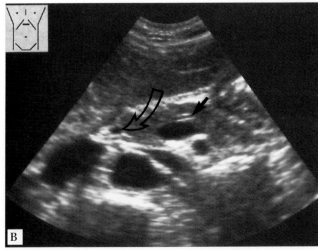

Fig. 15.18 Normal common duct in head of pancreas on transverse scans. A: Duct (open arrow) is within pancreatic substance (p). B: Duct (open arrow) is entering the duodenal papilla. (The pancreatic duct is also seen (solid arrow).)

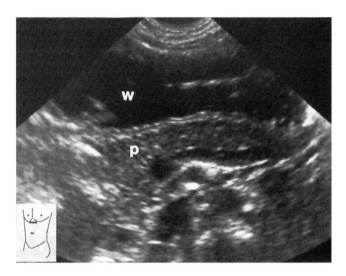

Fig. 15.19 Water load for pancreatic scanning. Water in the stomach (w) as an acoustic window improves visualisation of the pancreas (p).

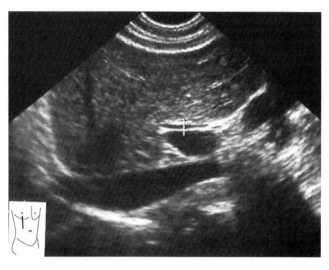

Fig. 15.20 Measurement of the common duct. Calipers on sharply defined walls of common duct.

common duct by displacing gas from the gastric antrum and duodenum in the left anterior oblique position, and it may also act as an acoustic window (Fig. 15.19).

Measurement of the common duct

The ability of ultrasound to discriminate between a normal and a dilated common duct is vital in the management of the jaundiced patient. This facility to distinguish between obstructive ('surgical') and non-obstructive ('medical') causes of jaundice depends on knowing the upper limit of normal for the duct diameter.

However, a clear value dividing normal from abnormal is not, in fact, easily attainable. In a normal population the values for the diameter of the common duct are distributed around a mean,[3] as happens with all biological measurements. The level at which the upper limit of normal is placed is a value judgement, and conventionally the '95% limit' or '2 standard deviations from the mean' are used. By definition, therefore, some normals fall outside the normal range, and conversely, some abnormals fall within it.

In the case of the ultrasound-derived measurement of common duct diameter there are particular factors to be considered:

1   Level of the measurement: the duct is most consistently demonstrated in its proximal portion via the right anterior oblique longitudinal view, and measurements are most often made just caudal to the porta hepatis.[14] Care must be taken not to let the indentation into the posterior wall of the duct, made by the right hepatic artery crossing between duct and portal vein, interfere with the measurement. Also, the duct usually widens slightly as it passes caudally in

the free edge of the lesser omentum and after it receives the cystic duct (Fig. 15.17).

2   The walls of the duct are highly reflective, and 'blooming' of the echoes from the walls may reduce the apparent duct lumen.[12,16] The overall gain and swept gain controls should be optimally adjusted to minimise this artefact (Fig. 15.20).

3   The cross-sectional shape of the duct is oval rather than circular, and thus measurements may differ according to which diameter is demonstrated on a particular scan plane (Fig. 15.21).[14]

4   In the elderly there is a generalised loss of elasticity of the tissues, and the normal duct diameter increases with advancing age.[17]

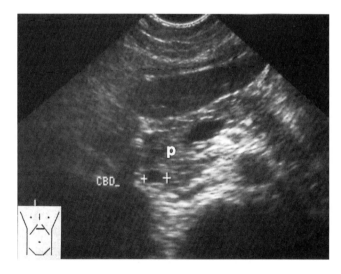

Fig. 15.21 Oval shape of common duct. False measurement of duct diameter due to oval shape in cross-section (p – pancreas).

5 The diameter of the duct is often increased in patients who have had a cholecystectomy. Ducts that were normal pre-operatively tend to remain normal postoperatively, whereas those that were acutely obstructed usually decrease in size postoperatively following stone removal or drainage. However, ducts that were chronically dilated, or in which there has been chronic infection, often remain permanently dilated after surgery or non-operative drainage, or may even increase slightly in diameter.[18-20] Inflammation presumably reduces the elasticity of the duct wall so that it becomes incapable of recoiling back down, and the resultant floppy duct distends with minimal pressure or volume increases as the duct assumes some of the original gallbladder reservoir function.[21,22]

Bearing all the above in mind, a useful working rule is that the diameter of the normal common duct, as measured on ultrasound scans, is less than 5 mm in its upper portion, although this figure can be increased to 6 mm for a measurement at its lower end, 8 mm in the elderly, and 10 mm in patients who have had a cholecystectomy.

Using the 'less than 5 mm' limit, the sensitivity of ultrasound for the diagnosis of extrahepatic obstruction has been shown to be 99%, with a specificity of 87%,[23] whereas moving the limit to 5 mm would have decreased the sensitivity to 94% without significantly altering the specificity.

Function studies

Although ultrasound scanning enables the display of excellent structural detail of the gallbladder, the images give little functional information. However, ultrasound can be used in combination with pharmacological agents so that the dynamics of gallbladder filling and emptying can be studied in both health and disease. Essentially the method consists of estimating gallbladder volume and monitoring that volume at regular intervals over a period of time.

Gallbladder contraction can be provoked by giving a standard 'fatty meal'. Gallbladder emptying dynamics have been studied in smokers, in pregnancy,[24] in patients with coeliac disease[25] and spinal cord injuries,[26] and in response to various drugs.

The response of the diameter of the common duct to a fatty meal has also been studied. The fatty meal causes the release of cholecystokinin from the duodenal mucosa and this promotes gallbladder contraction, relaxation of the sphincter of Oddi and an increase in the flow of bile from the liver. A normal bile duct either reduces in diameter or remains unchanged, but if there is partial or complete obstruction the diameter usually increases, though occasionally it remains unchanged.[27-30]

Endosonography

Endoscopic ultrasonography enables a high-frequency transducer to be placed in close proximity to the lower end of the bile duct and thus gives more detailed visualisation of lesions in this vicinity,[31] which are difficult to evaluate using conventional transabdominal ultrasound. A high-frequency ultrasound transducer is incorporated into a fully functional fibre-optic endoscope with both light and optical bundles and air/water channels, together with controllable tip movement. This specially adapted equipment is both difficult to use and expensive, and is therefore only used in a few centres.

Endosonography is significantly more sensitive, accurate and effective than either CT or transabdominal ultrasound in the evaluation of local spread of neoplastic obstructions[32] and in staging cholangiocarcinomas.

Intra-operative ultrasound

Intra-operative ultrasound scanning can assist the surgeon during biliary tract surgery. A high-frequency transducer of 7.5, 10 or even 12 MHz is placed directly in the operative field, and this technique is as accurate as peroperative cholangiography for the detection of common duct stones,[33] so that in some centres it has become established as a routine adjunct to peroperative cholangiography.[31] Care must be taken not to interpret air within the duct as stones.

Laparoscopic ultrasound

The increasing trend towards laparoscopic cholecystectomy has led to the development of adjunctive laparoscopic ultrasound. Like endosonography, this is a difficult technique to master and requires a specialised, flexible, high-frequency laparoscopic probe to evaluate the biliary anatomy, and in particular to examine the common duct for stones. Once learned, laparoscopic ultrasound has been shown to be highly sensitive and specific in evaluating the biliary tree,[34] and has the advantage of being quicker than operative cholangiography.

Gallbladder pathology

Ultrasound has been firmly established for many years as the primary imaging investigation in suspected gallbladder disease.[35] In patients who present with acute right upper quadrant pain ultrasound can demonstrate lesions of the gallbladder, and may show other causes for the pain. Cholescintigraphy, using a ^{99m}Tc-labelled derivative of iminodiacetic acid, is useful as a second-line test to confirm cystic duct obstruction, either when ultrasound has failed to show stones or when the origin of the symptoms remains in doubt in the presence of stones.

Stones

Advances in the range of therapies for gallstone disease place further demands on imaging techniques, and it is no longer enough simply to detect stones.[36] The selection of patients for the most appropriate therapy requires not only an assessment of cystic duct patency, but also detailed information concerning gallbladder and duct morphology, as well as characterisation and quantification of gallbladder contents.[37] Ultrasound is capable of providing most of these.[38,39]

The prevalence of gallstones in developed societies is approximately 10%, and as many as two-thirds of gallstone carriers are asymptomatic.[40,41] However, as the probability of developing biliary symptoms for subjects with silent stones is only 18% in 24 years,[42] the increasing use of ultrasound in patients with symptoms suggesting the presence of gallstones unmasks many previously undiagnosed stones, and thus creates ethical and economic dilemmas for physicians and health-care planners.[43]

The composition, size, shape and number of stones vary widely from patient to patient, presenting a wide range of ultrasound appearances.

Classic appearances

The most commonly encountered ultrasound appearance of a stone in the gallbladder is that of a highly reflective intraluminal structure which is gravity dependent and casts an acoustic shadow (Fig. 15.22). When all these features are present the diagnostic accuracy is 100%.[44] It is useful to analyse each of these ultrasound features more closely so that the limitations of the method are appreci-

ated, thus enabling scan technique and machine settings to be adjusted appropriately.

The size of a structure that can produce an echo from within the gallbladder lumen is not a limitation, as it has been shown that particles as small as 5–10 μm will produce echoes within bile.[45] Such tiny particles are not considered to be 'stones' and do not fulfil the diagnostic criteria given above, as they do not produce acoustic shadows.

The production of an acoustic shadow beyond a reflecting structure depends upon both the absorption and the reflection of sound by the structure, and the resulting shadow should be sharp and 'clean' (Fig. 15.23). This is in contrast to the shadowing beyond bowel gas, which is caused purely by sound reflection and is therefore usually less well defined and 'dirty' owing to reverberation artefacts (Fig. 15.24)[46] – a useful practical point in deciding whether shadows are due to gallstones or to bowel gas. Shadowing beyond a stone is not affected by the chemical composition of the stone, the presence of calcium within the stone or its shape and surface characteristics,[47] but rather is dependent upon the geometric relationship between the ultrasound beam and the stone.[48] The beam width needs to be as small as possible, as shadowing will not occur unless the stone occupies the full width of the beam (Fig. 15.25). Beam width is reduced by focusing methods and by using higher-frequency transducers (see Ch. 2).

A further practical consideration concerning the demonstration of stones in the gallbladder relates to signal processing methods.[49] Currently available TV display units have a limited dynamic range (less than 20 dB) and this necessitates the use of compression amplification. When this is combined with the use of time–gain compensation

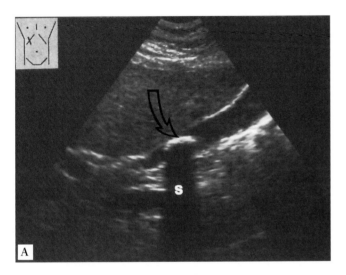
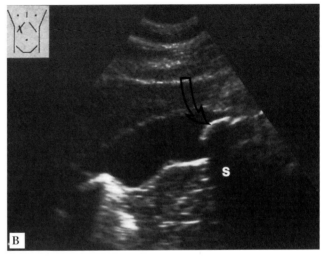

Fig. 15.22 Gallstones. 'Classic' appearances of stones in the gallbladder. **A:** With the patient supine there is an echo from the stone within the gallbladder lumen (arrow) and an acoustic shadow (s) distally. **B:** With the patient upright the stone (arrow) moves with gravity and drops into the fundus of the gallbladder.

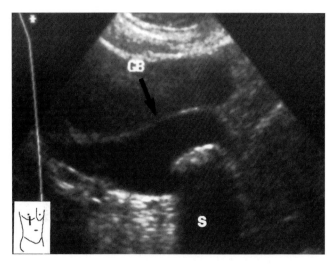

Fig. 15.23 Gallstone shadowing. 'Clean' shadowing (s). The acoustic shadow beyond the stone is free of reverberations.

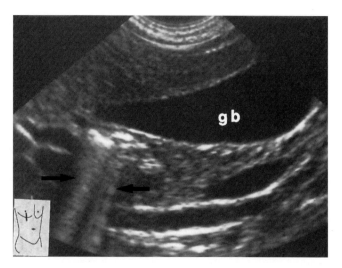

Fig. 15.24 Reverberative shadow. 'Dirty' shadowing. There are reverberation artefacts (arrows) distal to bowel gas (gb – gallbladder).

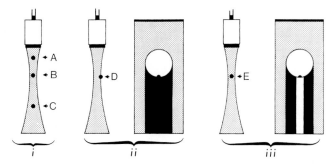

Fig. 15.25 Beam width and shadowing. Diagram to show the effect of beam width and incidence on the production of an acoustic shadow beyond a stone. (i) Stone B is in the focal zone of the beam and will give rise to an acoustic shadow, whereas stones A and C in the near and far fields of the beam are less likely to shadow (after Jaffe and Taylor).[21] (ii) and (iii) Diagrams to show the effect of positioning of a stone in relation to the beam; a linear array is viewed end-on on the left and in the scanning plane on the right. Stone D (ii) at the periphery of the beam will not occupy a sufficient proportion of the beam width to cast a shadow, but the same size stone E (iii) at the centre of the beam will shadow (after Filly et al.[20]).

curves, the distinction between acoustic shadow and surrounding tissues may be imperceptible.[50] This may be the most important limiting factor in real-life scanning, but good-quality modern equipment which is optimally adjusted should be capable of demonstrating gallbladder stones less than 1 mm in diameter (Fig. 15.26).

Contracted gallbladder

In the description of the 'classic' appearances of stones in the gallbladder it will be appreciated that the gallbladder lumen contains fluid bile within which the echoes reflected

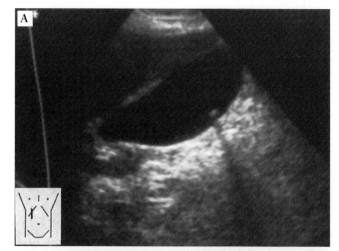

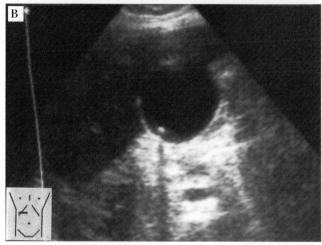

Fig. 15.26 Tiny stones with acoustic shadowing. A: Longitudinal scan. **B:** Transverse scan.

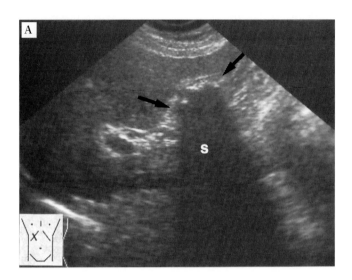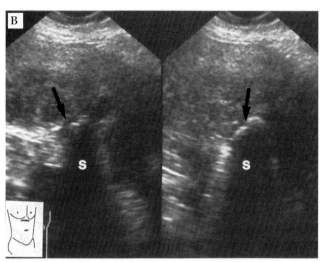

Fig. 15.27 **Contracted gallbladder full of stones** (arrows), with distal acoustic shadowing (s). **A:** Longitudinal scan. **B:** Transverse scans.

by the stone or stones can be detected. Where the lumen is totally filled by stones, or where the gallbladder wall has been chronically inflamed and become fibrotic, or where the cystic duct has been obstructed, there may be no fluid bile within the lumen.

Such 'contracted' or 'sclero-atrophic' gallbladders are now reliably recognised with modern equipment. In cases when the gallbladder lumen cannot be visualised distal acoustic shadowing may often be seen to emanate from the gallbladder fossa, representing the stone-filled lumen,[44] and the ability to locate the gallbladder fossa in different scan planes is crucial (Fig. 15.27).[51]

Refinement of the scanning technique can further improve the accuracy rates to almost 99%, using movement of the patient during the study[52] to observe differences in movement between bowel gas in the duodenum or hepatic flexure and a contracted gallbladder full of stones. Diagnostic specificity is also aided by the observation of the wall–echo–shadow (WES) triad,[53] otherwise known as the 'double-arc-shadow sign'.[54] This complex consists of the reflective anterior wall of the gallbladder separated by a thin echo-poor rim. The echo-poor line from the reflective anterior surface of the stone, which casts a complete acoustic shadow (Fig. 15.28) represents either a small amount of residual bile or an echo-poor portion of the thickened gallbladder wall.

Persistent acoustic shadowing emanating from the gallbladder fossa may also be produced by a porcelain gallbladder, which is the term given to calcification of the gallbladder wall.[55] This condition is associated with gallstones in over 95% of cases, but the particular importance of recognising it lies in the increased incidence of both gallbladder carcinoma and cholangiocarcinoma (in 10–20% of cases); prophylactic cholecystectomy is usually advised (see section on gallbladder carcinoma, p. 325).

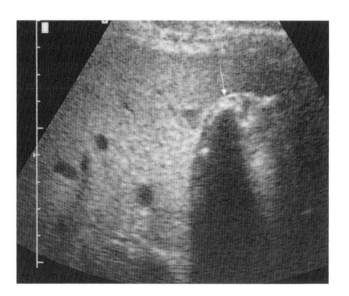

Fig. 15.28 **Double-arc shadow sign.** Echoes and acoustic shadow emanate from the gallbladder fossa (arrows).

Movement/layering/floating of stones

The gravity dependence of stones can be demonstrated by moving the patient during the ultrasound examination, usually by turning them into the left decubitus or right anterior oblique positions, but scans may also be performed with the patient sitting or standing. In this way previously hidden stones lying in the neck of the gallbladder may come into view, and the distinction between polyps and stones is facilitated (Figs 15.29 and 15.30).

Movement may also help when there are small stones from which it is proving difficult to demonstrate acoustic shadowing. If these stones can be collected into a group then the shadow may become more readily visible.[56]

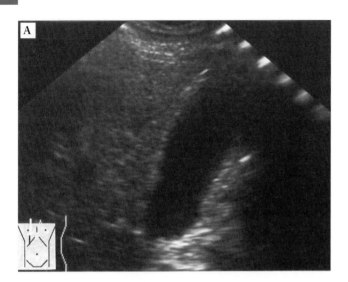

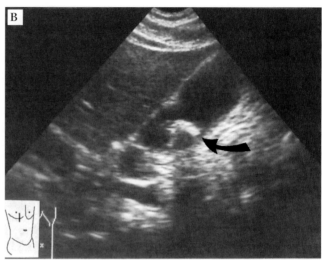

Fig. 15.29 Stone in the gallbladder. A: With the patient supine there is no evidence of any stone. **B:** A stone (arrowed) comes into view when the patient is turned right-side up.

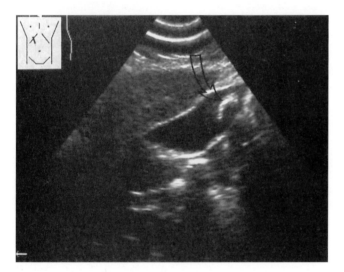

Fig. 15.30 Stone in the fundus. A stone (arrow) is clearly seen in the fundus of the gallbladder when the patient is scanned in the erect position.

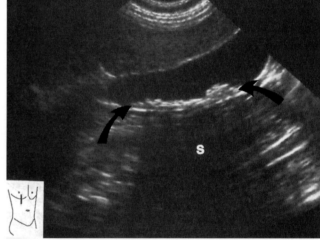

Fig. 15.31 Layered stones. A layer of stones on the posterior wall (arrows) is difficult to separate from the wall echoes, but note the distal shadowing (s).

Similarly, if small stones form a thin layer on the posterior wall of the gallbladder their echoes may erroneously be ascribed to the wall itself. Shadowing from small stones lying on the posterior wall of the gallbladder may be obscured by the high reflectivity of the wall itself or of the immediately adjacent bowel gas, causing a 'blooming' effect (Fig. 15.31). If such stones can be encouraged either to float across the gallbladder lumen or to clump together, the shadowing becomes obvious.

Difficulties can sometimes arise when stones float up to the anterior wall so that the gallbladder lumen is not visualised but, once again, movement of the patient is crucial in avoiding this pitfall (Fig. 15.32).

Milk of calcium bile is another instance where gravity dependence is an aid to ultrasound diagnosis. The appearances here are predominantly those of echoes and shadowing from the gallbladder fossa, but layering out of the milk of calcium is evident on the erect scans.[57,58]

Echogenic bile/biliary sludge

Non-shadowing gravity-dependent echoes within the gallbladder are variously referred to as 'biliary sludge' or 'echogenic bile'. Several pathological and physiological entities can result in these ultrasound appearances and, as neither of the above terms specifies a particular cause,

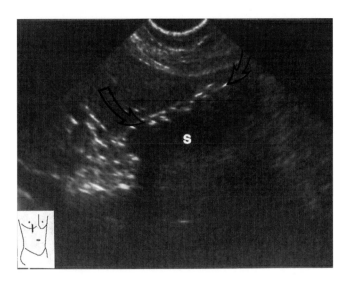

Fig. 15.32 Floating stones. The gallbladder lumen may be masked by the shadow (s) from stones (arrows) that float up to the anterior wall.

there is considerable confusion about the significance of these findings.

Echogenic bile may arise from pus or blood in the bile as a result of infection or trauma, or it may be seen in association with obvious stones in the gallbladder (Fig. 15.33).[59] In these cases the appearances are incontrovertibly pathological and, when taken in conjunction with the patient's history, physical signs and other ultrasound features, the diagnosis can be quite specific.

However, echogenic bile may also be seen when there is bile stasis in the absence of stone disease, and this may either follow biliary obstruction or occur for physiological reasons such as prolonged fasting,[60] in patients who are on parenteral nutrition[61] and after surgery on the gastro-

intestinal tract.[62] If the obstruction is relieved or if the gallbladder is rescanned after a normal diet has been resumed, the echoes will usually have disappeared from the bile. Occasionally the echoes may persist despite a normal HIDA scintiscan, and the significance of these findings has not yet been clarified (Fig. 15.34).

Some non-shadowing echoes within the gallbladder are caused by slice thickness artefacts. Clues that should alert the sonographer to this possibility include non-dependence on receiver gain and lack of change in height of debris between scans performed in transverse and longitudinal planes (Fig. 15.35).[63] Harmonic imaging helps to reduce artefactual echoes appearing within the gallbladder.

Occasionally non-shadowing echoes within the gallbladder may clump together, giving the so-called 'sludge balls' or 'tumefactive sludge' (Fig. 15.36). This may give rise to a diagnostic dilemma, as the appearances may mimic a soft tissue mass projecting into the gallbladder lumen, resulting in a false diagnosis of gallbladder tumour (Fig. 15.37).[64] Movement of the echoes with gravity should be the key to differentiating these conditions, but the bile in these cases may be thick and viscid so that movement of the echoes may be imperceptibly slow. A repeat scan with a normal diet in the interim should reveal the true nature of the problem.[65] Doppler signals are absent.

In vitro studies have shown that the echoes in 'biliary sludge' are caused by particles 5–10 μm in size, and chemical analysis reveals calcium bilirubinate granules together with some cholesterol crystals.[45] It has been postulated that the so-called 'sludge balls' may represent an early stage of the evolution of gallbladder stones,[66] but the relationship between the ability to form 'echogenic bile' on fasting and the lithogenicity of bile remains speculative at present.

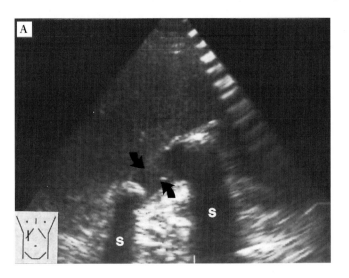

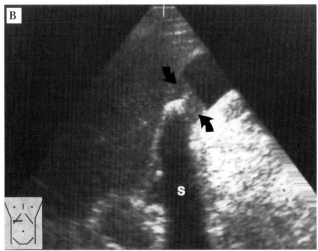

Fig. 15.33 Stones and echogenic bile. Stones giving rise to shadows (s) and non-shadowing echogenic bile (arrows). **A:** Longitudinal scan. **B:** Transverse scan.

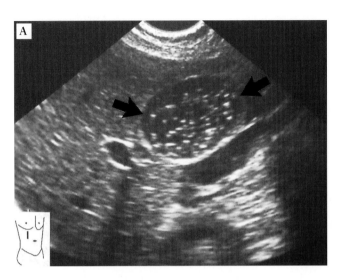

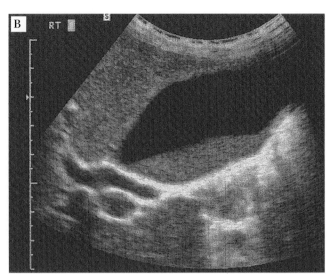

Fig. 15.34 Echogenic bile. A: In this patient who had been on intravenous feeding the gallbladder contains non-shadowing echogenic material. A rescan after a normal diet had been resumed showed identical appearances, but the patient was asymptomatic and both oral cholecystography and ^{99m}Tc-HIDA scans were normal. **B:** Gallbladder containing layering 'sludge' in a fasting patient.

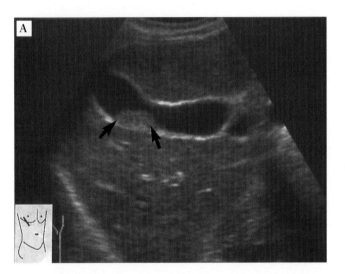

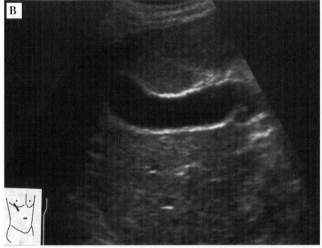

Fig. 15.35 False echogenic bile. A: Slice thickness artefact causing echoes within the gallbladder (arrows). **B:** The bile is echo-free after slight readjustment of the transducer angle.

Gallbladder wall thickening

In the fasting state the normal gallbladder is distended and has a wall thickness of 2 mm or less.[67] The normal anterior wall appears as a single, smooth, well defined reflecting structure, and its thickness can be measured accurately, whereas the posterior wall can be more difficult to measure because it is frequently in contact with air-containing bowel and the end-point is indistinct (Fig. 15.38).

When the gallbladder contracts in response to a fat-containing meal or the injection of cholecystokinin, the wall becomes thicker[68] and three distinct zones can then be identified: strongly reflecting outer and inner contours and an echo-poor intermediate layer (Fig. 15.38).[69]

The method of measuring gallbladder wall thickness is an important consideration as the ultrasound beam should be perpendicular to the wall to ensure that measurements are truly axial. This may mean that measurements of both anterior and posterior wall thicknesses cannot be made on the same scan section.

Minor angulation or decentring of the beam can cause 'pseudothickening' of the gallbladder wall,[70] and recognition of this artefact fuelled an interesting debate. It had been observed that the gallbladder wall appeared to be

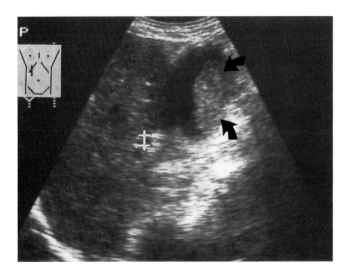

Fig. 15.36 **Tumefactive sludge** (arrows).

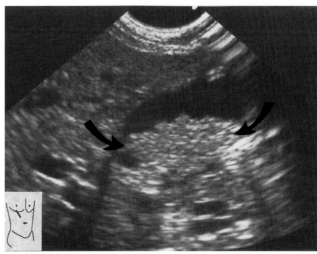

Fig. 15.37 **Lumpy bile.** Sludge giving the impression of a soft tissue mass (arrows), which led to an erroneous diagnosis of gallbladder carcinoma.

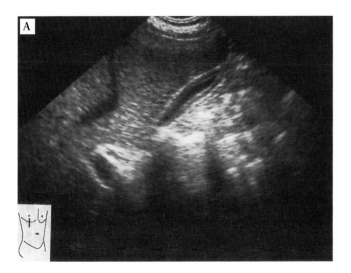

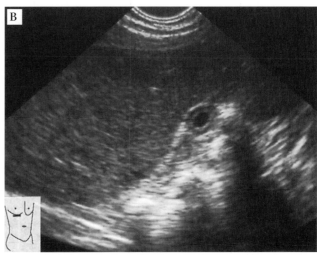

Fig. 15.38 **Non-fasting gallbladder.** Normal non-fasting gallbladder wall. **A:** Longitudinal scan. **B:** Transverse scan.

thickened in the presence of ascites (Fig. 15.39)[71] perhaps with oedema of the wall. Chronic alcoholics with hypoalbuminaemia have thickened gallbladder walls (Fig. 15.40), and in the majority of the cases there is no ascites in contact with the gallbladder.[72] It was therefore suggested that gallbladder wall thickening in the presence of ascites was a manifestation of underlying hypoalbuminaemia with a fluid shift from the intravascular to the extravascular space.

However, subsequent experience shows that gallbladder wall thickening can occur in ascites even when the serum albumin level is normal and care is taken over transducer angulation,[73] and that in these cases the wall thickening is caused by ascites *per se*, presumably owing to passive diffusion of fluid. In patients with cirrhosis, portal hypertension can give rise to thickening of the gallbladder wall – 'congestive cholecystopathy' due to venous dilatation – in the absence of either hypoalbuminaemia or ascites,[74] and colour or power Doppler can identify these varices.

The gallbladder wall thickens in response to a wide range of pathological processes (Fig. 15.41) (see Table 15.1) and this is thus a non-specific sign when used in isolation.[75] However, several of the conditions result in other ultrasound findings; the detection of gallbladder wall thickening may then provide useful contributory or confirmatory evidence.

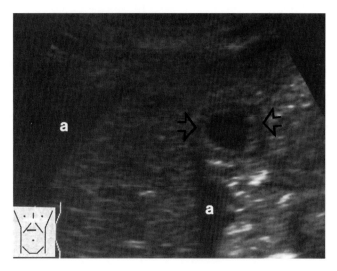

Fig. 15.39 Gallbladder in ascites. Thickened gallbladder wall (arrows) in the presence of ascites (a).

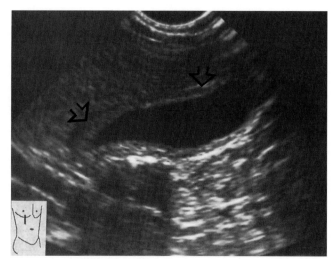

Fig. 15.40 Gallbladder wall in hypoalbuminaemia. Thickened gallbladder wall (arrows) in a patient with hypoalbuminaemia but no ascites.

Table 15.1 Causes of gallbladder wall thickening

Physiological
   Post-prandial

Inflammation
   Acute cholecystitis
   Chronic cholecystitis
   Sclerosing cholangitis[78]
   AIDS[79]
   Crohn's disease[80]

Non-inflammatory diseases
   Adenomyomatosis
   Carcinoma of gallbladder
   Leukaemia
   Multiple myeloma

Oedema of the gallbladder wall
   Ascites
   Hypoalbuminaemia
   Heart failure
   Portal hypertension
   Renal disease
   Malignant lymphatic obstruction[81]/lymphoma

Nearby inflammatory disease
   Acute viral hepatitis
   Alcoholic hepatitis[82]
   Acute pancreatitis
   Pericholecystic abscesses
   Hepatobiliary schistosomiasis[83]

Ultrasound signs may, of course, have uses other than purely diagnostic. In acute viral hepatitis gallbladder wall thickening has been shown to correlate well with the degree of liver cell necrosis and thus carries prognostic implications[76,77] (Fig. 15.42).

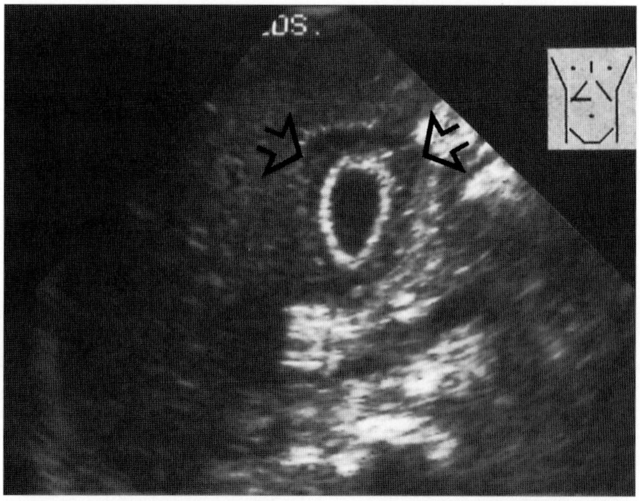

Fig. 15.41 Gallbladder in leukaemia. Grossly thickened gallbladder wall (arrows) in leukaemia.

Acute cholecystitis

A current therapeutic approach to patients who present with acute cholecystitis is to give immediate medical support in the form of analgesics and intravenous fluids, and antibiotics if necessary, and to perform a cholecystectomy as soon as the patient is fit for surgery, usually within the first 12–72 hours after admission.[84] This trend for urgent cholecystectomy demands that the diagnosis must be made quickly, and therefore for patients who present with acute right upper quadrant pain ultrasound is the initial imaging procedure of choice; it also enables a search to be made for other causes of the pain.[35]

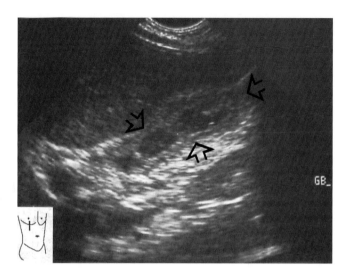

Fig. 15.42 Gallbladder in hepatitis. Thickened gallbladder wall (arrows) in acute viral hepatitis.

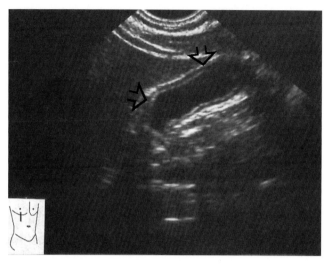

Fig. 15.43 Acute cholecystitis. Thickened gallbladder wall (arrows) with an echo-poor central zone due to acute cholecystitis.

Table 15.2 Ultrasound signs of acute cholecystitis

Major	Minor
Stones in gallbladder	Pericholecystic fluid
Oedema of gallbladder wall	Thickening of gallbladder wall
Gas in gallbladder wall	Intraluminal changes
Murphy's sign	Enlargement
	Round shape

There is no single ultrasound sign specific for the diagnosis of acute cholecystitis; rather there is a range of findings which are conveniently discussed as either 'major' or 'minor' signs (Table 15.2).

Most studies have indicated that the sensitivity for a major sign of acute cholecystitis is 81–86% and the specificity 94–98%. The addition of a minor sign increases the sensitivity of ultrasound to 90–98%.[85] Not reflected in these figures is the ability to diagnose non-biliary sources of right upper quadrant pain in as many as 35% of patients without gallbladder disease.[86]

Increased gallbladder wall thickness (Fig. 15.43) is well documented in acute cholecystitis[87,88] but, as discussed above, it is found in many other conditions and is thus a minor sign. However, more obvious oedema of the gallbladder wall, which is recognisable by either a continuous echo-poor rim around the gallbladder or by a focal echo-poor zone in the wall, is a major sign of acute cholecystitis, provided that other causes of oedema, such as hypoalbuminaemia, heart failure and other local inflammation, have been excluded (Fig. 15.44). The echo-poor zones probably represent the accumulation of oedema, inflammatory exudate and/or haemorrhage. It is most easily demonstrated between the liver and the anterior wall of the gallbladder, as the echo-poor bowel wall that is often

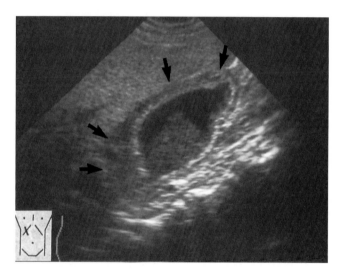

Fig. 15.44 Acute cholecystitis. Thickened gallbladder wall with an echo-poor 'halo' (arrows) due to acute cholecystitis. Note also the 'lumpy bile' giving echoes in the lumen.

adjacent to the posterior gallbladder wall may give a false positive 'halo sign'.[89]

Gallbladder tenderness is popularly known as the 'ultrasonic Murphy's sign',[90] but it does differ significantly from the clinical sign described by Murphy and modified by Moynihan.[91] In the clinical sign the examiner's left hand is placed on the costal margin so that the thumb lies over the fundus of the gallbladder. The thumb exerts moderate pressure and the patient is asked to take a deep breath. The sign is positive if the patient 'catches their breath' when the descending diaphragm causes the inflamed gallbladder to impinge on the thumb. A positive ultrasonic Murphy's sign is present when the tenderness is

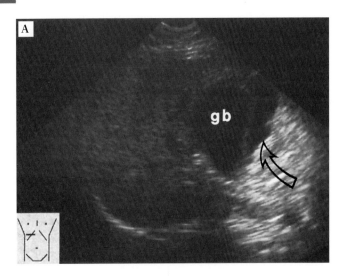
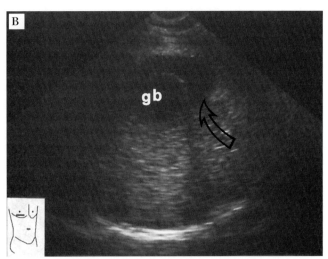

Fig. 15.45 Gangrene. Gangrenous gallbladder wall with small pericholecystic leak (arrow). A: Patient supine. B: Patient in right anterior oblique position (gb – gallbladder).

maximal over the ultrasonically located gallbladder,[92] thus ensuring that the pain is elicited only during image-verified deformation of the gallbladder.[68] The combination of stones in the gallbladder and a positive ultrasound Murphy's sign is highly specific for acute cholecystitis (92%).[93]

Acute cholecystitis may progress to gangrenous cholecystitis, which may perforate, resulting in a pericholecystic abscess (Figs 15.45 and 15.46) or peritonitis. The morbidity and mortality associated with this condition are considerably higher than with uncomplicated acute cholecystitis, and it is important to look for ultrasound signs that may expedite the diagnosis and emergency surgery. Marked irregularity or asymmetrical thickening of the

gallbladder wall reflect ulceration, haemorrhage, necrosis and intramural micro-abscesses.[94]

Empyema of the gallbladder is difficult to recognise on ultrasound because the typical finding of sludge (non-shadowing gravity-dependent echoes) may be caused by many processes other than debris or pus (Fig. 15.47).[95,96] Intraluminal membranes, caused by fibrinous strands of exudate and sloughing of the gallbladder mucosa, are features of gangrene of the gallbladder (Fig. 15.48).[97] Interestingly, only 33% of patients with gangrenous gallbladders have a positive ultrasonic Murphy's sign,[98] compared to the 95% prevalence in patients with acute non-gangrenous cholecystitis.[92] Presumably the lack of pain is due to necrosis of the nerves in the muscular and serosal layers of the gallbladder.

Pericholecystic fluid collections may be caused by localised peritonitis or by leaks from perforation of the gallbladder wall. These latter may vary in size and complexity, from a small bile collection as a result of a microperforation to a true pericholecystic abscess (Fig. 15.49).[99] The ultrasound appearances of such abscesses range from predominantly echo-free to predominantly highly reflective, although increased through transmission of sound remains apparent.[100]

Gas in the gallbladder wall – the hallmark of emphysematous cholecystitis – derives from gas-forming organisms in the bile, and is one of the major ultrasound signs of acute cholecystitis. It may be recognised by highly reflective areas within a thickened gallbladder wall, with shadowing and reverberations distally (Fig. 15.50).[101–103] There may also be gas within the gallbladder lumen, which may make it difficult to distinguish the gallbladder from a loop of bowel. Repositioning the patient may help, and the gas in the gallbladder wall may shift with gravity[104] and on real-time observation the gas in the lumen may be seen to

Fig. 15.46 Pericholecystic collection. The fluid within a pericholecystic leak contains non-shadowing echoes caused by pus (arrow).

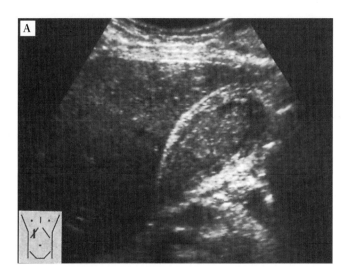 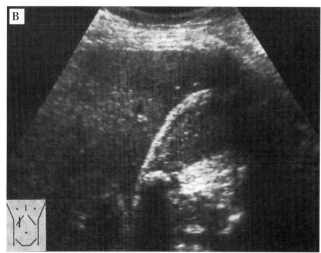

Fig. 15.47 Empyema of the gallbladder. A: Thickened wall and low-level echoes filling the lumen. **B:** The same case showing a stone in the neck of the gallbladder.

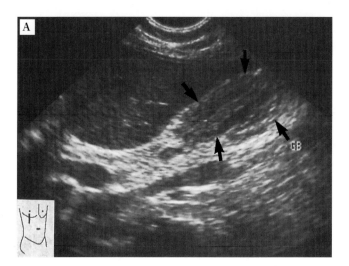 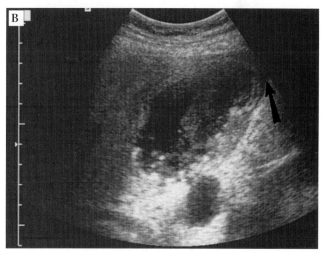

Fig. 15.48 Gangrenous cholecystitis. Gangrenous gallbladder wall and typical intraluminal membranes representing desquamated mucosa. **A:** Longitudinal scan. **B:** A rim of fluid (arrow) is forming around the fundus of this gallbladder.

'effervesce'.[105] Although this condition is rare it is important to recognise it because of its strong association with gangrene and perforation of the gallbladder.[106] Owing to the increasing use of high-resolution ultrasound in suspected biliary disease, however, the condition is being diagnosed with increasing frequency, and a spectrum of severity is now recognised, so that conservative treatment may be considered in some patients.[107] Emphysematous cholecystitis may occur without gallstones, usually in diabetics: it is postulated that ischaemia of the gallbladder wall may be a primary factor in such cases.

In 5–10% of cases acute cholecystitis is acalculous[108] and frequently occurs as a complication of a prolonged or severe illness, such as recent major surgery, burns, sepsis or prolonged hypotension (ischaemia may be the common factor), and in general debility and diabetes.[109] Histologically the changes in the gallbladder wall are similar to calculous cholecystitis, although gangrene and perforation are more common, presumably because of delayed diagnosis and treatment. The lack of stones and the inability to elicit the ultrasonic Murphy's sign in a comatose patient contribute to the diagnostic difficulty, although thickening of the gallbladder wall in association with a lack of response of the gallbladder to cholecystokinin, distension and the presence of sludge are helpful signs (Fig. 15.51).[110] Doppler may show hyperaemia in the

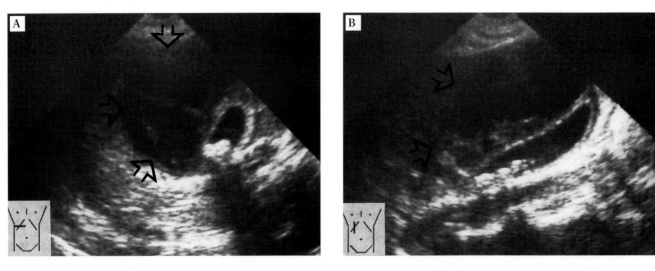

Fig. 15.49 Large pericholecystic abscess (arrows) extending into the liver from the thick-walled gallbladder, which is seen to contain stones. **A:** Longitudinal scan. **B:** Transverse scan.

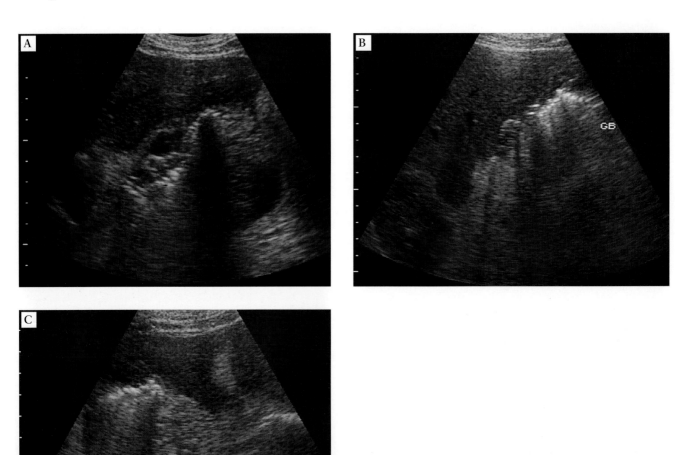

Fig. 15.50 Emphysematous cholecystitis. Thickened gallbladder wall containing areas of high reflectivity with distal shadowing due to gas. The gallbladder lumen is filled with echoes from infected bile. **A:** Longitudinal, **B:** transverse, **C:** transverse with patient in right anterior oblique position.

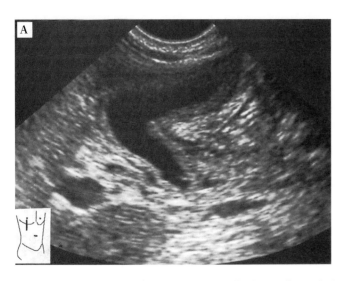
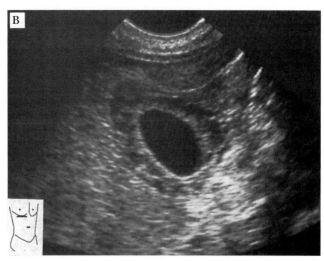

Fig. 15.51 Acalculous cholecystitis. Thickened gallbladder wall in acalculous cholecystitis. **A:** Longitudinal scan. **B:** Transverse scan.

gallbladder wall during the acute inflammatory phase, and failure of the gallbladder to change in size or shape on serial scans may imply cystic duct obstruction. Diagnostic specificity may be improved by ultrasound-guided percutaneous aspiration of the gallbladder, so that bacteria and/or leukocytes can be detected in the bile,[111] but initial enthusiasm for the technique has become tempered by the limitation that a negative result does not exclude acute cholecystitis.[112] This is only to be expected when it is remembered that only about half the patients who come to surgery for acute cholecystitis have infected bile from which aerobic or anaerobic organisms may be cultured.[84]

Chronic cholecystitis

Chronic cholecystitis, which may cause recurrent right upper quadrant pain, is almost always found in association with gallstones, although the exact pathogenesis is unclear and the 'chicken and egg' debate continues to rage. There is a chronic inflammatory cell infiltrate throughout all the layers of the wall, which becomes thickened with fibrosis in both the subserosal and the muscular layers, resulting in overall shrinkage. In this clinical context the ultrasonic demonstration of stones in the gallbladder, with or without thickening of the wall, is usually taken to be diagnostic, and has a sensitivity ranging from 90% to 98%, with specificity consistently in the 94–98% range (Fig. 15.52).[85]

Endoscopic retrograde cholangiography has been recommended on the rare occasion when ultrasound is negative but convincing symptoms persist.[35]

Hyperplastic cholecystoses

In some cases of chronic cholecystitis the epithelial lining of the gallbladder extends between the muscle bundles, giving

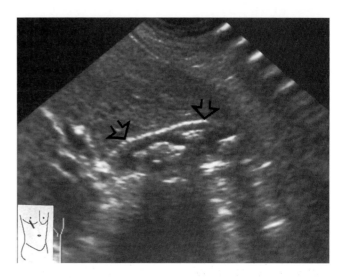

Fig. 15.52 Chronic cholecystitis with stones in a thick-walled gallbladder (arrows).

rise to deeply situated gland-like structures known as Rokitansky–Aschoff sinuses. When extensive these diverticula form numerous gland-like spaces lined by epithelial cells that extend throughout the gallbladder wall. A focal increase in wall thickness may result in localised narrowing of the gallbladder lumen, giving rise to the appearance of a stricture. The term 'cholecystitis glandularis proliferans' has been applied to this condition. However, these 'hyperplastic' changes in the gallbladder wall may occur in the absence of either gallstones or inflammatory infiltrates: the condition is then known as adenomyomatosis.[113] This is considered to be quite distinct from chronic cholecystitis and, although excessive intraluminal pressure has been suggested as the cause, its exact aetiology remains unclear.

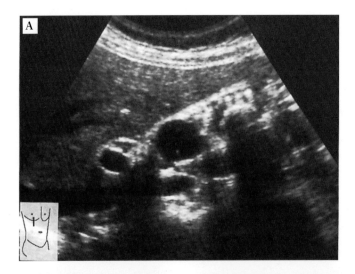

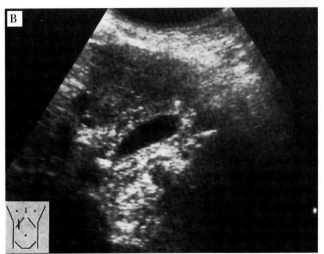
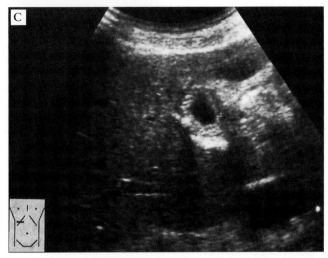

Fig. 15.53 Adenomyomatosis. A: Localised adenomyomatosis confined to the gallbladder fundus showing the typical 'diamond ring' appearance caused by concretions in the dilated sinuses. Note the solitary large gallstone. **B:** Generalised adenomyomatosis, longitudinal and **C:** transverse scan in another case.

The ultrasound features of adenomyomatosis are now well recognised.[114] There is diffuse or segmental thickening of the gallbladder wall, with intramural diverticula which may be echo-free if they contain fluid bile, or highly reflective if they contain bile concretions. Segmental and eccentric wall thickening produces mid-cavity strictures and the high-amplitude periluminal foci (caused by aggregates of solid bile elements in the Rokitansky–Aschoff sinuses) give a typical 'diamond ring' appearance on transverse sections (Fig. 15.53).[115]

The clinical significance of adenomyomatosis of the gallbladder is controversial as it may be found in asymptomatic individuals. However, many patients with adenomyomatosis do improve after cholecystectomy, especially if the symptoms were more suggestive of biliary colic than of vague dyspepsia, or if gallstones are found in association with the adenomyomatosis.[113]

The 'strawberry gallbladder' of cholesterolosis is another non-inflammatory condition of the gallbladder and is the result of the accumulation of lipids in the mucosa of the gallbladder wall. The resulting surface nodules are usually less than 1 mm in diameter and cannot therefore be recognised on ultrasound. However, larger polypoid excrescences forming cholesterol polyps sometimes develop, and these can be detected as small reflective foci attached to the wall of the gallbladder. They may be single or multiple, do not generally cast acoustic shadows, and do not move with changes in patient position (Fig. 15.54).[116]

The aetiology of cholesterolosis is not fully understood, although the mucosal changes might arise simply because of increased cholesterol uptake from bile containing extra cholesterol.[117] Although cholecystectomy is unlikely to benefit patients with vague dyspeptic symptoms, it may

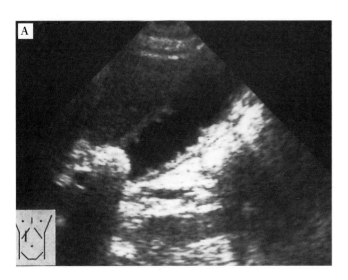 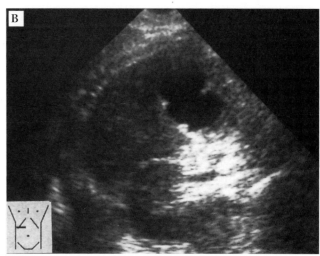

Fig. 15.54 Multiple cholesterol polyps projecting into the lumen of a gallbladder with a stone impacted in the neck. **A:** Longitudinal scan. **B:** Transverse scan.

help those in whom the history suggests biliary colic, or when there are associated gallstones.[113,117]

Polyps

Polyps of the gallbladder include pseudotumours such as inflammatory polyps, cholesterol polyps and adenomyomas, the localised form of adenomyomatosis. The typical ultrasound appearance is of a small reflective intraluminal structure which is fixed to the gallbladder wall and does not cast an acoustic shadow (Figs 15.55 and 15.56). Small reverberation artefacts may often be seen in the fluid posterior to the polyps. They are common and, in the absence of accompanying gallstones, are probably not clinically significant.

The commonest type of true benign neoplasm is the adenoma, which can be either sessile or papillary, and is usually solitary.[118] Adenomatous gallbladder polyps have been described in Peutz–Jeghers syndrome;[119] 10% are multiple, and 10% show evidence of carcinoma *in situ*.[120] Intestinal metaplasia can be found in large adenomas and may be a premalignant change[121] and, as in the intestinal tract, it is probably the larger adenomas that undergo malignant transformation. Adenomas are usually incidental findings, but they can cause biliary colic. The typical ultrasound appearance is of a soft tissue mass projecting into the gallbladder lumen. It remains fixed to the gallbladder wall despite patient movement and does not cast a true acoustic shadow, though edge shadowing can be confusing (Fig. 15.57). Because of the probability of an

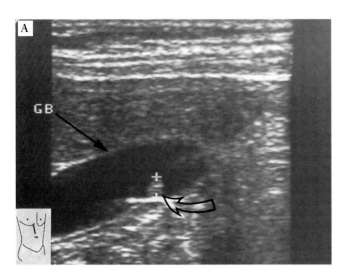 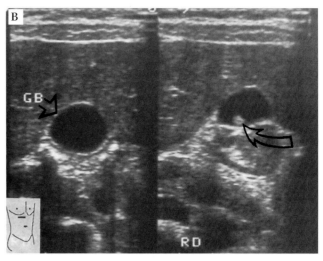

Fig. 15.55 Hyperplastic gallbladder polyp (curved arrows) in the gallbladder. **A:** Longitudinal scan. **B:** Transverse scans.

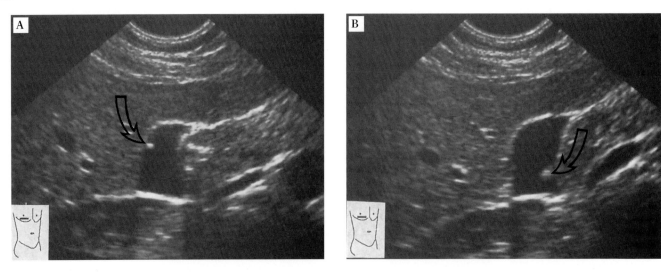

Fig. 15.56 **Two hyperplastic polyps** (arrows) within the same gallbladder. **A:** Transverse scan near the neck of the gallbladder. **B:** Transverse scan near the fundus.

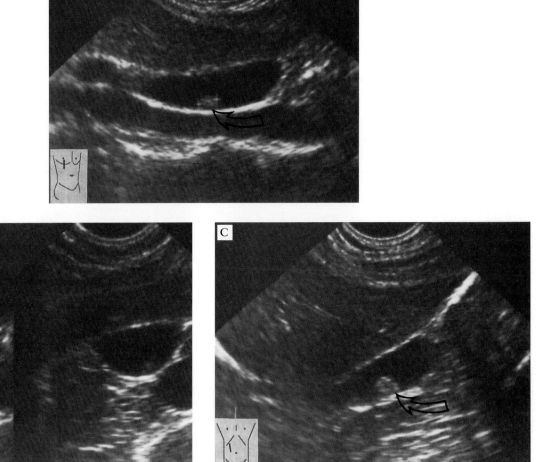

Fig. 15.57 **Adenomatous polyp** 7 mm in diameter (arrows). **A:** Longitudinal scan. **B:** Transverse scans. **C:** Scan with patient upright.

adenoma/carcinoma sequence, cholecystectomy is advisable, even for asymptomatic polyps.[122]

There are other benign neoplasms of the gallbladder, including fibroma, lipoma, myoma, carcinoid and haemangioma, but they are all extremely rare.[123]

Carcinoma

Carcinoma of the gallbladder is a highly malignant tumour characterised by early metastases and a rapidly downhill clinical course. It is the fifth most common malignancy of the gastrointestinal tract, comprising 1–3% of all cancers and affecting females four times as commonly as males; its prevalence increases with age. There is a correlation with gallstones (80–90%) and with chronic cholecystitis, suggesting that chronic inflammation of the gallbladder mucosa may result in a dysplasia which goes on to neoplastic transformation.

Diagnosis of this tumour is usually not made until local spread and metastases have occurred, but the ultrasound detection of gallbladder wall irregularities,[124] or of a complex reflective mass obliterating the gallbladder lumen,[125] may enable the diagnosis to be made pre-operatively.

The most common finding is of a large solid mass filling the gallbladder bed (Fig. 15.58).[126–129] This appearance is non-specific and the underlying nature of the mass has to be guessed at by the lack of visualisation of a separate gallbladder lumen or the presence of stones within the mass. The tumour may also form an irregular polypoid mass within the gallbladder lumen, or irregular thickening of the gallbladder wall which may be focal or diffuse, or a combination of the two. Local extension of the tumour into the adjacent liver is also readily identifiable with ultrasound,[130] but CT is still the method of choice for staging, particularly the detection of lymphatic and peritoneal spread.

Approximately 25% of patients with a porcelain gallbladder (calcification of the gallbladder wall) will have associated carcinoma, and the lesion may be obscured by the acoustic shadow arising from the calcified anterior wall. Differentiating a porcelain gallbladder from a gallbladder full of stones is important because of this high risk of malignancy. With careful scanning the non-calcified anterior wall of the gallbladder can be seen in the case of stones,[53,54] whereas the calcified posterior wall of a porcelain gallbladder may be seen, giving the diagnostic appearance of a biconvex curvilinear reflective structure (Fig. 15.59).[55] The development of a carcinoma within a porcelain gallbladder can be detected if there is local or diffuse thickening of the gallbladder wall external to the calcified portion, an eccentric mass arising from the gallbladder wall, or if there is evidence of biliary obstruction, porta hepatis or peripancreatic lymphadenopathy, or liver metastases.[89] Although the overall prognosis for this tumour remains bleak, with a mean survival of less than 5 months from the time of diagnosis, ultrasound may facilitate treatment of early and curable carcinomas by the fortuitous detection of tumours in patients who are asymptomatic or who have symptoms attributable to the coexistent stones.[131] In countries where the rate of cholecystectomy for cholelithiasis has increased, there has been a corresponding decrease in the mortality from gallbladder carcinoma.[132]

As with any other abdominal viscus, bloodborne metastases may find their way to the gallbladder – albeit rarely – and asymmetrical wall thickening or polypoid intraluminal masses may be indistinguishable from primary gallbladder cancer (Fig. 15.60).[133] Malignant melanoma is the

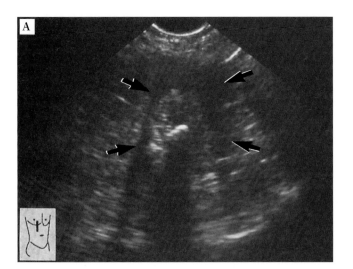 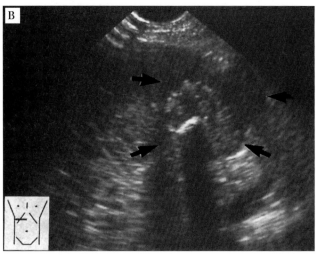

Fig. 15.58 Carcinoma of the gallbladder producing a large, ill-defined solid mass (arrows) in the gallbladder fossa – note the stone within the mass. **A:** Longitudinal scan. **B:** Transverse scan.

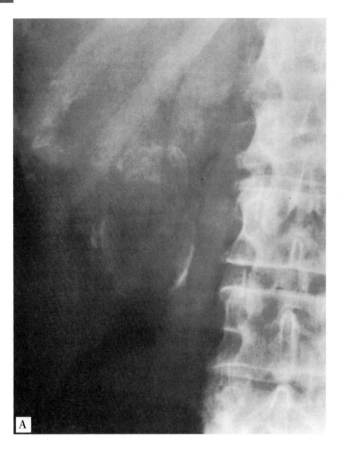

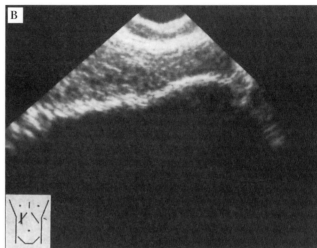

Fig. 15.59 Porcelain gallbladder. A: X-ray showing typical gallbladder wall calcification. **B:** Scan of gallbladder area showing total reflection of sound at the gallbladder wall. Figure courtesy of Dr A. E. A. Joseph.

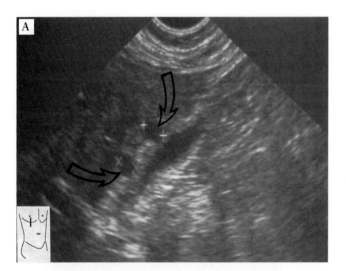

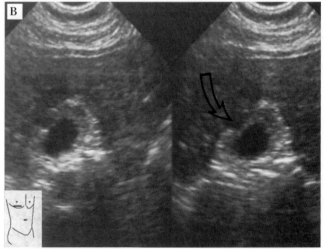

Fig. 15.60 Metastatic deposits (arrows) from an anaplastic lung primary are seen in the gallbladder wall as echo-poor nodules.
A: Longitudinal scan. **B:** Transverse scans. **C:** Metastases from malignant melanoma giving rise to a clearly defined, slightly heterogeneous soft tissue lesion arising from the gallbladder wall; oblique scan. **D:** Transverse scan.

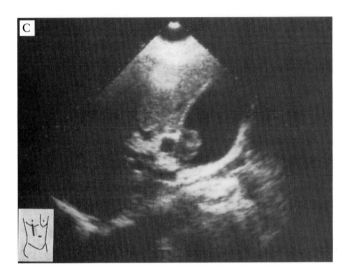

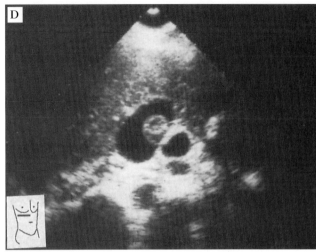

Fig. 15.60 C and D.

most common source of gallbladder metastases, which may be asymptomatic or simulate acute cholecystitis.[134]

Worms

Ascariasis

Infestation by the roundworm *Ascaris lumbricoides* is endemic in the Far East, CIS, Latin America and Africa, and worldwide is probably second only to gallstones as a cause of acute biliary symptoms. The adult worm is 15–50 cm long and some 5 mm thick, and lives mainly in the jejunum. It has a propensity to migrate up into the common bile duct, from where it may enter the gallbladder or the intrahepatic

bile ducts. It may then cause biliary colic or acute cholecystitis. Ultrasound scans demonstrate the worms in the common duct or gallbladder as single or multiple strips, coils, or amorphous fragments (Fig. 15.61).[135] The writhing movements of the living worm are striking on real-time scanning.

Clonorchiasis

Humans ingest the liver fluke *Clonorchis sinensis* by eating raw freshwater fish, and the disease is endemic in the Far East. The adult worms are some 5 mm in length and reside in the medium or small intrahepatic bile ducts, and occasionally also in the extrahepatic ducts and gall-

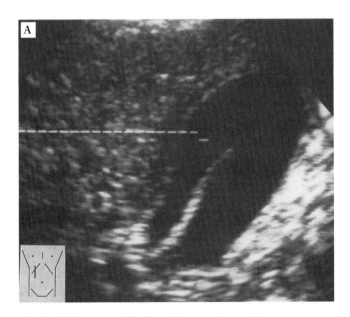

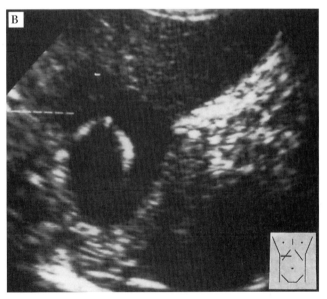

Fig. 15.61 Worms in gallbladder. A: Longitudinal and B: transverse scan showing a curved worm in the gallbladder lumen.

bladder. Intrahepatic duct dilatation and cholangitis are the main features of the disease and are the main ultrasound findings, but the parasites can be demonstrated in the gallbladder, where they cause floating or dependent discrete non-shadowing intraluminal reflective foci, which are fusiform in shape and measure 3–6 mm. Spontaneous movements of these structures have been observed on ultrasound, representing the movement of living worms. Thickening of the gallbladder wall has also been noted.[136]

Liver flukes

Adult fasciola worms have recently been observed within the gallbladder on ultrasound as irregular, linear reflective structures 20–30 mm long,[137] and similar findings have been documented in the gallbladder of a patient with *Opisthorchis viverrinii*.[138]

Hydrops

Enlargement of the gallbladder is a subjective judgement as the range of normal variations precludes precise ranges for the normal dimensions. The long axis measurement should not exceed 10 cm and the short axis 5 cm, but these figures are only a rough guide as many abnormally distended gallbladders are smaller than this, and some normal gallbladders are larger.

There are several conditions in which the gallbladder enlarges (e.g. diabetes, pregnancy,[139] and in response to narcotic and anticholinergic drugs),[140] but the term 'hydrops' is probably best reserved for gallbladders which are distended by blockage of the cystic duct, and in these the raised intraluminal pressure gives a more spherical and tense appearance (Fig. 15.62).

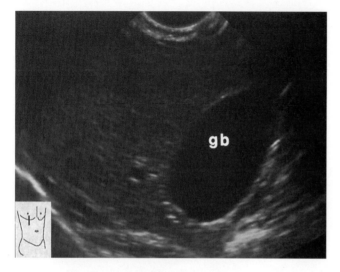

Fig. 15.62 Hydrops of the gallbladder due to mucocutaneous lymph node (Kawasaki) syndrome in a child aged 3 months.

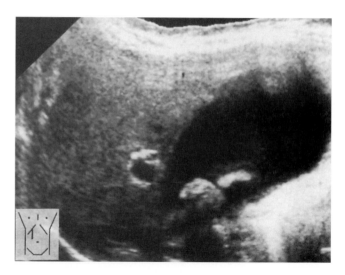

Fig. 15.63 Mucocele of the gallbladder. The gallbladder is distended, thin-walled, and contains stones.

Acute dilatation of the gallbladder may develop in children with typhoid, leptospirosis or other systemic infections.[141] It has also been reported in mucocutaneous lymph node (Kawasaki) syndrome,[142,143] Sjögren's disease[144] and systemic sclerosis.[145] Chronic dilatation may be due to stones in Hartman's pouch or the cystic duct, giving rise to a mucocele of the gallbladder (Fig. 15.63).

Microgallbladder

If the gallbladder measures less than 3 × 1 cm in the fasting state it is classified as a microgallbladder, and this occurs in approximately 30% of patients with cystic fibrosis.[146] The gallbladder usually contains colourless viscid mucus – 'white bile' – and the cystic duct may be atrophic or occluded with mucus. There is an increased incidence of gallstones in cystic fibrosis because of a combination of factors, which include loss of bile salts because of malabsorption, increased biliary lipid composition and bile stasis; thickening of the gallbladder wall may develop if secondary cholecystitis occurs (Fig. 15.64).[147]

Bile duct pathology

Jaundice

Jaundice is caused by an increase in the serum bilirubin level above the normal range of 1–15 mg/l (1.7–25 μmol/l). When the increase is mild its presence may only be detected on biochemical analysis of the blood, but when the bilirubin level rises sufficiently there is a clinically detectable yellow discoloration of the skin, sclerae and mucous membranes. The pathological mechanisms that give rise to jaundice

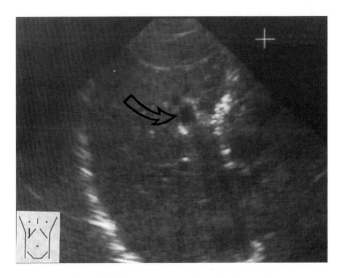

Fig. 15.64 Microgallbladder (arrow) in a fasted patient with cystic fibrosis.

can be classified into three main groups: haemolytic (or pre-hepatic), hepatocellular (or hepatic) and obstructive.

The haemolytic nature of jaundice is readily apparent from haematological and biochemical blood tests, and imaging has little part to play in diagnosis or management.

There are many causes of hepatocellular jaundice, most of which are diagnosed on biochemical, serological or histological examinations of the blood or liver, but some cause structural changes in the liver which may be detectable on ultrasound. The ultrasonographic features of parenchymal liver diseases, such as the various types of hepatitis and cirrhosis, of primary and secondary malignant disease of the liver, and of inflammatory processes such as pyogenic liver abscess, are discussed in Chapters 10, 11 and 12. Ultrasound may suggest the cause of hepatocellular jaundice and it can be used to guide a needle for a diagnostic aspiration or biopsy (see Ch. 7).

Obstructive jaundice results from a block in the pathway between the site of bile conjugation in the liver cells and the entry of bile into the duodenum through the ampulla. The block may be intrahepatic, at the biochemical, cellular or canalicular level, or extrahepatic in the bile ducts. It is this latter group of causes that are referred to as surgical jaundice, to simplify their distinction from all other causes of jaundice, which are then referred to as medical.

Although the cause can often be diagnosed on the basis of a careful history and examination, the differing managements of medical and surgical jaundice make early differential diagnosis essential. Conventional blood tests usually confirm the presence of cholestasis (obstruction), but provide little or even misleading information about the site of obstruction and its cause. A variety of techniques for visualising the biliary tree is now available and, because some are expensive and some involve risks, it is important that patients are investigated in a sensible and rational way.[148] Ultrasound scores highly on the grounds of safety, simplicity, cost and accuracy, and has therefore come to be universally regarded as the best initial imaging procedure.[149]

Ultrasound is very accurate in diagnosing surgical jaundice, detecting dilatation of the intrahepatic or extrahepatic biliary tree in 85–95% of patients with proven obstruction,[150–156] and has a high positive predictive value for obstruction, with false positive findings in less than 5%. It is also highly accurate at defining the level of obstruction, although the exact cause may be diagnosed in only about a third of patients.

Obstruction may occur without duct dilatation (see below) and thus there is a false negative rate of up to 25% in patients with gallstone jaundice in most of the early published series,[157] although more recently the reported sensitivity for the detection of choledocholithiasis has increased to over 80%.[158,159] These results are attributable to improvements in equipment and to meticulous scanning technique.

Bile duct dilatation

The ultrasound diagnosis of obstructive or surgical jaundice depends upon the detection of bile duct dilatation.

The normal bile ducts within the liver are generally too small to be visualised on ultrasound, although progressive improvements in spatial resolution reveal fine ductal structures in 'easy to scan' subjects. The larger main right and left bile ducts can be identified as tubular structures running anterior and parallel to the right and left branches of the portal vein, and measure up to 2 mm in diameter in the non-dilated system (Fig. 15.65).[160,161] The diameter of the normal common duct at the porta hepatis should be less than 5 mm,[162,163] increasing slightly (less than 6 mm) as the duct runs caudally in the free edge of the lesser omentum[164] and within the head of the pancreas. The diameter of the non-obstructed duct does increase with age,[165] after cholecystectomy,[166–168] or if there has been previous obstruction.[169]

Dilatation of the intrahepatic bile ducts results in one or more of the following ultrasound findings:

1   parallel channel sign,
2   double-barrel shotgun sign,
3   stylet sign,
4   'too many tubes' in the liver,
5   stellate pattern near the porta,
6   increased sound transmission distal to ducts.

The 'parallel channel'[170] and 'double-barrelled shotgun'[171] signs depend upon the bile ducts dilating to become equal to or greater than the diameter of the adjacent portal vein branch. When scanned along their long axes these structures are seen as two parallel channels, whereas in cross-section the appearance is apparently that of a double-barrelled shotgun (Fig. 15.66). When the parallel channels occur in a

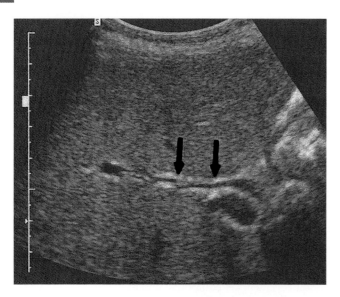

Fig. 15.65 Normal intrahepatic bile duct. Right hepatic duct (arrows) seen running anterior to right branch of portal vein.

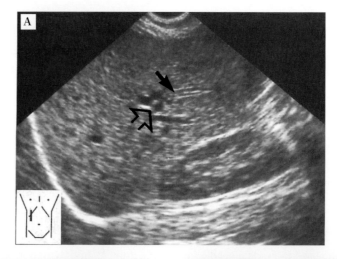

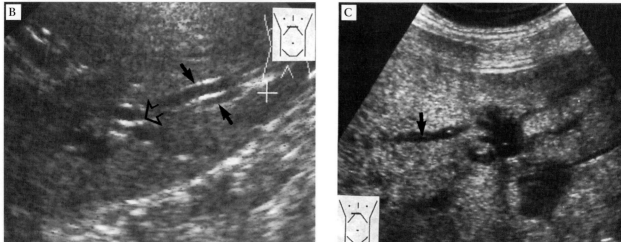

Fig. 15.66 Dilated intrahepatic bile duct. 'Parallel channel' (arrows), and 'double-barrelled shotgun' (open arrows) signs. A: Longitudinal scan. B: Transverse scan (magnified). C: Stylet sign; the linear echoes (arrow) represent the interface between the dilated bile duct and the adjacent portal vein.

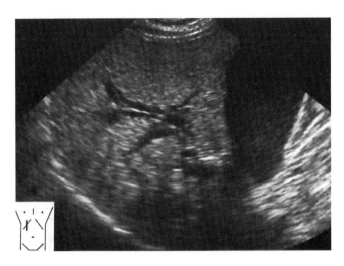

Fig. 15.67 **Dilated intrahepatic bile ducts** – 'too many tubes' within the liver. Note the distended gallbladder with echogenic bile.

a characteristic stellate pattern. This is in contrast to the branching pattern of the portal veins, which has a more orderly arrangement whereby the peripheral branches all take origin from the main right and left branches (Fig. 15.68).[174]

Finally, the fluid in the dilated bile ducts is clear bile and ultrasound is transmitted without attenuation. With the time–gain compensation (swept gain) set to compensate for the liver's attenuation, increased through-transmission of sound (enhancement) is seen beyond dilated ducts but not beyond the intrahepatic blood vessels (Fig. 15.69). Although this sign is useful when distinguishing dilated ducts from blood vessels, the patchy enhancement beyond the dilated bile ducts disturbs the normally uniform echo pattern of the liver parenchyma, so that it becomes difficult to detect small metastatic lesions with confidence.

fatty liver the outer walls may be masked by the high reflectivity of the liver parenchyma. In such a case all that is seen is the interface between the vein and the duct, giving rise to the 'stylet' sign (Fig. 15.66C).[172]

In a patient with dilated intrahepatic ducts there is an immediate overall impression of 'too many tubes' in the liver, and when the scans are carefully analysed it can be seen that these tubes do not correspond to arteries or veins, and must therefore be bile ducts (Fig. 15.67).[173] Colour Doppler is useful in making the distinction between dilated ducts, which do not display flow, and hypertrophied hepatic arteries, which may produce a similar appearance to the parallel channel sign in portal hypertension.

The branching pattern of the intrahepatic bile duct system converges towards the porta hepatis, and this gives

Obstruction without dilatation

Unfortunately, complete reliance upon the ultrasound detection of duct dilatation to detect obstruction leads to a false negative diagnosis in some cases, as it has been well documented that obstruction may occur without dilatation.[175–178] If the obstruction is of recent onset the ducts may not have had time to dilate, despite the onset of jaundice.[179] Rescanning after an interval of a couple of days may well detect these cases, and is recommended if the ultrasound findings do not fit with the clinical impression.

It is possible to detect stones in non-dilated ducts on ultrasound, but a negative scan in suspicious clinical circumstances should lead to further investigations, such as CT scanning or direct cholangiography via the percutaneous trans-hepatic or endoscopic retrograde routes.[148,159]

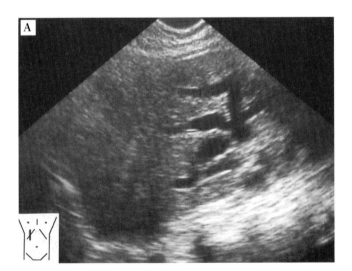

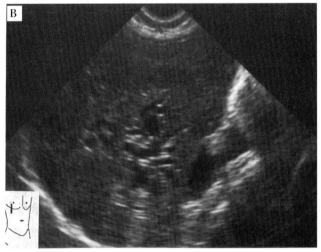

Fig. 15.68 **Dilated intrahepatic bile ducts** – 'stellate branching pattern'. A: Patient supine. B: Patient in right anterior oblique position.

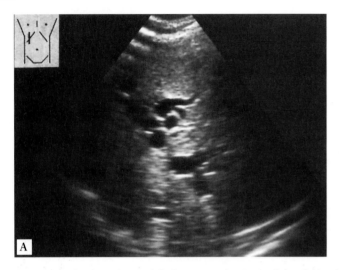 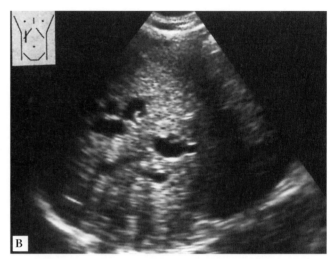

Fig. 15.69 Dilated intrahepatic bile ducts. A: 'Enhancement beyond dilated ducts' results in **B:** patchy echo texture within liver.

Other causes of obstruction without dilatation are encasement of the common duct by tumour[177] or fibrosis of the duct wall, as in sclerosing cholangitis[151,180] and, in chronic hepatitis or cirrhosis, dilatation of intrahepatic ducts may be impossible owing to rigidity of the surrounding liver parenchyma.

Although direct cholangiography remains the 'gold standard' for the exclusion of biliary obstruction, adjuncts to ultrasound scanning, such as fatty meal sonography[181–184] and endosonography,[185] offer improved accuracy and significantly lessen the false negative rate.

Dilatation without jaundice

Ultrasound detection of biliary dilatation may precede the onset of clinically detectable jaundice[186–188] in several different clinical settings:

1   when segments of the intrahepatic biliary tree are obstructed by tumour while other parts remain unobstructed,
2   when stones in the common duct cause a ball-valve effect, the intermittent relief of obstruction allows clearance of the bile so that jaundice may not develop,
3   in chronic incomplete or slowly progressive obstruction, such as may be caused by tumour in the head of the pancreas or chronic pancreatitis, the wider extrahepatic portions of the biliary tree dilate more, in keeping with Laplace's law.

These pathological conditions must be differentiated from the non-pathological dilatation of the common duct with increasing age[165] and from post-cholecystectomy dilatation;[165–167] fatty meal sonography may again prove helpful.[181–184] However, it should also be noted that although the serum bilirubin may not be elevated, so that the patient remains anicteric, the serum level of alkaline phosphatase is more sensitive and is almost always raised if the duct dilatation is pathological, and this finding should aid the decision to proceed to CT or direct cholangiography.[188]

Rapid changes in duct diameter

The diameter of the common duct may respond rapidly to both physiological and pathological changes in intraductal pressure,[189–191] and thus the ultrasound measurement of duct calibre at any one time may not convey the entire picture. The walls of the extrahepatic ducts are composed mainly of elastic fibres and connective tissue, with little or no smooth muscle.[192] The stretch potential of the elastic fibres permits duct dilatation, and the elastic recoil of the fibres is responsible for return of the duct to normal size after relief of an obstruction.

An increase in the volume of bile within the biliary system results in increased intraductal pressure and the common duct dilates.[193] The bile volume is controlled by the balance between bile production (choleresis) and bile outflow, which is itself controlled in health by the tone of the sphincter of Oddi and the reservoir function of the gallbladder.

After cholecystectomy choleresis may cause dilatation of the common duct, particularly when it has been subject to previous obstruction and dilatation. Furthermore, it is apparent that an abrupt increase in bile duct volume caused by the direct injection of contrast medium into the bile duct at cholangiography may result in an assessment of duct diameter that is significantly discrepant from the preceding ultrasound scan.[191,194]

Gallbladder distension

Courvoisier's law states that 'if in a jaundiced patient the gallbladder is enlarged, it is not a case of stone impacted in the common duct, for previous cholecystitis which existed when the stone was in the gallbladder, must have rendered the gallbladder fibrotic and incapable of dilatation'.[195] We now know that, as with all rules in medicine, there are exceptions to this law: stones can form *de novo* in the common duct, leaving the gallbladder wall in pristine condition; there may be double impaction of stones when the stone in the cystic duct causes a distended gallbladder and the stone in the common duct causes jaundice (Fig. 15.70); or there may be a pancreatic calculus impacted at the ampulla, obstructing both bile and pancreatic ducts.

However, whenever duct dilatation is encountered, it is useful to assess the degree of distension of the gallbladder as this may offer a clue to the level of the obstructing lesion. A distended gallbladder suggests a low common duct obstruction, whereas an empty gallbladder is consistent with obstruction above the level of the cystic duct insertion. The possibility of dual pathology must always be considered, however, and the gallbladder findings ust be regarded as supportive rather than of primary importance.

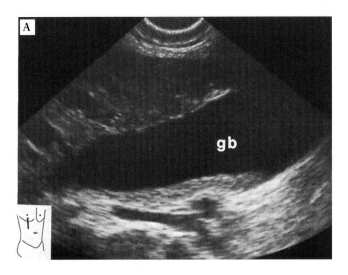

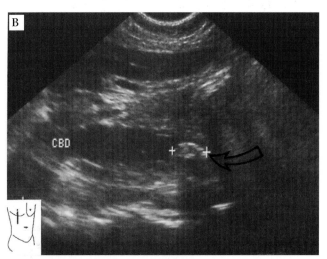

Fig. 15.70 Choledocholithiasis. A: Distended gallbladder (gb) due to **B:** a stone (arrow) obstructing the common duct (CBD). **C:** Confirmed on ERCP.

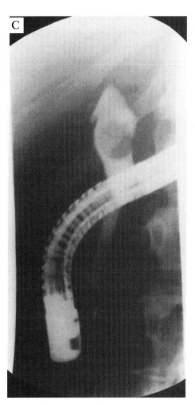

Choledocholithiasis

Early, disappointing sensitivity rates of around 33% for the detection of stones in the bile duct[196–199] have been replaced by sensitivities of 75–80%[159,199,200] because of improved scanning techniques and considerable developments in the resolution of equipment.

Choledocholithiasis occurs in approximately 15% of patients with stones in the gallbladder,[201] but may also occur in the absence of cholelithiasis, and may be found in as many as 4% of post-cholecystectomy cases,[202] many of whom will present with abdominal symptoms without jaundice.[169]

The classic clinical presentations of choledocholithiasis include biliary colic, jaundice and fluctuating fever – Chariot's triad. However, one or more of these components is often absent, the clinical features depending upon the varying degrees of bile duct obstruction, inflammation and infection present in any individual case.

There are several explanations for the low sensitivity of ultrasound in the diagnosis of choledocholithiasis:

1   Gas in the first and second parts of the duodenum interferes with the ultrasound demonstration of the common duct, which accounts for the finding that stones in the proximal portion of the duct are detected very much more often than stones in the distal portion (Fig. 15.71).[158,199]

2   Lack of dilatation of common ducts that contain stones, even in the presence of obstruction, is now well recognised[177,178] and may occur in as many as 25% of acutely obstructed ducts (Fig. 15.72).[197,203] Explanations for this phenomenon include the so-called 'ball-valve effect',[197] whereby the intermittent nature of the obstruction prevents the intraductal

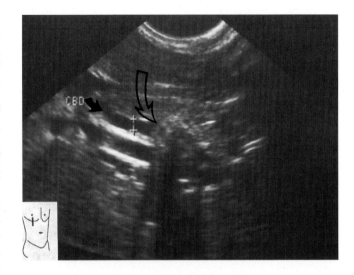

Fig. 15.72 Stone in non-dilated duct. Stone (open arrow) within a normal-calibre common duct (CBD, solid arrow) (4 mm).

pressure from rising sufficiently to cause dilatation, and the lag between onset of obstruction and onset of dilatation.[179]

3   The absence of a bile pool around stones in the duct impairs the ability of the ultrasonographer to spot the stones. The contrast between the reflectivity of solid stone and the echo-free nature of fluid bile that is so useful in the diagnosis of stones in the gallbladder is often absent, as the stones are in direct contact with the highly reflective walls of the duct and the adjacent gas-containing bowel. A particularly embarrassing situation can arise when the duct is completely full of stones, giving rise to a highly reflective structure with distal acoustic shadowing which is misdiagnosed as bowel gas (Fig. 15.73).

4   As many as 10% of common duct stones lack a distal acoustic shadow,[198,204,205] especially when they are at the lower end of the duct (Fig. 15.74). This phenomenon may be due to the differing composition of common duct stones (compared to gallbladder stones) – some are merely conglomerations of soft sludge – or to technical factors such as gain settings, transducer frequency and focusing, and reflection/refraction of sound by the curved walls of the duct. Non-shadowing stones in the duct cannot be distinguished from other intraluminal pathology such as blood clot, tumour or parasitic infestation.

5   Gas in the bile duct may give ultrasound appearances identical to those of stones, i.e. high reflectivity and acoustic shadowing emanating from within the duct lumen (Fig. 15.75), and may obscure the presence of stones. The gas is usually widely distributed throughout the intrahepatic biliary ducts and is

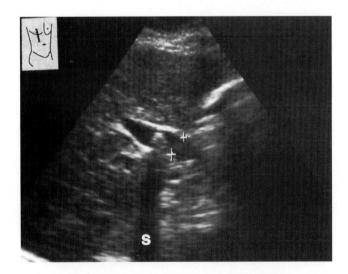

Fig. 15.71 Choledocholithiasis. Stone in the dilated common duct casting acoustic shadow (s).

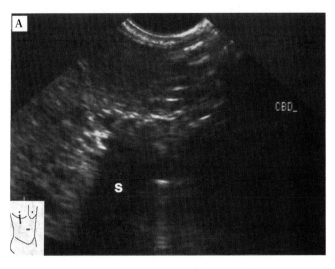

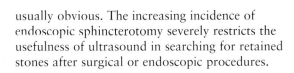

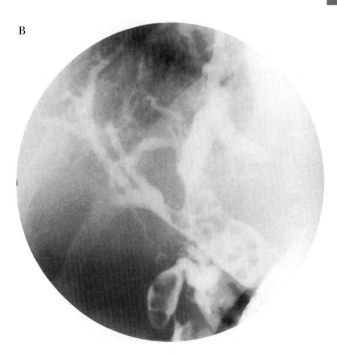

Fig. 15.73 Stones filling the lumen of the common duct. A: Longitudinal scan with patient in right anterior oblique position (s – shadow). **B:** ERCP shows duct full of stones.

usually obvious. The increasing incidence of endoscopic sphincterotomy severely restricts the usefulness of ultrasound in searching for retained stones after surgical or endoscopic procedures.

Developments in equipment and transducer technology now permit the demonstration of small stones within minimally dilated or even normal-calibre ducts, as long as the scanning technique is meticulous. It is important to scan the common duct in both longitudinal and transverse planes (Fig. 15.76), to move the patient into both right and left anterior oblique (Fig. 15.77), as well as upright and semi-upright positions, and to use water in the stomach and duodenum, all in an effort to demonstrate pathology in the common duct. An important clue to a calculous aetiology of biliary obstruction is the disproportionate dilatation of the extrahepatic biliary tree compared to the intrahepatic ducts. When this is noted the search for a calculus should be even more diligent. However, despite all these efforts approximately 30% of common duct stones are missed, mainly because they are impacted in the lower end of the common duct where they are hidden by the duodenum (Fig. 15.78).

Bile duct neoplasms

Benign tumours of the bile ducts are extremely rare; they include papillomas, adenomas, cystadenomas and granular cell myoblastomas.[204,206–209] Papillomas and solid adenomas appear as solid, non-shadowing intraluminal masses, whereas cystadenomas are multiloculated cystic masses that usually occur in young females. These latter originate from the bile duct epithelium but usually do not communicate with the biliary tree. The differential diagnosis includes echinococcal cysts, cystic metastases, abscesses, partially liquefied haematomas and hepatic artery aneurysms.

Primary malignant tumours of the bile ducts – cholangiocarcinomas – although rare, are much more common than benign tumours and their incidence is thought to be increasing. They may develop at any level within the biliary tree, and when they involve the confluence of the left and right hepatic ducts at the porta hepatis they are referred to as Klatskin tumours, following his original description in 1965.[210] The ultrasound features of cholangiocarcinomas have been well documented,[211–217] although the frequency with which these signs are detected varies greatly, depending upon the site and size of the tumour.

Dilatation of the biliary tree can be followed down to the point of obstruction, where it may be possible to detect a solid, poorly reflective mass which, if large enough, can be seen to have a heterogeneous internal echo pattern and ill-defined margins (Fig. 15.79). Occasionally an intraluminal mass is detected (Fig. 15.80), whereas in other cases thickening of the walls of the bile duct may be the only evidence of a tumour (Fig. 15.81). These ultrasound signs are a direct representation of the gross pathology, as these tumours can vary from large solid masses to lesions that infiltrate the submucosa with a thickness of only a few millimetres, when they may be undetectable to both palpation by the surgeon and naked eye inspection by the pathologist. It is this latter form of cholangiocarcinoma that presents on ultrasound as biliary dilatation without a detectable mass, possibly with some increased reflectivity and thickening of the duct wall, and is thus extremely difficult to diagnose.

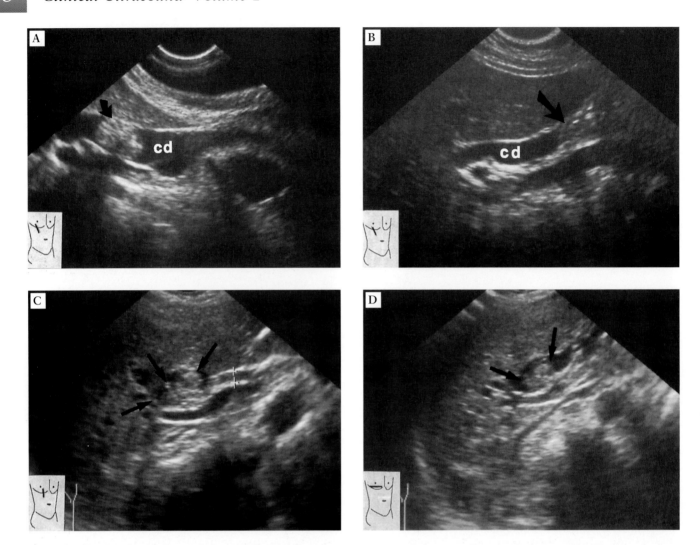

Fig. 15.74 No shadowing from stones within the common duct. A: Stone (arrow) in mid-duct. **B:** Stone (arrow) at lower end of duct (cd – common duct). **C and D:** Longitudinal and transverse scans in another patient. The calculus (arrows) is producing a mass effect in the common duct.

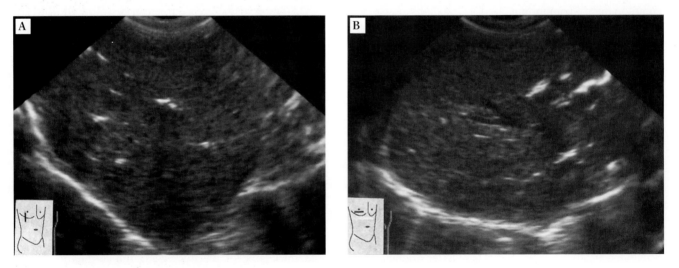

Fig. 15.75 Gas in the bile ducts. A: Longitudinal and **B:** transverse scans showing gas in intrahepatic bile ducts.

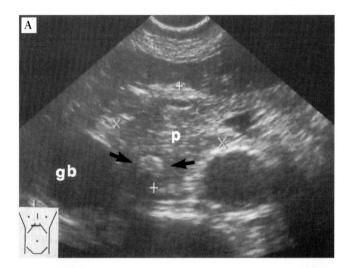

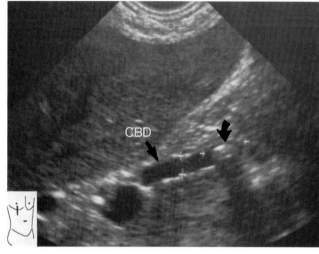

Fig. 15.77 Stone in the common bile duct. Stone (curved arrow) seen in common duct (CBD) only on the right anterior oblique view.

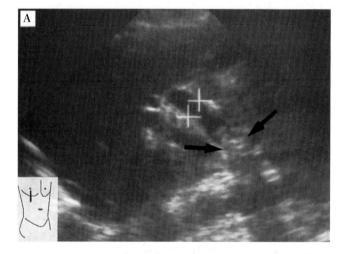

Fig. 15.76 Stone in the lower end of the common bile duct. A: Stone (arrows) identified within the lower end of common duct in a swollen head of pancreas (p) on transverse scan (gb – gallbladder). **B:** Confirmed on ERCP.

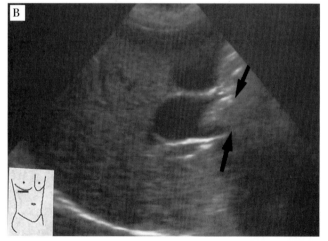

Fig. 15.78 Stone in the common bile duct. Stones (arrows) impacted within the lower end of the common duct. **A:** Longitudinal scan. **B:** Transverse scan in a different patient.

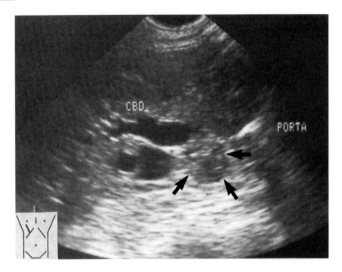

Fig. 15.79 **Klatskin tumour** (arrows) obstructing the common duct (CBD).

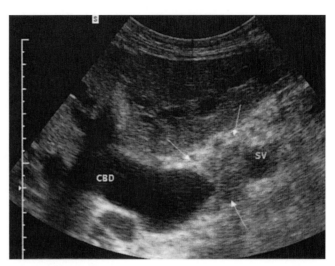

Fig. 15.80 **Cholangiocarcinoma** – intraluminal mass (arrows) (cbd – common duct).

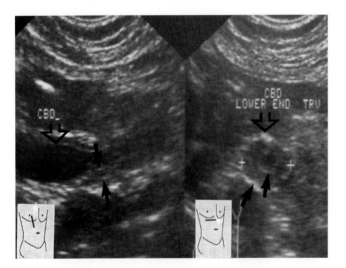

Fig. 15.81 **Cholangiocarcinoma** – thickening of walls (solid arrows) of common duct seen on both longitudinal and transverse scans.

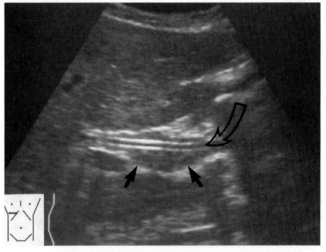

Fig. 15.82 **Cholangiocarcinoma** (solid arrows) has become visible after insertion of a stent (open arrow).

The ultrasound visibility of these tumours may increase after a biliary stent has been inserted (percutaneous or endoscopic) (Fig. 15.82), and it is often then possible to visualise the lesion sufficiently well to permit ultrasound-guided biopsy. However, cholangiocarcinomas have a fibrous nature, making it difficult to obtain samples adequate for cytological confirmation via fine-needle aspiration, so that a cutting biopsy for a histological sample is often necessary.

The role of ultrasound extends beyond the diagnosis of cholangiocarcinoma to assessment of operability by demonstrating evidence of spread of the tumour. Direct invasion to involve surrounding structures, such as the portal vein, hepatic artery and liver substance, as well as metastatic spread to regional lymph nodes, are both demon-strable on ultrasound (Fig. 15.83), which has been shown to be more accurate than CT scanning in this respect.[215]

As well as metastasising to the liver, cholangiocarcinomas may be multifocal and may be indistinguishable from hepatic metastatic disease on ultrasound, and from sclerosing cholangitis on cholangiography owing to the multiple strictures in the biliary tree.

Other tumours obstructing the bile ducts

The bile ducts may be obstructed by intrahepatic tumour, enlarged lymph nodes at the porta hepatis, carcinoma of the head of the pancreas, and ampullary tumours.

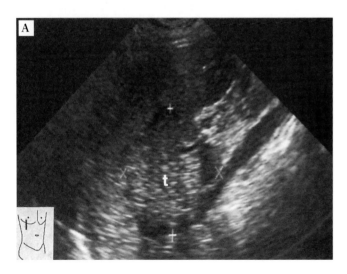

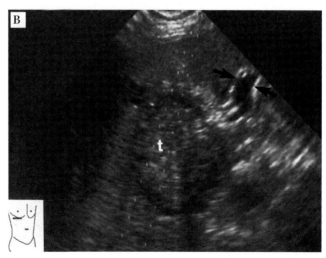

Fig. 15.83 Cholangiocarcinoma (t) invading liver and occluding portal vein (arrows). **A:** Longitudinal scan. **B:** Transverse scan with biopsy lines in place.

The lymph nodes at the porta hepatis are not usually demonstrable on ultrasound unless enlarged. Because of their proximity to the confluence of the right and left hepatic ducts, and their distribution along the length of the common duct, the bile ducts may be compressed and obstructed by lymphomatous or metastatic disease in the nodes. The nodal nature of a mass at the porta hepatis is usually obvious on ultrasound by carefully observing the interfaces that indicate that the tumour is composed of several discrete masses, and although it is true that lymphoma usually results in large nodes that are particularly poorly reflective, biopsy is required for accurate distinction between lymphoma and metastases (most frequently from the colon, stomach, pancreas and breast) (Fig. 15.84).

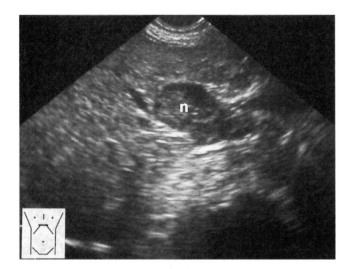

Fig. 15.84 Lymph node mass (n) at porta hepatis (Hodgkin's disease).

Enlargement of the head of the pancreas, whether from inflammation or malignancy, may compress the lower end of the common duct as it traverses the gland. Acute pancreatitis may cause transient extrahepatic duct dilatation but does not usually result in intrahepatic duct dilatation (Fig. 15.85), whereas the fibrous stricturing of the common duct in chronic pancreatitis may be indistinguishable from malignant disease both on ultrasound and at surgery. Carcinomas of the head of the pancreas are characteristically echo-poor solid masses into which the dilated common duct can be followed (Fig. 15.86) (see Ch. 16). The detection of coexisting pancreatic duct dilatation provides useful confirmatory evidence of pancreatic pathology, and 'ultrasonic double duct dilatation' may be caused by chronic pancreatitis, impacted pancreatic and biliary calculi and ampullary carcinoma, as well as by pancreatic carcinoma. Ultrasound is highly sensitive for duct dilatation but has less specificity than the ERCP sign of 'double duct obstruction', which is almost invariably due to pancreatic carcinoma (Fig. 15.87).

Ampullary carcinoma is difficult to identify on ultrasound. The findings of dilatation of the common duct with a normal head of pancreas should raise the suspicion of this tumour, especially if pancreatic duct dilatation is also detected. The diagnosis must be made endoscopically and it is important that it is not overlooked, as these tumours often present early with jaundice (owing to their strategic location) and radical surgery offers a good chance of cure.

Choledochal cysts

Choledochal cysts usually present in children or young adults and are discussed more fully in Chapter 48. The ultrasound appearances are usually of massive cystic dilatation of the extrahepatic common duct, although the

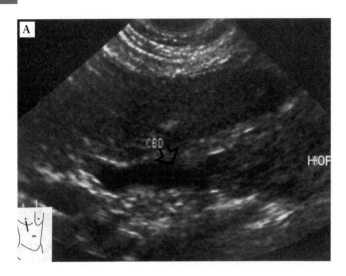 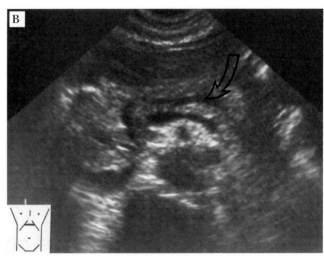

Fig. 15.85 Dilated common duct due to acute pancreatitis. A: Longitudinal scan. B: Transverse scan showing dilated pancreatic duct (curved arrow) (HOP – head of pancreas).

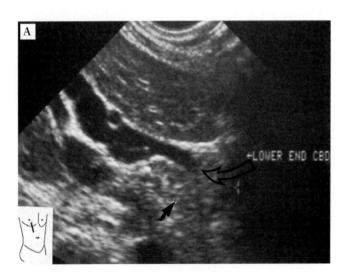 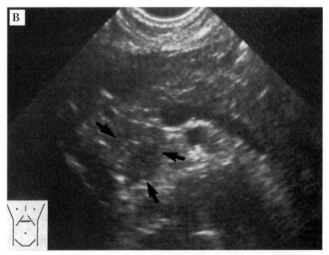

Fig. 15.86 Dilated common duct due to pancreatic carcinoma (solid arrows). A: Longitudinal scan. B: Transverse scan.

main intrahepatic ducts may be affected.[218–221] The underlying anomaly is thought to be an abnormal insertion of the common duct into the distal pancreatic duct, resulting in reflux of pancreatic secretions into the common duct that causes fibrotic structuring and obstruction to the biliary tree.[222,223] The condition is more common in females and Orientals, and presents with jaundice, fever and pain (due to cholangitis) with a palpable right upper quadrant mass (Fig. 15.88). As well as recurrent cholangitis, complications include stone formation with progression to biliary cirrhosis and portal hypertension, and an increased incidence of cholangiocarcinoma. The differential diagnosis includes other fluid-filled masses such as hepatic cyst and pancreatic pseudocyst, enteric duplica-

tion, hepatic artery aneurysm[224] and echinococcal disease (Fig. 15.89). The diagnosis may be confirmed by ^{99m}Tc-HIDA scintigraphy, when excretion of radioactivity into the cyst confirms its continuity with the biliary system.

Caroli's disease

Caroli's disease – congenital cystic dilatation of the intrahepatic bile ducts,[225] otherwise known as communicating cavernous ectasia of the intrahepatic ducts[226] – is an autosomal recessive disorder in which ultrasound scanning reveals multiple cyst-like spaces throughout the liver substance (Fig. 15.90).[227,228] These 'cysts' are seen on cholangiography to communicate with the dilated intrahepatic

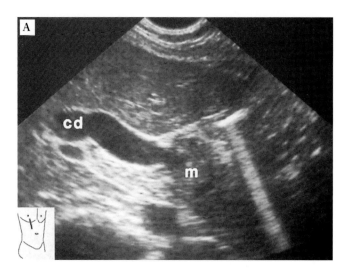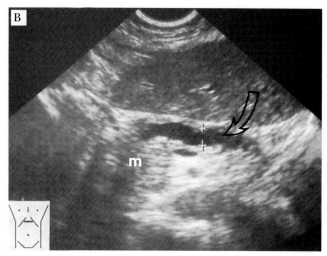

Fig. 15.87 Double duct obstruction due to pancreatic carcinoma (m). **A:** Longitudinal scan (cd – common duct). **B:** Transverse scan (arrow – pancreatic duct).

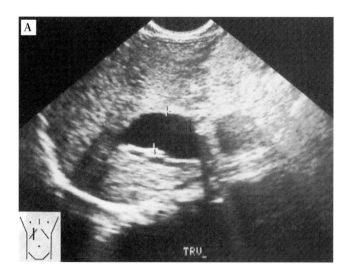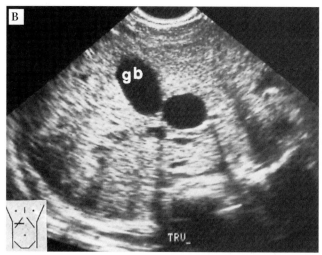

Fig. 15.88 Choledochal cyst. A: Longitudinal scan. **B:** Transverse scan showing aneurysmally dilated common duct in a young child.

biliary tree, but the extrahepatic bile ducts are usually unaffected. Stones often form within the cysts or dilated ducts, giving rise to attacks of cholangitis which may lead to pyogenic liver abscesses. There may be an association with renal tubular ectasia or other forms of cystic kidney disease, and there is a rather uncertain relationship to congenital hepatic fibrosis, in which there is bile duct proliferation and multiple strictures with proximal cystic dilatation[229] – also in association with renal cystic disease, usually of the infantile polycystic type. Caroli himself classified the condition into two types: the pure form without hepatic fibrosis or portal hypertension, and a second type associated with congenital hepatic fibrosis.[230]

The differential diagnosis includes severe biliary dilatation due to any of the other causes of biliary obstruction, polycystic disease of the liver (in which the cysts do not communicate with the bile ducts or each other), and congenital hepatic fibrosis. Other non-invasive imaging tests, such as ^{99m}Tc-HIDA scanning, may help in diagnosis[231] but, as alluded to above, it has been speculated that Caroli's disease, polycystic disease and congenital hepatic fibrosis are all parts of the same spectrum,[226] and hence cholangiography and even liver biopsy may be needed for a specific diagnosis.

Oriental cholangiohepatitis

Recurrent pyogenic cholangitis, also known as oriental cholangiohepatitis, is endemic in southeast Asia and is characterised by recurrent attacks of cholangitis. It is

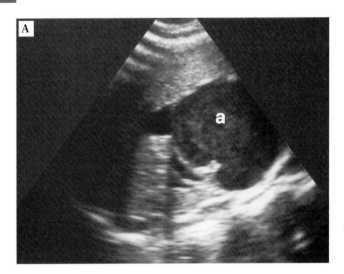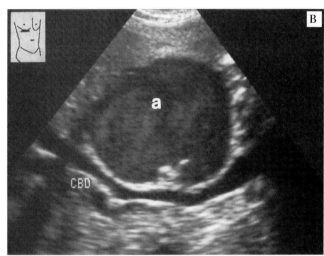

Fig. 15.89 Hepatic artery aneurysm (a) obstructing the common duct. **A:** Longitudinal scan. **B:** Transverse scan. Note the low-level echoes within the aneurysm, due to blood clot in this case.

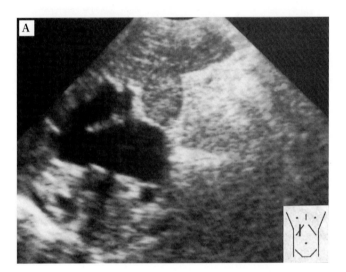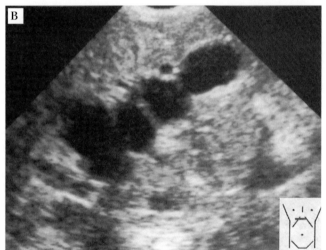

Fig. 15.90 Caroli's disease. A: and **B:** Cystic dilatation of the biliary tree in a child, subsequently shown to be Caroli's disease.

caused by peribiliary fibrosis which leads to bile duct strictures, and is probably caused by the adult worms of the *Chlonorchis sinensis* liver fluke which are ingested by man in raw freshwater fish. However, the parasites are not found in all patients with the clinical condition, and some authorities question the causal relationship.

The ultrasound features consist of massively dilated bile ducts with multiple strictures, the common duct being most frequently involved, followed by the left then the right hepatic ducts. The parasites may be identified within the ducts[232] and also within the gallbladder.[233] There are often bilirubinate stones within the ducts; these are often soft and sludge-like. In most patients there is secondary bacterial infection with *Escherichia coli* in the bile. Gas-

forming organisms may cause pneumobilia and there is an increased incidence of cholangiocarcinoma, presumably as a result of chronic irritation leading to metaplasia. All these pathological processes result in a complex ultrasonographic picture,[232–235] and although ultrasound may be of considerable value in screening for the disease and in suggesting the diagnosis, cholangiography is needed for full evaluation.

Biliary ascariasis

As described earlier in this chapter (p. 327), the roundworm *Ascaris lumbricoides* is an extremely common cause of biliary pathology worldwide. The worms infest the small

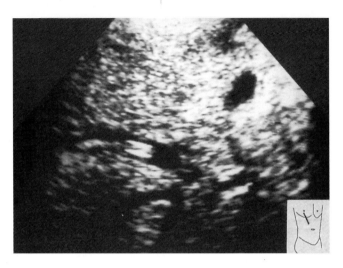

Fig. 15.91 *Ascaris* **worm in biliary tract.** Oblique view of common hepatic duct showing the typical 'tramline' appearance of *Ascaris* in the duct.

bowel, but can migrate up the common bile duct and may enter the gallbladder and intrahepatic ducts. Biliary colic is common, but jaundice, ascending cholangitis and parasitic liver abscesses occur occasionally.

The worm may be seen as a non-shadowing reflective linear structure within the lumen of the common duct (Fig. 15.91), and multiple worms may produce a spaghetti-like appearance. The digestive tract of the worm may be visualised as an echo-free tubular structure within the worm and as a bull's eye appearance on transverse scan,[236] and movement of the worms in the common duct and gallbladder may be observed.[237] The diagnosis is confirmed by isolating the worms or their eggs from the stool, and medical treatment is usually effective in eradicating the infestation.

Sclerosing cholangitis

Sclerosing cholangitis predominantly affects young men and may be idiopathic or associated with inflammatory bowel disease. Histologically there is non-specific inflammation of the bile duct walls and the ultrasound findings are of dilatation of the intrahepatic bile ducts, which may be confined to one or more segments or lobes depending upon the anatomical location of the strictures.[238] Thickening of the wall of the common duct has been reported (Fig. 15.92),[180] but the findings are not specific and the differential diagnosis includes cholangiocarcinoma and other causes of ascending cholangitis.

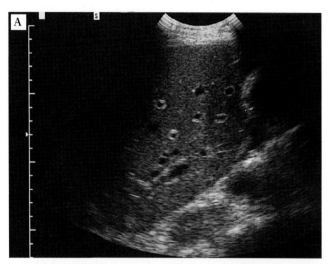

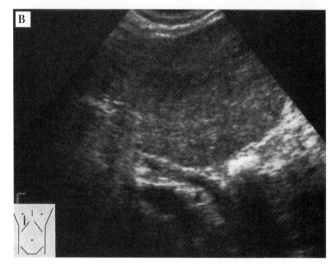

Fig. 15.92 **Sclerosing cholangitis. A:** Increased reflectivity of intrahepatic portal tracts. **B:** There is irregular mucosal thickening in the common duct.

REFERENCES

1 Finberg H J, Birnholz J C. Ultrasound evaluation of the gallbladder wall. Radiology 1979; 133: 693–698

2 Taylor K J W, Carpenter D A. The anatomy and pathology of the porta hepatis demonstrated by gray scale ultrasound. JCU 1975; 3: 117–119

3 Parulekar S G. Evaluation of common bile duct size. Radiology 1979; 133: 703–707

4 Edell S. A comparison of the 'Phrygian cap' deformity with bistable and gray scale ultrasound. JCU 1978; 6: 34–35

5 Sukov R J, Sample F, Sarti D A, Whitcomb M J. Cholecystosonography – the junctional fold. Radiology 1979; 133: 435–436

6 Cooperberg P L, Gibney R G. Imaging of the gallbladder, 1987. Radiology 1987; 163: 605–613

7 Marchal G, Kint E, Nijssens M, Baert A L. Variability of the hepatic arterial anatomy: a sonographic demonstration. JCU 1981; 9: 377–381

8 Berland L L, Lawson T L, Foley W D. Porta hepatis: sonographic discrimination of bile ducts from arteries with pulsed Doppler with new anatomic criteria. AJR 1982; 138: 833–840

9 Marchal G, Van de Voorde P, Van Dooren W, Ponette E, Baert A. Ultrasonic appearance of the filled and contracted normal gallbladder. JCU 1980; 8: 439–442

10 Filly R A, Moss A A, Way L W. In vitro investigation of gallstone shadowing with ultrasound tomography. JCU 1979; 7: 255–262

11 Jaffe C C, Taylor K J W. The clinical impact of ultrasonic beam focusing patterns. Radiology 1979; 131: 469–472

12 Dewbury K C. Visualisation of normal biliary ducts with ultrasound. Br J Radiol 1980; 53: 774–780

13 Lewandowski B J, Winsberg F. Gallbladder wall thickness distortion by ascites. AJR 1981; 137: 519–521

14 Behan M, Kazam E. Sonography of the common bile duct: value of the right anterior oblique view. AJR 1978; 130: 701–709

15 Laing F C, Jeffrey R B, Wing V W, Nyberg D A. Biliary dilatation: defining the level and cause by real time ultrasound. Radiology 1986; 160: 39–42

16 Sauerbrei E E, Cooperberg P L, Gordon P, Li D, Cohen M M, Burhenne H J. The discrepancy between radiographic and sonographic bile duct measurements. Radiology 1980; 137: 751–755

17 Wu C-C, Ho Y-H, Chen C-Y. Effect of aging on common bile duct diameter: a real time sonographic study. JCU 1984; 12: 473

18 Graham M F, Cooperberg P L, Cohen M M, Burhenne H J. The size of the normal common hepatic duct following cholecystectomy: an ultrasonic study. Radiology 1980; 135: 137–139

19 Mueller P R, Ferrucci J T Jnr, Simeone J F et al. Post-cholecystectomy bile duct dilatation: myth or reality? AJR 1981; 136: 355

20 Wedmann B, Borsch G, Coenen C, Paassen A. Effect of cholecystectomy on common bile duct diameters; a longitudinal prospective ultrasonographic study. JCU 1988; 16: 619–624

21 Glazer G M, Filly R A, Laing F C. Rapid change in caliber of the non-obstructed common duct. Radiology 1981; 140: 161–162

22 Mueller P R, Ferrucci J F, Simeone J F, van Sonnenberg E, Hall P D A, Wittenberg J. Observations on the distensibility of the common bile duct. Radiology 1982; 142: 467–472

23 Cooperberg P L, Li D, Wong P, Cohen M M, Burhenne H J. Accuracy of common duct size in the evaluation of extrahepatic biliary obstruction. Radiology 1980; 135: 141–144

24 Braverman D Z, Johnson M L, Kern F. Effects of pregnancy and contraceptive steroids on gallbladder function. N Engl J Med 1980; 302: 362–364

25 Delamarre J, Capron J-P, Joly J-P et al. Gallbladder inertia in celiac disease: ultrasonographic demonstration. Dig Dis Sci 1984; 29: 876–877

26 Nino-Murcia M, Burton M, Chang P, Stone J, Perkash I. Gallbladder contractility in patients with spinal cord injuries: a sonographic investigation. AJR 1990; 154: 521–524

27 Simeone J F, Mueller P R, Ferrucci J T et al. Sonography of the bile ducts after a fatty meal: an aid in the detection of obstruction. Radiology 1982; 143: 211–215

28 Wilson S A, Gosink B B, vanSonnenberg E. Unchanged size of a dilated common bile duct after a fatty meal: results and significance. Radiology 1986; 160: 29–31

29 Simeone J F, Butch R J, Mueller P R et al. The bile ducts after a fatty meal: further sonographic observations. Radiology 1985; 154: 763–768

30 Darweesh R M A, Dodds W J, Hogan W J et al. Fatty meal sonography for evaluating patients with suspected partial common duct obstruction. AJR 1988; 151: 63–68

31 Amouzal P, Palazzo L, Amouzal G et al. Endosonography: promising method for diagnosis of extrahepatic cholestasis. Lancet 1989; ii: 1195–1198

32 Tio T L. Endosonography in gastroenterology. Berlin: Springer Verlag, 1988

33 Lane R J, Glazer G. Intra-operative B-mode ultrasound scanning of the extrahepatic biliary system and pancreas. Lancet 1980; ii: 334–337

34 Machi J, Tateishi T, Oishi A J et al. Laparoscopic ultrasonography versus operative cholangiography during laparoscopic cholecystectomy: review of the literature and a comparison with open intraoperative ultrasonography.

35 Health and Policy Committee, American College of Physicians. How to study the gallbladder. Ann Intern Med 1988; 109: 752–754

36 Simeone J F, Mueller P R, Ferrucci J T. Non-surgical therapy of gallstones: implications for imaging. Am J Radiol 1989; 152: 11–17

37 Lees W R, Kellett M J. Gallbladder stones: new roles for the radiologist. Clin Radiol 1989; 40: 561–563

38 Bellamy P R, Hicks A. Assessment of gallbladder function by ultrasound: implications for dissolution therapy. Clin Radiol 1988; 39: 511–512

39 Mathieson J R, So C B, Malone D E, Becker C D, Burhenne H J. Accuracy of sonography for determining the number and size of gallbladder stones before and after lithotripsy. AJR 1989; 153: 977–980

40 Barbara L. Epidemiology of gallstone disease: the 'Sirmione Study'. In: Capocaccia L, Ricci G, Angelico F, Angelico M, Attili A F, eds. Epidemiology and prevention of gallstone disease. Lancaster: MTP Press, 1984; 23–25

41 GREPCO. Prevalence of gallstone disease in an Italian adult female population. Am J Epidemiol 1984; 119: 796–805

42 Gracie W A, Ransohoff D F. The natural history of silent gallstones: the innocent gallstone is not a myth. N Engl J Med 1982; 307: 798–800

43 Dowling R H. Epidemiology and medical treatment of cholesterol gallstones: recurrence, post-dissolution management and the future. In: Capocaccia L, Ricci G, Angelico F, Angelico M, Attili A F, eds. Epidemiology and prevention of gallstone disease. Lancaster: MTP Press, 1984: 116–128

44 Crade M, Taylor K J W, Rosenfield A T, de Graaf C S, Minihan P. Surgical and pathologic correlation of cholecystosonography and cholecystography. AJR 1978; 131: 227–229

45 Filly R A, Allen B, Minton M J, Bernhoft R, Way L W. In vitro investigation of the origin of echoes within biliary sludge. JCU 1980; 8: 193–200

46 Sommer F G, Taylor K J W. Differentiation of acoustic shadowing due to calculi and gas collections. Radiology 1980; 135: 399

47 Carroll B A. Gallstones: in vitro comparison of physical, radiographic and ultrasonic characteristics. AJR 1978; 131: 223–226

48 Filly R A, Moss A A, Way L W. In vitro investigation of gallstone shadowing with ultrasonic tomography. J Clin Ultrasound 1979; 7: 255

49 Jaffe C C, Taylor K J W. The clinical impact of ultrasonic beam focusing patterns. Radiology 1979; 131: 469–472

50 Taylor K J W, Jacobson P, Jaffe C C. Lack of an acoustic shadow on scans of gallstones: a possible artefact. Radiology 1979; 131: 463–464

51 Callen P W, Filly R A. Ultrasonographic localisation of the gallbladder. Radiology 1979; 133: 693–698

52 Conrad M R, Leonard J, Landay M J. Left lateral decubitus sonography of gallstones in the contracted gallbladder. AJR 1980; 134: 141–144

53 MacDonald F R, Cooperberg P L, Cohen M M. The WES triad – a specific sign of gallstones in the contracted gallbladder. Gastrointest Radiol 1981; 6: 39–41

54 Ratpopoulos V, D'Orsi C, Smith E, Reuter K, Moss L, Kleinman P. Dynamic cholecystosonography of the contracted gallbladder: the double-arc-shadow sign. AJR 1982; 138: 275–278

55 Kane R A, Jacobs R, Katz J, Costello P. Porcelain gallbladder: ultrasound and CT appearance. Radiology 1984; 152: 137–141

56 Crow H C, Bartrum R J, Foote S R. Expanded criteria for the ultrasonic diagnosis of gallstones. JCU 1976; 4: 289

57 Love M B. Sonographic features of milk of calcium bile. J Ultrasound Med 1982; 1: 325–327

58 Chun G H, Deutsch A L, Scheible W. Sonographic findings in milk of calcium bile. Gastrointest Radiol 1982; 7: 371–373

59 Conrad M R, Janes J O, Dietchy J. Significance of low level echoes within the gallbladder. AJR 1979; 132: 967–972

60 Simeone J F, Mueller P R, Ferrucci J T, Harbin W P, Wittenberg J. Significance of non-shadowing focal opacities at cholecystosonography. Radiology 1980; 137: 181–185

61 Messing B, Bories C, Kunstlinger F, Bernier J J. Does total parenteral nutrition induce gallbladder sludge formation and lithiasis? Gastroenterology 1983; 84: 1012–1019

62 Bolondi L et al. Early detection of biliary sludge and gallstones after surgery of the GI tract. In: Barbara L, Dowling R H, Hofman A F, Roda E, eds. Recent advances in bile acid research. New York: Raven Press, 1985: 281–285

63 Goldstein A, Madrazo B L. Slice thickness artefacts in gray scale ultrasound. JCU 1981; 9: 365–375

64 Anastasi B, Sutherland G R. Biliary sludge ultrasonic appearance simulating neoplasm. Br J Radiol 1981; 54: 679–681

65 Fakhry J. Sonography of tumefactive biliary sludge. AJR 1982; 139: 717–719

66 Britten J S, Golding R H, Cooperberg P L. Sludge balls to gallstones. J Ultrasound Med 1984; 3: 81–82

67 Engel J M, Deitch E A, Sikkema W. Gallbladder wall thickness: sonographic accuracy and relation to disease. AJR 1979; 134: 907–909

68 Finberg H J, Birnholtz J. Ultrasound evaluation of the gallbladder wall. Radiology 1979; 133: 693–698

69 Marchal G, Van de Voorde P, Van Dooren W, Ponette E, Baert A. Ultrasonic appearance of the filled and contracted normal gallbladder. JCU 1980; 8: 439–442

70 Lewandowski B J, Winsberg F. Gallbladder wall thickness distortion by ascites. AJR 1981; 137: 519–521

71 Sanders R C. The significance of sonographic gallbladder wall thickening. JCU 1980; 8: 143–146

72 Fiske C E, Laing F C, Brown T W. Ultrasonographic evidence of gallbladder wall thickening in association with hypoalbuminemia. Radiology 1980; 135: 713–716

73 Ralls P W, Quinn M F, Juttner H U, Halls J M, Boswell W D. Gallbladder wall thickening: patients without intrinsic gallbladder disease. AJR 1981; 137: 65–68

74 Saverymuttu S H, Grammatopoulos A, Meanock C I, Maxwell J D, Joseph A E A. Gallbladder wall thickening (congestive cholecystopathy) in chronic liver disease: a sign of portal hypertension. Br J Radiol 1990; 63: 922–925

75 Shlaer W J, Leopold G R, Scheible F W. Sonography of thickened gallbladder wall: a non-specific finding. AJR 1981; 136: 337–339

76 Maudgal D P, Wansborough Jones M H, Joseph A E A. Gallbladder abnormalities in acute infectious hepatitis. Dig Dis Sci 1984; 29: 257–260

77 Juttner H-U, Ralls P W, Quinn M F, Jenney J M. Thickening of gallbladder wall in acute hepatitis: ultrasound demonstration. Radiology 1982; 142: 465–466

78 Brandt D J, MacCarty R L, Charbonneau J W, LaRusso N F, Wiesner R H, Ludwig J. Gallbladder disease in patients with primary sclerosing cholangitis. AJR 1988; 150: 571–574

79 Romano A J, vanSonnenberg E, Casola G et al. Gallbladder and bile duct abnormalities in AIDS: sonographic findings in eight patients. AJR 1988; 150: 123–127

80 McClure J, Banerjee S S, Schofield P S. Crohn's disease of the gallbladder. J Clin Pathol 1984; 37: 516–518

81 Carroll B A. Gallbladder wall thickening secondary to focal lymphatic obstruction. J Ultrasound Med 1983; 2: 89–91

82 Laudanna A A, Ferreyra N P, Cerri G G, Bettarello A. Thickening of the gallbladder wall in alcoholic hepatitis verified by ultrasonographic examination. Scand J Gastroenterol 1987; 22: 521–524

83 Cerri G G, Alves V, Magalhaes A. Sonography in hepatobiliary schistosomiasis. Radiology 1984; 153: 777

84 Bouchier I A D. New drugs: gallstones. Br Med J 1990; 300: 592–597

85 Marton K I, Doubilet P. How to image the gallbladder in suspected cholecystitis. Ann Intern Med 1988; 109: 722–729

86 Laing F C, Federle M P, Jeffrey R B, Brown T W. Ultrasonic evaluation of patients with acute right upper quadrant pain. Radiology 1981; 190: 449–455

87 Handler S J. Ultrasound of gallbladder wall thickening and its relation to cholecystitis. AJR 1979; 132: 581–585

88 Marchal G J F, Casaer M, Baert A L, Goddeeris P G, Kerremans R, Fevery J. Gallbladder wall sonolucency in acute cholecystitis. Radiology 1979; 133: 429–433.

89 Kane R A. The biliary system. In: Kurtz A B, Goldberg B B, eds. Gastrointestinal ultrasonography. New York: Churchill Livingstone, 1988: 75–137

90 Sherman M, Ralls P W, Quinn M, Halls J, Keats J B. Intravenous cholangiography and sonography in acute cholecystitis: prospective evaluation. AJR 1980; 135: 311–313

91 Clain A. Hamilton Bailey's physical sign in clinical surgery, 14th edn. Bristol: Wright, 1967

92 Ralls P W, Halls, J, Lapin S A, Quinn M F, Morris U L, Boswell W. Prospective evaluation of the sonographic Murphy sign in suspected acute cholecystitis. JCU 1982; 10: 113–115

93 Ralls P W, Colletti P M, Lapin S M et al. Real time sonography in suspected acute cholecystitis. Radiology 1985; 155: 767

94 Jeffrey R B, Laing F C, Wong W, Callen P W. Gangrenous cholecystitis: diagnosis by ultrasound. Radiology 1983; 148: 219–221

95 Kane R A. Ultrasonographic diagnosis of gangrenous cholecystitis and empyema of the gallbladder. Radiology 1980; 134: 191–194

96 Jenkins M, Golding R H, Cooperberg P L. Sonography and computed tomography of haemorrhagic cholecystitis. AJR 1983; 140: 1197–1198

97 Wales L R. Desquamated gallbladder mucosa: unusual sign of cholecystitis. AJR 1982; 139: 810–811

98 Simeone J F, Brink J A, Mueller P R et al. The sonographic diagnosis of acute gangrenous cholecystitis: importance of the Murphy sign. AJR 1989; 152: 289–290

99 Bergman A B, Neiman H L, Kraut B. Ultrasonographic evaluation of pericholecystic abscesses. AJR 1979; 132: 201–203

100 Madrazo B L, Francis I, Hricak H, Sandler M A, Hudak S, Gitschlag K. Sonographic findings in perforation of the gallbladder. AJR 1982; 139: 491–496

101 Hunter N D, Macintosh P K. Acute emphysematous cholecystitis: an ultrasonic diagnosis. AJR 1980; 134: 592–593

102 Blaquiere R M, Dewbury K C. The ultrasound diagnosis of emphysematous cholecystitis. Br J Radiol 1982; 55: 114–116

103 Parulekar S G. Sonographic findings in acute emphysematous cholecystitis. Radiology 1982; 145: 117–119

104 Bloom R A, Fisher A, Pode D, Asaf Y. Shifting intramural gas: a new ultrasound sign of emphysematous cholecystitis. J Clin 1984; 12: 40–42

105 Nemcek A A, Gore R M, Vogelzang R L, Grant M. The effervescent gallbladder: a sonographic sign of emphysematous cholecystitis. AJR 1988; 150: 575–577

106 Bloom R A, Libson E, Lebensart P D et al. The ultrasound spectrum of emphysematous cholecystitis. JCU 1989; 17: 251–256

107 Gill K S, Chapman A H, Weston M J. The changing face of emphysematous cholecystitis. Br J Radiol 1997; 70: 986–991

108 Deitch E A, Engel J M. Acute acalculous cholecystitis: an ultrasonic diagnosis. AJR 1981; 142: 290–242

109 Shuman W P, Rogers J V, Ruydd T G, Mack L A, Plumley T, Larson E B. Low sensitivity of sonography and cholescintigraphy in acalculous cholecystitis. AJR 1984; 142: 531–534

110 Mirvis S E, Vainright J R, Nelson A W et al. The diagnosis of acute acalculous cholecystitis: a comparison of sonography, scintigraphy, and CT. AJR 1986; 147: 1171–1175

111 McGahan J P, Walter J R. Diagnostic percutaneous aspiration of the gallbladder. Radiology 1985; 155: 619–622

112 McGahan J P, Lindfors K K. Acute cholecystitis: diagnostic accuracy of percutaneous aspiration of the gallbladder. Radiology 1988; 167: 669–671

113 Berk R N, van der Vegt J H, Lichtenstein J E. The hyperplastic cholecystoses: cholesterolosis and adenomyomatosis. Radiology 1983; 146: 595–601

114 Raghavendra B N, Subramanyam B R, Balthazar E J, Horii S C, Megibow A J, Hilton S. Sonography of adenomyomatosis of the gallbladder: radiologic-pathologic correlation. Radiology 1983; 146: 747–752

115 Fowler R C, Reid W A. Ultrasound diagnosis of adenomyomatosis of the gallbladder: ultrasonic and pathological correlation. Clin Radiol 1988; 39: 402–406

116 Price R J, Stewart E T, Foley W D, Dodds W J. Sonography of polypoid cholesterolosis. AJR 1982; 139: 1197

117 Jacyna M R, Bouchier I A D. Cholesterolosis: a physical cause of 'functional' disorder. Br Med J 1987; 295: 619–620

118 Carter S J, Rutledge J, Hirsch J H. Papillary adenoma of the gallbladder: ultrasonic demonstration. JCU 1978; 6: 433

119 Foster D R, Foster D B E. Gallbladder polyps in Peutz-Jeghers syndrome. Postgrad Med J 1980; 56: 373–376

120 Niv Y, Kosakov K, Shcolnik B. Fragile papilloma (papillary adenoma) of the gallbladder. A cause of recurrent biliary colic. Gastroenterology 1986; 91: 999–1001

121 Kozuka S, Kurashina M, Tsubone M, Hachisuka K, Yasui A. Significance of intestinal metaplasia for the evolution of cancer in the biliary tract. Cancer 1984; 54: 2277–2285

122 Williamson R C N. Acalculous disease of the gallbladder. Gut 1988; 29: 860–872

123 Majeski J A. Polyps of the gallbladder. J Surg Oncol 1986; 32: 16–18

124 Olken S M, Bledsoe R, Newmark H. The ultrasonic diagnosis of primary carcinoma of the gallbladder. Radiology 1978; 129: 481–482

125 Crade M, Taylor K J W, Rosenfield A T et al. The varied ultrasonic character of gallbladder tumour. JAMA 1979; 241: 2195–2196

126 Yeh H-C. Ultrasonography and computed tomography of carcinoma of the gallbladder. Radiology 1979; 133: 167–173

127 Dalla Palma L, Rizzatto G, Pozzi-Mucelli R S, Bazzocchi M. Grey scale ultrasonography in the evaluation of carcinoma of the gallbladder. Br J Radiol 1980; 53: 662–667

128 Yum H Y, Fink A H. Sonographic findings in primary carcinoma of the gallbladder. Radiology 1980; 134: 693–696

129 Ruiz R, Teyssou H, Fernandez N et al. Ultrasonic diagnosis of primary carcinoma of the gallbladder: a review of 16 cases. JCU 1980; 8: 489–495

130 Bach A M, Loring L A, Hann L E et al. Gallbladder cancer: can ultrasonography evaluate extent of disease? J Ultrasound Med 1998; 17: 303–309

131 Koga A, Yamauchi S, Izumi Y, Hamanaka N. Ultrasonographic detection of early and curable carcinoma of the gallbladder. Br J Surg 1985; 72: 728–730

132 Diehl A K, Beral V. Cholecystectomy and changing mortality from gallbladder cancer. Lancet 1981; ii: 187–189

133 Phillips G, Pochaczevsky R, Goodman J, et al. Ultrasound patterns of metastatic tumours in the gallbladder. JCU 1982; 10: 379

134 Bundy A L, Richie W G M. Ultrasonic diagnosis of metastatic melanoma presenting as acute cholecystitis. JCU 1982; 10: 285

135 Schulman A, Loxton A J, Heydenrych J J, Abdurahman K E. Sonographic diagnosis of biliary ascariasis. AJR 1982; 139: 485–489

136 Lim J H, Ko Y T, Lee D H, Kim S Y. Clonorchiasis: sonographic findings in 59 proved cases. AJR 1989; 152: 761–764

137 Bassily S, Iskander M, Youssef F G, El-Masry N, Bawden M. Sonography in diagnosis of fascioliasis. Lancet 1989; i: 1270–1271

138 Wong R K, Peura D A, Mutter M L, Heit H A, Birns M T, Johnson L F. Hemobilia and liver flukes in a patient from Thailand. Gastroenterology 1985; 88: 1958–1963

139 Braverman D Z, Johnson M L, Kern F Jr. Effects of pregnancy and contraceptive steroids on gallbladder function. N Engl J Med 1980; 302: 362

140 Kane R A. Ultrasonographic evaluation of the gallbladder. Crit Rev Diagn Imaging 1982; 17: 107

141 Cohen E K, Stringer D A, Smith C R, Daneman A. Hydrops of the gallbladder in typhoid fever as demonstrated by sonography. JCU 1986; 14: 633–635

142 Slovis T L, Hight D W, Philippart A I, Dubois R S. Sonography in the diagnosis and management of hydrops of the gallbladder in children with mucocutaneous lymphnode syndrome. Pediatrics 1980; 65: 789–794

143 Koss J C, Coleman B G, Mulhern C B et al. Mucocutaneous lymph node syndrome with hydrops of the gallbladder diagnosed by ultrasound. JCU 1981; 9: 477–479

144 Tanaka K, Shimada M, Hattori M, Utsunomiya T, Oya N. Sjogren's syndrome with abnormal manifestations of the gallbladder and central nervous system. J Pediatr Gastroenterol Nutr 1985; 4: 148–151

145 Copeman P W M, Medd W E. Diffuse systemic sclerosis with abnormal liver and gallbladder. Br Med J 1967; 3: 353–354

146 Wilson-Sharp R C, Irving H C, Brown R C, Chalmers D M, Littlewood J M. Ultrasonography of the pancreas, liver, and biliary system in cystic fibrosis. Arch Dis Child 1984; 59: 923–926

147 Wilson-Sharp R C, Irving H C. Abdominal ultrasonography in cystic fibrosis. Français d'Echographie 1985; 3: 191–200

148 Scharsschmidt B F, Goldberg H I, Schmid R. Approach to the patient with cholestatic jaundice. N Engl J Med 1983; 308: 1515–1519

149 Lunderquist A. The radiology of jaundice. Clin Gastroenterol 1989; 3: 387–406

150 Taylor K J W, Rosenfield A T. Grey scale ultrasonography in the differential diagnosis of jaundice. Arch Surg 1977; 112: 820–825

151 Sample W F, Sarti D A, Goldstein L I, Weiner M, Kadell B M. Gray-scale ultrasonography of the jaundiced patient. Radiology 1978; 128: 719–725

152 Vallon A G, Lees W R, Cotton P B. Gray-scale ultrasonography in obstructive jaundice. Gut 1979; 20: 51–54

153 Koenigsberg M, Wiener S N, Walzer A. Accuracy of sonography in the differential diagnosis of obstructive jaundice: a comparison with cholangiography. Radiology 1979; 133: 157–165

154 Dewbury K C, Joseph A E A, Hayes S, Murray C. Ultrasound in the evaluation and diagnosis of jaundice. Br J Radiol 1979; 52: 276–280

155 Wild S R, Cruikshank J G, Fraser G G M, Copland W A, Grieve D C. Grey-scale ultrasonography and percutaneous transhepatic cholangiography in biliary tract disease. BMJ 1980; 281: 1524–1526

156 Haubek A, Pedersen J H, Buscharth F, Gammelgaard J, Hancke S, Willumsen L. Dynamic sonography in the evaluation of jaundice. AJR 1981; 136: 1071–1074

157 Ruddell W S J. Ultrasound in biliary tract disease. BMJ 1981; 282: 311

158 Laing F C, Jeffrey R B, Wing V W, Nyberg D A. Biliary dilatation: defining the level and cause by real time ultrasound. Radiology 1986; 160: 39–42

159 Lindsell D R M. Ultrasound imaging of pancreas and biliary tract. Lancet 1990; 335: 390–393

160 Dewbury K C. Visualisation of normal biliary ducts with ultrasound. Br J Radiol 1980; 53: 774–780

161 Bressler E L, Rubin J M, McCracken S. Sonographic parallel channel sign: a reappraisal. Radiology 1987; 164: 343–346

162 Cooperberg P L. High resolution real time ultrasound in the evaluation of the normal and obstructed biliary tract. Radiology 1978; 129: 477–480

163 Cooperberg P L, Li D, Wong P, Cohen M M, Burhenne H J. Accuracy of common hepatic duct size in the evaluation of extrahepatic biliary obstruction. Radiology 1980; 135: 141–144

164 Parulekar S G. Evaluation of common bile duct size. Radiology 1979; 133: 703–707

165 Wu C-C, Ho Y-H, Chen C-Y. Effect of aging on common bile duct diameter: a real time sonographic study. JCU 1984; 12: 473

166 Graham M F, Cooperberg P L, Cohen M M et al. The size of normal common hepatic duct following cholecystectomy: an ultrasonic study. Radiology 1980; 135: 137

167 Mueller P R, Ferrucci J T Jr, Simeone J F et al. Postcholecystectomy bile duct dilatation: myth or reality? AJR 1981; 136: 355

168 Wedmann B, Borsch G, Coenen C, Paassen A. Effect of cholecystectomy on common bile duct diameters; a longitudinal prospective ultrasonographic study. JCU 1988; 16: 619–624

169 Ruddell W S J, Ashton M G, Lintott D J, Axon A T R. Endoscopic retrograde cholangiography and pancreatography in investigation of post-cholecystectomy patients. Lancet 1980; i: 444–447

170 Weill F, Eisencher A, Zeltner F. Ultrasonic study of the normal and dilated biliary tree: 'shot-gun sign'. Radiology 1978; 127: 221

171 Conrad M R, Landay M J, Janes J O. Sonographic 'parallel channel' sign of biliary tree enlargement in mild to moderate obstructive jaundice. AJR 1978; 130: 279

172 Ingram C, Joseph A E A. The stilette sign: the appearance of dilated ducts in the fatty liver. Clin Radiol 1989; 40: 257–258

173 Laing F C, London L A, Filly R A. Ultrasonographic identification of dilated intrahepatic bile ducts and their differentiation from portal venous structures. JCU 1978; 6: 90

174 Taylor K J W, Rosenfield A T, De Graaff C S. Anatomy and pathology of the biliary tree as demonstrated by ultrasound. In: Taylor K J W, ed. Diagnostic ultrasound in gastrointestinal disease. Clinics in diagnostic ultrasound. Edinburgh: Churchill Livingstone, 1979: 103–121

175 Muhletaler C A, Gerlock A J, Fleischer A C, James A E. Diagnosis of obstructive jaundice with non-dilated bile ducts. AJR 1980; 134: 1149–1152

176 Thomas J L, Zornoza J. Obstructive jaundice in the absence of sonographic biliary dilatation. Gastrointest Radiol 1980; 5: 357–360

177 Beinart C, Efremidis S, Cohen B, Mitty H A. Obstruction without dilatation. JAMA 1981; 245: 353–356

178 Greenwald R A, Pereiras R, Morris S J, Schiff E R. Jaundice, choledocholithiasis, and a non-dilated common duct. JAMA 1978; 240: 1983–1984

179 Fried A M, Bell R M, Bivins B A. Biliary obstruction in a canine model: sequential study of the sonographic threshold. Invest Radiol 1981; 16: 317–319

180 Carroll B A, Oppenheimer D A. Sclerosing cholangitis: sonographic demonstration of bile duct wall thickening. AJR 1982; 139: 1016

181 Simeone J F, Mueller P R, Ferrucci J T et al. Sonography of the bile ducts after a fatty meal: an aid in detection of obstruction. Radiology 1982; 143: 211–215

182 Simeone J F, Butch R J, Mueller P R et al. The bile ducts after a fatty meal: furthur sonographic observations. Radiology 1985; 154: 763–768

183 Wilson S A, Gosink B R, vanSonnenberg E. Unchanged size of a dilated common bile duct after a fatty meal; results and significance. Radiology 1986; 160: 29–31

184 Darweesh R M A, Dodds W J, Hogan W J et al. Fatty meal sonography for evaluating patients with suspected partial common duct obstruction. AJR 1988; 151: 63–68

185 Amouyal P, Palazzo L, Amouyal G et al. Endosonography: promising method for diagnosis of extrahepatic cholestasis. Lancet 1989; ii: 1195–1198

186 Weinstein D P, Weinstein B J, Brodmerkel G J. Ultrasonography of biliary tract dilatation without jaundice. AJR 1979; 132: 729–734

187 Weinstein B J, Weinstein D P. Biliary tract dilatation in the non-jaundiced patient. AJR 1980; 134: 899

188 Zeman R, Taylor K J W, Burrell M I et al. Ultrasonic demonstration of anicteric dilatation of the biliary tree. Radiology 1980; 134: 689

189 Glazer G M, Filly R A, Laing F C. Rapid change in calibre of the non-obstructed common duct. Radiology 1980; 140: 161–162

190 Scheske G A, Cooperberg P L, Cohen M M et al. Dynamic changes in the caliber of the major bile ducts, related to obstruction. Radiology 1980; 135: 215–216

191 Mueller P R, Ferrucci J T Jr, Simeone J F. Observations on the distensibility of the common bile duct. Radiology 1982; 142: 467–472

192 Mahour G H, Wakim K G, Soule E H et al. Structure of the common bile duct in man. Ann Surg 1967; 166: 91–94

193 Schein C F, Beneventano T C. Choledochal dynamics in man. Surg Gynecol Obstet 1968; 126: 591–596

194 Sauerbrei E E, Cooperberg P L, Gordon P, Li D, Cohen M M, Burhenne H J. The discrepancy between radiographic and sonographic bile duct measurements. Radiology 1980; 137: 751–755

195 Clain A. Hamilton Bailey's physical signs in clinical surgery, 14th edn. Bristol: Wright, 1967

196 Gross B H, Harter L P, Gore R M et al. Ultrasonic evaluation of common bile duct stones; prospective comparison with endoscopic retrograde cholangiopancreatography. Radiology 1983; 146: 471–474

197 Cronan J J, Mueller P R, Simeone J F et al. Prospective diagnosis of choledocholithiasis. Radiology 1983; 146: 467–469

198 Einstein D M, Lapin S A, Ralls P W, Halls J M. The insensitivity of sonography in the detection of choledocholithiasis. AJR 1984; 142: 725–728

199 Laing F C, Jeffrey R B, Wing V W. Improved visualisation of choledocholithiasis by sonography. AJR 1984; 143: 949–952

200 Dong B, Chen M. Improved sonographic visualisation of choledocholithiasis. JCU 1987; 15: 185–190

201 Way L W, Sleisenger M H. Biliary obstruction, cholangitis, and choledocholithiasis. In: Sleisenger M H, Fordtran J S, eds. Gastrointestinal disease. Philadelphia: W B Saunders, 1983; 1389–1403

202 Glenn F. Postcholecystectomy choledocholithiasis. Surg Gynecol Obstet 1972; 134: 249–252

203 Laing F C, Jeffrey R B. Choledocholithiasis and cystic duct obstruction: difficult ultrasonographic diagnosis. Radiology 1983; 146: 475–479

204 Kane R A. The biliary system. In: Kurtz A B, Goldberg B B, eds. Gastrointestinal ultrasonography. Clinics in diagnostic ultrasound. Edinburgh: Churchill Livingstone, 1988: 75–137

205 Dewbury K C, Smith C L. The misdiagnosis of common bile duct stones with ultrasound. Br J Radiol 1983; 56: 625–630

206 Carroll B A. Biliary cystadenoma and cystadenocarcinoma: gray scale ultrasound appearance. JCU 1978; 6: 337–340

207 Bondstam S, Kivilaakse E O, Standetskjold-Nordenstam C-G M, Holmstrom T, Hastebaeka J. Sonographic diagnosis of a bile duct polyp. AJR 1980; 135: 610–611

208 Stanley J, Vujic I, Schabel S I, Gobien R P, Reines H D. Evaluation of biliary cystadenoma and cystadenocarcinoma. Gastrointest Radiol 1983; 8: 245–258

209 Marchal G, Gelin J, Van Steenbergen W V et al. Sonographic diagnosis of intraluminal bile duct neoplasm; a report of 3 cases. Gastrointest Radiol 1984; 9: 329–333

210 Klatskin G. Adenocarcinoma of the hepatic duct at its bifurcation within the porta hepatis. Am J Med 1965; 38: 241–256

211 Dillon E, Peel A L G, Parkin G J S. The diagnosis of primary bile duct carcinoma (cholangiocarcinoma) in the jaundiced patient. Clin Radiol 1981; 32: 311–317

212 Meyer D G, Weinstein B J. Klatskin tumors of the bile ducts: sonographic appearance. Radiology 1983; 148: 803–804

213 Subramanyam B R, Raghavendra B N, Balthazar E J et al. Ultrasonic features of cholangiocarcinoma. J Ultrasound Med 1984; 3: 405

214 Marchan L, Muller N L, Cooperberg P L. Sonographic diagnosis of Klatskin tumors. AJR 1986; 147: 509

215 Gibson R N, Yeung E, Thompson J N et al. Bile duct obstruction; radiologic evaluation of level, cause and tumour resectability. Radiology 1986; 160: 43–47

216 Karstrup S. Ultrasound diagnosis of cholangiocarcinoma at the confluence of the hepatic ducts (Klatskin tumours). Br J Radiol 1988; 61: 987–990

217 Yeung E Y C, McCarthy P, Gompertz R H, Benjamin I S, Gibson R N, Dawson P. The ultrasonographic appearances of hilar cholangiocarcinoma (Klatskin tumours). Br J Radiol 1988; 61: 991–995

218 Filly R A, Carlsen E N. Choledochal cyst: report of a case with specific ultrasonographic findings. JCU 1979; 4: 7–10

219 Reuter K, Raptopoulos V D, Cantelmo N, Fitzpatrick G, Hawes H L E. The diagnosis of a choledochal cyst by ultrasound. Radiology 1980; 136: 437–438

220 Han B K, Babcock D S, Gelfand M H. Choledochal cyst with bile duct dilatation; sonography and ^{99m}Tc IDA cholescintigraphy. AJR 1981; 136: 1075–1079

221 Kangarloo H, Sarti D A, Sample W F et al. Ultrasonographic spectrum of choledochal cysts in children. Pediatr Radiol 1980; 9: 15

222 Kimura K, Ohto M, Ono T et al. Congenital cystic dilatation of the common bile duct: relationship to anomalous pancreaticobiliary ductal union. AJR 1977; 128: 571–577

223 Jona J Z, Babitt D P, Starshak R J, Laporta A J, Glicklich M, Cohen R D. Anatomic observations and etiologic and surgical considerations in choledochal cyst. J Pediatr Surg 1979; 14: 315–320

224 Filly R A, Freimanis A K. Thrombosed hepatic artery aneurysm – report of a case diagnosed echographically. Radiology 1970; 97: 629–630

225 Caroli J, Spoupaut R, Kossakowski J, Plocker I, Paradowska M. La dilatation polykistique congénitale des voies biliaires interhépatiques: essai de classification. Semin Hosp Paris 1958; 34: 488–495

226 Mujahed Z, Glenn F, Evans J. Communicating cavernous ectasia of the intrahepatic bile ducts (Caroli's disease). Am J Radiol 1971; 113: 21–26

227 Bass E M, Funston M R, Shaff M I. Caroli's disease: an ultrasound diagnosis. Br J Radiol 1977; 50: 366–369

228 Mittelstaedt C A, Volberg F M, Fischer G J et al. Caroli's disease: sonographic findings. AJR 1980; 134: 585–587

229 Rosenfield A T, Siegel N J, Kappelman N B, Taylor K J W. Gray scale ultrasonography in medullary cystic disease of the kidney and congenital hepatic fibrosis with tubular ectasia: new observations. AJR 1977; 129: 297–303

230 Caroli J. Disease of intrahepatic bile ducts. Israel J Med Sci 1968; 4: 213–215

231 Imai Y, Watanabe M D, Kondo Y, Nakanishi M D. Caroli's disease: its diagnosis with non-invasive methods. Br J Radiol 1981; 54: 526–528

232 Morikawa P, Ishida H, Niizawa M, Komatsu M, Arakawa H, Masamune O. Sonographic features of biliary clonorchiasis. JCU 1988; 16: 655–658

233 Lim J H, Ko Y T, Lee D H, Kim S Y. Clonorchiasis: sonographic findings in 59 proved cases. AJR 1989; 152: 761–764

234 Ralls P W, Colletti P M, Quinn M F et al. Sonography in recurrent oriental pyogenic cholangitis. AJR 1981; 136: 1010

235 Federle M P, Cello J P, Laing F C, Jeffrey R B. Recurrent pyogenic cholangitis in Asian immigrants. Radiology 1982; 143: 151

236 Schulman A, Loxton A J, Heydenrych J J, Abdurahman K E. Sonographic diagnosis of biliary ascariasis. AJR 1982; 139: 485–489

237 Cerri G C, Leite G J, Simoes J B et al. Ultrasonographic evaluation of ascaris in the biliary tract. Radiology 1983; 146: 753–754

238 Doyle T C A, Roberts-Thomson I C. Radiological features of sclerosing cholangitis. Australas Radiol 1983; 27: 163

16

The pancreas

David O Cosgrove

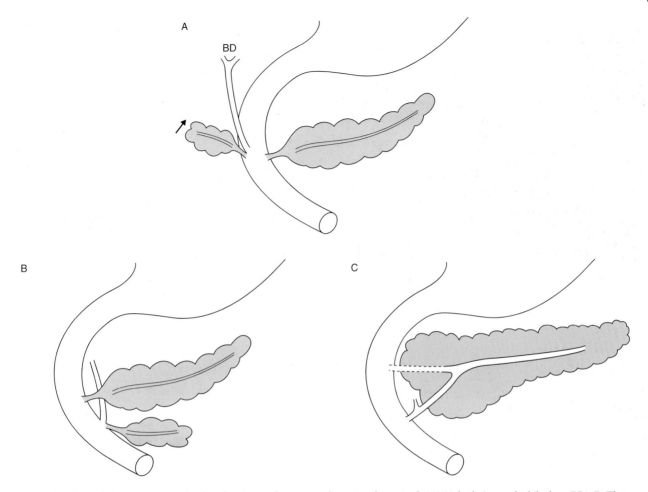

Fig. 16.5 Embryology of the pancreas. A: The dorsal and ventral (arrow) anlagen are shown in their initial relation to the bile duct (BD). **B:** The ventral pancreas lies adjacent to the dorsal segment following its migration around the duodenum. **C:** The normal adult configuration. The head of the pancreas has components from both the dorsal and ventral anlagen, whereas the uncinate process derives exclusively from the ventral anlage.

wall, the small intestine and even the spleen and gall-bladder can all contain ectopic tissue.

The commonest form of pancreatic ectopia is the annular pancreas (Fig. 16.6).[3] Pancreatic tissue encircles the bowel, usually the second part of the duodenum, lying within the muscularis mucosa.[4] Patients present early in life (50% in the first year) with proximal small bowel obstruction. Sometimes only partial encirclement is seen, and these patients may be symptom free. Annular pancreas is thought to be persistence of part of the ventral pancreas and is associated with duodenal atresia, malrotations, tracheo-oesophageal fistulae and imperforate anus.[5]

Pancreas divisum

In a small percentage of cases (1–5%) dorsal and ventral anlagen fail to fuse and their duct systems remain separate;

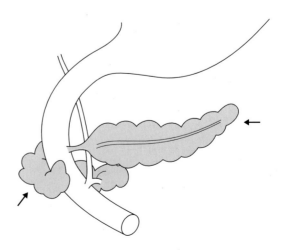

Fig. 16.6 Annular pancreas:. The ventral anlage (arrow) encircles the duodenum and may lead to obstruction.

this is termed 'pancreas divisum', an anomaly that is most often diagnosed by ERCP.[6,7] On cannulation of the duct of Wirsung, contrast only fills the ventral segment of the gland – the accessory duct of Santorini must be cannulated separately to delineate the pancreatic body and tail. It can also be recognised with high-resolution ultrasound (Figs 16.7 and 16.8).

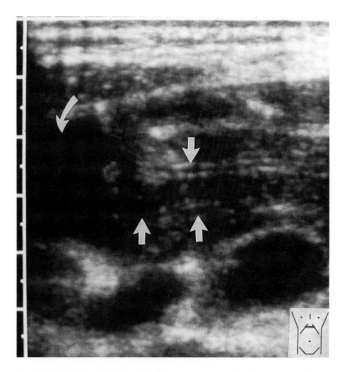

Fig. 16.7 Pancreas divisum. The two non-communicating pancreatic ducts (arrows) open into the fluid-filled duodenum (curved arrow).

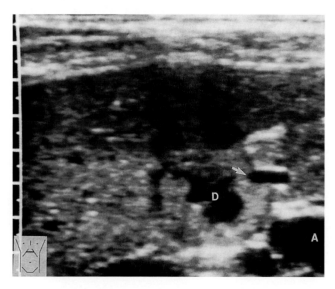

Fig. 16.8 Pancreas divisum. A dilated duct of Santorini (arrow) at its opening into the duodenum (D). A – aorta.

Pancreas divisum is thought to predispose to pancreatitis of the dorsal segment because of inadequate drainage.[6] However, despite pancreatic duct pressure monitoring the precise association remains uncertain.

Cysts

Solitary or multiple congenital cysts may be found in the pancreas, either as isolated lesions or as part of adult dominant polycystic kidney disease (see Ch. 22) or the von Hippel–Lindau syndrome. In cystic fibrosis the cysts contain inspissated secretions.

Ultrasound appearances

The normal pancreas is homogeneous with a reflectivity greater than or equal to the adjacent liver.[8] Correlation with CT shows that variations in reflectivity probably relate to the degree of fatty infiltration that occurs along the pancreatic septa[9] (Fig. 16.9). After 60 years of age fatty accumulation in pancreatic tissues is common; it is also increased in the obese, in patients on corticosteroids and in Cushing's disease.[10] On CT the lobular architecture of the pancreas is exaggerated, whereas on ultrasound the more reflective gland blends with the surrounding retroperitoneal fat, so that its size may be overestimated. Intralobular fat can also contribute to pancreatic reflectivity: the portion of the gland derived from the ventral pancreas (uncinate and posterior part of the head) is relatively echo poor in 25% of subjects, and this correlates with a lack of intraparenchymal fat cells on histology[11] (Fig. 16.10). It is important to recognise that this is a normal variant and not an echo-poor lesion: the characteristic position, lack of mass effect or of Doppler changes are helpful features.

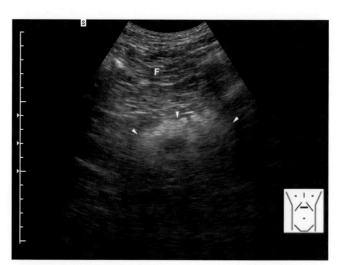

Fig. 16.9 Fatty infiltration. In this obese subject the pancreas is highly reflective with a feathered anterior margin (arrowheads). This is a normal variant. F – fat (subcutaneous).

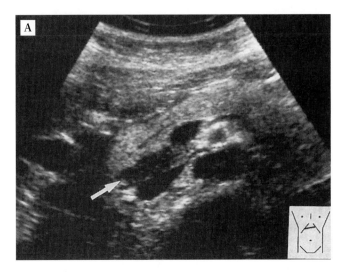 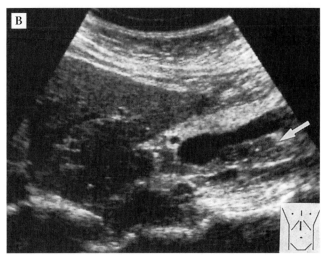

Fig. 16.10 Normal ventral pancreas. A: Transverse and **B:** longitudinal scans. The decreased reflectivity of the ventral pancreas (arrows) compared with the rest of the gland is shown.

The maximum AP diameters on ultrasound of the head and body have been measured as 25 and 15 mm,[12,13] and the maximum for the tail is 35 mm. However, pancreatic measurements may not be very useful in clinical practice because of the wide normal variations, particularly relating to the distribution of the volume of the pancreas between the head and body–tail regions: some subjects seem to have a 'top-heavy' gland, whereas in others the tail is relatively large.[14] In one study, the classic superior curving of the tail was only seen in 50% of normals.[15] Clinical assessment must have regard for the aggregate size and, in practice, the shape is more useful: a pancreas that has lost the tapering portion at its neck is under suspicion of being enlarged.

The variations in size of the normal pancreas are partly age related. The fact that the pancreas tends to atrophy with age must be borne in mind: a pancreas of normal size for a young patient may represent a diffusely enlarged gland in an elderly patient. Not all pancreatic disease increases the gland's size: for instance, in diabetes mellitus the pancreas may be smaller than normal.[16]

Pancreatic duct

With modern ultrasound equipment the duct can be visualised in almost 90% of patients as a tubular structure with reflective walls. It is best assessed in the body of the pancreas, where it lies perpendicular to the ultrasound beam and has a relatively straight course.[17] The duct dilates with age, but in subjects younger than 60 years its maximum diameter should be no more than 3 mm. Duct enlargement occurs in a wide range of pancreatic diseases.

In equivocal cases a stress test using secretin to stimulate the exocrine pancreas may be useful: in the fasting state the normal duct has a diameter of 1 mm, and this dilates to 2.7 mm 3 minutes after secretin injection.[18] If the duct is obstructed, dilatation is more marked following secretin stimulation.[19]

Ultrasound techniques

Several different ultrasound methods may be used to visualise the pancreas. Although transabdominal scanning with B-mode or Doppler is the conventional way to image the pancreas, endoscopic and intra-operative ultrasound can also be used to advantage.

Transabdominal ultrasound

Techniques to overcome the barrier of intestinal gas include an overnight fast (to ensure an empty stomach) and imaging the head and body of the pancreas through the left lobe of the liver, which is improved with the patient upright because the gassy bowel falls inferiorly.[20] Displacement of intervening bowel gas by gentle but firm pressure with the ultrasound probe is often sufficient alone to achieve adequate access to the pancreas: the main practical requirement is patience!

The pancreatic tail can often be detected through the spleen, where the splenic vessels form a useful landmark, and a fluid load is helpful in producing an acoustic window through the stomach.[21] Up to 500 ml of any non-gassy fluid may be used, and one of the chopped cellulose preparations (e.g. SonoRx, Bracco, Milan) has been shown to offer better visualisation than water.[22] The fluid is given with the patient lying on the left side, to fill the gastric fundus. Scanning is delayed a few minutes to allow the fluid to settle. The body and tail of the gland are best seen in this position, and turning the patient on to the right side allows fluid to pass into the antrum and duodenum, facilitating examination of the head and uncinate process. In the fasted patient the fluid load in the stomach may all spill into the duodenum within a few minutes while the patient is in this position. Duodenal paralysis greatly enhances visualisation of the ampulla and ventral segment of the pancreas, but is not often required.[23]

Doppler

Doppler studies are an integral part of the ultrasound examination of the abnormal pancreas. Frequencies of 2.5–5 MHz are used, with a high-pass filter to reduce the effects of vessel wall and other non-vascular movements. The normal Doppler time velocity (spectral) waveform signals for all the major intra-abdominal vessels have been well documented.[24] Although understanding of abnormal signals is incomplete, changes in the time–velocity waveform do reflect the effect of pancreatic disease on surrounding vasculature (Fig. 16.11). Colour Doppler complements spectral Doppler with useful anatomical information on the relationship of masses to blood vessels, and this is useful in tumour staging and gauging resectability.[25–27]

Endoscopic ultrasound

Endoscopic ultrasound is another way to improve acoustic access to the pancreas.[28,29] Conventional duodenoscopes have been modified to incorporate an ultrasound trans-

ducer at or near their tip. Linear array systems have a smaller field of view than radial transducers, which produce a 360° image. The latter are shorter and therefore impede scope flexibility to a lesser degree. They are covered by a rubber balloon which, when distended with fluid, ensures good contact with the bowel wall for sound transmission. As with intra-operative scanning the close proximity of the target organ to the transducer allows a high-frequency transducer to be used, and they are capable of resolution of the order of 0.2 mm.

After distension of the bowel with air the scope is passed under visual control to the third part of the duodenum. The air is then removed, the balloon distended and the scope slowly withdrawn. The head of the pancreas and uncinate process can be imaged through the duodenal wall, the body and neck through the gastric antrum, and the tail through the stomach body. Resolution is much better than with transabdominal scanning, so that small lesions not previously seen may be identified (Figs 16.12 and 16.13). It is more sensitive in identifying peri-pancreatic adenopathy and a better assessment of ductal anatomy can be made; this technique is the most specific diagnostic method currently available, next to biopsy.[30]

An extension of this approach is to use miniature transducers that can be passed into the pancreatic duct to study its detailed morphology, particularly in chronic pancreatitis and intraductal tumours.[31]

Intraoperative ultrasound

For intra-operative ultrasound linear array probes of up to 10 MHz are used to provide good resolution of structures close to the probe face. The transducer may be gas sterilised, but covering with a sterile plastic drape or sheath is

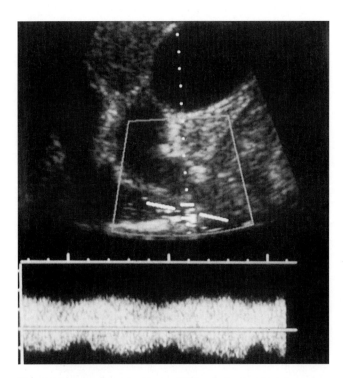

Fig. 16.11 Spectral Doppler. Trace of high-velocity flow in the portal vein at a stenosis produced by a compressing pancreatic mass. Note the reversed flow component indicating flow disturbance.

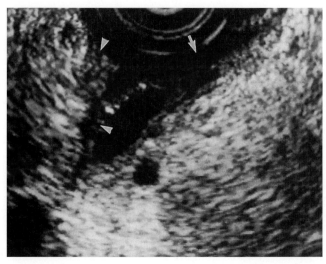

Fig. 16.12 Ampullary tumour. Endoscopic ultrasound showing tumour invading the bile duct (arrowheads) and duodenal wall (arrow).

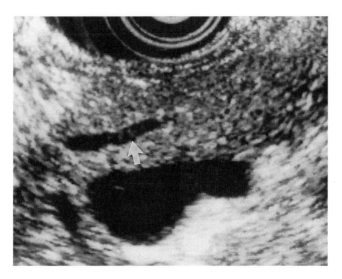

Fig. 16.13 Duct dilatation. Endoscopic ultrasound image of a minimally dilated pancreatic duct (arrow).

more practical and generally satisfactory. The surgically exposed pancreas is examined directly. To improve superficial resolution the lesser sac may be part-filled with saline and the probe held just above the tissue surface.[32–34]

Manipulation of the probe is best performed by the radiologist, who is more familiar with ultrasound landmarks. If possible the patient should be scanned from the right side. Many intra-operative probes have a very short focus and the scanning technique should aim to bring the target into the focal zone. Intra-operative ultrasound is of value in searching for small tumours, such as insulinomas, and in defining the pancreatic anatomy, particularly of the ductal system, prior to surgery. Small calculi, cysts and vascular abnormalities are well demonstrated.

Acute pancreatitis

An accepted international definition of acute pancreatitis is 'an acute condition typically presenting with abdominal pain and usually associated with raised pancreatic enzymes in blood or urine, due to inflammatory disease of the pancreas.' The vagueness of this definition reveals the poverty of our understanding of the underlying pathology.[35]

Aetiology and clinical features

The incidence of alcoholic pancreatitis is increasing in most countries in the west. Nevertheless, over 60% of cases in the UK are caused by gallstones, and these patients are more likely to die, probably because of early bacterial contamination of necrotic pancreatic tissue.[36,37] The mumps virus, hyperlipidaemia and hypercalcaemia can all cause acute pancreatitis, and although many other aetiologies are listed in the medical literature these are relatively uncommon and clinically unimportant, being based largely on single case reports.

Many different experimental models of acute pancreatitis have been constructed but only three features of relevance to the disease in humans can be derived from animal studies: reflux of bile or duodenal contents into the pancreatic duct system; an increase in intraduct pressure; and bacterial contamination of the interstitial spaces of the pancreatic parenchyma. The most consistent experimental cause is elevation of the pressure in the pancreatic duct system. Above a pressure of $60\,\mathrm{cmH_2O}$ the basement membranes of the alveoli rupture, allowing duct contents to escape into the interstitium. This alone is enough to cause acute pancreatitis, but the presence of bile or duodenal content, particularly enterokinase, accelerates enzyme activation. Bacterial contamination leads to early infection of necrotic material.

The mechanism of alcohol induction of pancreatitis remains subject to debate (see below).

Most of our knowledge of the progress of acute pancreatitis is based on radiological studies; the separation of acute pancreatitis into acute interstitial and necrotising varieties is of practical value. Acute interstitial pancreatitis (AIP) is a mild disease characterised by rapid recovery and complete restitution of the pancreas to normal, whereas in necrotising pancreatitis there is irreversible destruction of the gland; it may be subclassified as mild (<50% of the pancreas necrosed) or severe. Mortality is much higher in the severe form.[4]

Histopathological studies of acute pancreatitis are difficult to perform because of the rapid autolysis that occurs after death. Despite this, all cases of severe and long-standing pancreatitis show a common feature: large and confluent foci of peripancreatic fat necrosis. These foci extend along the interstitial septa into the parenchyma of the pancreas itself, and are associated with necrosis of contiguous acini.

Venous thrombosis, haemorrhage and infarction characterise advanced parenchymal damage; involvement of the parenchyma is irregular, with necrosis often being very localised. These observations suggest that acute pancreatitis advances mainly through the progression of fat necrosis across the surface of the gland, with subsequent patchy vascular damage leading to infarction.[38] This theory is consistent with the available imaging evidence, where glandular tissue can appear well perfused with normal architecture in the first 24 hours, patchy or confluent necrosis only becoming evident beyond 48 hours.

Despite the increasing incidence of acute pancreatitis, mortality rates have steadily reduced over the past 10 years. This improvement can be attributed to improved metabolic maintenance (particularly with total parenteral nutrition), better management of patients in respiratory failure, and active radiological monitoring of acute pancreatitis and its complications, especially the detection of pancreatic necrosis or abscess, leading to earlier intervention.

The diagnosis of acute pancreatitis is usually made on clinical grounds, together with a serum amylase elevated above 1000 IU/l. However, even in severe pancreatitis the rise in serum amylase may be transitory and unrecorded, so that the diagnosis may be unclear. The majority of patients recover with conservative management. Imaging studies are not needed at this stage, but it is very important that an ultrasound scan of the gallbladder and biliary tree be performed during recovery to detect gallstones. Over 30% of patients with gallstone pancreatitis will have further attacks within 6 months, and the recurrences are often more severe. Virtually all these can be prevented by interval cholecystectomy. The scan is best performed immediately prior to discharge, when visualisation is better than during the acute stage because of meteorism.

Two clinical methods are commonly used for early assessment of the severity of acute pancreatitis. A cumulative score of clinical features on admission factors in age (over 55 years), white blood cell count (>16 000), blood glucose (>10 mmol/l), serum LDH (>700 IU) and AST (>250 units). Other important prognostic factors within the first 48 hours of admission are a rising blood urea nitrogen (BUN) >5 mg%, PaO_2<60 mm/mg and a serum calcium <2 mmol/l. Prognostic factor analysis provides a reliable method of identifying patients at risk of severe disease early in the course of the illness. Alternatively, a simple analysis of peritoneal lavage fluid has been proposed. This can be performed at the bedside and has similar accuracy in discriminating severe from mild pancreatitis. Dark-coloured fluid with the appearance of prune juice is a strong indication of pancreatic necrosis with extension of the inflammatory process into the peritoneal cavity. Radiological grading methods based on morphological criteria have also been developed (see below).

Complications following AIP are uncommon, but significant pseudocysts can follow even mild attacks and should be excluded by ultrasound or CT scanning prior to discharge.[39]

Ultrasound appearances

Mild acute interstitial pancreatitis (AIP) causes swelling of the parenchyma of the gland, which may be focal or lobular in distribution. Oedema accumulating in the peripancreatic fat spaces leads to reduction in the echo intensity and there may also be fluid in the lesser sac or adjacent peritoneal recesses (Figs 16.14 to 16.16). The duct system is compressed.

Ultrasound is highly specific in the diagnosis of AIP, typically showing pancreatic enlargement, a generalised reduction in parenchymal reflectivity and a relative increase in the reflectivity of the walls of a normal or narrowed duct system. Colour Doppler frequently shows hyperaemia in and around the poorly reflective regions of

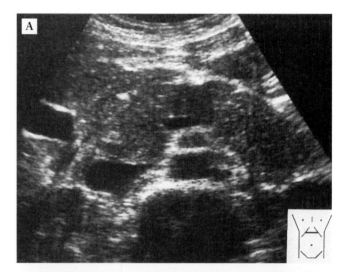

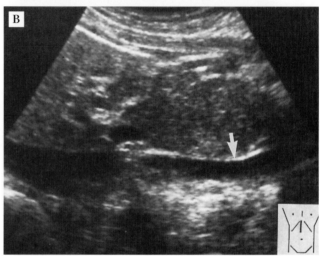

Fig. 16.14 Mild acute interstitial pancreatitis. A: Transverse section. **B:** Longitudinal section. There is generalised enlargement of the gland with a slightly heterogeneous parenchyma and an overall reduction in reflectivity. Note the indentation of the cava (arrow) by the swollen pancreatic head in B.

acute pancreatitis. Small fluid accumulations are easy to recognise, but oedema in the surrounding fat may obscure the pancreatic boundaries. It is important to note that the changes in mild AIP may be focal: patchy oedema or necrosis can be confined to one or more individual pancreatic lobules, which are 7–8 mm in diameter and divided from one another by fine fibrous septa. Intrapancreatic oedema may render the septa visible as thin, bright lines radiating from the centre to the periphery of the gland. Focal interstitial pancreatitis sometimes produces an echo-poor mass that is difficult to distinguish from a tumour.

CT is less sensitive in showing the intrapancreatic changes in mild AIP but demonstrates the effects on the surrounding tissues better.[40] Oedema in peripancreatic fat results in a density midway between fat and fluid, and

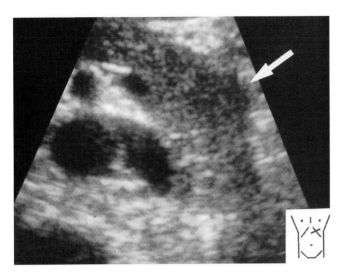

Fig. 16.15 Focal acute interstitial pancreatitis. A single lobule is enlarged and reduced in reflectivity (arrow).

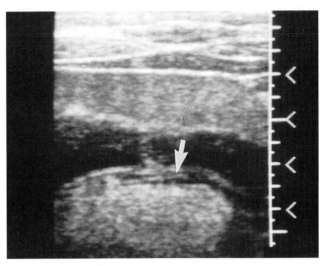

Fig. 16.16 Moderate acute interstitial pancreatitis. The pancreas is swollen, with a small fluid collection in the lesser sac (arrow).

small fluid collections are easily recognised. Thickening of the peritoneum and Gerota's fascia suggests retroperitoneal inflammation, but if these are the sole features on CT they do not necessarily indicate the presence of active pancreatic disease.[41]

For patients with clinically severe acute pancreatitis the initial ultrasound examination should concentrate on the biliary tree to exclude gallstone disease as a remediable cause; significant dilation (CBD >6 mm) is an indication for urgent endoscopy and biliary sphincterotomy, with removal of any choledochal stones.[42–44]

A scan of the pancreas performed too early in the disease process may be misleading, as the gland can appear to be remarkably normal in the first 24 hours. Later it typically appears bulky and echo poor, and peripancreatic collections may be identified. Meteorism, abdominal tenderness and other problems of the acute abdomen often preclude satisfactory ultrasound visualisation, although scans of the head and tail of the pancreas can usually be obtained through the flanks (Figs 16.17 and 16.18). There are no useful ultrasound features that allow a distinction between necrotising and non-necrotising pancreatitis. Virtually all patients with clinically significant acute pancreatitis develop peripancreatic fluid collections in the first week of the disease, but only a few form true pseudocysts.[45] These track along the tissue planes, especially in the anterior pararenal space, where they give a striated pattern to the retroperitoneal fat tissue and may collect in the lesser sac. They are the precursors of pseudocysts.

Complications of acute pancreatitis

The important complications of acute pancreatitis are:

- biliary obstruction;

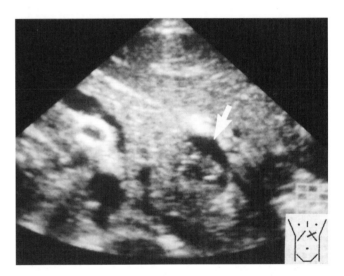

Fig. 16.17 Focal necrotising pancreatitis. A small focus of parenchymal necrosis in the tail is associated with leakage of juice into the peripancreatic fat space (arrow).

- obstruction to the gastrointestinal tract;
- pancreatic ascites;
- renal obstruction;
- aneurysm formation;
- pseudocyst formation.

Most of these are minor and transient and require no active intervention, but aneurysms can cause fatal haemorrhage. They take 2–3 weeks to develop and should be searched for by colour Doppler scanning in any case of severe pancreatitis.[46,47]

Pseudocysts are collections of pancreatic fluid with a high amylase content, surrounded by a fibrous wall. They develop in up to 50% of patients 2–3 weeks after a severe

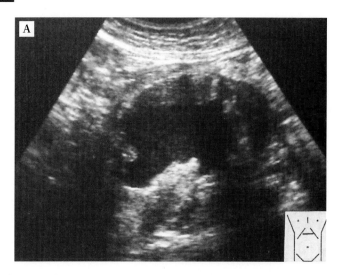

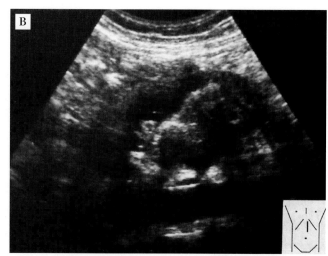

Fig. 16.18 Severe necrotising pancreatitis. A: Transverse section. **B:** Longitudinal section. The pancreas has been replaced by a heterogeneous mass with no discernible anatomical features.

attack of acute pancreatitis (Figs 16.19 and 16.20) and are usually easy to delineate with ultrasound as fluid spaces with no or only low-level internal echoes. Sometimes they are multiloculated. The wall thickens as the cyst matures, and this is a useful guide to plan the timing of surgery (Figs 16.21 to 16.23); eventually they may calcify. The surgical and radiological literature is replete with descriptions of chronic pseudocysts which have dissected through various tissue planes to unusual locations. With prompt diagnosis and early treatment few cysts are now allowed time to dissect into remote locations, and the vast majority lie close to the pancreas, most in the lesser sac. Rarely a pseudocyst may rupture into the peritoneal space, when its digestive enzymes produce severe acute peritonitis.

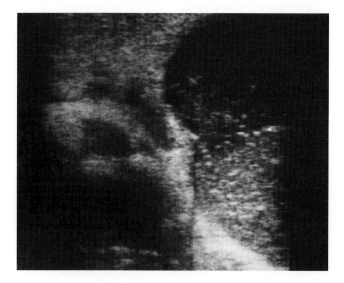

Fig. 16.19 Infected pseudocyst. An intra-operative scan showing low-level echoes in the cavity.

In the early stages pseudocysts may regress and disappear, but if there is no improvement by 6 weeks,[48] percutaneous drainage is required and can be curative. With non-communicating cysts drainage ceases promptly after evacuation and the catheter can be safely removed after a few days, following a check ultrasound.[20] If the cyst communicates with the duct system, pancreatic juice continues to flow at 30–200 ml daily. The communication may be demonstrated by ERCP which, though ordinarily contraindicated in the presence of a pseudocyst, carries minimal risk of rupture with a drainage catheter in situ.[49]

Pseudocysts arising in the tail of the pancreas lie close to the spleen and its pedicle so that splenic vein thrombosis and splenic infarction are common complications. Both may be demonstrated with colour Doppler. The thrombosis may extend to include the superior mesenteric and portal veins. Subsequently gastric varices may develop and the patient may re-present with a haematemesis. Damage to the splenic artery by a pseudocyst is the most common cause of aneurysm formation.

Sepsis is a major causes of death in pancreatitis.[50] Others include cholangitis (especially when the biliary tree is obstructed), infected pancreatic necrosis and infection of the peripancreatic spaces.[51] Cholangitis cannot be diagnosed reliably with ultrasound, but abscesses in the pancreas or infection of pseudocysts produce cavities with irregular walls. However, as these appearances may be part of non-infective pancreatitis aspiration of fluid for culture is needed, and this can be guided by ultrasound or CT. Gas, the telltale sign of an infected collection, is uncommon in acute pancreatitis (about 10%).[52] The demonstration of organisms on an immediate Gram stain (about 50% of cases) is an indication for urgent surgery.

Percutaneous catheter drainage of infected pancreatic necrosis is rarely effective because of the viscid nature of

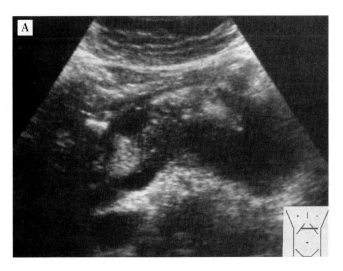
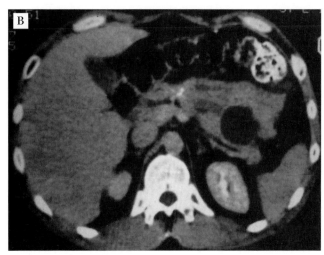

Fig. 16.20 Acute pancreatitis. A: Ultrasound, **B:** CT of a complex phlegmon arising from the tail of the pancreas and extending into the splenic pedicle. There is a small associated pseudocyst.

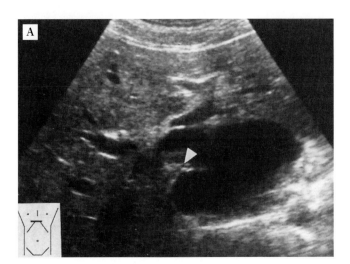
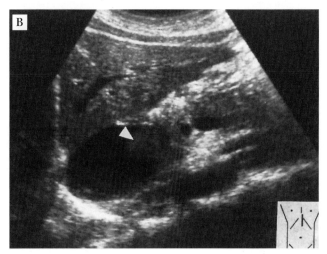

Fig. 16.21 Pseudocyst. A: Transverse, **B:** longitudinal scans in the upper abdomen show a small pseudocyst above the pancreas, probably lying in the lesser sac. The wall is thin (indicating that it is recent) and irregular in parts (arrowheads).

the fluid, although percutaneous lavage may have some value. However, infection of a pseudocyst or a peripancreatic space is a less urgent complication which does not always require formal surgical intervention and can often be managed solely by catheter drainage.[53] Complications include haemorrhage, which is usually self-limiting, and empyema. However, resolution is often slow (up to 6 months) and cutaneous or enteric fistulae may develop.

Traumatic pancreatitis

Severe pancreatic trauma produces the typical ultrasonic features of acute pancreatitis with an enlarged, dark gland.[54] Because the duct is usually disrupted, large pseudo-

cysts often form. With penetrating injuries the disruption can occur at any point, and there is usually also traumatic necrosis (Fig. 16.24).[21] In blunt injuries the neck of the pancreas is most vulnerable and the duct tears where it is compressed against the aorta and spine; it is the commonest cause of pancreatitis in the paediatric age group.[55] Even complete transection of the pancreas can be clinically silent until pancreatic ascites or a large pseudocyst develops. Distal pancreatectomy is required if there has been complete disruption of the main pancreatic duct, and a pancreatogram is essential in planning surgery. As with communicating pseudocysts, percutaneous decompression of the fluid collection improves the general wellbeing of the patient and allows a contrast study of the distal pancreas.

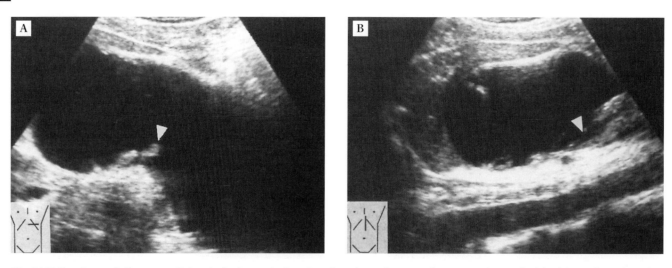

Fig. 16.22 Pseudocyst. A: Transverse, **B:** longitudinal scans in the epigastrium show a large pseudocyst extending to the left of the midline, along the lie of the lesser sac. Note the debris in the sac (arrowheads); its walls are thicker than in the case illustrated in Figure 16.21.

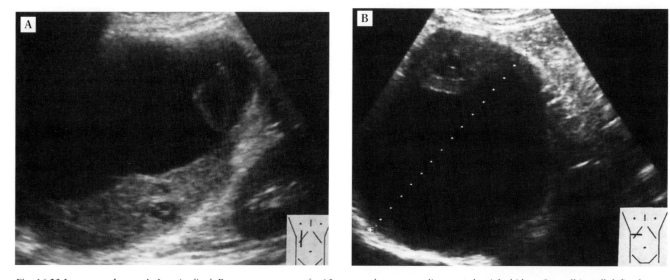

Fig. 16.23 Large pseudocyst. A: Longitudinal, **B:** transverse scans of a 15 cm pseudocyst extending over the right kidney. Its wall is well defined.

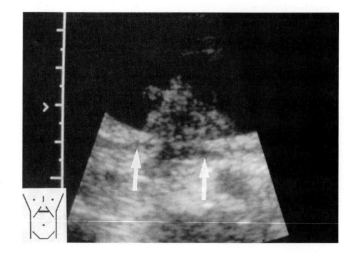

Fig. 16.24 Traumatic pancreatitis. A transverse view through the cyst shows a blood clot attached at the point of disruption of the gland. The main pancreatic duct can be seen to run through the disrupted segment (arrows).

Relapsing pancreatitis

Repeated attacks of acute pancreatitis are common in patients with gallstones and in cases of untreated hypercalcaemia and hyperlipidaemia, but the concept of a relapsing form of acute pancreatitis as originally proposed in Marseilles in 1960 is no longer recognised as a distinct entity.[56] Acute pancreatitis can also occur as an exacerbation of chronic pancreatitis. It is the latter that has caused most of the confusion in classification. Recurrent attacks of acute pancreatitis in patients with underlying chronic pancreatitis vary from bouts of abdominal pain to full-blown attacks of pancreatitis.

The ultrasonic features are a variable mixture of acute and chronic changes with a heterogeneous gland of irregular outline and calcifications. In mild or early cases careful ultrasonography usually reveals a focus of reduced reflectivity, which may be confined to a portion of the pancreas or even to a single lobule and is often associated with a small collection, either within or around the pancreas. These foci of acute pancreatitis are usually hypervascular on colour Doppler. Similar bouts of focal acute pancreatitis may follow percutaneous biopsy procedures and pancreatography if the injection pressure has been too high.

Obstructive pancreatopathy

Pancreatic fibrosis and atrophy of the parenchyma follow partial or complete obstruction of the main pancreatic duct. On histology this is a desmoplastic reaction most commonly seen surrounding infiltrating pancreatic carcinomas, but also found with any intraduct lesion that interferes with the free flow of pancreatic juice.[57] The lesion may be a small tumour (e.g. a neurofibroma or smooth muscle tumour) or heterotopic pancreatic tissue infiltrating the major or minor papilla, and is often obscured by the surrounding fibrosis so that it can be difficult to find, even in a resected specimen.

Many cases of pancreatitis secondary to congenital abnormalities of the pancreas have their origin in incomplete drainage. Pancreas divisum has an incidence of approximately 6%, but is seen in a higher proportion of patients with acute pancreatitis or duct obstruction. Careful ultrasonography often reveals the main pancreatic continuing towards the cranial and ventral aspect of the duodenal loop, a sign of dominant drainage via the duct of Santorini (Figs 16.25 and 16.26). The pancreas divisum anomaly can modify the distribution of disease. For example, in gallstone pancreatitis only the ventral pancreas may be affected, whereas because drainage via the minor papilla is more precarious, obstructive pancreatopathy may be confined to the dorsal portion.

Other congenital anomalies of pancreatic drainage are rare and, with the exception of the annular pancreas, usually asymptomatic. Drainage of the annular pancreas

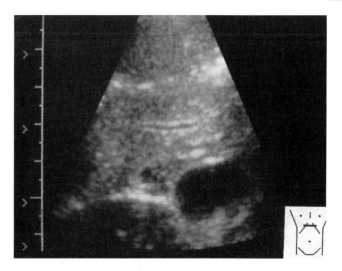

Fig. 16.25 Pancreas divisum. Transverse section through the head of the pancreas. The duct runs ventral to the more usual course.

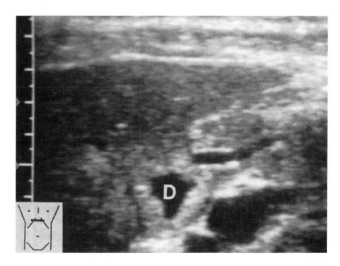

Fig. 16.26 Obstructive pancreatopathy. There is dilatation of the dorsal duct caused by poor drainage via the accessory papilla. The duct is visible as it enters the fluid-filled duodenum (D).

may be so poor that it results in pancreatic fibrosis, with subsequent duodenal stenosis.

Chronic pancreatitis

Chronic pancreatitis is a relatively uncommon disease whose incidence varies from 0.2% to 3% in autopsy series. It seems to have become more common in the past 20 years, probably as a result of increased alcohol consumption, though its pathogenesis is still a matter of debate.[58] Alcohol may cause direct parenchymal damage or operate by precipitating protein secretions so that ducts are obstructed.[57,59] The features of advanced chronic pancreatitis are irregular scarring of the pancreatic parenchyma (typically on a lobular scale), strictures of the main pancreatic duct and stenosis of the side branches (usually at their junctions with the main duct). Intraductal protein plugs are a common finding, and these frequently calcify in severe disease. Many cases show focal necrosis with intrapancreatic pseudocyst formation.

The ultrasound changes of chronic pancreatitis are best understood in the light of its evolution.[60] In early disease parenchymal damage with fibrosis, irregularities of the main pancreatic duct and an increase in bulk of the pancreatic parenchyma predominate. The pancreas has an inhomogeneous echo texture with a beaded duct and pseudocysts. In more severe cases the parenchymal fibrosis becomes confluent and progresses to form strictures in the main pancreatic duct, with upstream dilatation (leading to intraduct calcifications) and inflammation extending to surrounding retroperitoneal structures (Figs 16.27 and 16.28). The pancreas shrinks with advancing fibrosis and calcifications may be extensive, especially in the alcoholic type.

Chronic pancreatitis may be a focal disease involving small segments of pancreatic tissue. The descriptive term 'groove pancreatitis' has recently been proposed for the common type of focal pancreatitis, which affects the segment of pancreas lying between the common bile duct and the duodenum. This may result in dense focal fibrosis, indistinguishable from a desmoplastic tumour on ultrasound.[61]

A combination of imaging techniques is required to demonstrate all of these features and allow a grading scheme[35] (Table 16.1). Pancreatography is the most sensitive to duct changes and is generally regarded as the most specific method of diagnosis.[62,63] CT is not sensitive to chronic pancreatitis unless there is calcification, major duct dilatation or cyst formation. High-resolution ultrasonography is capable of demonstrating parenchymal changes involving the main pancreatic duct, and under good conditions of visualisation can demonstrate the side branches. However, it is notorious for being operator and patient dependent and has a lower success rate than CT in visualising the entire pancreas (Fig. 16.29).

Table 16.1 Grading of chronic pancreatitis

Ultrasound and CT signs of chronic pancreatitis:
Main duct dilated (>4 mm)
Gland enlarged (2 x N)
Cavities (<10 mm)
Irregular ducts
Focal acute pancreatitis
Parenchymal heterogeneity
Duct wall echoes increased
Irregular head/body contours

		ERCP	Ultrasound and CT
1.	Normal	Quality study demonstrating whole gland to be normal	
2.	Equivocal	< 3 abnormal branches	One sign only
3.	Mild	> 3 abnormal branches	Two or more signs
4.	Moderate	Abnormal main duct and branches	Two or more signs
5.	Marked	Abnormal main duct and branches, with one or more of: large cavities (> 10 mm) gross gland enlargement (> 2 x N) intraduct filling defects or calculi duct obstruction, stricture or gross irregularity contiguous organ invasion	

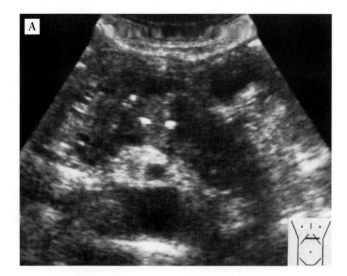
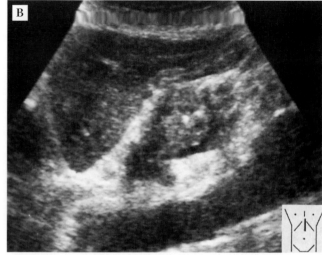

Fig. 16.27 Calcific pancreatitis. A: Transverse, **B:** longitudinal section of a moderately enlarged pancreas with multiple highly reflective foci representing calcification.

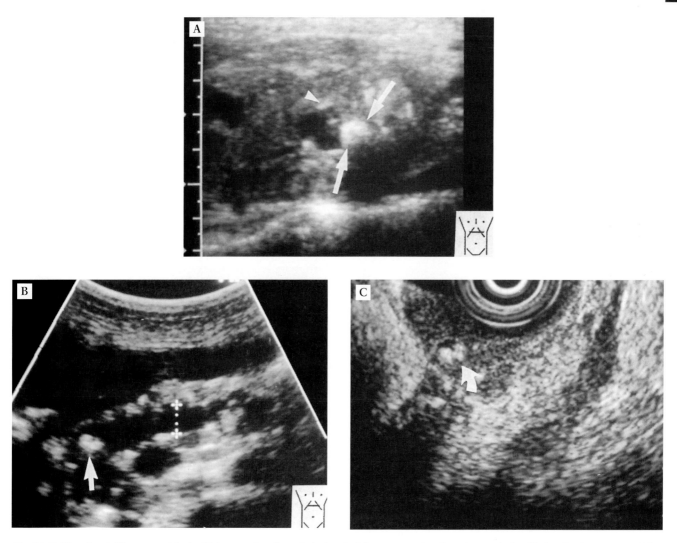

Fig. 16.28 Chronic calcific pancreatitis. A: Oblique section through the head of the pancreas showing a large calculus dilating the duct (arrows). The whole gland is bulky, with small calculi within the parenchyma (arrowhead). **B:** Transverse section through the pancreatic body shows an obstructing calculus (arrow) causing duct dilatation (7 mm). The surrounding parenchyma is atrophic. **C:** Endoscopic ultrasound scan showing small calculi within the duct in the ventral segment (arrow). Note the difference in reflectivity between the ventral segment and the surrounding dorsal gland.

Complications of chronic pancreatitis

The main complications of chronic pancreatitis are pseudocyst formation, biliary obstruction, portal vein thrombosis and duodenal obstruction. Pseudocysts in this condition are almost always secondary to complete duct obstruction by a calculus, and rarely respond to conservative measures or percutaneous drainage.[53]

The peribiliary fibrosis of chronic pancreatitis typically leads to the classic 'rat-tail' stricture in the distal common bile duct, but short strictures indistinguishable from their malignant equivalent are frequently seen. Evidence of previous portal vein fibrosis is commonly seen on colour Doppler imaging, with visualisation of varices or portal venous collaterals after occlusion of the main portal vein.

The portal vein thrombosis has usually been clinically silent, with full physiological compensation via collaterals. Local high-velocity flow can often be demonstrated by spectral or colour Doppler in regions where the vein is compressed.

Pancreatic tumours

Carcinoma of the pancreas accounts for 10% of all cancers of the digestive system and is the fifth commonest cause of cancer-related death in the USA. Adenocarcinoma, the commonest type, is highly lethal, with a 5-year survival of only 1–2%, though this improves to 10% if radical resection has been achieved.[64,65] The outlook for some of the rarer types is better. Its incidence has increased sharply over

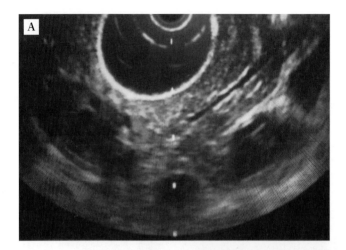

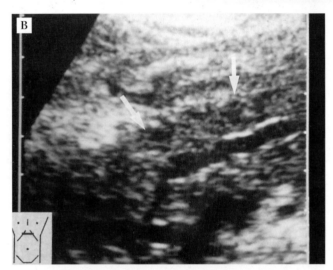

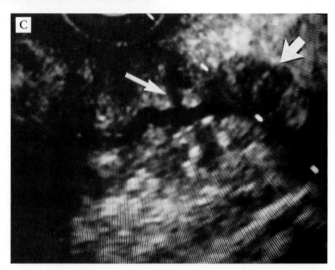

Fig. 16.29 Chronic pancreatitis. A: Endoscopic ultrasound of mild chronic pancreatitis. The parenchyma is normal but there is an increase in the reflectivity of the walls of the main duct. **B:** A section through the head and mid-body showing a dilated duct with irregularly reflective walls. The parenchyma contains some echo-poor lobules (arrows). **C:** Moderate chronic pancreatitis. An endoscopic scan shows dilatation of the main duct and of a side branch (arrow) which drains a poorly reflective lobule. Another inflamed lobule is seen with prominent intralobular septa (broad arrow). Highly reflective foci are seen throughout the parenchyma.

recent years: in England and Wales it has doubled since 1930. Despite advances in imaging techniques, attempts at early diagnosis have been unsuccessful and less than 10% of cases are suitable for resection. The overall mean survival time from presentation remains unchanged, at 6 months.

Pancreatic cancer is more common in men (male to female ratio of 1.5:1), but over the years this difference has decreased. The incidence of pancreatic cancer is age related, being uncommon below 45 but becoming increasingly common with age, and markedly so in the seventh and eighth decades. There is no significant geographical distribution and no important genetic, familial or social class factors have been identified.[66] An association between pancreatic cancer and smoking has been estab-

lished, but no other carcinogens have been convincingly defined.[67] Chronic alcoholism, a western diet and pre-existing diabetes mellitus have been implicated as aetiological factors in some studies, but the evidence for all of these remains inconclusive.

The most common presentation is with weight loss, abdominal pain and jaundice. Often these symptoms have been present for several months.[68] Pain is most often epigastric and radiates to the back in 60% of patients. Jaundice occurs at some time in the condition in 90% of cases and is progressive, although initially it may fluctuate in severity.

Primary non-endocrine pancreatic tumours can be classified by their cell type into ductal, acinar and connective tissue types (Table 16.1). Metastases constitute up to 7%

of pancreatic tumours in some studies, lymphoma being the most common.

Ductal adenocarcinoma

Ductal adenocarcinoma is the commonest type of pancreatic malignancy and most epidemiological research data relate to this type of lesion. On surgical specimens the majority of tumours range between 1.5 and 5 cm, the larger lesions being more typical of tumours that do not obstruct the bile and pancreatic ducts and so present later.[69] Its doubling time of around 60 days means that the tumour has been present for over 5 years before it can be

detected by current imaging techniques. Ductal hyperplasia is frequently seen in tissue adjacent to tumours of ductal origin, whereas this is not the case with acinar cell carcinomas. This, and evidence from mucin histochemistry, points to atypical ductal hyperplasia as a precancerous lesion in the development of ductal adenocarcinoma.[70]

Pancreatic cancer arises in the head of the pancreas in 61% of cases, the body in 13%, the tail in 5%, and in combination in 21%. Dilatation of the pancreatic and/or bile ducts is readily demonstrated (Figs 16.30 and 16.31), so that tumours as small as 1 cm can be identified in the head of the pancreas and the presence of even smaller lesions inferred, especially when both duct systems are

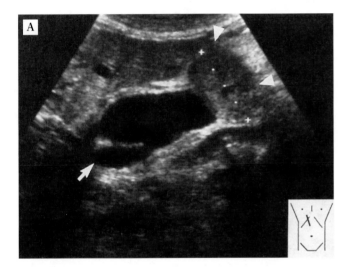
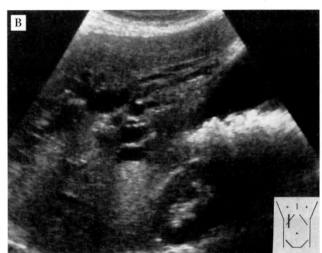

Fig. 16.30 Pancreatic carcinoma. A: A 4 cm echo-poor mass (arrowheads) is obstructing the lower end of the common bile duct. A dilated cystic duct (arrow) is also seen. **B:** Scan through the right lobe of the liver showing the dilated biliary tree and gallbladder, which contains incidental calculi. Gallbladder calculi are very common and must not be assumed to be the cause of the obstruction.

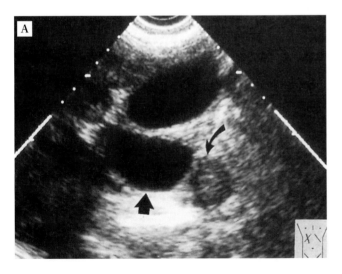
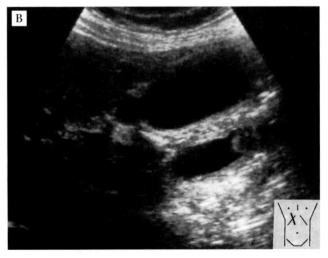

Fig. 16.31 Pancreatic carcinoma. A: A markedly dilated common bile duct (arrow) ends in a small, irregular pancreatic tumour (curved arrow). The gallbladder is also shown. **B:** A similar tumour extending into the lumen of the duct.

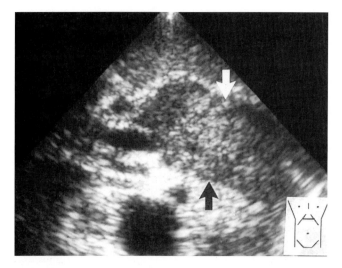

Fig. 16.32 Pancreatic carcinoma. The whole of the pancreatic tail is expanded by tumour (arrows).

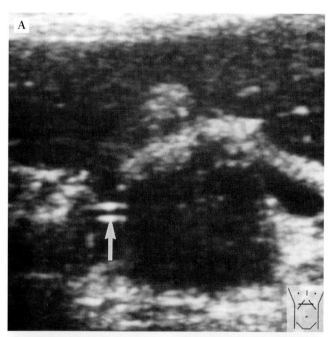

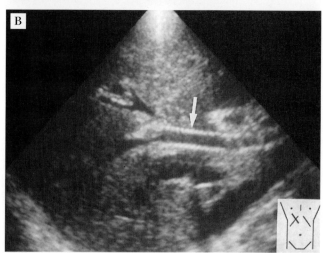

Fig. 16.33 Pancreatic carcinoma. A: A biliary stent (arrow) has been placed through the tumour. **B:** An expanding metal stent (arrow) is shown in the common hepatic duct.

dilated – the 'double-duct sign'.[1] Tumours elsewhere in the gland are harder to detect and may only be manifest by a change in the overlying pancreatic contour (Fig. 16.32).

Surgical excision offers the only cure for carcinoma of the pancreas, but is possible in less than 10% of cases. Relative contraindications to resection include tumours larger than 3 cm, site other than the head, invasion of the portal vein or retroperitoneum and the presence of metastases (nodal and hepatic being the most frequent). Unresectable tumours may be treated with chemotherapy or radiotherapy; results are, however, disappointing, with mean survival prolonged by only around 6 months. More useful is palliation of the troublesome pruritis and jaundice by stenting or by surgical bypass (Fig. 16.33). Ultrasound is useful for follow-up of these patients to assess biliary duct dilatation and drainage, and also to monitor tumour growth and spread.

Ultrasound appearances

The majority of pancreatic cancers are seen as a poorly reflective mass that is usually highly attenuating, perhaps because of their high connective tissue content, which may constitute over 99% of the total mass. Small tumours are homogeneous because their uniform internal structure presents few interfaces to the ultrasound beam (Fig. 16.34). Larger lesions are more heterogeneous because their internal structure becomes increasingly disorganised (Fig. 16.35), but uniformly strongly reflective adenocarcinomas are rare. The tumour is usually well defined with irregular or lobulated margins. Pre-existing chronic pancreatitis,[73] surrounding inflammation, a multifocal carcinoma or a tumour of similar reflectivity to the surrounding parenchyma may all impair tumour definition on ultrasound.

Indirect signs are also useful. If the pancreatic duct becomes obstructed it initially dilates smoothly with atrophy of the surrounding parenchyma. (Fig. 16.36), but further dilatation results in elongation of the duct (associated with shrinkage of the parenchyma) that leads to kinking of the main pancreatic duct[74] and the 'chain of lakes' appearance. Bile duct dilatation is a common and important feature (see Ch. 15).

In staging pancreatic carcinoma, tumour size and location, invasion of surrounding tissues, lymph node involvement and the presence of metastases must be assessed (Figs 16.37 and 16.38). Tumour size is taken as

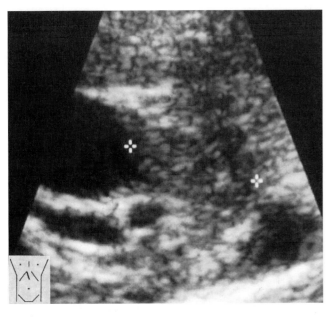

Fig. 16.34 Pancreatic carcinoma. A 2 cm tumour (calipers) is shown obstructing the common bile duct.

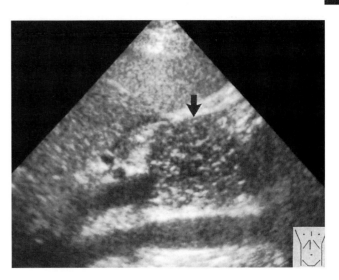

Fig. 16.35 Highly reflective pancreatic carcinoma. This tumour is heterogeneous with widespread areas of increased reflectivity, unlike the common poorly reflective type.

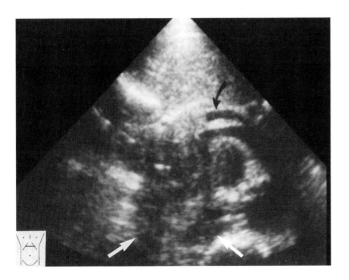

Fig. 16.36 Pancreatic carcinoma. The large tumour is infiltrating posteriorly into the retroperitoneum (arrows). The pancreatic duct is dilated (curved arrow).

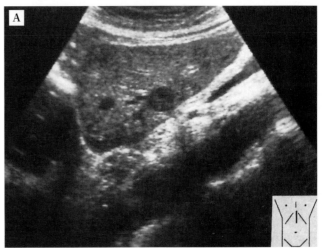

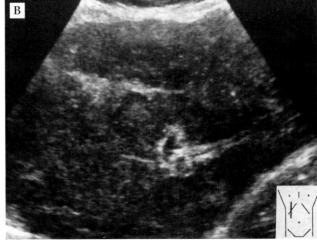

Fig. 16.37 Liver metastasis. Small, poorly reflective metastases from a carcinoma of the pancreas (same patient as in Figure 16.28B).

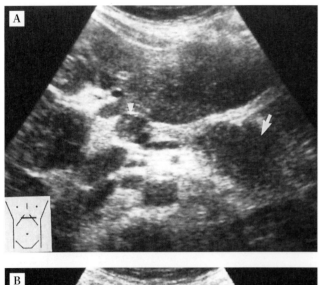

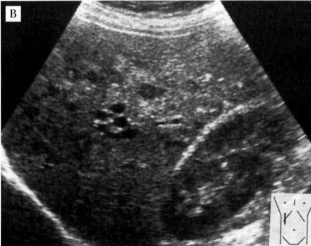

Fig. 16.38 Metastases. A: Transverse scan showing a poorly defined carcinoma in the pancreatic body (arrow) and an enlarged peripancreatic node (arrowhead). **B:** Multiple liver metastases in the same patient.

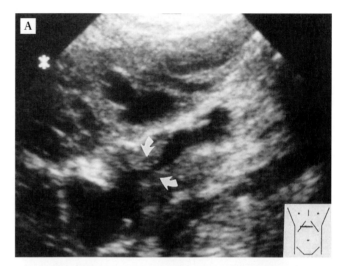

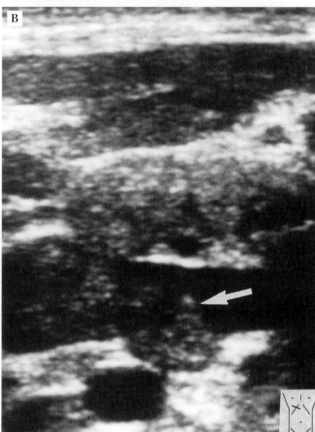

Fig. 16.39 Splenic/portal vein involvement. A: Pancreatic tumour compressing the portal vein (arrows). **B:** Pancreatic tumour invading through the wall of the portal vein (arrow).

the maximum transverse diameter and is an important prognostic indicator, lesions smaller than 2 cm carrying a more favourable outlook.[75] Whether a tumour is surrounded by parenchyma, is adjacent to the capsule, or has actually breached the capsule must be assessed.[76] As local invasion continues infiltration of the duodenum often occurs, distorting its mucosal outline and leading eventually to complete obstruction. Invasion of retroperitoneal fat occurs early, with tumour tracking along perineural sheaths and lymphatics (Fig. 16.33).

Retroperitoneal invasion fixes the pancreas to the adjacent blood vessels (splenic and portal veins), which it may then invade (Fig. 16.39). Tumour may extend up to or invade the vessel wall or even obstruct its lumen. Vascular invasion may be detected on grey-scale ultrasound as distortion of the vessel structure, but it is better evaluated with Doppler studies (Fig. 16.40). Flow in the hepatic and gastroduodenal arteries may also be affected by a pancreatic tumour. Typically these vessels become encased by tumour, resulting in stenosis. Early spread to surrounding lymph nodes is common. Nodes in the pancreaticoduode-

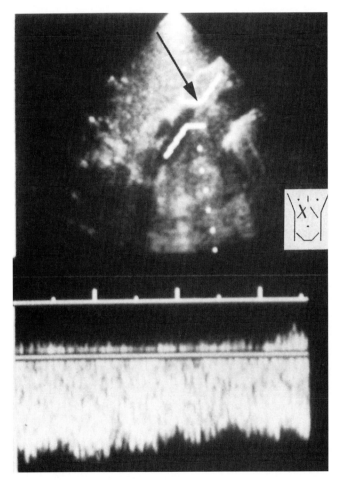

Fig. 16.40 Doppler of portal vein stenosis. Duplex Doppler study of high flow velocity in the portal vein just distal to a stenosis produced by tumour invading through the vein wall (arrow).

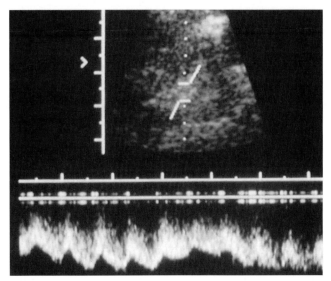

Fig. 16.41 Tumour Doppler signal. Continuous flow pattern recorded from within a heterogeneous pancreatic tumour.

nal region, the inferior pancreatic body, the hepatoduodenal region and coeliac axis may all be involved. Metastases and ascites are only seen at a late stage.

Pancreatic carcinomas can affect blood flow in several ways. Involvement of the portal vein by tumour is common, occurring in 65% of pancreatic and 40% of bile duct tumours. Compression of the vein may be obvious on colour Doppler and produces a high-velocity jet through the narrowed area, with vortices causing chaotic or turbulent flow distal to the stenosis (Fig. 16.37).[26] The Doppler sonogram shows spectral broadening, in extreme cases with signals above and below the baseline. Invasion of the vessel wall produces local flow disturbances. Portal vein occlusion obliterates the Doppler signal, but collateral vessels may be demonstrated and flow may persist through small channels around the occlusion.[77] Without the use of colour Doppler an occlusion may be missed because fresh thrombus is very poorly reflective.[78] Doppler offers the advantage over angiography of providing an assessment of the haemodynamic disturbances at the same time as the

surrounding soft tissue anatomy. In addition to changes in the surrounding vasculature, characteristic tumour Doppler signals have been detected from neoplastic lesions, including pancreatic tumours (Fig. 16.41).[79]

Invasion and occlusion of the hepatic artery can be demonstrated with colour Doppler and the sensitivity is as good as contrast CT, so that if invasion is found on ultrasound a follow-up CT scan may not be necessary for preoperative staging.[27]

The neovascularisation associated with neoplasia is well documented. Strickland[80] described tumour vessels as wandering, with no diminution in calibre. Histologically these tumour vessels are thin walled with little smooth muscle.[81,82] Flow is characteristically slow and with low distal impedance, depicted on the Doppler spectrum as continuous forward flow throughout diastole. Also seen are high-frequency Doppler shift signals, thought to represent arteriovenous shunts in the tumour. These signatures of malignancy may be more easily recognised after microbubble enhancement.[83]

Differential diagnosis

The most important differential diagnosis is from focal chronic inflammation (Fig. 16.42) but other lesions, such as non-endocrine tumours, metastatic tumours (Fig. 16.43), malignant islet cell tumours and acute focal inflammation, also must be considered.[73,84] The demonstration of cysts, calcification or irregular duct dilatation favours chronic pancreatitis; however, an underlying malignancy may be impossible to exclude. In acute biliary obstruction, focal inflammation typically affects the pancreatic head to form an echo-poor mass that is indistinguishable from a ductal carcinoma. Rarely adenocarcinomas are predominantly

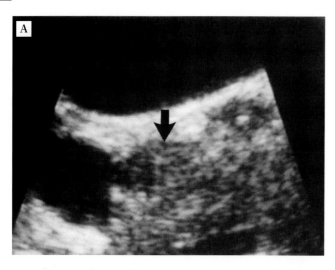

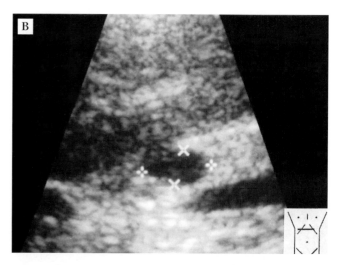

Fig. 16.42 Focal pancreatitis. A: An inflammatory mass involving the pancreatic head (arrow). No evidence of malignancy was found on biopsy and the patient remained well on follow up. **B:** A small, well defined poorly reflective area is seen in the pancreatic head. Tubercle bacilli were cultured from a biopsy of this lesion.

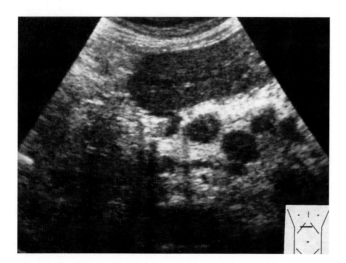

Fig. 16.43 Metastases to the pancreas. Multiple metastases to the pancreas in a patient with melanoma.

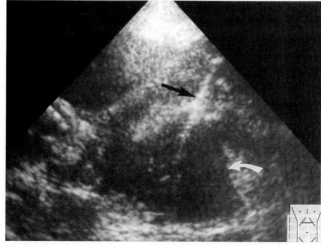

Fig. 16.44 Pancreatic biopsy. The tract from a percutaneous biopsy (arrow) of a pancreatic mass (curved arrow) is still seen up to 1 minute after the biopsy needle has been removed.

cystic and cannot be distinguished from mucinous cystic neoplasms. Pancreatic lymphoma may be large, multifocal, and is not usually associated with massive or widespread lymphadenopathy. It usually has very low-level echoes. Endocrine tumours are often small with a reflective capsule.

Histological diagnosis is important for determining management, especially because both inflammation and malignancy of some other histological types carry a much better prognosis than adenocarcinoma. Fine-needle aspiration for cytology has been widely used since its introduction at the beginning of the 1970s. Although false positives are rare, the sensitivity of the method is disappointing

at around 75%.[85,86] This low detection rate is probably partly explained by the extensive desmoplastic reaction that pancreatic tumours excite: the fibrous tissue may deflect the biopsy needle, leading to a sampling error. TruCut tissue biopsies using the Biopty® Gun give better specimens, and biopsies directed by endoscopic ultrasound are also more reliable (Fig. 16.44).[87]

Comparison of ultrasound and CT

Both ultrasound and CT are excellent imaging methods for pancreatic carcinoma (Fig. 16.45).[40] In a patient with

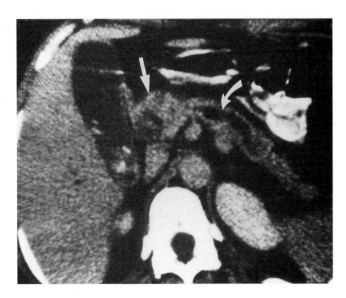

Fig. 16.45 Pancreatic tumour. CT showing a tumour in the head of the pancreas (arrow) with dilatation of the pancreatic duct (curved arrow).

suspected pancreatic malignancy the sensitivity of ultrasound for detecting a pancreatic mass is of the order of 90%, approaching 98% with high-resolution equipment and good technique.[88] This is limited by the small number of technical failures, where overlying bowel gas or patient obesity prevent adequate visualisation of the pancreatic tail. Ultrasound is the best means of assessing the biliary tree in suspected biliary obstruction, and in some 90% of patients both the level and cause of obstruction can be defined.[89]

Ultrasound is also useful in staging pancreatic malignancy, with a high accuracy for predicting non-resectability, although prediction of resectability is less good.[90] The addition of Doppler and endoscopic ultrasound might improve this.[26] The advantages of CT include fewer technical failures and its ability to detect other abdominal abnormalities.[40] The pancreatic tail is more reliably seen on CT, although in thin patients fascial planes around the pancreatic head may be difficult to define. Using current-generation CT scanners and state of the art techniques, the positive predictive value for tumour resectability is 78% and for non-resectability 100%.

Other non-endocrine tumours

Giant cell carcinoma

Bizarre giant tumour cells and sarcomatous cells characterise this lesion. The cells are anaplastic with marked pleomorphism. Epithelial glandular elements and mucin may also be present.[91,92] Patients present late and by this stage the tumour is often a large echo-poor mass with a necrotic centre and metastases have occurred. The prognosis is poor, with median survival around 2 months.

Adenosquamous carcinoma

This is a mixture of adeno- and squamous carcinoma, probably arising from a stem cell capable of differentiating into both.[93] On ultrasound they are similar to ductal adenocarcinomas, though if the squamous components predominate they may undergo necrosis to form large cystic regions.[94] The prognosis is slightly worse than average for pancreatic cancers.

Mucinous adenocarcinoma

This well recognised tumour is characterised by marked mucin production.[95,96] It consists of well differentiated clumps of columnar epithelium lying within mucinous spaces which are echo free, and it tends to form in the body or tail of the pancreas.[97] Calcification may be seen. The pancreatic duct may be dilated and contain mucin of varying reflectivity (Fig. 16.46). ERCP demonstrates the mucin as filling defects and typically shows mucus flowing from a patulous papilla.[98] The prognosis is relatively good, with long survival after pancreatectomy.

Micro-adenocarcinoma

Microadenocarcinomas are often large and elicit less desmoplastic reaction than do ductal adenocarcinomas. They are composed of solid cellular regions with fine fibrous septa. The cells have uniform nuclei and form small mucin-filled glands.[98] This tumour presents in a slightly younger age group than do ductal adenocarcinomas; survival is poor.

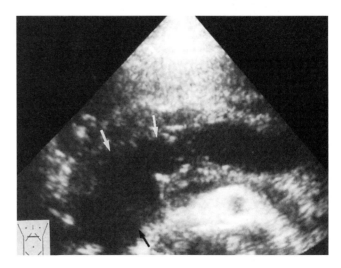

Fig. 16.46 Intraductal mucinous adenocarcinoma. The poorly reflective material filling the pancreatic duct is mucin secreted by the tumour (arrows).

Mucinous cystic neoplasms

These cystic tumours are now thought of as frankly or potentially malignant at presentation. They occur predominantly in middle-aged women and the majority are located in the body or tail of the pancreas (Fig.16.47).[99] They are irregular in shape, with a smooth outline. Unilocular or multilocular, the cysts are lined by columnar epithelium and their surface often displays shaggy excrescences. On ultrasound the cystic elements can be clearly identified, with internal septa and nodular or papillary projections. Mucinous tumours are usually cured by complete resection, and even if this is not possible the prognosis is much better than for ductal adenocarcinoma. The mucinous duct ectatic type is a variant, occurring predominantly in the head and uncinate process. It is caused by localised dilatation of a duct side branch.

Microcystic adenoma

The other main cystic pancreatic neoplasm is the microcystic adenoma. It is a well defined, vascular tumour composed of innumerable small cysts with a fibrous stroma that may partially calcify (Fig. 16.48). It is non-invasive but may compress adjacent structures.[100] If the cysts are small (2 mm or less) the lesion is predominantly reflective; however, if they are larger it is seen as a multiloculated cystic mass.

Pancreatoblastoma

This rare tumour arises in the ventral pancreas; it affects children under 7 years of age, and is thought to result from

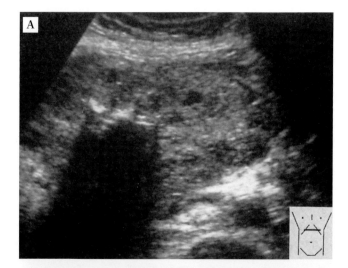

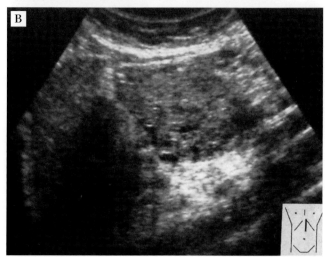

Fig. 16.48 Microcystic adenoma. A well defined heterogeneous tumour containing numerous very small cysts, together with a central region of calcification that casts an acoustic shadow.

a failure in organogenesis.[101] The tumours are often large and composed of sheets of epithelial cells interspersed with mesenchymal tissue. They appear on ultrasound as well defined, predominantly reflective masses.

Anaplastic carcinoma

This group of undifferentiated malignant tumours is similar clinically to ductal adenocarcinomas. On ultrasound they appear as large solid tumours.

Acinar cell carcinoma

These lesions are solid grey tumours with necrotic centres. Acinar formation occurs. Survival is similar to that with ductal adenocarcinomas.

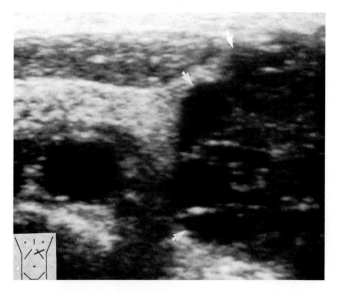

Fig. 16.47 Mucinous cystic tumour. The multicystic mass in the pancreatic tail (arrows) is the typical pattern of a mucinous cystic neoplasm.

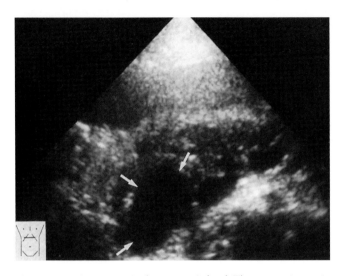

Fig. 16.49 Benign tumour in the pancreatic head. The tumour (arrows) is well defined, poorly reflective and homogeneous.

Benign tumours (Fig.16.49), papillary cystic tumours and tumours of connective tissue origin are all very rare.

Endocrine tumours

At least five types of islet cell are found in the normal pancreas, each producing a distinct peptide or amine: β cells produce insulin; α cells glucagon; δ cells somatostatin; F cells pancreatic polypeptide; and enterochromaffin cells serotonin.[76] Tumours may arise from each of these cell types but, in addition, pancreatic endocrine tumours may develop from tissues found in the fetal pancreas or other glands; for example, gastrinoma, VIPoma and tumours producing combinations of different peptides all occur.

Insulinoma is the commonest pancreatic endocrine tumour and, in contrast to other tumours described, is almost always benign.[102] Gastrinoma is the second most common; 60% or more are malignant.[103] Insulinoma, gastrinoma, glucagonoma and VIPoma all produce recognisable clinical syndromes as a result of their excess hormone production. These symptoms mean that they present much earlier than do other pancreatic tumours, and so they are usually small, often less than 1.5 cm. Somatostatinomas and pancreatic polypeptidomas produce few if any clinical symptoms and at presentation the tumour bulk may be considerable.

Localisation of islet cell tumours can be extremely difficult because of their small size.[102] Several imaging techniques may be required, including ultrasound, ERCP, CT, MRI and angiography with venous sampling. Ultrasound is used as the initial localising investigation and has an important role as an intra-operative guide for the surgeon. Most published data relate to insulinomas: 90% of these tumours are small, well defined oval masses with a homogeneous, poorly reflective pattern. In young patients

(under 30 years of age) the normal pancreas is relatively echo poor, so that the tumour is difficult to distinguish from normal parenchyma (Figs 16.50 and 16.51). Detection rates for small insulinomas with modern equipment and techniques compare favourably with both CT and angiography (all approximately 60%). The pancreatic tail remains an area of particular difficulty. Endoscopic and intra-operative ultrasound are better at detecting these

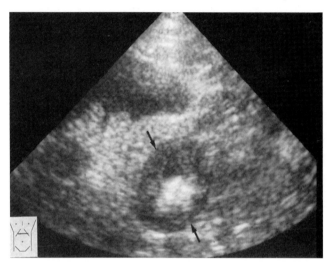

Fig. 16.50 Benign neuro-endocrine tumour. The mass in the pancreatic head (arrows) proved to be a benign neuro-endocrine tumour. The central area of high reflectivity represents calcification.

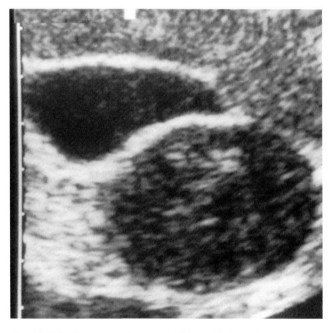

Fig. 16.51 Benign pancreatic tumour. This well defined, homogeneous and poorly reflective tumour remained unchanged during several years follow-up.

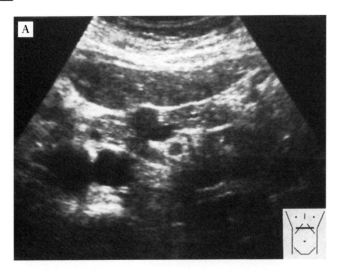

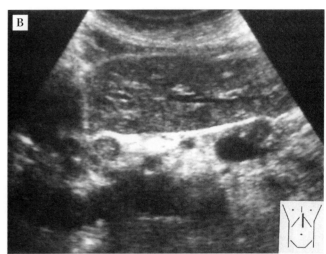

Fig. 16.52 Insulinoma. A. Longitudinal and **B:** transverse scans. The lesion is detectable by virtue of its lower reflectivity compared to the adjacent parenchyma and the distortion of the gland outline.

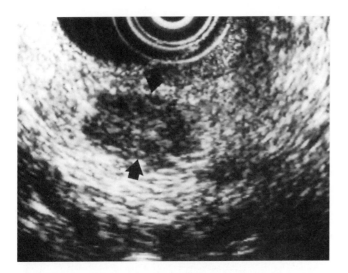

Fig. 16.53 Insulinoma. Endoscopic ultrasound showing a small, poorly reflective tumour in the pancreatic head (arrows).

lesions[104] (Figs 16.52 and 16.53). The relation of the tumour to pancreatic blood vessels and the duct can be demonstrated, helping the surgeon decide whether enucleation is safe or whether partial pancreatectomy is required. Experience with endoscopic and intra-operative ultrasound for gastrinomas has been disappointing, as these are frequently multiple, extremely small and may even be extrapancreatic.

Pancreatic transplantation

A variety of techniques have been explored for transplanting the pancreas, some using implants of cellular separations. The most successful have been transplantation of the intact gland with a part of the duodenum, which is anastomosed into the fundus of the urinary bladder.[105] This procedure is often combined with a renal transplant in diabetics with end-stage nephropathy.

The same spectrum of complications as afflict renal transplants can occur, and ultrasound is useful in defining collections and vascular anastomotic problems using B-mode and Doppler, respectively. Rejection and pancreatitis cannot be detected with ultrasound.[84]

REFERENCES

1 Lees W R. Pancreatic ultrasonography. Clin Gastroenterol 1984; 13: 763–789
2 The pancreas, The Pancreas, 1989, Gray's anatomy: Williams, P L, Warwick, R, Dyson, M, Bannister, L H.
3 Ravitch M M. The pancreas in infants and children. Surg Clin North Am 1975; 55: 377–385
4 Hyden W H. The true nature of annular pancreas. Ann Surg 1963; 157: 71–77
5 Seifert G. Congenital anomalies. In: Kloppel G, Heitz P U, eds. Pancreatic pathology.
6 Cotton P B. Congenital anomaly of pancreas divisum as a cause of obstructive pain and pancreatitis. Gut 1980; 21: 105–108
7 Varshney S, Johnson C D. Pancreas divisum. Int J Pancreatol 1999; 25: 135–141
8 Filly R A, London S S. The normal pancreas: acoustic characteristics and frequency of imaging. J Clin Ultrasound 1979; 7: 121–124
9 Marks V, Filly R, Callen P. Ultrasonic evaluation of normal pancreatic echogenicity and its relation to fat deposition. Radiology 1980; 137: 457–459
10 Gupta A, Arenson A, Mckee J. Effect of steroid ingestion on pancreatic echogenicity. JCU 1987; 15: 171–174
11 Donald J, Shorvon P, Lees W. A hypoechoic area within the head of the pancreas. Clin Radiol 1990; 41: 337–338
12 Niederau C, Sonnenberg A, Muller J, Erkenbrecht J, Scholten T, Fritsch W. Sonographic measurements of the normal liver, spleen, pancreas and portal vein. Radiology 1983; 149: 537–540
13 De Graff C, Taylor K J W, Simmonds B, Rosenfield A. Gray scale echography of the pancreas. Reevaluation of normal size. Radiology 1978; 129: 157–161

14 Terruzzi V, Radaelli F, Spinzi G C, Imperiali G, Minoli G. Congenital short pancreas. Report of a new case observed during the course of a recurrent acute pancreatitis. Ital Gastroenterol Hepatol 1998; 30: 199–201

15 Neumann C H, Hessel S J. CT of the pancreatic tail. AJR 1980; 35: 741–745

16 Goldberg B. The pancreas. Clin Diagn Ultrasound 1988; 23: 165–193

17 Bryan P. Appearance of normal pancreatic duct. JCU 1982; 10: 63–66

18 Bolondi L, Gaiani S, Casanova S, Testa P, Priori P, Labo G. Improvement of pancreatic ultrasound imaging after secretin administration. Ultrasound Med Biol 1983; 9: 497–501

19 Glaser J. Clinical perspectives of a sonographic secretin test. Zeitschr Gastroenterol 1997; 35: 579–583

20 Lee J K T, Stanley R J, Melson G L, Sagel S S. Pancreatic imaging by ultrasound and computed tomography: a general review. Radiol Clin North Am 1979; 16: 105–117

21 Warren P, Garret W, Kossoff G. The liquid filled stomach: an ultrasonic window to the upper abdomen. JCU 1978; 6: 295–302

22 Lev-Toaff A S, Langer J E, Rubin D L et al. Safety and efficacy of a new oral contrast agent for sonography: a phase II trial. Air. AJR 1999; 173: 431–436

23 Simon C, Hoffmann V, Richter G M, Seelos R, Senninger N, Kauffmann G W. Hydrosonography of the pancreas. Initial results of a pilot study. Radiologe 1996; 36: 389–396

24 Taylor K, Burns P, Woodcock J, Wells P. Blood flow in deep abdominal and pelvic vessels: ultrasonic pulsed Doppler analysis. Radiology 1985; 154: 487–493

25 Yassa N A, Yang J, Stein S, Johnson M, Ralls P. Gray-scale and color flow sonography of pancreatic ductal adenocarcinoma. JCU 1997; 25: 473–480

26 Casadei R, Ghigi G, Gullo L et al. Role of color Doppler ultrasonography in the preoperative staging of pancreatic cancer. Pancreas 1998; 16: 26–30

27 Tomiyama T, Ueno N, Tano S, Wada S, Kimura K. Assessment of arterial invasion in pancreatic cancer using color Doppler ultrasonography. Am J Gastroenterol 1996; 91: 1410–1416

28 Machi J, Schwartz J H, Zaren H A, Noritomi T, Sigel B. Technique of laparoscopic ultrasound examination of the liver and pancreas. Surg Endosc 1996; 10: 684–689

29 Caletti G, Fusaroli P. Endoscopic ultrasonography. Endoscopy 1999; 31: 95–102

30 Catalano M F, Lahoti S, Alcocer E, Geenen J E, Hogan W J. Dynamic imaging of the pancreas using real-time endoscopic ultrasonography with secretin stimulation. Gastrointest Endosc 1998; 48: 580–587

31 Furukawa T, Oohashi K, Yamao K et al. Intraductal ultrasonography of the pancreas: development and clinical potential. Endoscopy 1997; 29: 561–569

32 Charboneau J, Gorman B, Reading C, James M, Grant C. Intraoperative ultrasonography of pancreatic endocrine tumours. Clin Diagn Ultrasound 1987; 23: 123–134

33 Cerri L M, Cerri G G. Intraoperative ultrasonography of liver, bile ducts and pancreas. Revi Paul Med 1996; 114: 1196–1207

34 Kubota K, Noie T, Sano K, Abe H, Bandai Y, Makuuchi M. Impact of intraoperative ultrasonography on surgery for cystic lesions of the pancreas. World J Surg 1997; 21: 72–76; discussion 77

35 Samer M, Cotton P B. Classification of pancreatitis. Gut 1984; 25: 756–759

36 Imrie C W, White S. A prospective study of acute pancreatitis. Br J Surg 1975; 62: 490–494

37 Trapnell J E, Duncan E H L. Patterns of incidence in acute pancreatitis. Br Med J 1975; 2: 179–183

38 Banks S, Wie L, Gersten M. Risk factors in acute pancreatitis. Am J Gastroenterol 1983; 78: 637–640

39 Donovan P J, Sanders R C, Siegelman S S. Collections of fluid after pancreatitis: evaluation by computed tomography and ultrasonography. Radiol Clin North Am 1982; 20: 653–665

40 Choi Y H, Rubenstein W A, Ramirez De Arellano E, Intriere L, Kazam E. CT and US of the pancreas. Clin Imag 1997; 21: 414–440

41 Freeny P C. Computed tomography of the pancreas. Clin Gastroenterol 1984; 13: 791–818

42 Safrany L, Cotton P B. A preliminary report: urgent duodenoscopic sphincterotomy for acute gallstone pancreatitis. Surgery 1981; 89: 424–428

43 Sugiyama M, Atomi Y. Acute biliary pancreatitis: the roles of endoscopic ultrasonography and endoscopic retrograde cholangiopancreatography. Surgery 1998; 124: 14–21

44 Uomo G, Visconti M, Manes G, Calise F, Laccetti M, Rabitti P G. Nonsurgical treatment of acute necrotizing pancreatitis. Pancreas 1996; 12: 142–148

45 Sarti D A. Rapid development and spontaneous regression of pancreatic pseudocysts documented by ultrasound. Radiology 1977; 125: 789–793

46 Dirks K, Schuler A, Lutz H. An unusual cause of gastrointestinal hemorrhage: pseudoaneurysm of the gastroduodenal artery in chronic pancreatitis. Zeitschr Gastroenterol 1999; 37: 489–493

47 Waslen T, Wallace K, Burbridge B, Kwauk S. Pseudoaneurysm secondary to pancreatitis presenting as GI bleeding. Abdom Imag 1998; 23: 318–321

48 Bradley E, Clements L. Spontaneous resolution of pseudocysts. Am J Surg 1976; 129: 23–28

49 Mosca F. [The percutaneous drainage of pancreatic pseudocysts]. Ann Ital Chir 1999; 70: 173–176

50 Uhl W, Isenmann R, Buchler M W. Infections complicating pancreatitis: diagnosing, treating, preventing. New Horizons 1998; 6: S72–79

51 Ranson J H C. Acute pancreatitis: pathogenesis, outcome and treatment. Clin Gastroenterol 1984; 13: 843–863

52 Vernacchia F S, Jeffrey R B, Federle M P et al. Pancreatic abscess: predictive value of early abdominal CT. Radiology 1987; 162: 435–438

53 Freeny P C, Lewis G P, Marks W M. Percutaneous catheter drainage of infected pancreatic fluid collections. Radiology 1986; 161: 89

54 Yoshii H, Sato M, Yamamoto S et al. Usefulness and limitations of ultrasonography in the initial evaluation of blunt abdominal trauma. J Trauma 1998; 45: 45–50; discussion 50–51

55 Cabrera R, Otero H, Blesa E, Jimenez C, Nunez R. [Pancreatic pseudocyst. Review of 22 cases]. Chir Ped 1997; 10: 49–53

56 Singer M V, Gyr G E, Sarles H. Revised classification of pancreatitis. Report on the second international symposium on the classification of pancreatitis in Marseille, France, 28–30 March 1984. Gastroenterology 1985; 89: 683–690

57 Sahel J, Sarles H, Chronic calcifying pancreatitis and obstructive pancreatitis – two entities. In: Gyr K, Singer MV, Sarles H, eds. Pancreatitis: concepts and classification. Amsterdam: Elsevier, 1984: 47–49

58 Ito T, Nakano I, Koyanagi S et al. Autoimmune pancreatitis as a new clinical entity. Three cases of autoimmune pancreatitis with effective steroid therapy. Dig Dis Sci 1997; 42: 1458–1468

59 Klopel G, Adler G, Kern H F. Pathomorphology of acute pancreatitis in relation to its clinical course and pathogenesis. In: Malfertheiner P et al. eds. Diagnostic procedures in pancreatic disease. Berlin: Springer-Verlag, 1997

60 Nagata A, Homma T, Tamai K et al. A study of chronic pancreatitis by serial endoscopic pancreatography. Gastroenterology 1981; 81: 884–891

61 Nix G, Schmitz P. Diagnostic features of chronic pancreatitis. Diagn Imag 1981; 50: 130–137

62 Cotton P B, Lees W R, Vallon A G, Cottone M, Croker J R, Chapman M. Grey-scale ultrasonography and endoscopic pancreatography in pancreatic diagnosis. Radiology 1980; 134: 453–459

63 Kataoka K, Yamane Y, Kato M, Kashima K. Diagnosis of chronic pancreatitis using noninvasive tests of exocrine pancreatic function – comparison to duodenal intubation tests. Pancreas 1997; 15: 409–415

64 Howard T J. Pancreatic adenocarcinoma. Curr Probl Cancer 1996; 20: 281–328

65 Appelros S, Borgstrom A. Incidence, aetiology and mortality rate of acute pancreatitis over 10 years in a defined urban population in Sweden. Br J Surg 1999; 86: 465–470

66 Russel R C G. Carcinoma of the pancreas and ampulla of Vater. In: Misiewicz JS, Pounder RE, Venebles CW, eds. Diseases of the gut and pancreas. Oxford: Blackwell Scientific, 1993

67 Wynder E L. An epidemiological evaluation of the causes of cancer of the pancreas. Cancer Res 1975; 35: 2228–2233

68 Puchalski Z, Ladny J R, Polakow J, Razak H, Deeb A. Diagnosis and surgical treatment of pancreatic carcinoma. Roczniki Akademii Medycznej W Bialymstoku 1996; 41: 210–217

69 Malagelada J R. Pancreatic cancer: an overview of epidemiology, clinical presentation and diagnosis. Mayo Clin Proc 1979; 54: 459–467

70 Chien J, Baithun S I, Ramsay M. Histogenesis of pancreatic cancer: a study based on 248 cases. J Pathol 1985; 146: 65–76

71 Van Heerden J A. Pancreatic resection for carcinoma of the pancreas. World J Surg 1984; 8: 880–888

72 Gunderson L L, Martin J K, Kirols L K. Intraoperative and external beam irradiation ± 5FU for locally advanced pancreatic carcinoma. Int J Radiat Oncol Biol Phy 1987; 13: 319–329

73 Yamaguchi K, Chijiiwa K, Saiki S, Nakatsuka A, Tanaka M. 'Mass-forming' pancreatitis masquerades as pancreatic carcinoma. Int J Pancreatol 1996; 20: 27–35

74 Ohto M, Saotome N, Saisho H et al. Real time ultrasonography of the pancreatic duct: application to percutaneous pancreatic ductograph. AJR 1980; 134: 647–652

75 Birk D, Fortnagel G, Formentini A, Beger H G. Small carcinoma of the pancreas. Factors of prognostic relevance. Hepatobiliary Pancreat Surg 1998; 5: 450–454

76 Kloppel G, Maillet B. Classification and staging of pancreatic non-endocrine tumours. Radiol Clin North Am 1989; 27: 105–119

77 Kane R A, Katz S G. The spectrum of sonographic findings in portal hypertension; a subject review and new observations. Radiology 1982; 142: 453–458

78 Kitamra T, Tanaka S. Evolution of ultrasonographic diagnosis for early cancer. Nippon Rinsho. JPN Clin Med 1996; 54: 1236–1240

79 Taylor K J W, Ramos I, Carter D, Morse S S, Shower D, Fortune K. Correlation of Doppler ultrasound tumor signals with neovascular morphological features. Radiology 1988; 166: 57–62

80 Strickland B. The value of angiography in the diagnosis of bone tumour. Br J Radiol 1959; 32: 705–713

81 Vaupel P. Blood flow, oxygenation, tissue pH distribution and bioenergetic state of tumors. Ernst Schering Research Foundation No 23. Berlin: Schering AG, 1994

82 Folkman J. Angiogenesis in cancer, vascular, rheumatoid and other disease. Nature Med 1995; 1: 27–31

83 Bhutani M S, Hoffman B J, van Velse A, Hawes R H. Contrast-enhanced endoscopic ultrasonography with galactose microparticles: SHU508 A (Levovist). Endoscopy 1997; 29: 635–639

84 Aideyan O A, Foshager M C, Benedetti E, Troppmann C, Gruessner R W. Correlation of the arterial resistive index in pancreas transplants of patients with transplant rejection. AJR 1997; 168: 1445–1447

85 Hanke S, Holm H H, Koch F, Ultrasonically guided puncture of solid pancreatic mass lesions. In: Interventional ultrasound. Copenhagen: Munksgaard. 1985; 100–105

86 Di Stasi M, Lencioni R, Solmi L et al. Ultrasound-guided fine needle biopsy of pancreatic masses: results of a multicenter study. Am J Gastroenterol 1998; 93: 1329–1333

87 Suits J, Franzee R, Erickson R A. Endoscopic ultrasound and fine needle aspiration for the evaluation of pancreatic masses. Arch Surg 1999; 134: 639–642; discussion 642–643

88 Lees W R, Vallon A G, Denyer M E. Prospective study of ultrasonography in pancreatic disease. Br Med J 1979; 1: 162–164

89 Ormson M J, Charboneau J W, Stephens D H. Sonography in patients with a possible pancreatic mass on computed tomography. AJR 1987; 148: 551–555

90 Campbell J P, Wilson S R. Pancreatic neoplasm: how useful is evaluation with ultrasonography? Radiology 1988; 167: 341–344

91 Cubilla A L, Fitzgerald P J. Cancer (non-endocrine) of the pancreas (a suggested classification). Mayo Clin Pro 1979; 54: 449–458

92 Watanabe M, Miura H, Inoue H et al. Mixed osteoclastic/pleomorphic-type giant cell tumor of the pancreas with ductal adenocarcinoma: histochemical and immunohistochemical study with review of the literature. Pancreas 1997; 15: 201–208

93 Serafini F, Rosemurgy A S, Carey L C. Squamous cell carcinoma of the pancreas. Am J Gastroenterol 1996; 91: 2621–2622

94 Freeny P. Radiology of the pancreas. Curr Opin Radiol 1989; 1: 81–93

95 Torresan F, Casadei R, Solmi L, Marrano D, Gandolfi L. The role of ultrasound in the differential diagnosis of serous and mucinous cystic tumours of the pancreas. Eur J Gastroenterol Hepatol 1997; 9: 169–172

96 Takada T, Yasuda H, Amano H, Yoshida M, Hijikata H, Takada K. An introduction to mucin-producing tumors of the pancreas: why they deserve more attention. Hepato-Gastroenterology 1998; 45: 1967–1972

97 Zamboni G, Scarpa A, Bogina G et al. Mucinous cystic tumors of the pancreas: clinicopathological features, prognosis, and relationship to other mucinous cystic tumors. Am J Surg Pathol 1999; 23: 410–422

98 Friedman A C, Edmonds P R. Rare pancreatic malignancies. Radiol Clin North Am 1989; 27: 177–190

99 Buetow P C, Rao P, Thompson L D. From the archives of the AFIP. Mucinous cystic neoplasms of the pancreas: radiologic-pathologic correlation. Radiographics 1998; 18: 433–449

100 Procacci C, Graziani R, Bicego E et al. Serous cystadenoma of the pancreas: report of 30 cases with emphasis on the imaging findings. J Comput Assist Tomogr 1997; 21: 373–382

101 Chun Y, Kim W, Park K, Lee S, Jung S. Pancreatoblastoma. J Pediatr Surg 1997; 32: 1612–1615

102 Lo C Y, van Heerden J A, Thompson G B, Grant C S, Soreide J A, Harmsen W S. Islet cell carcinoma of the pancreas. World J Surg 1996; 20: 878–883; discussion 884

103 Kisker O, Bastian D, Bartsch D, Nies C, Rothmund M. Localization, malignant potential, and surgical management of gastrinomas. World J Surg 1998; 22: 651–657; discussion 657–658

104 Kuzin N M, Egorov A V, Kondrashin S A, Lotov A N, Kuznetzov N S, Majorova J B. Preoperative and intraoperative topographic diagnosis of insulinomas. World J Surg 1998; 22: 593–597; discussion 597–598

105 Kahl A, Venz S, Keske U et al. Magnetic resonance imaging and Levovist-enhanced color and power Doppler imaging in the follow-up of pancreas transplants in patients after combined pancreas and kidney transplantation. Transplan Proc 1998; 30: 246–247

17

The spleen

Christian Görg

The basics of splenic sonography

Because of its protected situation in the left upper quadrant of the abdomen, clinical evaluation of a normal spleen is often unsatisfactory. The simplicity of this technique, its availability, the ease with which it can be repeated, the lack of exposure to ionising radiation and the possibility of bedside examination using mobile equipment have made sonography the primary method of examination of upper abdominal organs in many centres. Splenic scintigraphy, while useful for the functional information it provides, is too inaccurate for size assessment and involves exposure to radiation. CT scanning is very useful and in many situations, for example in abdominal trauma, is the preferred imaging test for the spleen. MRI generally does not contribute significant additional information.

Indications

The most common indications for a splenic ultrasound are:

1. size assessment,
2. diagnosis and follow-up of splenomegaly (e.g. infectious disease, diseases of the lymphatic system, myeloproliferative disorders, haemolytic anaemias, congestive splenomegaly and storage diseases),
3. diagnosis and follow-up of splenic masses (e.g. lymphomas, infarcts, cysts, tumours, calcification, abscesses, rupture),
4. changes in the splenic vasculature using Doppler (e.g. splenic vein thrombosis, perisplenic portosystemic shunt, aneurysm of the splenic artery, intrasplenic pseudo-aneurysm, arteriovenous fistula),
5. for the categorisation of vague pain and/or abnormal findings on palpitation of the left upper quadrant,
6. to guide in diagnostic and therapeutic intervention (e.g. abscesses, symptomatic cysts).

The spleen should always be evaluated as part of a complete upper abdominal scan.

Embryology

The spleen arises as a mesenchymal mass between the layers of the dorsal mesentery around the fifth week of embryonic development and soon attains its characteristic shape (Fig. 17.1). In the fetus it is divided into lobes which usually fuse before birth. Lack of or incomplete fusion results in polysplenia, accessory spleens and lobulation or septation of the mature spleen (Fig. 17.2). Polysplenia may be associated with complex congenital anomalies of thoracic and abdominal organs.[1]

Through the rotation of the stomach, the base of the dorsal mesentery meets and fuses with the posterior peritoneum near the left kidney, thus forming the short

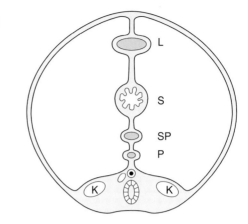

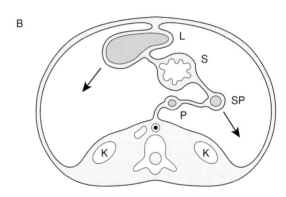

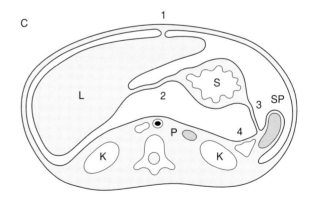

Fig. 17.1 Embryology of the spleen A: Cross-section through the liver (L), stomach (S), spleen (SP), and the pancreas (P) at the end of the fifth week of embryonic development. K – kidney. B: Displacement of the liver (L) to the right in the mesentery, while the spleen (SP) and the pancreas (P) are displaced to the left in the dorsal mesentery.
C: Cross-section showing the fusion of the dorsal mesentery with the peritoneum of the dorsal abdominal wall. 1 – falciform ligament, 2 – hapatgastric ligament, 3 – gastrosplenic ligament, 4 – splenorenal ligament.

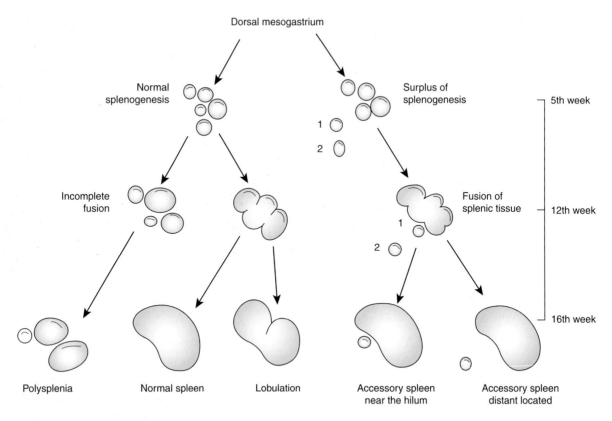

Fig. 17.2 Embryonic genesis of splenic variants.

residual mesenteric root, the so-called splenorenal ligament. The splenic artery enters this ligament, though it is
predominantly retroperitoneal. In rare cases, fusion of the
dorsal mesentery with the peritoneum does not take place
so that the spleen is attached by a mesentery of varying
length and it is abnormally mobile, the 'wandering
spleen'.[2,3]

Topographical anatomy

The spleen lies in the upper left quadrant of the abdominal
cavity between the ninth and twelfth ribs, usually with its
long axis parallel to the tenth rib (Fig. 17.3). It is normally
coffee bean shaped. The convex diaphragmatic surface is
smooth and may extend below the rib cage (Fig. 17.4).
The upper pole of the spleen is directed dorsally toward
the spine. The concave visceral splenic surface lies adjacent
to the posterior wall of the stomach and superior to the
upper pole of the left kidney. Inferiorly, the spleen lies
close to the left colonic flexure (Fig. 17.5). Parts of the
pancreatic tail extend to the splenic hilum, in which the
splenorenal ligament lies. Here, the splenic vein lies superior to the tail of the pancreas. The splenic artery first runs
along the cranial border of the pancreas, then enters the
hilum, usually as several branches (Figs 17.6 and 17.7).

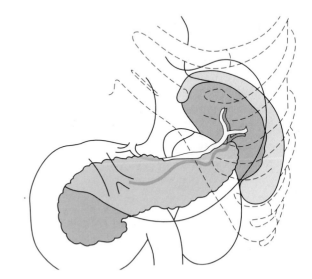

Fig. 17.3 Relations of the spleen. Schematic diagram of the relative
positions of the spleen to the pancreas, the stomach and the kidney.

The entire spleen, except for the hilum, is surrounded
by peritoneum. The gastrosplenic ligament extends toward
the stomach and may sometimes be demonstrated if there

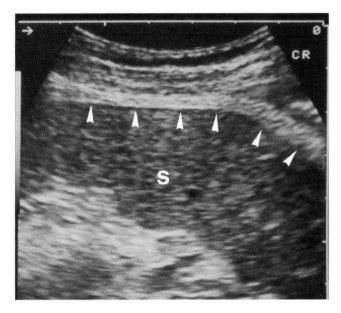

Fig. 17.4 Splenic scan in longitudinal section showing the caudally extended contact of the convex (diaphragmatic) surface of the spleen (arrowheads) with the left crus of the diaphragm. S – spleen

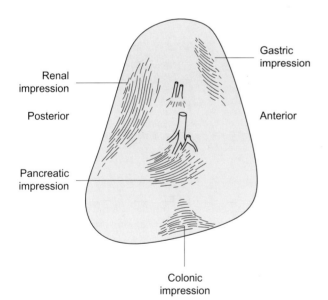

Fig. 17.5 Schematic diagram of the medial surface of the spleen.

Gastric impression

Renal impression

Posterior

Anterior

Pancreatic impression

Colonic impression

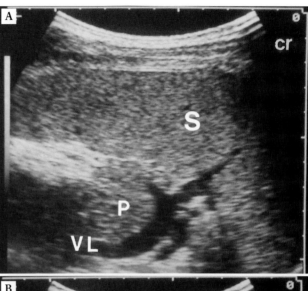

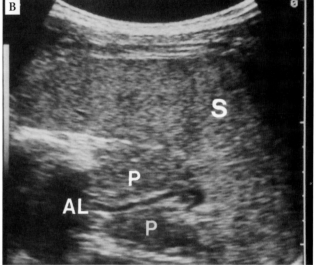

Fig. 17.6 The splenic vessels. A: The splenic vein (VL) courses caudally across the pancreatic tail (P) from the hilum. **B:** The splenic artery (AL) runs through pancreatic tissue (P) to the spleen

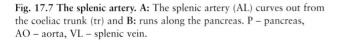

Fig. 17.7 The splenic artery. A: The splenic artery (AL) curves out from the coeliac trunk (tr) and **B:** runs along the pancreas. P – pancreas, AO – aorta, VL – splenic vein.

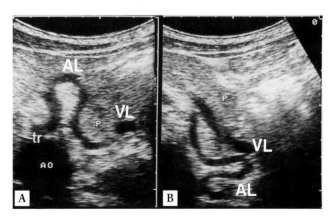

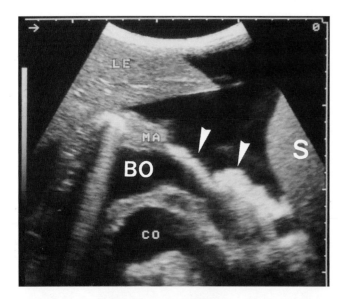

Fig. 17.8 Upper abdominal cross-section demonstrating ascites. The gastrosplenic ligament is revealed (arrowheads). LE – liver, MA – stomach, BO – Bursa omentalis, CO – confluence of the superior mesenteric and splenic veins, S – spleen.

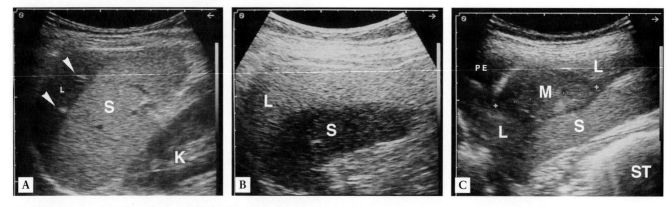

Fig. 17.9 Liver overlying the spleen. A: If the left lobe of the liver is extensive, its tip may lie over the spleen separating it from the left hemidiaphragm. Usually the liver appears to be less reflective than the spleen (arrowheads in A) but if the liver is fatty **B:** the pattern is reversed. Masses such as metastases in this part of the liver may indent the spleen (**C**). K – kidney, L – liver, M – metastasis, PE – pleural fluid, ST – stomach.

is ascites (Fig. 17.8). If the left lobe of the liver is enlarged, it may come in contact with the diaphragmatic surface of the spleen (Fig. 17.9).

Examination technique

Splenic examination is carried out with the patient in the supine or decubitus position with the left arm raised in order to spread the intercostal spaces. The transducer is placed parallel to the ribs in the tenth or eleventh intercostal spaces in the left mid-axillary line and a search for the best window carried out. In this manner, and at maximum expiration, it is often possible to demonstrate the entire spleen as far as the diaphragm. If air-filled lung tissue is displaced by pleural fluid, or if there is ascites, the visualisation of the convex diaphragmal splenic surface may be improved due to the better transmission of sound

through liquids. The upper pole of a small spleen may be difficult to assess (Fig. 17.10).

The spleen is only poorly accessible from a posterior approach while the colon or the stomach are interposed when scanning it from anterior and subcostal approaches.

A sector transducer is optimal for intercostal scanning as it avoids rib shadowing. Depending on the phase of respiration, the spleen moves over the left kidney: this is often helpful in the differentiation of perisplenic masses from retroperitoneal processes. Usually, the splenic capsule cannot be visualised separately on ultrasound.

Normal features and normal variants

Splenic size is most accurately assessed in an intercostal section when its maximum length may be measured. The

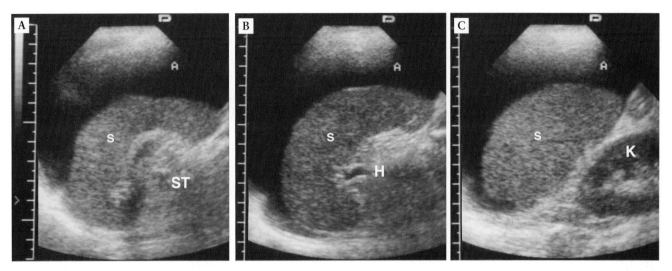

Fig. 17.10 The spleen in ascites. Longitudinal intercostal scans of the spleen (S) in a patient with ascites (A) showing the complex shape of the concave, hilar surface of the spleen. **A:** Scan directed ventrally showing the gas-filled stomach (St). **B:** Intermediate plane of section showing the hilum (H). **C:** Dorsally directed plane of section showing the kidney (K).

transverse diameter is measured vertically from the hilum to the apex of the splenic curvature (Fig. 17.11). Although additional measurements of splenic width for the calculation of organ volume, as well as the calculation of the two-dimensional sectional area, do show a correlation with measured splenic weight, they have not become used routinely.[4,5]

A length of 11 cm or less and a width of 5 cm or less is considered normal (Fig. 17.12). Depending on age (ado-

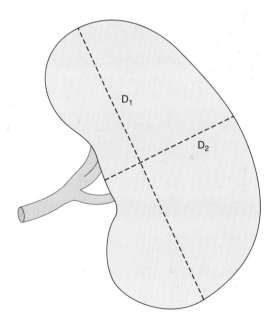

Fig. 17.12 Splenic size assessment with maximum length (D1) and thickness (D2) measurements.

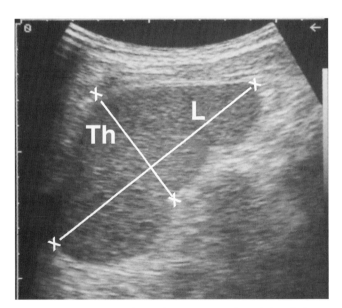

Fig. 17.11 Measurement of the spleen. L – maximum pole length, Th – thickness.

lescents)[6] and constitution (asthenic build), a somewhat greater polar length accompanied by a smaller width is also considered normal (Fig. 17.13); short, plump spleens may be found in pyknic patients. With increasing age, splenic volume decreases (Fig. 17.14).[7]

The spleen has a crescent moon or a coffee bean shape, but this is variable dependent on the tomographic plane (Fig. 17.10). While the surface of the outer, convex border

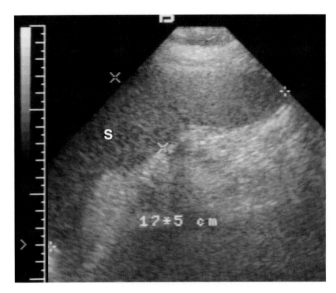

Fig. 17.13 **Elongated spleen in an asthenic subject,** interpreted as a normal variant.

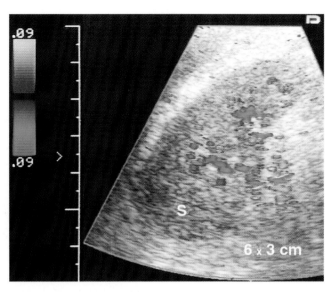

Fig. 17.14 **Colour Doppler scan of a small spleen** in an elderly subject with normal vascularisation.

is usually smooth, the visceral surface is usually bumpy with intervening indentations representing the positions of the embryological components of the spleen (Fig. 17.15).[8] This nodularity can be mistaken for masses originating from neighbouring visceral organs. Clefts and septations may even arise on the diaphragmatic surface of the spleen (Figs 17.16 to 17.18). In rare cases, complete septation

with separate vessels from the splenic hilum (polysplenia) may be observed (Fig. 17.19). An abnormal lobulation of the entire organ is rare (Fig. 17.20). The importance of normal variants lies mainly in the differential diagnosis of scarring following infarction or trauma (Fig. 17.21).

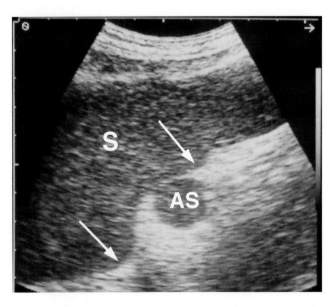

Fig. 17.15 **The concave hilar surface of the spleen** often has an indented appearance (arrows). Note the incidentally found accessory spleen (AS) in the typical position.

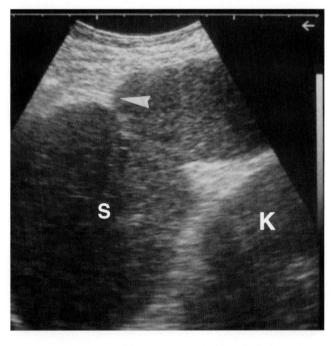

Fig. 17.16 **Indentations of the spleen** (arrowhead) on both the convex and concave surfaces. K – kidney.

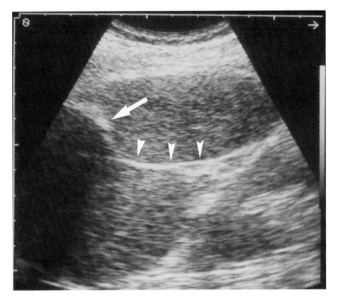

Fig. 17.17 **Retraction and septation of fibrous tissue** originating from the hilum (arrowheads); calcification on the convex side of the spleen (arrow).

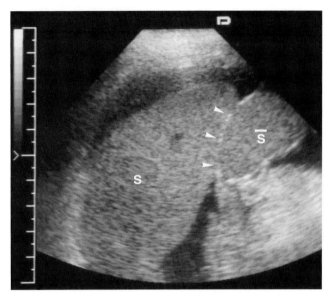

Fig. 17.18 **An incomplete septation of the spleen** is displayed as a reflective band (arrowhead).

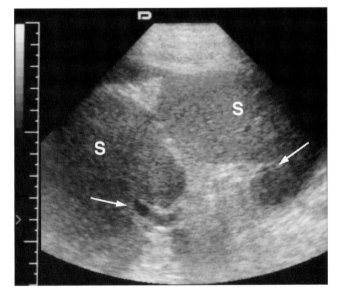

Fig. 17.19 **Complete septation of the spleen** with separate hilar vessels (arrows).

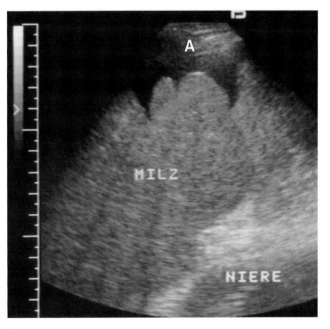

Fig. 17.20 **Marked lobulation of the convex surface of the spleen.** A – ascites, MILZ – spleen, NIERE – kidney.

The echo pattern of a normal spleen is very homogeneous and similar in reflectivity to normal liver, but more reflective than normal renal cortex (Fig. 17.22). The architecture of the spleen is characterised by a radiating pattern of segmental arteries and veins (Fig. 17.23). The main trunk of the splenic vein is a guide in finding the pancreatic tail using the spleen as an acoustic window (Figs 17.24 and 17.25).

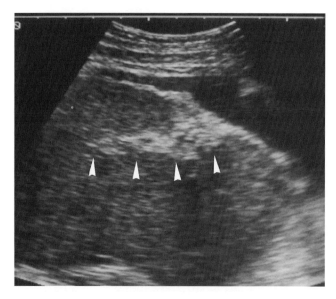

Fig. 17.21 **Reflective band of connective tissue** on the convex surface of the spleen (arrowheads).

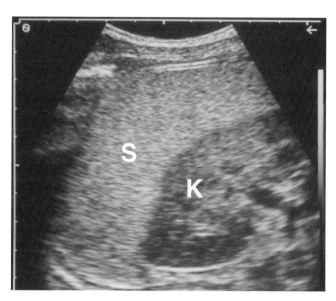

Fig. 17.22 **Normal splenic tissue** (S) has a slightly higher parenchymal reflectivity than healthy renal tissue (K).

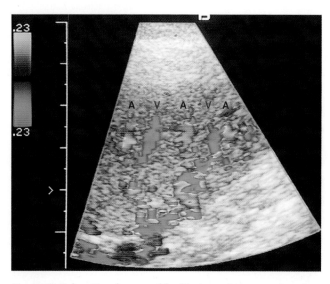

Fig. 17.23 **Colour Doppler scan of fan-like intrasplenic parenchymal vessels.** V – veins, A – arteries.

Aberrations during fusion of the splenic primordium are responsible for the frequency accessory spleens (approximately 10% on autopsy studies), though many are too small to be detected on ultrasound (Figs 17.15 and 17.26).[1,9] The majority (80%) are solitary and localised in the hilar region. In a study of 20 patients, their average diameter was 1.2 cm.[9] The clinical relevance

of this measurement is in the differential diagnosis of other masses such as lymph nodes, tumours of the pancreatic tail and adrenal masses (Fig. 17.27). In addition to the typical location and almost invariable spherical shape of accessory spleens, their homogeneous echo texture is useful diagnostically. The vascular trunk of an accessory spleen can be visualised in some two-thirds of cases (Fig. 17.28).[9,10] Definitive diagnosis may require isotope scintigraphy or a liver-specific microbubble study (see Vol. 1, Ch. 5).[11]

After a splenectomy, pre-existing accessory spleens may undergo compensatory hypertrophy (Fig. 17.29). Ectopic splenic tissue may be congenital or result from intentional or unintentional traumatic or surgical autotransplantation (Fig. 17.30). In an intentional autotransplantation, splenic tissue is reimplanted into the omentum and is seen sonographically as irregular masses of variable echogenicity. Occasionally afferent vessels may be demonstrated with colour Doppler.[10] Here also, a definite diagnosis may be possible only with a splenic scintigram[12] (Fig. 17.31).

Diffuse and focal abnormalities of splenic parenchyma

Splenomegaly

The causes of splenomegaly are extremely varied (Table 17.1) and ultrasound cannot usually offer a precise diagnosis, either by eye or using computer-assisted techniques.[13–16] The spleen is usually homogeneous in texture; its echogenicity is assessed by comparison with the renal

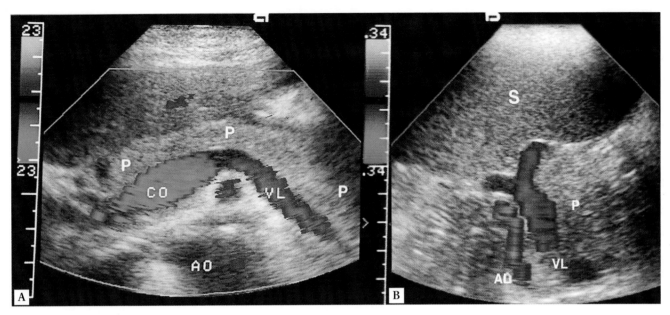

Fig. 17.24 Colour-Doppler scan of the splenic vein A: near the head and body of the pancreas and B: in the area of the pancreatic tail (right). AO – aorta, CO – confluence, P – pancreas, AL – splenic artery, VL – splenic artery.

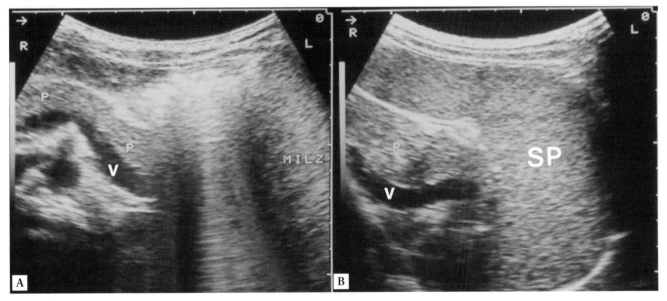

Fig. 17.25 The spleen as a window for the pancreas. A: Upper abdominal cross-section showing the splenic vein (V) and pancreas (P); the pancreatic tail is obscured by gas in the stomach. R – right, L – left, Milz – spleen. B: Left lateral cross-section of the upper abdomen showing the pancreatic tail, the spleen (SP) acting as an acoustic window.

cortex. Despite some variation in different diseases, an assessment of splenic size does provide some differential diagnostic clues. Mild to moderate splenomegaly occurs in infections, in portal hypertension and in acute leukaemia. More marked enlargement is characteristic of lymphoma, haemolytic anaemia, storage disorders and infectious mononucleosis. Extreme splenomegaly is observed in myelofibrosis and the later stages of chronic myeloid leukaemia, as well as in the advanced stages of low-grade malignant lymphomas. In such cases, the spleen may be too large to be measured with ultrasound (Fig. 17.32).

Viral or bacterial infections cause moderate spleno-megaly and occasionally slight inhomogeneity of the splenic parenchyma without clearly definable focal lesions

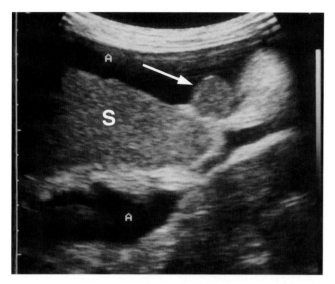

Fig. 17.26 Unusual position of an accessory spleen (arrow) on the convex surface of the spleen. A – ascites.

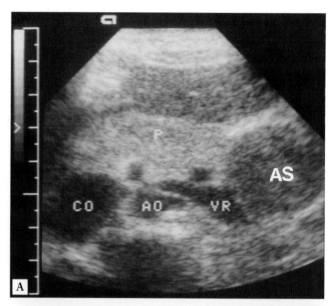

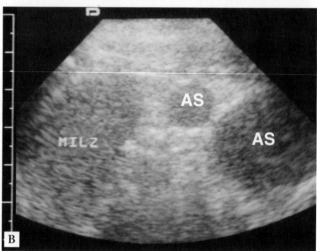

Fig. 17.27 Splenunculi. A: Accessory spleen (AS) close to the pancreatic tail. CO – confluence of splenic and superior mesenteric veins, AO – aorta, VR – renal vein. **B:** Two splenunculi (AS) close to the spleen (Milz).

Table 17.2 Typical ultrasound features of the main diseases of the spleen

Common	Rare
Echo-free splenic lesions	
Dysontogenetic cyst	Metastasis
Secondary cyst	Pseudo-aneurysm
Parasitic cyst	Lymphangioma
Abscess	Haemangioma
Haemorrhage	Hamartoma
	Infarct
Echo-poor splenic lesions	
lymphoma	Metastasis
Infarct	Tuberculosis
Abscess	Sarcoidosis
	Immunological disease
	Amyloidosis
	Histoplasmosis
	Infiltrate of leukaemia
	Micro-abscesses
Reflective splenic lesions	
Haemangioma	Haemangiosarcoma
Hamartoma	Haemorrhage
	Abscess
	Metastasis
	Infiltrate of malignant lymphoma
	Lipid storage disease
	Extramedullary haematopoiesis
	Peliosis
	Spherocytosis
	Schistosomiasis

Table 17.1 Potential causes of splenomegaly

1 Acute and chronic systemic infection
   Infectious mononucleosis, varicella, hepatitis, AIDS, sepsis, endocarditis, typhus, tuberculosis, malaria, toxoplasmosis, leishmaniasis, candidiasis, brucellosis
2 Portal hypertension, liver cirrhosis, portal vein thrombosis, splenic vein thrombosis, splenic arteriovenous fistula, Budd–Chiari syndrome, congestive heart failure.
3 Haemolytic anaemia
   Pernicious anaemia, spherocytosis, thalassaemia, sickle cell anaemia
4 Malignant haematological diseases
   Leukaemia, myeloproliferative syndromes, myelodysplastic syndromes, non-Hodgkin's lymphoma, Hodgkin's disease, malignant histocytosis, systemic mastocytosis
5 Immunological diseases
   Systemic connective tissue diseases, autoimmune cytopenias
6 Varia Amyloidosis, Wegener's granulomatosis, sarcoidosis, haemochromatosis, lipid storage disease

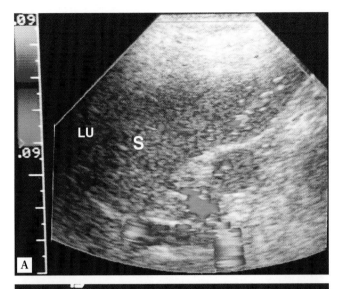

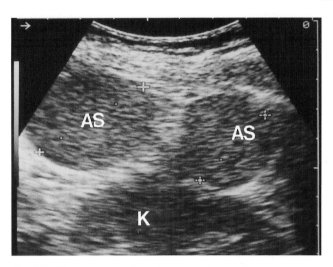

Fig. 17.29 Two accessory spleens (AS) seen 10 years after a post-traumatic splenectomy. K – kidney.

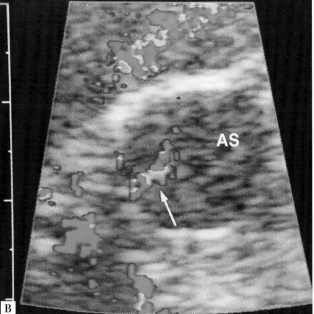

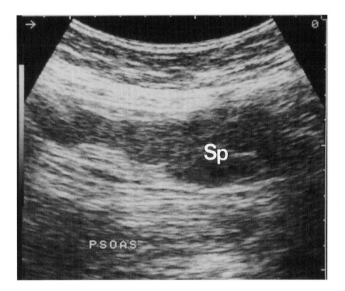

Fig. 17.28 Colour Doppler scans of an accessory spleen showing the hilar vessels (arrow) of the accessory spleen.

Fig. 17.30 Splenosis. A well-defined lobulated poorly reflective mass over the left psoas muscle indicates splenosis (SP) (see also Fig. 17.31).

(Fig. 17.33). In isolated cases, especially in infectious mononucleosis, extreme splenomegaly may be seen. The splenomegaly may take several months to regress (Fig. 17.34). In rare cases, when splenic volume increases rapidly, spontaneous haemorrhage or rupture after minor trauma may occur (Fig. 17.35).

The spleen is usually enlarged in cirrhosis of the liver with portal hypertension.[17,18] A normal-sized spleen does not, however, rule out portal hypertension. Varices and collateral veins may be demonstrated in the splenic hilum

(Fig. 17.36). There is no useful correlation between splenomegaly and the severity of the cirrhosis.[19] Doppler flow measurements of the portal and the splenic veins show no correlation with splenic size.[19]

The normal spleen is characterised by a high diastolic flow velocity with low impedance indices. A resistance index (RI) of approximately 0.50 and a pulsatility index (PI) of approximately 0.70 are considered normal (Fig. 17.37). In patients with cirrhosis and portal hypertension they show no relation to splenic size though the measurements may

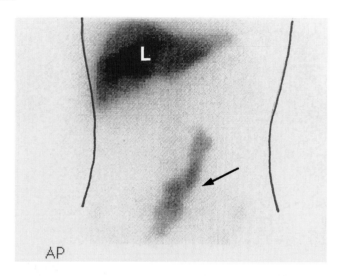

Fig. 17.31 Splenosis. Splenic scintigraphy using 270 mBq TC99m-MDP. Physiological concentration within the liver (L) and an increased concentration in the lower abdomen is seen 20 min after injection. Scintigram taken after a splenectomy demonstrating functioning splenic tissue (arrow) (splenosis) reimplantated in the major omentum.

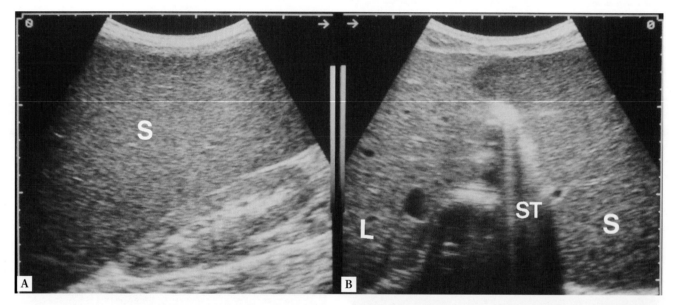

Fig. 17.32 Massive enlargement of the spleen. A: Extreme splenomegaly (S) in chronic lymphatic leukaemia; the exact length is difficult to determine with ultrasound. **B:** So-called 'kissing' phenomena of liver (L) and spleen (S) in extreme hepatosplenomegaly. ST – stomach.

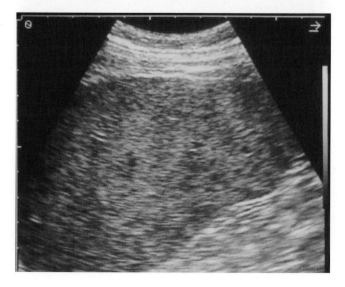

Fig. 17.33 Mild splenomegaly and uncharacteristic structural inhomogeneity of the spleen in florid ulcerative colitis.

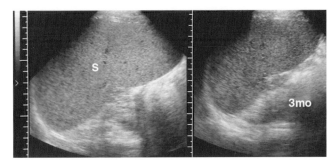

Fig. 17.34 **Splenomegay sonographic follow-up.** Splenomegaly caused by infectious mononucleosis. Splenic size returns to normal over a period of 3 months.

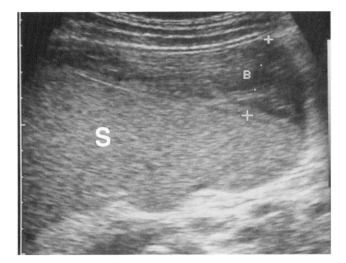

Fig. 17.35 **Subcapsular haematoma** (B) resulting from a spontaneous splenic rupture in infectious mononucleosis. S – spleen.

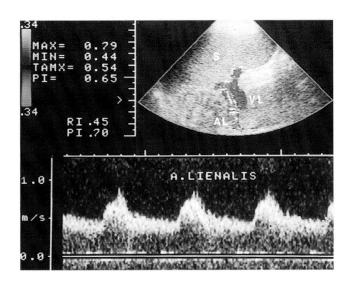

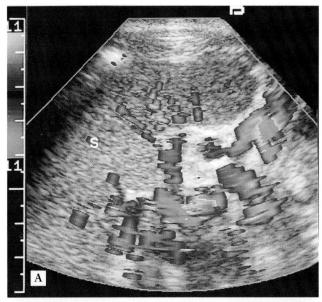

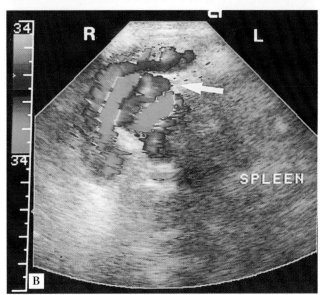

Fig. 17.36 **Portal hypertension. A:** Colour Doppler of enlarged hilar vessels and **B:** pronounced varices (arrow) in cirrhosis with portal hypertension.

Fig. 17.37 **Normal flow profile of the splenic artery** (RI 0.45, PI 0.70).

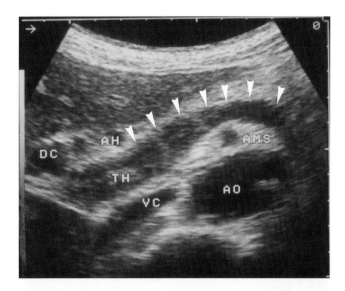

Fig. 17.38 Splenic vein thrombosis – recent. Upper abdominal cross-section of a recent splenic vein thrombosis (arrowheads). AH – hepatic artery, AMS – superior mesenteric artery, AO – aorta, DC – bile duct, TH – thrombosis, VC – vena cava.

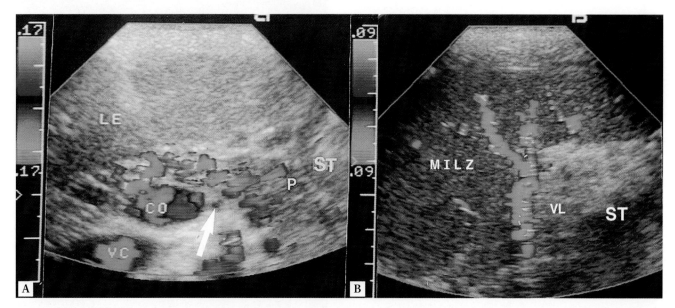

Fig. 17.39 Splenic vein thrombosis. Colour Doppler scans of long-standing splenic vein thrombosis. **A:** The splenic vein cannot be seen in the region of the confluence (arrow) and is replaced by peripancreatic collaterals. LE – liver, VC – vena cava, P – pancreas. **B:** The splenic vein (VL) is clearly seen in close proximity to the hilum. ST – stomach, MILZ – spleen.

be higher than those from subjects with healthy livers and normal splenic size.[20]

Splenomegaly occurs in approximately 60% of cases of splenic vein thrombosis. A normal-sized spleen, therefore, does not rule out splenic vein thrombosis.[21] Sonographically, splenic vein thrombosis is seen as a homogeneous, reflective band of variable width (Fig. 17.38). Unless there is recanalisation, no colour Doppler signals can be obtained from the thrombus and Doplper is useful for demonstrating collaterals (Fig. 17.39).

Splenomegaly is usually marked in myeloproliferative disorders,[22] especially myelofibrosis and in chronic myeloid leukaemia it is a prognostic factor.[23,24] The assessment of splenic size in high-grade lymphoma does not reliably predict splenic involvement and, in particular, a normal-appearing spleen does not rule out splenic involvement. In low-grade lymphoma, particularly chronic lymphatic leukaemia (CLL), hairy cell leukaemia and immunocytoma, splenomegaly is usually a sign of splenic involvement, even if the splenic echo texture is homogeneous.[25] The detection of splenomegaly in CLL carries a worse prognosis.[26]

Splenomegaly is not a reliable indicator of involvement with Hodgkin's disease: approximately one-third of all

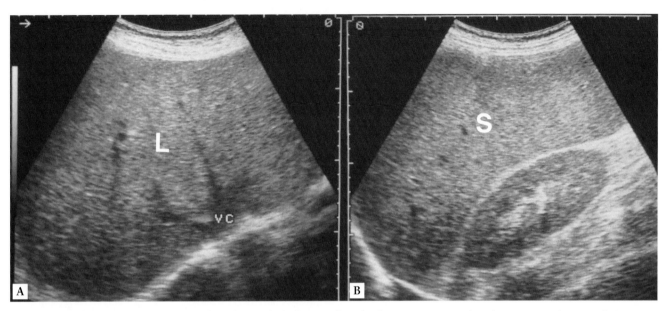

Fig. 17.40 Hodgkin's disease. A: Hepatomegaly and **B:** marked splenomegaly with a homogeneous parenchymal texture; in such cases, splenic involvement must be assumed despite homogeneous texture. L – liver, VC – vena cava, S – spleen.

infiltrated spleens are of normal size.[27] There is a loose relationship between splenic size and degree of infiltration in Hodgkin's disease, unlike in most forms of non-Hodgkin's lymphoma.[28] With marked splenic enlargement (>400 g), lymphoma involvement is almost invariable even if the echo texture is homogeneous[29] (Fig. 17.40). Based on

pathological-anatomical studies, splenic involvement may be assumed when liver involvement is diagnosed, despite a sonographically homogeneous and normal-sized spleen[28] (Fig. 17.41). The low diagnostic accuracy of sonography (and also of CT) means that staging laparotomy is usually required.[30]

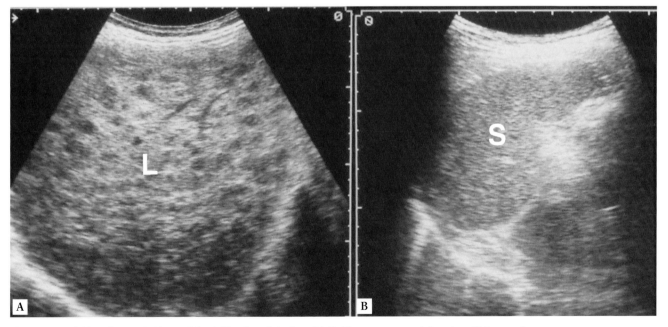

Fig. 17.41 Hodgkin's disease. A: Fine nodular infiltration of the liver (L). **B:** The appearance of the spleen (S) is normal.

Focal splenic lesions

Focal lesions of the spleen are rare (about 0.2%).[31,32] As in the liver, focal lesions of the spleen are characterised with respect to reflectivity, size and number.[31] The differential diagnosis generally requires additional clinical information. When necessary a firm diagnosis can be obtained from an ultrasound-guided fine needle biopsy.[31,33]

Primary malignant tumours

Primary malignancies of the spleen including haemangiosarcomas, are extremely rare.[34,35] They are seen as inhomogeneous, often reflective masses that may also be partially cystic,[33,36,37] a type of tumour that may rupture (ca. 30%).

Primary lymphomas are also rare (<1% of lymphomas) and, by definition, occur only when lymphoma involvement is limited to the spleen and the hilar nodes[38] (Fig. 17.42). This type of lymphoma can be cured by splenectomy.[39] The sonographic pattern is the same as that for secondary splenic involvement.[40]

Splenic metastases

Splenic metastases are found in some 7% of post-mortems of patients with metastatic carcinomas,[41] while on ultrasound approximately 8% of all splenic lesions have been found to be metastases.[31] The tortuous splenic artery as well as the special immunological micro-environment of the spleen may

be responsible for the spleen's resistance to metastatic involvement.[42] Splenic metastases like liver metastases, may be described by their reflectivity compared with the splenic parenchyma as echo-free (Fig. 17.43), poorly reflective (the most common) (Fig. 17.44), highly reflective (Fig. 17.45), or complex.[43] Reflective metastases are the least common[33,44] and target lesions are less common than in the liver[45] (Fig. 17.46). Larger metastases may undergo central necrosis; small metastases may only show as diffuse inhomogeneity of

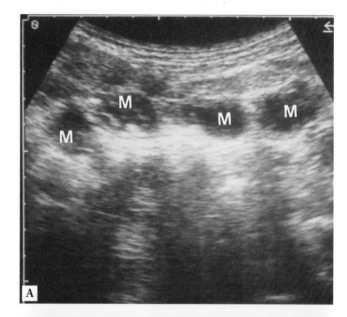

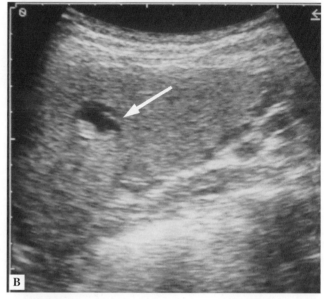

Fig. 17.43 Cystadenocarcinoma of the ovary. A: Upper abdominal cross-section showing multiple peritoneal metastases (M). **B:** Intrasplenic, predominantly cystic metastasis (arrow).

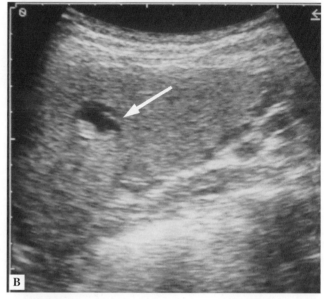

Fig. 17.42 Lymphoma. Poorly reflective mass (M) with pronounced vascularisation of the margins; histologically confirmed primary splenic lymphoma.

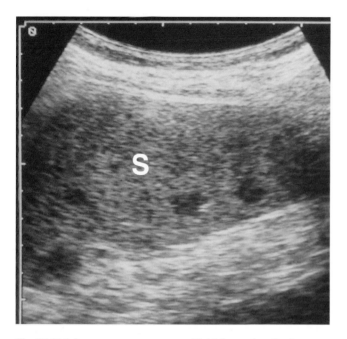

Fig. 17.44 Leiomyosarcoma metastases. Multiple poorly reflective splenic metastases in leiomyosarcoma. S – spleen.

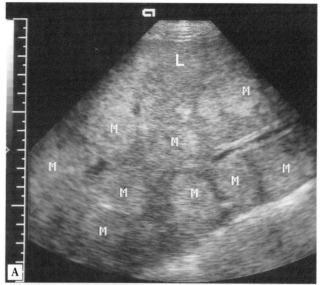

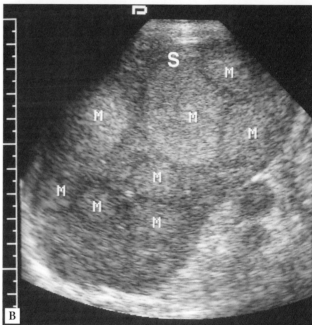

Fig. 17.45 Carcinoid tumour. A: Reflective metastases of the liver (M) and **B:** spleen (S). M – metastases.

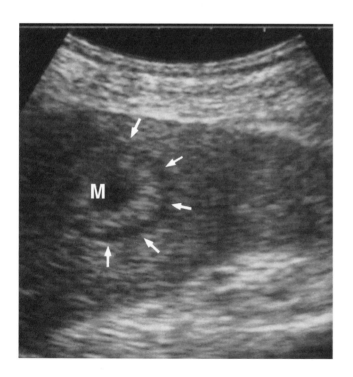

Fig. 17.46 Splenic metastases. Reflective mass (M) with liquefied centre and poorly reflective margins ('Halo' sign) (arrows) due to splenic metastases of a colorectal carcinoma.

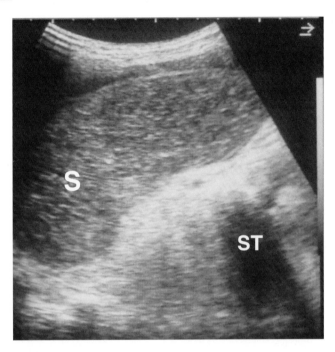

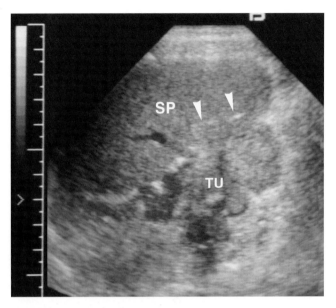

Fig. 17.49 Neuroendocrine tumour of the pancreatic tail (TU) (VIPOMA) with direct invasion (arrowheads) of the spleen (SP).

Fig. 17.47 Small nodular metastates in adenocarcinoma, confirmed at autopsy. ST – stomach, S – spleen.

the splenic tissue (Fig. 17.47). Since splenic involvement is usually a very late manifestation of metastatic disease, sonographic follow-up is sufficient to determine whether or not the lesion is malignant (Fig. 17.48).

It is important to distinguish direct tumour invasion of the spleen by carcinomas of the pancreatic tail (Fig. 17.49), colon and stomach (Fig. 17.50) from

haematogenous metastases. Complications such as bowel perforations covered by splenic parenchyma, abscesses or splenic haemorrhage may be observed (Fig. 17.51). Tumours of the lung or diaphragm occasionally invade the diaphragm and infiltrate the spleen (Fig 17.52) and the spleen may be involved in patients with peritoneal carcinomatosis (Figs 17.53 and 17.54).[46]

Secondary lymphoma of the spleen

The frequency of splenic involvement in disseminated malignant lymphoma is difficult to assess. Depending on the length of illness and the biological behaviour of different lymphoma types, splenic involvement may be found in 30–60% of these patients.[28] It is manifest as splenomegaly, perhaps with focal or diffuse parenchymal lesions. However, lymphomatous involvement cannot be ruled out by normal size and homogeneous texture.

Lymphoma of the spleen is the most common cause of focal lesions making up nearly 40% of all focal splenic lesions in one ultrasound series.[31] Five patterns may be differentiated (Fig. 17.55). Diffuse involvement is the most difficult to detect and is the reason why ultrasound, along with other imaging modalities, has such a low sensitivity for splenic lymphoma (Figs 17.56 and 17.57). The liver can be a useful reference as it usually has a uniform echo texture (Fig. 17.58).

Sonography has a sensitivity of over 90% and a specificity of 96% in the diagnosis of focal parenchymal lesions.[47] With the low incidence of focal involvement of

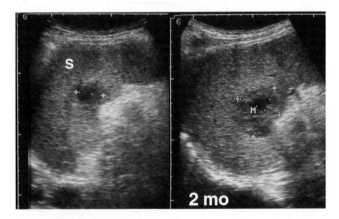

Fig. 17.48 Splenic metastases. Sonographic follow-up. A: A poorly reflective rounded lesion near the hilum found in a patient with colonic cancer B: had enlarged at the 2-month follow-up and therefore was thought to be a metastasis (M). S – spleen.

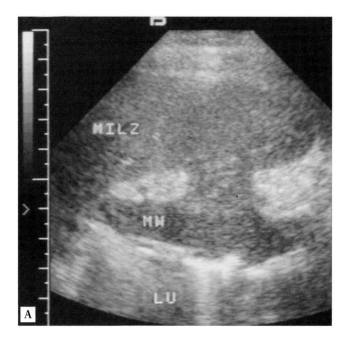

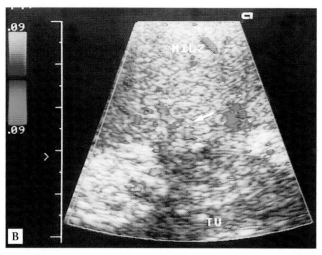

Fig. 17.50 Gastric carcinoma. A: Thickening of the gastric wall (MW) in a gastric carcinoma that has spread directly to the splenic hilum. **B:** On Doppler the continuity of vasculature between the mass and the spleen can be discerned (arrow). LU – lumen, MILZ – spleen.

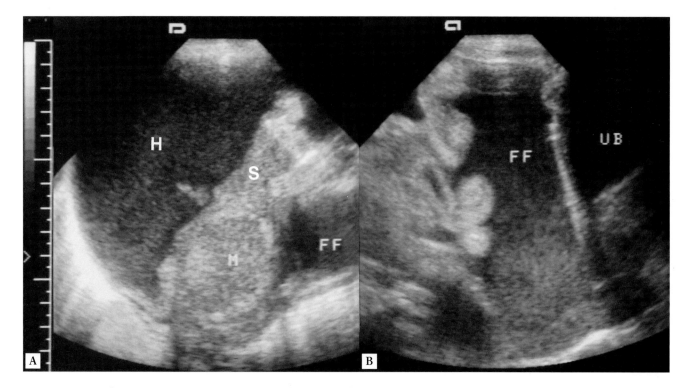

Fig. 17.51 Haemorrhagic metastasis. A: Spontaneous intrasplenic haemorrhage (H) of metastasis (M) from a squamous cell carcinoma of the floor of the mouth. Note the free fluid in the hilum (FF) and **B:** in the pouch of Douglas. Fine needle aspiration yielded blood. UB – urinary bladder.

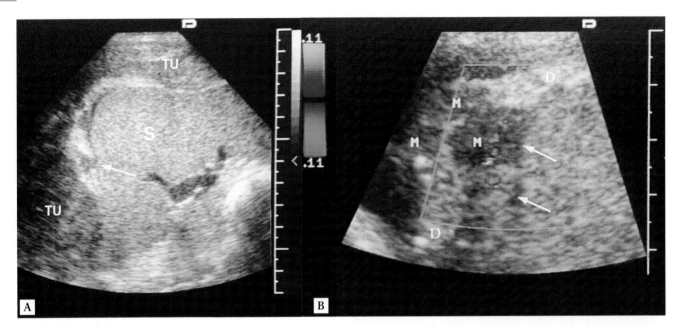

Fig. 17.52 Carcinoma of the bronchus. A: Patient with an advanced blastoma of the left lung showing trans-diaphragmatic invasion of the spleen by tumour (TU). **B:** Vessels indicate perfused tumour tissue (arrow). M – metastases, D – diaphragm.

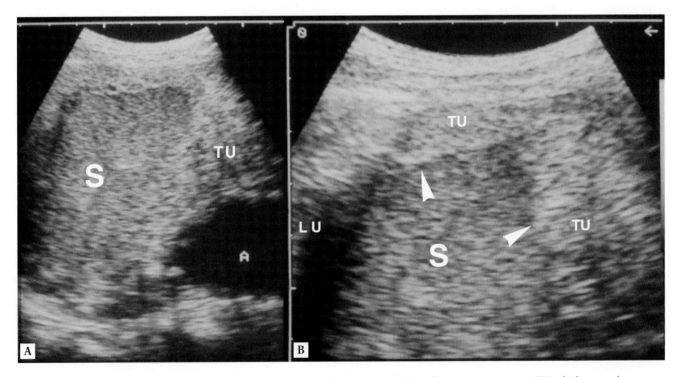

Fig. 17.53 Ovarian carcinoma. A: Peritoneal spread of ovarian cancer with ascites (A) and **B:** reflective tumour masses (TU) which cannot be separated from the spleen (S) (arrowheads). LU – lung.

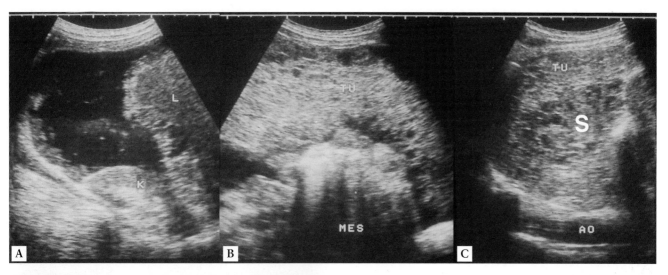

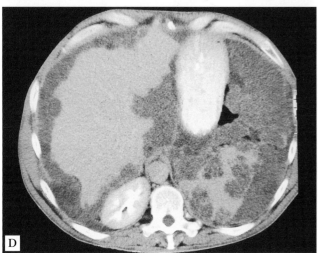

Fig. 17.54 Carcinoma of the colon. A: Peritoneal carcinoma in a patient with a mucinoid adenocarcinoma of the colon with ascites and perihepatic infiltration. B: Tumour infiltration of the omentum and C: perisplenic (TU) and splenic infiltration (S). L – liver, K – kidney, MES – mesentery, CR – cranial. D: Abdominal CT confirms peritoneal carcinoma and splenic infiltration.

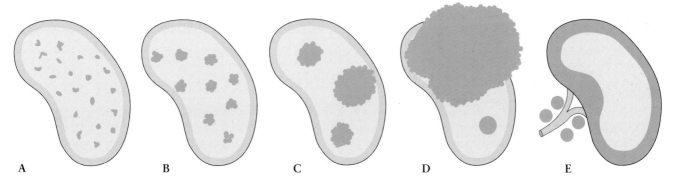

Fig. 17.55 Lymphoma. Schematic diagram of the sonographic pattern of splenic involvement in malignant lymphoma. A: Diffuse infiltration, B: small nodular infiltration (largest lesion <3 cm²), C: large nodular infiltration (largest lesion >3 cm²), D: bulky tumour, E: perisplenic infiltration.

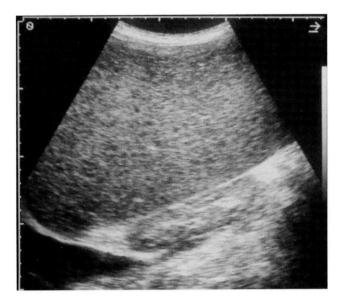

Fig. 17.56 Lymphoma. Splenomegaly with an altered texture in mantle zone cell lymphoma.

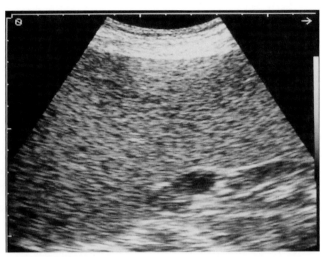

Fig. 17.57 Leukaemia. Splenomegaly with a finely altered texture in chronic lymphatic leukaemia.

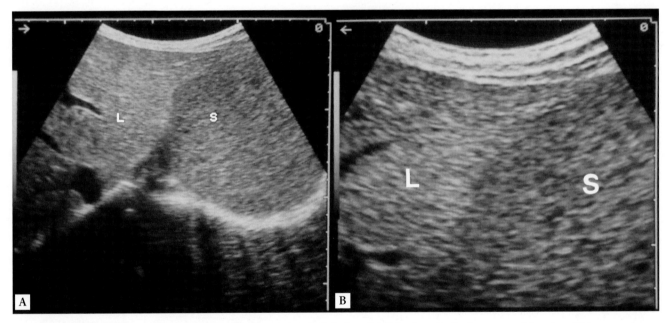

Fig. 17.58 Leukaemia. Hepatosplenomegaly caused by chronic lymphatic leukaemia; slight alteration in the texture of the spleen (S) in comparison to the liver (L) is seen, indicating diffuse splenic involvement.

the spleen in lymphoma, the demonstration of a poorly reflective lesion in a patient with lymphoma may be considered diagnostic of splenic involvement[48] and confirmation by fine needle puncture is unnecessary.[49] Colour Doppler images show sparse vascularisation that penetrates into the mass (Fig. 17.59). Highly reflective lesions are rare in lymphoma[50] (Figs 17.60 and 17.61) and the

pathological correlation is unclear, though heterogeneity is more often found in large lesions (Fig. 17.62). Reflective lymph nodes in patients with malignant lymphoma have been correlated with fatty tissue and fibrosis.[51] In correspondence with the macroscopic findings,[28] non-Hodgkin's lymphoma of low grade, as well as Hodgkin's lymphoma, tend to have a diffuse or nodular type of

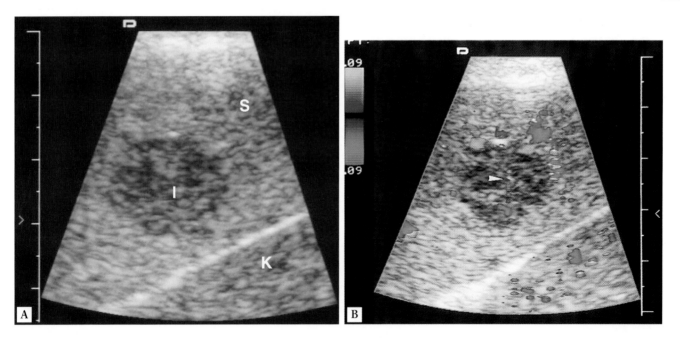

Fig. 17.59 Lymphoma. A: A poorly reflective lymphomatous lesion (l) in Hodgkin's disease. **B:** The colour Doppler study shows sparse vascularisation (arrowhead). K – kidney, S – spleen.

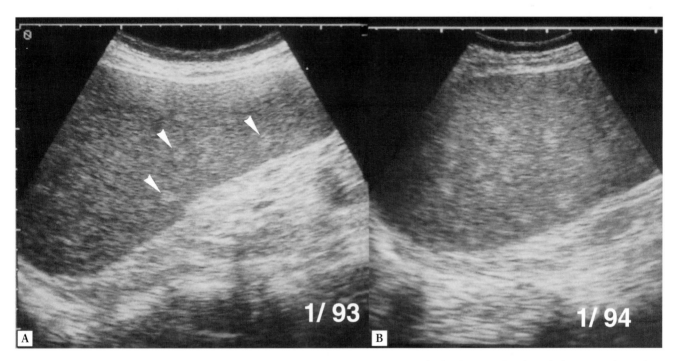

Fig. 17.60 Leukaemia. Sonographic follow-up. A: Small, isolated, reflective splenic lesions (arrowheads) seen in lymphatic leukaemia; **B:** the number of reflective lesions increases over time. Autopsy confirmed small nodular splenic involvement.

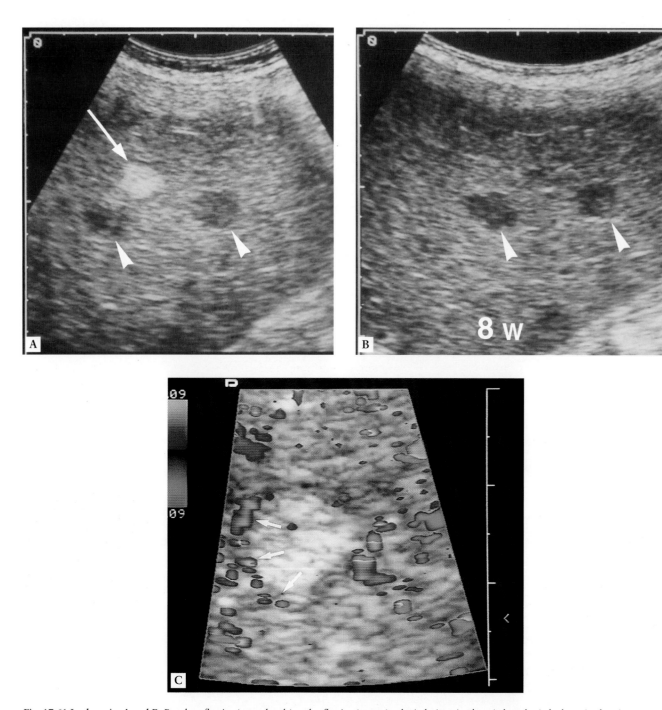

Fig. 17.61 Leukaemia. A and B: Poorly reflective (arrowheads) and reflective (arrow) splenic lesions in chronic lymphatic leukaemia showing regression of the reflective lesions during treatment. **C:** Doppler sonogram of a reflective splenic lesion in malignant lymphoma with peripheral vascularisation (arrows).

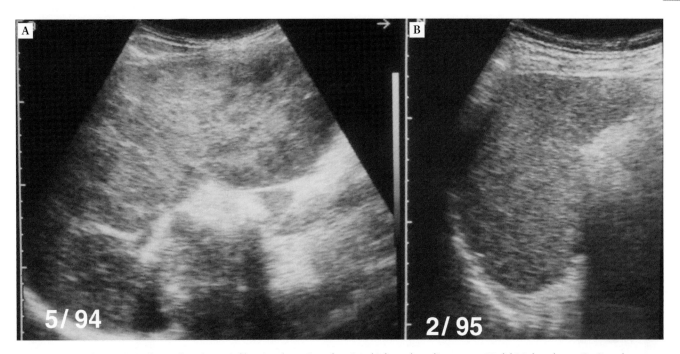

Fig. 17.62 Lymphoma. A: Reflective lymphoma infiltrating the entire spleen in a high-grade malignant non-Hodgkin's lymphoma. **B:** Complete regression after 10 months of treatment.

infiltration, while high-grade non-Hodgkin's lymphoma tends to form larger focal masses (Figs 17.63 to 17.66).[48] Perisplenic infiltration typically extends from the hilum (Figs 17.67 and 17.68) but thoracic lymphoma may infiltrate through the diaphragm and penetrate the splenic capsule (Figs 17.69 and 17.70). Only in rare cases does splenic infiltration lead to splenic haemorrhage (Fig. 17.71), rupture (Figs 17.72 and 17.73) or infarction.

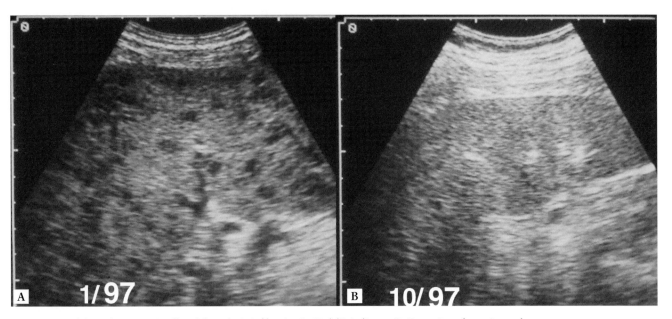

Fig. 17.63 Hodgkin's disease. A: Small nodular splenic infiltration in Hodgkin's disease. **B:** Formation of scar tissue after treatment.

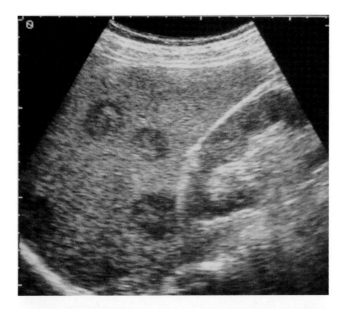

Fig. 17.64 Lymphoma. Multiple poorly reflective nodules in the spleen in non-Hodgkin's lymphoma.

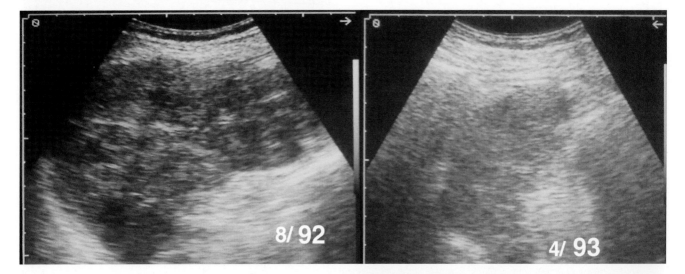

Fig. 17.65 Hodgkin's disease. Lymphoma infiltration in Hodgkin's disease and complete regression after 8 months of treatment.

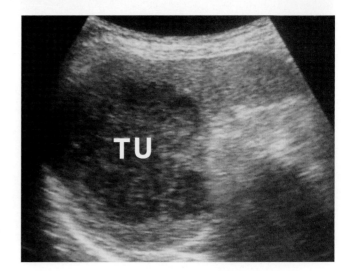

Fig. 17.66 Lymphoma. A large, solitary, poorly reflective tumour (TU) in high-grade malignant lymphoma.

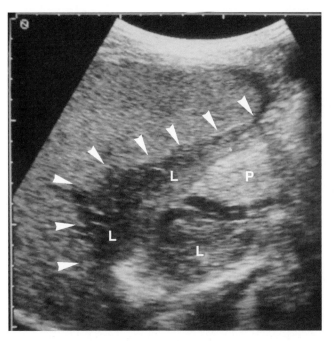

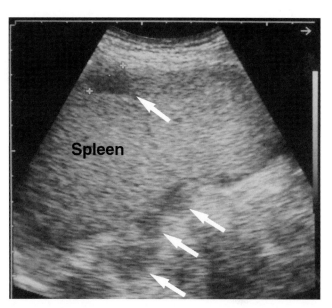

Fig. 17.67 Lymphoma. Poorly reflective lymphatic tissue (L) which stretches, garland-like, from the splenic hilum and surrounds the spleen (arrowheads). P – pancreas.

Fig. 17.68 Lymphoma. Perisplenic, poorly reflective nodular tumour (arrow) in high-grade malignant lymphoma.

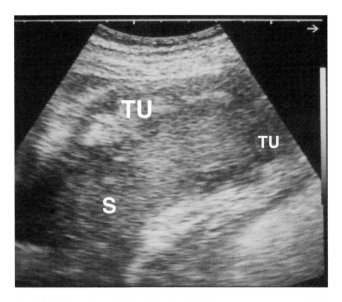

Fig. 17.69 Lymphoma. Perisplenic mixed reflective tumour masses (TU) in high-grade malignant lymphoma; the surface of the spleen (S) is no longer clearly distinguishable.

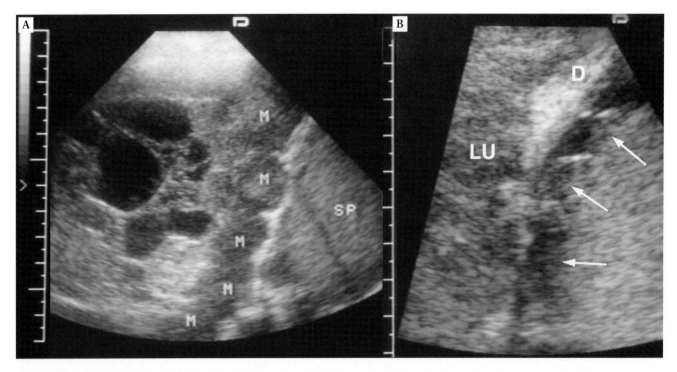

Fig. 17.70 Lymphoma. A: Tumour invasion of the left thoracic cavity in high-grade malignant lymphoma. Lymphomatous, string-of-beads infiltration of the diaphragm by the lymphoma (M) **B:** Image of a thoracic tumour (LU) with diaphragmatic (D) involvement and tumour nodules on the surface of the spleen (arrows).

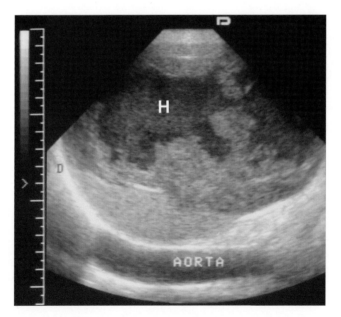

Fig. 17.71 Lymphoma. Splenic involvement in high-grade lymphoma which has resulted in liquefaction of the tumour, or hidden intraparenchymal haemorrhage (H). D – diaphragm.

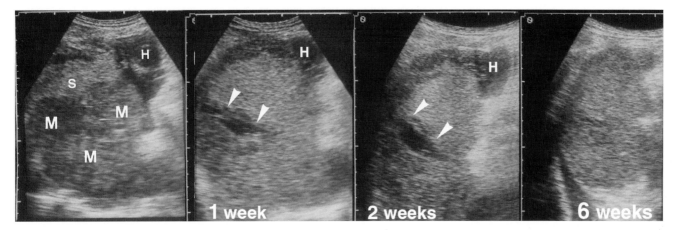

Fig. 17.72 Lymphoma. Large, nodular splenic infiltration (M) exceeding beyond the margins of the organ in malignant lymphoma complicated by a subcapsular haematoma (H); with treatment, the infiltration regresses and the laceration of the parenchyma (arrowheads) is visualised during follow-up. Complete healing is the final stage. S – spleen.

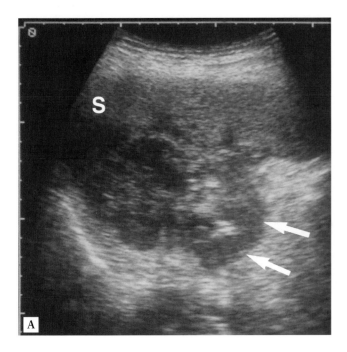

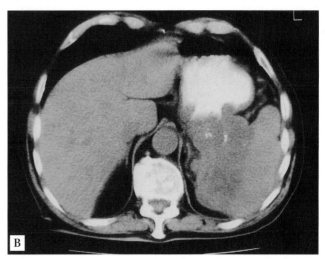

Fig. 17.73 Gastric lymphoma. A: Large, complex intrasplenic mass which cannot be separated from the stomach (arrow) in a locally infiltrating primary gastric lymphoma, surgically confirmed. **B:** Abdominal CT confirming tumoral invasion of the spleen. S – spleen.

Primary benign tumours of the spleen

The rare benign tumours of the spleen are usually incidental findings during an abdominal scan. They include haemangiomas, hamartomas and lymphangiomas.[52] The fundamental importance of ultrasound and other cross-sectional imaging techniques lies in differenting them from malignancies or other reflective intrasplenic masses. The final diagnosis usually requires additional tests.

Haemangiomas are the most common with an incidence at autopsy between 0.03% and 14%.[53,54] They are tumours of the epithelium of the vascular sinuses and are more commonly cavernous in pattern than capillary. Haemangiomas may be solitary or multiple. They normally grow slowly but rupture in up to 25% of cases.[53] Anaemia, thrombocytopenia and coagulopathy (Kasabach–Merrit syndrome) may occur with very large haemangiomas.[55] Sarcomatous degeneration has been documented.[54]

On ultrasound two patterns may be differentiated: predominantly smooth, well-defined, homogeneous, reflective, usually rounded lesions (Fig. 17.74); and complex lesions with poorly reflective sometimes echo-free areas and occasionally also shadowing from calcification

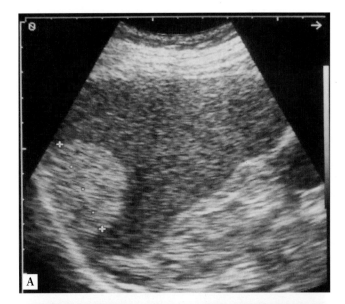

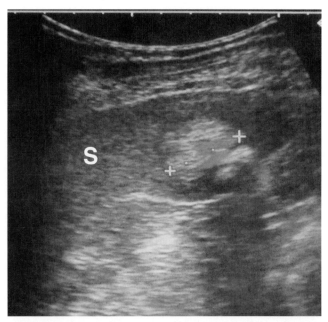

Fig. 17.75 Haemangioma. Seen as a reflective rounded mass with slight calcification. S – spleen.

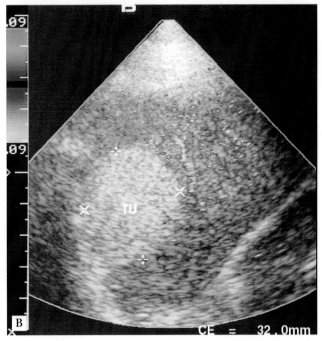

Fig. 17.74 Haemangioma. A: Reflective rounded splenic nodule. CT suggested a haemangioma. **B:** Colour Doppler sonogram of the splenic haemangioma (TU) shows no signals ('silent tumour').

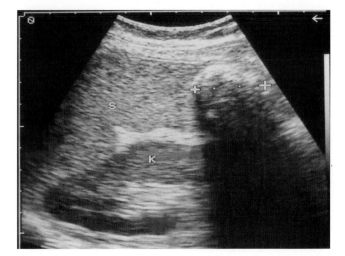

Fig. 17.76 Haemangioma. A crescent moon-shaped, highly reflective mass with distal shadowing consistent with a calcified haemangioma. K – kidney, S – spleen.

(Figs 17.75 and 17.76). These patterns correlate with a homogeneous vessel pattern and fluid areas (comprising haemorrhage and sometimes serous fluid) respectively.[55] Cystic haemangioma is a rare variant.[56]

Hamartomas have been reported occasionally, usually as incidental findings.[57,58] Usually solitary, in rare cases they are generalised (tuberous sclerosis, Wiskott–Aldrich syndrome).[52] They consist of normal splenic tissue. Sonographically, the tumour is displayed as homogeneous and more reflective than the surrounding splenic tissue (Figs 17.77 and 17.78). They are well defined and, like haemangiomas, lack colour Doppler signals.[59] In rare cases, they may also be displayed as poorly reflective vascular masses (Fig. 17.79). Cystic hamartomas have also

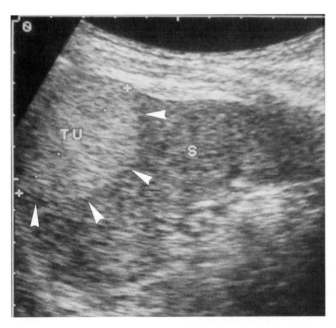

Fig. 17.77 Hamatoma. Reflective mass (TU) in the spleen (S): a hamartoma (splenoma) was found on histology after surgery.

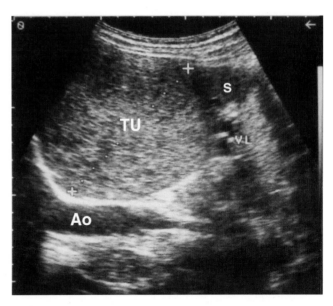

Fig. 17.78 Hamatoma. Large, solid, reflective splenic tumour (TU), histologically confirmed as a splenic hamartoma (splenoma). VL – splenic vein, AO – aorta, S – spleen.

been documented.[60] Lymphangiomas are extremely rare.[61] They are seen sonographically as honeycomb cystic lesions in an enlarged spleen.[62,63]

Splenic cysts and pseudocysts

Splenic cysts are benign lesions with an incidence of less than 0.1%.[64] They include true cysts (developmental, epidermoid and dermoid), pseudocysts (non-epithelial cysts) and echinococcal cysts.[65]

Parasitic splenic cysts are rare and are observed in less than 2% of all patients with echinococcal disease.[66] Such cysts are usually echo-free and daughter cysts may be present. Intracystic membrane formation, hydatid sand, solid components and calcification have been documented (Fig. 17.80).[67]

True splenic cysts are epithelialised. The theory that these originate as mesothelial cysts which arose through an embryonic dispersal of splenic tissue during fusion is increasingly gaining support.[68,69] Sonographically, they appear as well-defined, smooth-walled, echo-free lesions which show increased through transmission of ultrasound (Fig. 17.81). Features such as reflective separations (Fig. 17.82), internal echoes (Fig. 17.83), sedimentation (Fig. 17.84), tissue sequestering and wall calcification (Figs 17.85 to 87) may be observed. The cyst contents may be watery and clear, or brackish-brown in colour if there has been a haemorrhage.

Pseudocysts are, by definition, not epithelialized. They are found with pancreatitis,[70] splenic trauma,[71] (Fig. 17.88)

infarction[72] (Fig. 17.89) and metastases.[73] Differentiation between true splenic cysts and pseudocysts is impossible with imaging: in a series of 52 patients with non-parasitic splenic cysts (24 true cysts, 28 pseudocysts), no difference was found between the two types with respect to size, internal reflectivity or cystic contents, though wall calcification was observed more frequently in pseudocysts.[69]

The treatment of splenic cysts generally depends on whether they are symptomatic, which, in turn, depends on their size. Cysts <5 cm may be kept under observation but larger formations usually require surgery, which is designed to preserve as much healthy splenic tissue as possible.[74] Ultrasound-guided catheter drainage[75] with sclerosing agents[76–78] is increasingly becoming an alternative (Chapter 4 and Fig. 17.90). Cyst rupture[79] and cystic carcinoma[80] are documented complications.

Splenic abscesses

In autopsy studies, the incidence of splenic abscesses is 0.14–7%.[81] Splenic abscesses accounted for 4% of sonographically diagnosed splenic lesions in one medical patient population.[31] Macro-abscesses are discussed separately from micro-abscesses.

The sonographic features of macro-abscesses are extremely varied. In addition to lesions that are purely cystic (Fig. 17.91), poorly reflective (Fig. 17.92) as well as predominantly reflective abscesses (Fig. 17.93), may be encountered. This wide spectrum of ultrasound features

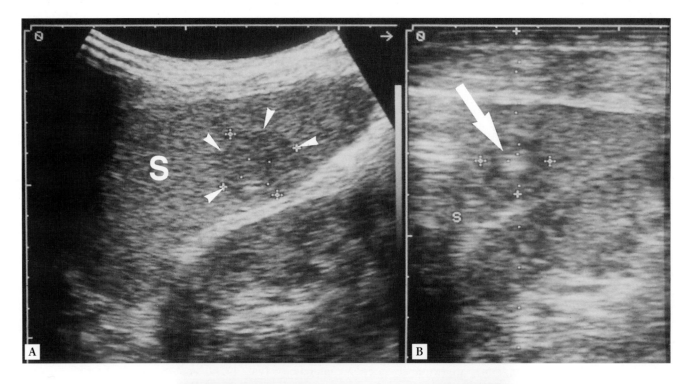

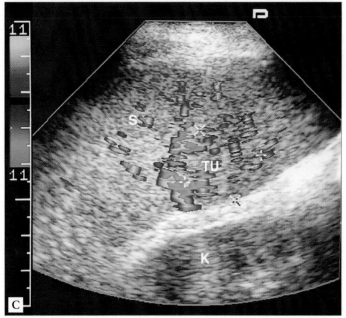

Fig. 17.79 Needle biopsy A: An almost isoechoic splenic tumour (arrowheads). **B:** Fine needle aspiration puncture of the focus. The tip of needle (arrow) lies within the mass. On histology the tissue was normal splenic tissue, suggesting a splenoma. The tumour remained constant over 5 years. **C:** Doppler demonstrating marked vascularization (TU). S – spleen.

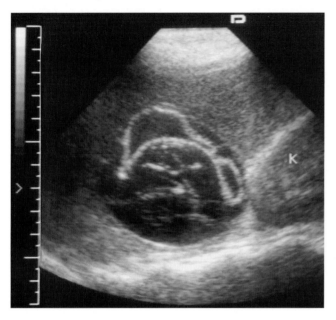

Fig. 17.80 Echinococcus cyst showing separation of the cyst wall to form the waterlily sign. K – kidney.

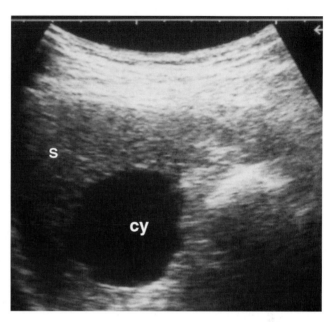

Fig. 17.81 Splenic cyst. Echo-free lesion represents a splenic cyst (cy). S – spleen.

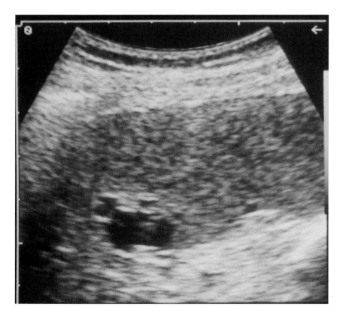

Fig. 17.82 Splenic cyst with multiple internal septations.

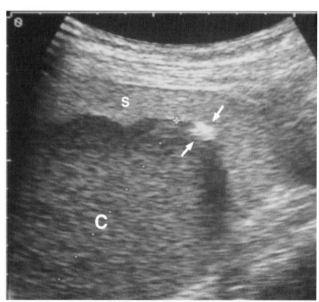

Fig. 17.83 Poorly reflective splenic cyst (C) with mobile echoes ('snowstorm effect') and a calcific focus (arrows). S – spleen.

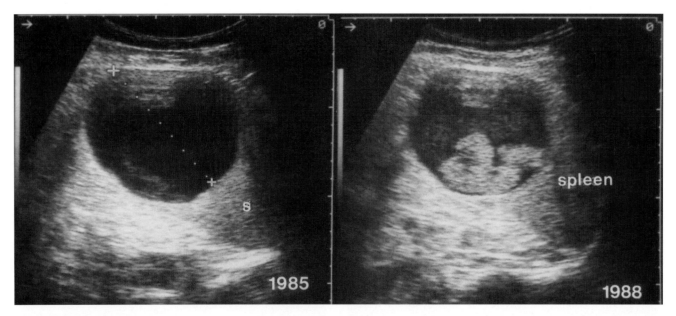

Fig. 17.84 Splenic cyst. Sonographic follow-up. Asymptomatic solitary splenic cyst; at routine follow-up it was found to contain clumps of internal reflective material presumably resulting from intracystic haemorrhage. S – spleen.

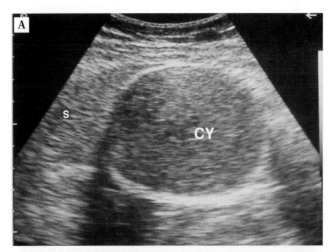

Fig. 17.85 Splenic cyst. A: Large, isoechogenic splenic cyst (CY) with calcified margins. **B:** Abdominal CT confirming a calcified cyst. S – spleen.

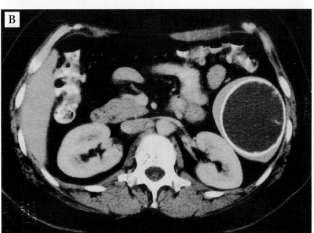

Fig. 17.86 Calcified cyst. The round, ring-shaped, highly reflective structure with dorsal shadowing is a calcified splenic cyst.

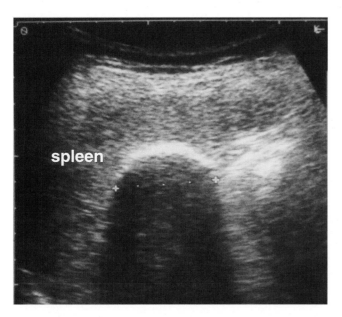

Fig. 17.87 Calcification. Sickle-shaped calcification with dorsal shadowing confirmed splenic cyst on CT.

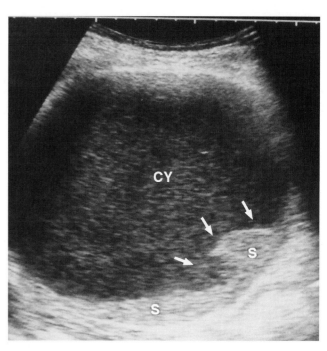

Fig. 17.88 Post-traumatic cyst. Blunt abdominal trauma 1 year ago has led to the formation of a large pseudocyst (CY); laboratory findings showed thrombocytosis (>1000 000/mm³) the arrows mark splenic tissue (S).

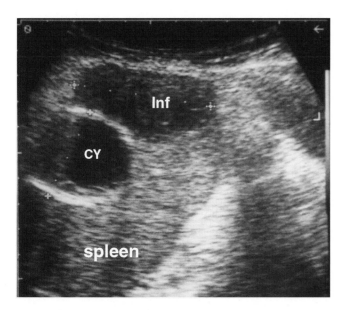

Fig. 17.89 Calcified splenic cyst (cy) adjacent to a poorly reflective splenic infarct (Inf); the cystic lesion is most probably due to pseudocyst formation following a previous splenic infarct.

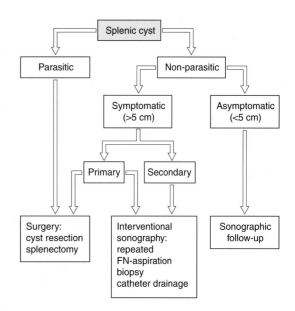

Fig. 17.90 Therapeutic procedures in splenic cysts.

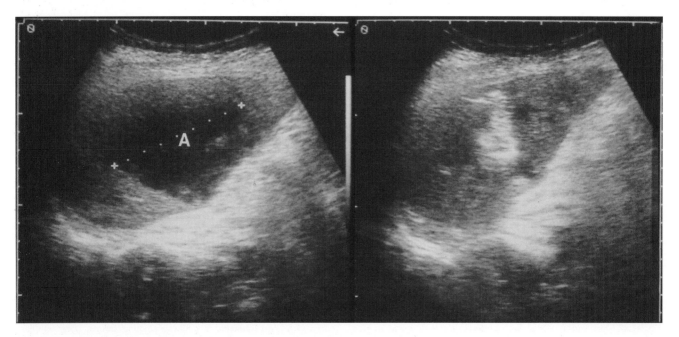

Fig. 17.91 Splenic abscess (A). Percutaneous fine needle aspiration yielded 115 ml of pus; following instillation of an antibiotic solution, the space was seen to contain reflective structures due to gas bubbles.

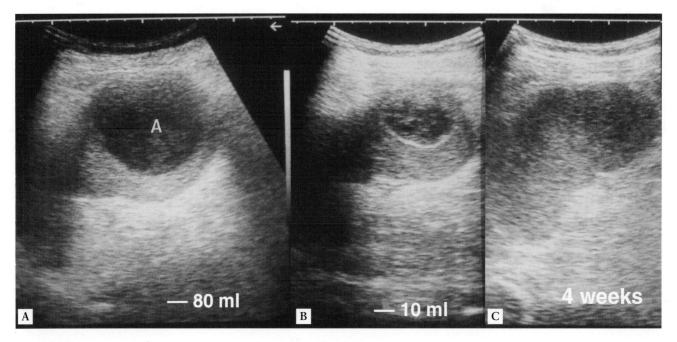

Fig. 17.92 Splenic abscess (A). **A:** Complete healing of a poorly reflective splenic abscess was documented, **B** and **C:** after two drainage procedures.

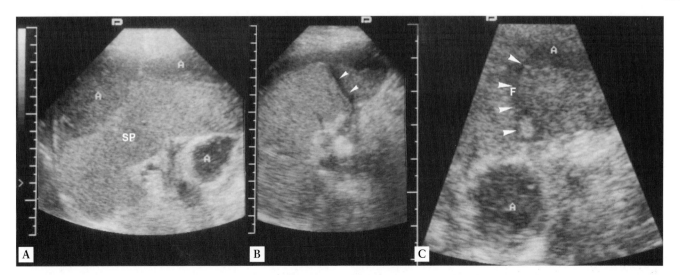

Fig. 17.93 Perisplenic abscess. A: Perisplenic abscess (A) including one at the hilum. **B:** The two abscess cavities are joined by a neck (arrowheads). **C:** Fluctuation of abscess material through the fistula (F) when compressed by the transducer. Sp – spleen.

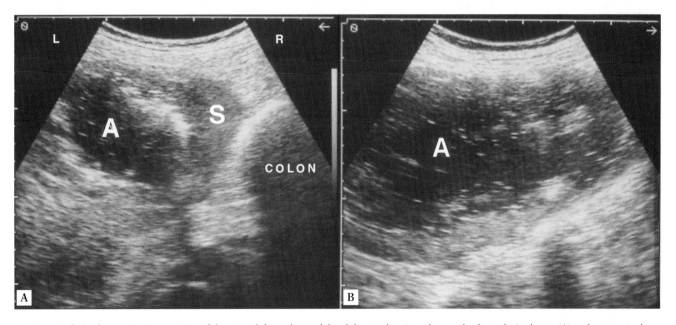

Fig. 17.94 Splenic abscess. A: Cross-section of the upper left quadrant of the abdomen showing a large, echo-free splenic abscess (A) and pronounced reflectivity due to gas-forming bacteria in lymphatic leukaemia. S – spleen. **B:** Image of an abscess (A) that involves almost the entire spleen. A splenectomy was performed.

often makes it impossible to diagnose splenic abscesses based on sonographic findings alone. Microbubbles due to gas-producing bacteria may be detected and are a patho-gnomonic feature (Fig. 17.94). Common causes are:

1 haematogenous pyogenic infections such as bacterial endocarditis,
2 primary or secondary infected splenic infarctions or splenic haematomas,

3 infections of neighbouring organs (such as pancreatitis (Fig. 17.93), or perforated gastric carcinomas (Fig. 17.95).

Splenic abscesses carry a high mortality rate if left untreated,[82] making early diagnosis and treatment high priorities. Percutaneous drainage is now the management of choice, repeated aspiration being recommended for abscesses <10 cm (Figs 17.91 and 17.92) and catheter

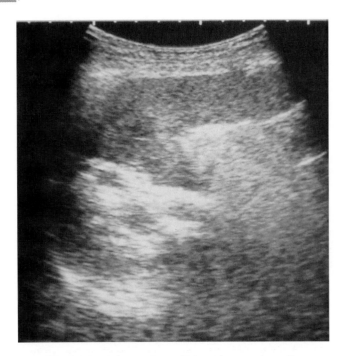

Fig. 17.95 Gastric carcinoma. Intrasplenic gas in a gastric carcinoma that has penetrated into the spleen and led to the development of a splenic abscess.

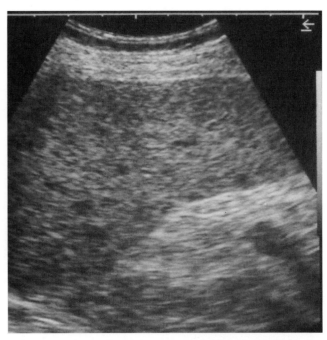

Fig. 17.96 Candida. Multiple, poorly reflective candida micro-abscesses in malignant lymphoma; the lesions arose after high-dose chemotherapy and an antibiotic-resistant fever.

drainage for abscesses >10 cm in diameter.[83] Splenectomy is rarely required.

Micro-abscesses of the spleen and liver are rare and are seen, for the most part, in immunosuppressed patients especially after chemotherapy or bone marrow transplantation for myeloproliferative disorders.[84] Aetiologically, candida infection[85–87] is the most common. Chronic leukocytopenia and septic fever despite antibiotic therapy are predisposing factors. Sonographically, splenic micro-abscesses are seen as multiple, mostly poorly reflective foci 0.5–2 cm in size, some of which may be considered 'target' lesions with a small reflective central dot (Fig. 17.96).[86] The differentiation of this type of poorly reflective focus from the small nodular infiltrations of malignant lymphomas or leukaemia is difficult but serial scans during antimicrobial treatment to document response is helpful (Fig. 17.97), and in a few cases ultrasound-guided fine needle biopsy is necessary for diagnostic confirmation.

Splenic infarct

Splenic infarction is relatively common[31] and predominantly results from thrombo-embolism of splenic artery branches (Fig. 17.98). It may also occur as a complication of myeloproliferative syndromes, diseases of the lymphatic system, sepsis (especially endocarditis) and in sickle cell anaemia.[72,88] Occasionally, in children with thalassaemia major and signs of hypersplenism, therapeutic partial ligation of the splenic artery is carried out to produce splenic infarction.[89] Infarction may be painless or may produce pain that is generalised or localised to the left upper quadrant of the abdomen.

Splenic infarction may be demonstrated on ultrasound as altered texture.[90,91] Acute splenic infarction at about 24 hours is seen as a well-defined, wedge-shaped, poorly reflective lesion.[91] The shape of the infarct depends on the plane of section (Figs 17.99 and 17.100) but always extends to the surface of the spleen. The size and number of infarcted areas is variable. With colour Doppler, the infarct is defined by the absence of Doppler signals in comparison to normal splenic tissue (Fig. 17.101).[92]

Chronic recurrent infarction, as is characteristic of homozygous sickle cell anaemia, produces focal poorly reflective and reflective lesions, sometimes with calcification (Figs 17.102 and 17.103) and progressive shrinkage of the spleen, leading ultimately to autosplenectomy.[88,93,94] Marked reduction in vascularity of a scarred spleen may be demonstrated with colour Doppler (Figs 17.104 and 17.105). The broad spectrum of sonographic features of splenic infarctions described in the literature is, in part, attributable to the fact that retrospective determination of the age of an infarct is not possible.[90]

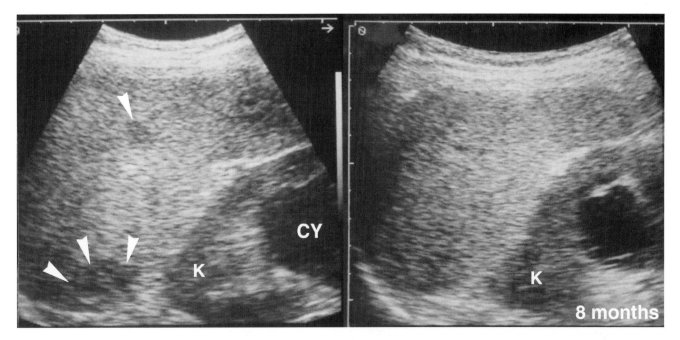

Fig. 17.97 Candida. Multiple, poorly reflective candida abscesses in myeloid leukaemia with complete regression after antimycotic treatment. K – kidney, CY – renal cyst.

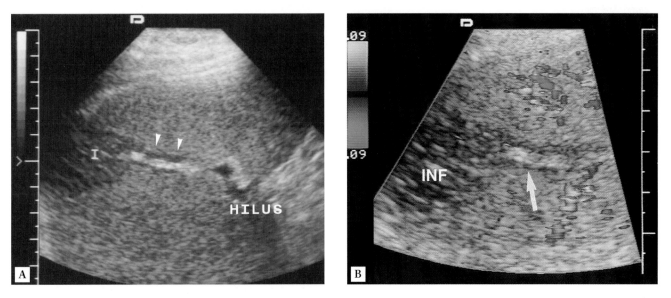

Fig. 17.98 Splenic infarct. A: Splenic infarct in a patient with lung cancer showing reflective thrombus in a vessel (arrowheads) leading to the wedge-shaped infarct (I). **B:** On colour Doppler the ischaemic infact (INF) and the lack of signals in the vessel (arrow) are shown.

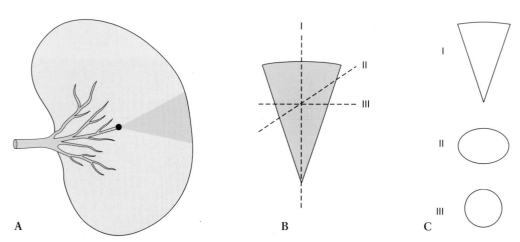

Fig. 17.99 Splenic infarct. A: Schematic diagram of an arterial occlusion that has led to a wedge-shaped splenic infarct (circular cone). **B:** Diagram of various sectional planes of the circular cone. **C:** Shapes that result from scanning through various sectional planes of the circular cone.

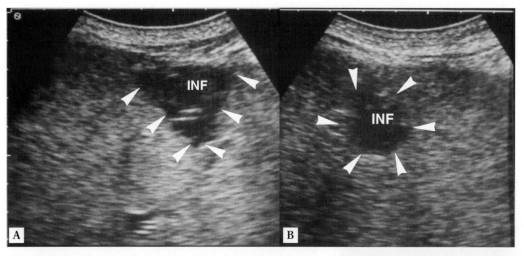

Fig. 17.100 Splenic infarct. A: A characteristically wedge-shaped splenic infarct (INF) (arrowheads) with its base on the surface of the spleen. **B:** From a slightly different angle, the same splenic infarct (INF) is seen as a rounded shape (arrowheads).

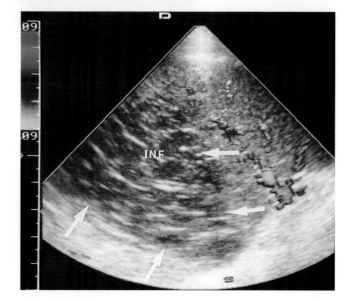

Fig. 17.101 Splenic infarct. A large, wedge-shaped avascular splenic infarct (INF) (arrows).

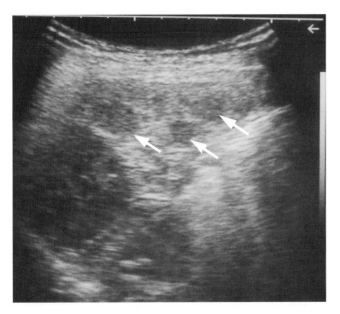

Fig. 17.102 A scarred spleen following multiple infarcts (arrows) caused by homozygotic sickle-cell anaemia.

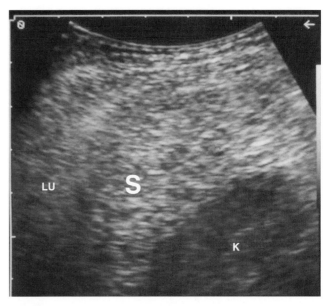

Fig. 17.103 Shrunken spleen. The texture of this shrunken spleen (S), in homozygotic sickle-cell anaemia (scarred spleen), is inhomogeneous and slightly reflective. K – kidney, LU – lung.

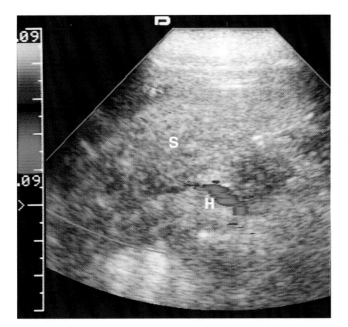

Fig. 17.104 Scarred spleen. Colour Doppler study of a scarred spleen in homozygotic sickle-cell anaemia demonstrates scanty flow. H – hilum.

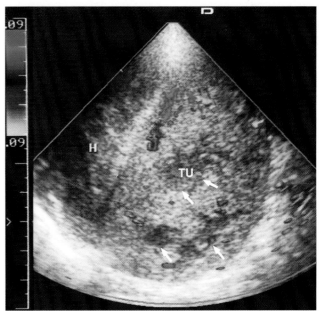

Fig. 17.105 Splenic infarct. A reflective tumour of the spleen with poorly reflective areas (TU) and an adjacent subcapsular haematoma (H). On colour Doppler, vessels were shown within the mass. Splenectomy was performed and demonstrated recurrent splenic infarcts.

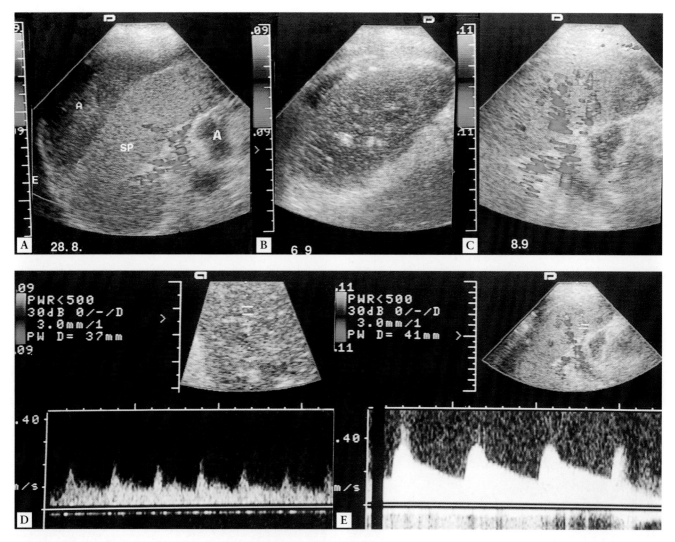

Fig. 17.106 Splenic infarct. A spleen with temporary occlusion of its artery by an abscess of the splenic hilum during an acute episode of chronic, recurrent pancreatitis. **A:** Spleen and the hilar vessels. **B:** Thrombocytosis developed and the spleen became poorly reflective without definite demonstration of splenic colour flow signals. **C:** Spontaneous revascularisation of the spleen occurred and the platelet count returned to normal. **D:** Bypass circulation in response to occlusion of the splenic artery with a 'nutritive' blood supply most likely via collaterals. **E:** A regular flow profile of the intraparenchymal arteries near the hilum is seen after a spontaneous reopening of the splenic artery. A – abscess, SP –Spleen, E – Pleural effusion

The entire spleen may become infarcted in acute splenic thrombosis, for example in torsion of the splenic pedicle or in acute pancreatitis. The entire spleen becomes poorly reflective (Fig. 17.106). In haemorrhagic infarction, the parenchyma is heterogeneous with irregular poorly reflective zones.[95]

The healing process is characterised by increasing reflectivity and shrinkage of the infarct (Fig. 17.107). Occasionally a healed infarct is seen as a focal reflective region (Fig. 17.108) or as calcification (Fig. 17.109).

Eighty percent of infarcts heal without complications[72] (Fig. 17.110) but liquefaction (Fig. 17.111) and haemorrhage may occur, either subcapsular (Fig. 17.112) or with bleeding into the peritoneum (Fig. 17.113). Pseudoaneurysms or arteriovenous fistulae may be demonstrated on colour Doppler (Fig. 17.114). Liquefaction of the infarct may regress completely (Fig. 17.115), persist as a cyst (Fig. 17.89), or may become superinfected and form an abscess. Depending on clinical need, fine needle aspiration may be used for diagnosis or therapy.

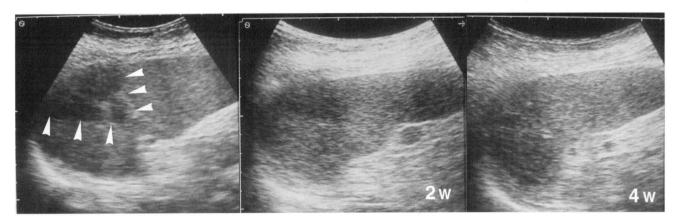

Fig. 17.107 Splenic infarct. A wedge-shaped, poorly reflective splenic infarct (arrowheads) showed complete healing over the course of 4 weeks.

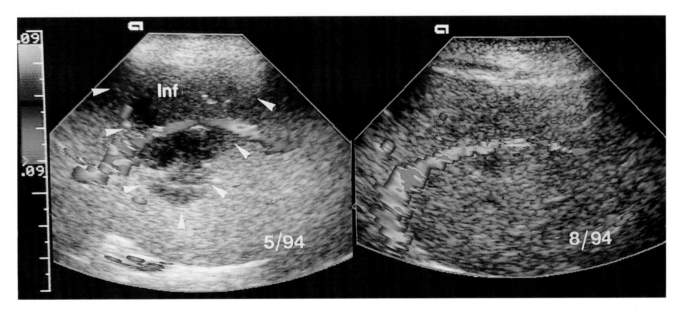

Fig. 17.108 Splenic infarct (Inf) (arrowheads) in chronic myeloid leukaemia showing an intact vessel in an otherwise 'avascular' infarct area; as the infarct heals, slight structural inhomogeneity becomes apparent.

Splenic trauma

The commoner traumatic splenic rupture should be differentiated from idiopathic or spontaneous splenic rupture.

Because of its position, immobility and soft consistency, the spleen is the organ most frequently injured in blunt abdominal trauma (up to 35%).[96,97] The diagnosis is frequently made using imaging such as ultrasound and more particularly CT.[98–101] Sonography is a quick, non-invasive method of examination in primary diagnosis[102] and is the method of choice for the detection of free abdominal fluid.[103] However, it is inferior to CT in the demonstration of splenic damage.[104] Modern management

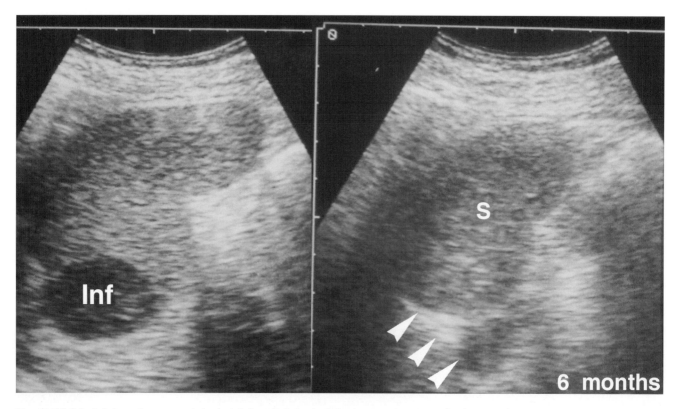

Fig. 17.109 Splenic infarct. A new, rounded splenic infarct (Inf) that heals leaving scar tissue (arrowheads). S – spleen.

Fig. 17.112 Splenic infarct. A splenic infarct (INF) with a subcapsular haematoma (H) in chronic myeloid leukaemia during a blastic crisis heals almost completely.

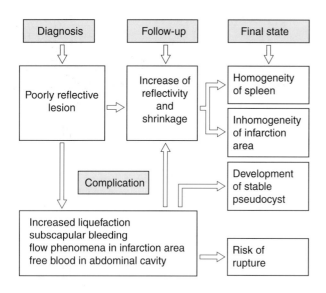

Fig. 17.110 Splenic infarct. US characteristics, follow-up and complications of splenic infarction.

Fig. 17.113 Splenic infarct. A: A characteristically wedge-shaped (arrowheads) splenic infarct (Inf) in endocarditis; **B:** free fluid (FF) diagnosed as blood was demonstrated in the lower abdomen despite a sonographically intact splenic surface. HB – urinary bladder. S – spleen.

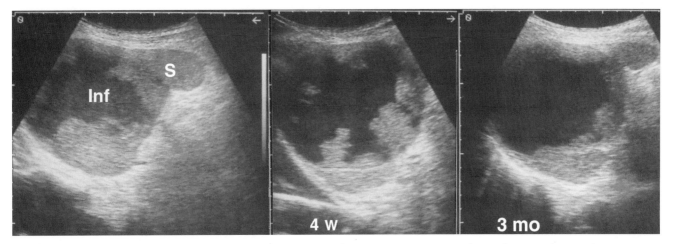

Fig. 17.111 **Splenic infarct.** A liquefied splenic infarct (Inf) in endocarditis showing progression to a pseudocyst after 3 months. S – spleen.

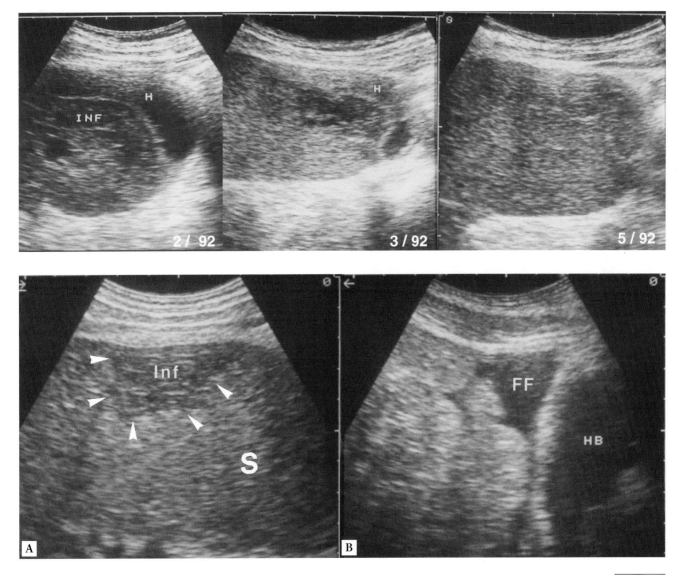

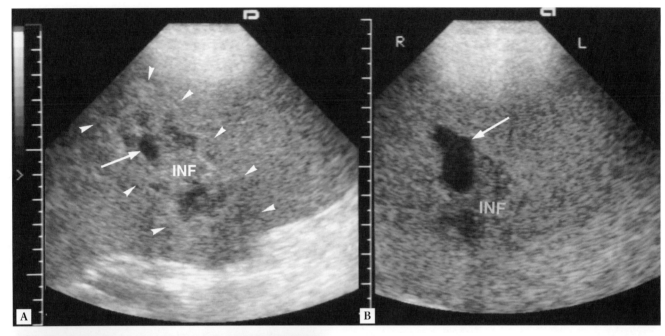

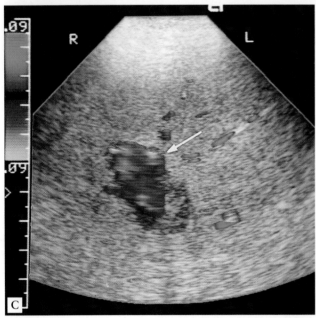

Fig. 17.114 Splenic infarct. A: Splenic infarct (INF) in chronic myeloid leukaemia (arrowheads) **B:** An adjacent echo-free zone (arrow) is seen adjacent to the infarct (INF). **C:** A colour Doppler image of a splenic infarct showing that this was an intrasplenic pseudo-aneurysm (arrow).

strives to preserve the spleen where possible, depending, among other factors, on the degree of splenic damage, for which various grading systems have been developed.[98,105] The decision to opt for conservative management depends chiefly on clinical features and laboratory results rather than on imaging findings.[106] Sonographic follow-up at short intervals has proven to be very helpful in this situation.[107]

Signs of splenic trauma that may be sonographically demonstrated include:[100,101]

1. free abdominal fluid (perisplenic, perihepatic) in the pouch of Douglas (Fig. 17.116),
2. fluid between the splenic parenchyma and splenic capsule indicating a subcapsular splenic rupture (Fig. 17.117).

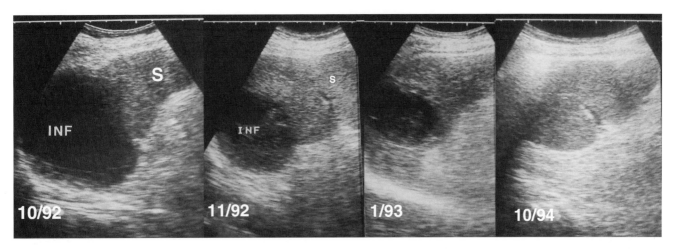

Fig. 17.115 **Splenic infarct. Sonographic follow-up.** A liquefied splenic infarct (INF) in aortic valve endocarditis heals almost entirely. S – spleen.

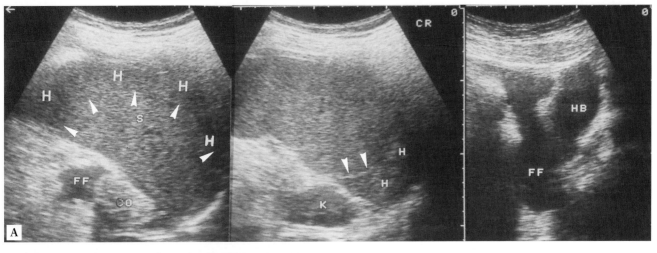

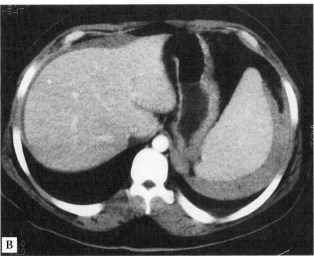

Fig. 17.116 **Splenic rupture. A:** Splenic rupture with subcapsular haemorrhage (H) that is difficult to demarcate on ultrasound; arrowheads mark the surface of the spleen (S). There was free fluid (FF) in the pouch of Douglas and in the hilum of the spleen. **B:** An abdominal CT confirms the development of a perisplenic haematoma. K – kidney, HB – urinary bladder.

Destruction of splenic parenchyma is seen as an irregular texture or splenic lacerations of varying degrees (Figs 17.118 and 17.119). It is important to note that haemoperitoneum is usually echo-free, though layering may be seen (Fig. 17.120). The amount of blood found at surgery can be estimated from the thickness of the layer in the hepatorenal recess.[108]

Subcapsular splenic rupture is usually displayed as a crescentic collection in the region of the convex border. Recent haemorrhages may be reflective or have the same reflectivity as intact splenic tissue and therefore are easily overlooked.[109,110] (Fig. 17.116). Occasionally, enlargement of the left lobe of the liver may mimic a subcapsular collection (Fig. 17.9).[111] Increasing loss of reflectivity of the haematoma may be observed in follow-up examinations.

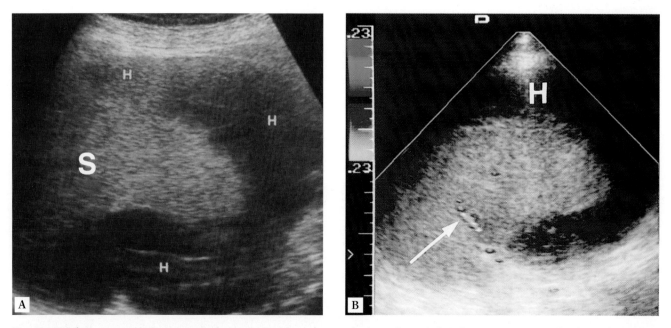

Fig. 17.117 Splenic rupture. A: Spontaneous splenic rupture with a pronounced subcapsular perisplenic haematoma (H) arrowheads – surface of the spleen (S) in low-grade malignant non-Hodgkin's lymphoma. **B:** A color Doppler image showing intact vascularisation of the splenic hilum (arrow).

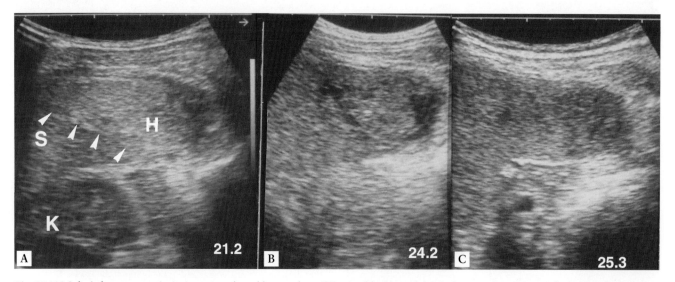

Fig. 17.118 Splenic haematoma. A: An intraparenchymal haemorrhage (H) caused by blunt abdominal trauma is seen as a reflective region in the medial portion of the spleen. The arrowheads mark the margins of the haemorrhage. **B and C:** The haemorrhage healed almost completely.

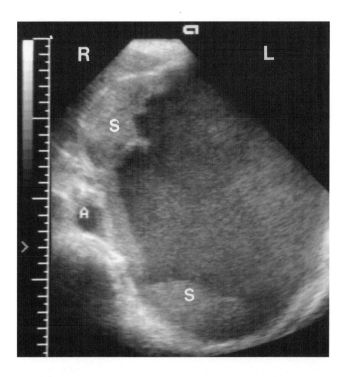

Fig. 17.119 **Spontaneous intrasplenic haemorrhage** accompanied by pseudocyst formation. A – aorta, S – spleen, R – right, L – left.

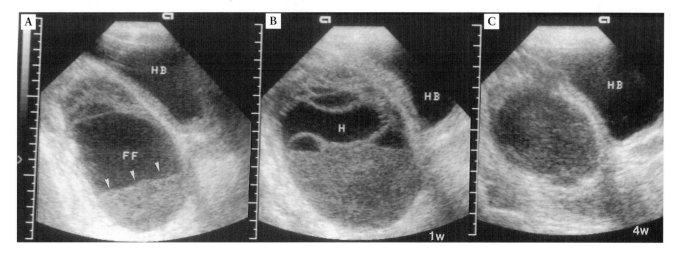

Fig. 17.120 **Splenic rupture. A:** Blood (FF) retrieved by fine needle puncture from the pouch of Douglas exhibited sedimentation (arrowheads). **B:** One week after splenic rupture, increasing septation and absorption is seen. **C:** A small haematoma remnant is still present after 4 weeks. HB – urinary bladder. H – haematoma.

A rare complication of splenic trauma is pseudo-aneurysm (14%);[112] these may be regarded as a special form of occult splenic rupture and can be diagnosed using colour Doppler. They may be a precursor of delayed rupture into the abdominal cavity, as may subcapsular rupture, which has been reported in up to 15% of cases.[96,113]

Recent intraparenchymal haemorrhage is seen as a reflective, variably well-defined lesion[110] or merely as an irregularly defined inhomogeneity of splenic texture (Fig. 17.118). Because of its low sensitivity to intra-parenchymal damage, ultrasound may fail to demonstrate the source of intraperitoneal haemorrhage. Large intra-splenic haemorrhages mimic pseudocysts (Fig. 17.119).

Infectious mononucleosis is the most important cause of spontaneous (idiopathic) splenic rupture, which occurs in 0.2–0.5% of cases, most frequently in the second or third week.[95] Spontaneous splenic rupture has also been

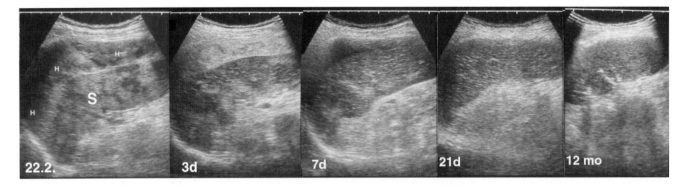

Fig. 17.121 Splenic rupture. Spontaneous rupture of the spleen (S) in a kidney transplant patient with acute varicella infection; the subcapsular haematoma (H) is reflective at first, later echo-free, and is absorbed within 21 days leaving scar tissue as a reflective band in the splenic hilum.

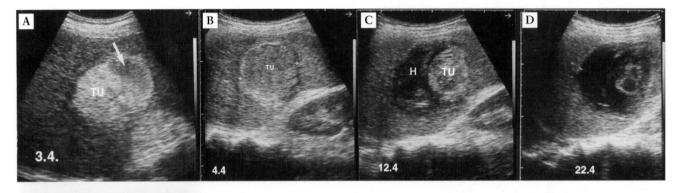

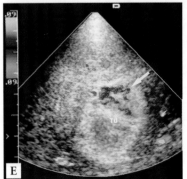

Fig. 17.122 Splenic haemorrhage. A non-traumatic intraparenchymal splenic haemorrhage (TU) in acute myeloid leukaemia first seen as **A:** reflective, then **B:** poorly reflective and **C** and **D:** finally as a cystic space. The arrow points to the mobile echoes during real-time examination. The patient underwent a splenectomy and histological examination confirmed splenic rupture. **E:** Colour Doppler image of a non-traumatic intraparenchymal splenic haemorrhage (TU). Isolated mobile echoes during active bleeding were seen in the cranial area (arrow) of the spleen.

reported in infectious diseases causing splenomegaly (varicella (Fig. 17.121), rubella, malaria, endocarditis, echinococcosis) and haematological diseases (acute leukaemia (Fig. 17.122), malignant lymphoma, chronic myeloid leukaemia), and in other diseases such as pancreatitis, splenic vein thrombosis, splenic peliosis, fibrinolysis therapy (Fig. 17.123) and splenic infarction.[107,114,115,116]

Whether or not so-called 'trivial trauma' is responsible for spontaneous splenic rupture is controversial. Rare cases of spontaneous splenic rupture in patients with healthy spleens have been reported.[117] Similar to traumatic splenic rupture, intrasplenic pseudo-aneurysm is an occasional complication of spontaneous splenic rupture (Figs 17.124 and 17.125).

Splenic calcification

Calcification in the spleen is seen as solitary (Fig. 17.126) or multiple highly reflective structures (Fig. 17.127). Typically, a complete or partial acoustic shadowing is observed. The ultrasound findings do not allow definitive classification and this is generally unimportant since no treatment is needed.[118] Focal calcification may also develop in the scar after infarctions and in haematomas,

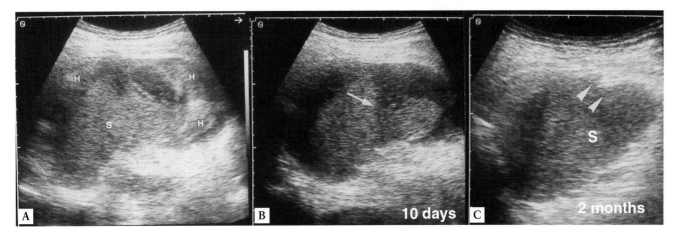

Fig. 17.123 Splenic rupture. A: Spontaneous splenic rupture with a reflective haemorrhage (H) occurring after systemic fibrinolysis; **B:** the arrow marks the tear in the parenchymal tissue. **C:** The healing process leads to scarring and retractions at the spleen's surface (arrowheads). S – spleen.

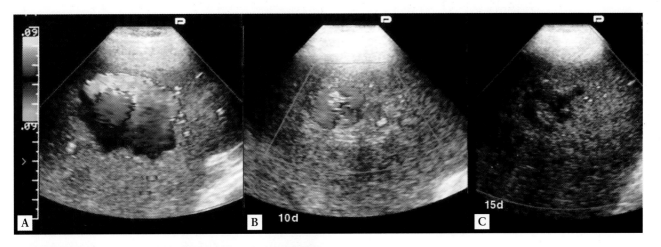

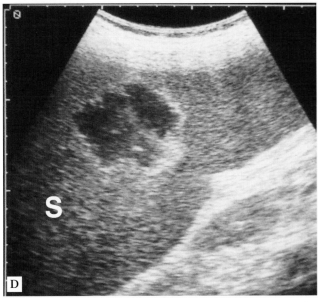

Fig. 17.124 Splenic pseudo-aneurysm. A: A poorly reflective mass exhibiting intralesional flow on grey scale in a non-traumatic intrasplenic pseudo-aneurysm. **B:** Follow-up of colour Doppler images of a patient with an intrasplenic pseudo-aneurysm and chronic myeloid leukaemia **C:** showing partial thrombosis and **D:** complete spontaneous thrombosis after 15 days.

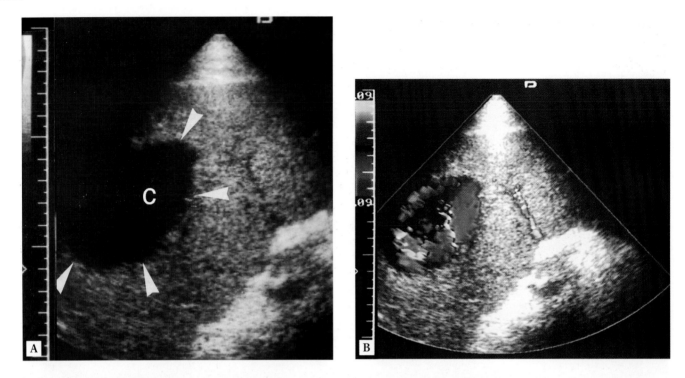

Fig. 17.125 Splenic pseudo-aneurysm. A: An incidentally diagnosed pseudo-aneurysm seen as a homogeneous cyst-like lesion (C) (arrowheads) exhibiting flow phenomena on grey scale scanning. **B:** The flow is well seen on colour Doppler; splenectomy was performed.

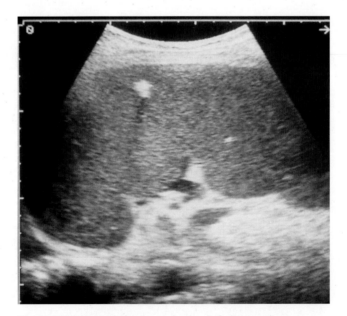

Fig. 17.126 Splenic calcification. A focal, calcified, intrasplenic structure with faint distal shadowing in an asymptomatic patient.

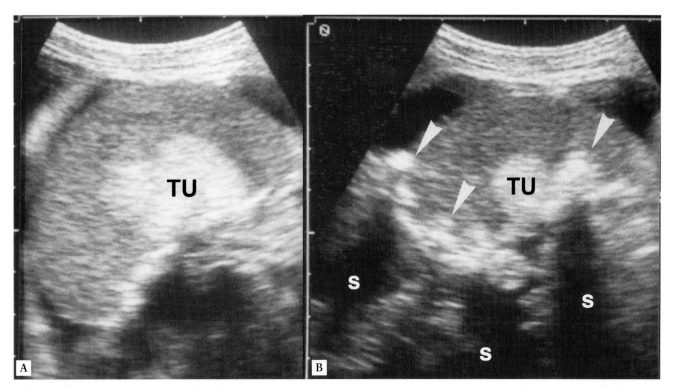

Fig. 17.127 Haemangioma. A: The reflective mass (TU) in the hilar area is most probably a haemangioma. **B:** Multiple calcifications (arrowheads) in chronic renal failure. S – shadowing.

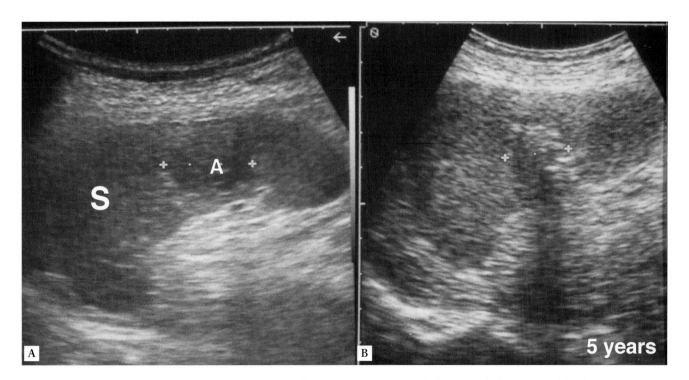

Fig. 17.128 Calcification in a splenic abscess. A: Small poorly reflective splenic abscess; **B:** calcification in the former area of the abscess is seen after twice undergoing aspiration drainage. S – spleen.

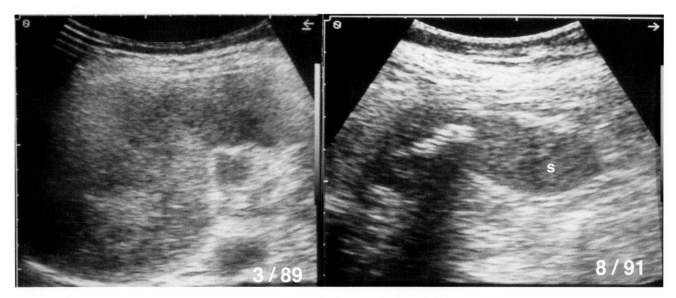

Fig. 17.129 Lymphoma. A diffuse structural inhomogeneity of the entire spleen in malignant lymphoma heals after treatment leaving scar tissue. S – spleen.

abscesses (Fig. 17.128) are rarely in lymphoma after treatment[119] (Fig. 17.129). Calcification may be dystrophic, for example, renal insufficiency (Fig. 17.130). The walls of splenic cysts may calcify. Calcified foci may arise particularly as a result of haemorrhage in larger haemangiomas[120] and in recurrent splenic infarction (Fig. 17.131). Occasionally, such a spleen is seen merely as a linear calcification sickle, as is typical of homozygotic sickle cell anaemia.[88]

Fine, diffusely scattered reflectors produce a 'starry sky' pattern in the spleen (Fig. 17.132). This pattern is seen after infections such as tuberculosis, brucellosis, sarcoidosis, aspergillosis, candidia and pneumocystis,[121] and in amyloidosis and lupus erythematosus.[122]

Calcification of vessel walls predominantly affects the splenic hilum (Figs 17.133 and 17.134), but sometimes is seen throughout the splenic parenchyma; its aetiology usually remains unclear but it must be distinguished from

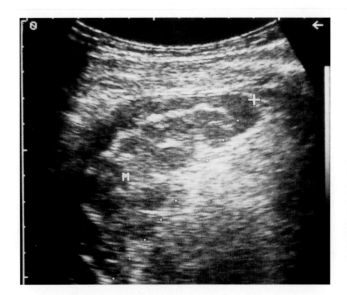

Fig. 17.130 Dystrophic calcification. Garland-like calcification of splenic parenchyma in chronic renal insufficiency requiring dialysis. M – spleen.

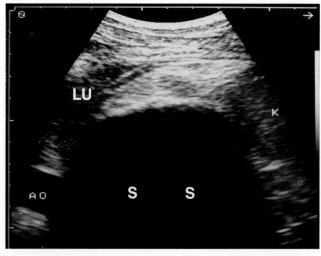

Fig. 17.131 Sickle-cell anaemia. The scarred spleen of a patient with sickle-cell anaemia is sonographically seen as a reflective spleen with intrasplenic sickle-shaped calcifications. K – kidney, S – shadowing, LU – lung, AO – aorta.

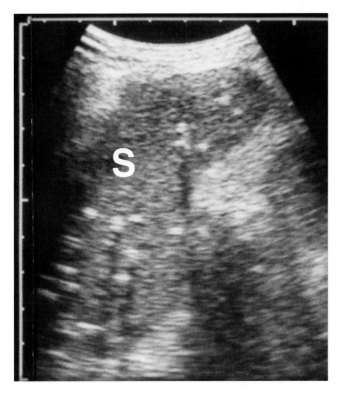

Fig. 17.132 Miliary tuberculosis. A 'starry sky' patterned calcification of the spleen (S) is seen after miliary tuberculosis.

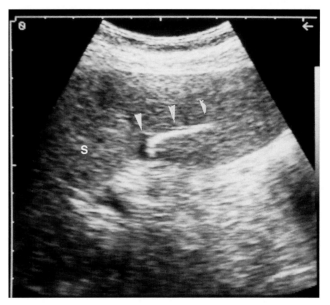

Fig. 17.133 Calcified splenic artery. The elongated, highly reflective structure within the splenic hilum (arrowheads) represents calcification of the splenic artery. S – spleen.

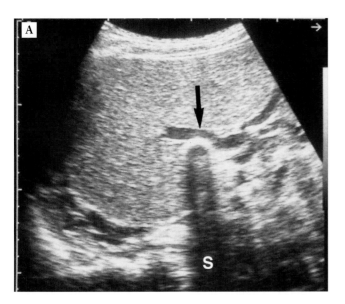

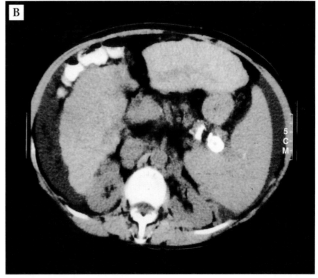

Fig. 17.134 Calcified aneurysm. A: The sickle-shaped calcification (arrow) within the splenic hilum with dorsal shadowing (S) represents a calcified aneurysm of the splenic artery. **B:** Abdominal CT confirms a calcified aneurysm of the splenic artery in the splenic hilum.

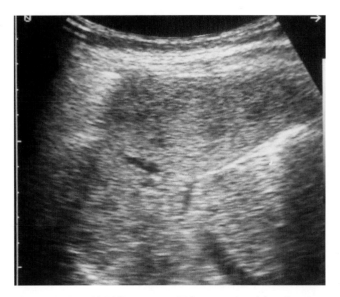

Fig. 17.135 Sarcoid. Diffuse structural inhomogeneity of the spleen in sarcoidosis

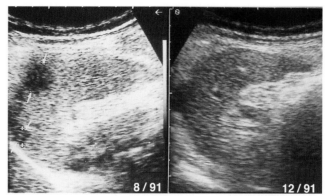

Fig. 17.136 Sarcoid. The formation of poorly reflective, rounded lesions (arrow) within the spleen in sarcoidosis with complete regression after treatment.

the above types of calcification. In rare cases, calcification of the vessel walls has been found in portal hypertension.[123,124]

Differential diagnostic overview

A classification based on the typical ultrasound features of the main diseases of the spleen is given in Table 17.1. Most poorly reflective intrasplenic masses may be diagnosed from their ultrasonic and clinical features (abscesses, haemorrhage, infarction, metastases) supported by laboratory data (echinococcosis, abscesses) or through guided biopsy (abscesses). AV fistulae and pseudo-aneurysms may be demonstrated with colour Doppler.[101] The rare cystic tumours such as lymphangiomas, haemangiomas or haematomas are usually diagnosed only after splenectomy.[56,60,61]

Most poorly reflective intrasplenic masses may be classified according to their aetiology based on the sonographic and clinical features (lymphoma, infarctions, abscesses). Diffuse inhomogeneity and the development of nodular foci may occur in infectious and granulomatous diseases: sarcoidosis (Figs 17.135 and 17.136), tuberculosis (Figs 17.137 and 17.138), Wegener's disease (Fig. 17.139) and amyloidosis (Fig. 17.140).[125–127] Frequently, the tentative diagnosis is confirmed by sonographic demonstration of regression during therapy. Fine needle puncture is only rarely needed. Myeloproliferative disorders (osteomyelofibrosis, chronic myelocytic leukaemia, polycythaemia) occasionally produce poorly reflective lesions (Figs 17.141 and 17.142).

Experience has shown that reflective splenic lesions pose the greatest difficulties for differential diagnosis.[118] The majority of incidentally diagnosed reflective splenic

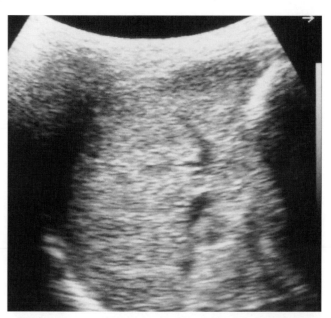

Fig. 17.137 Military tuberculosis. Diffuse structural inhomogeneity of the spleen in conjunction with military tuberculosis.

foci are benign. No change in size is observed on follow-up ultrasound and haemangioma is most likely, but the diagnosis remains speculative. Reflective foci have been documented in myeloproliferative syndromes and in haemolytic anaemia (Figs 17.143 and 17.144). In most cases, these foci are the result of extramedullary haematopoiesis[128–130] but occasionally haemorrhage may form reflective lesions[131] (Fig. 17.145). Reflective lesions are the most common focal splenic abnormality in storage diseases[132,133] (Figs 17.146 and 17.147) and have also been documented in infectious diseases.[134]

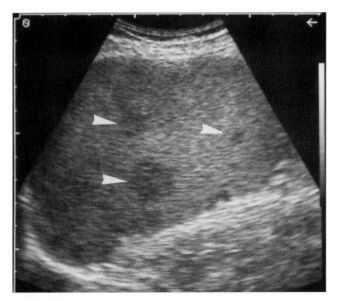

Fig. 17.138 Military tuberculosis. Multiple, poorly reflective, rounded intrasplenic lesions (arrowheads) due to miliary tuberculosis.

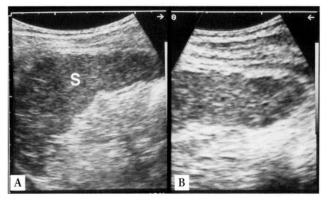

Fig. 17.139 Wegener's granuloma. A: Diffuse structural inhomogeneity of the spleen caused by Wegener's granulomatosis. B: The surface of the spleen is markedly irregular, indicating small nodular infiltrations.

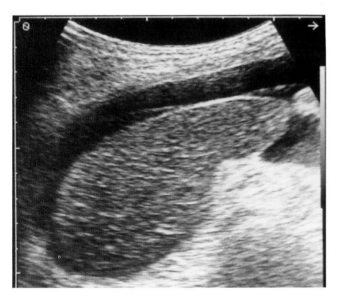

Fig. 17.140 Amyloidosis. Slightly inhomogeneous, poorly reflective parenchymal texture in amyloidosis. Splenic involvement was confirmed by autopsy.

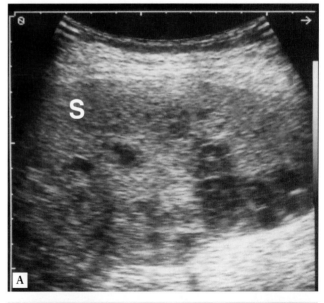
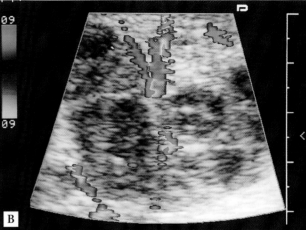

Fig. 17.141 Chronic myeloid leukaemia. A: Multiple, poorly reflective lesions in chronic myeloid leukaemia during a blast crisis. B: Colour Doppler shows no vascularisation. The aetiology of the lesions was not established.

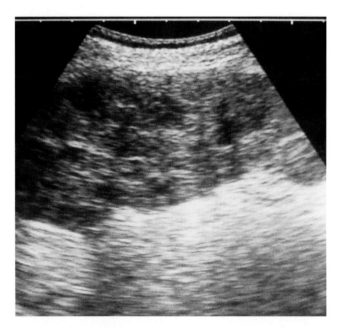

Fig. 17.142 Polycythemia. Marked structural inhomogeneity and poorly reflective lesions in polycythemia vera.

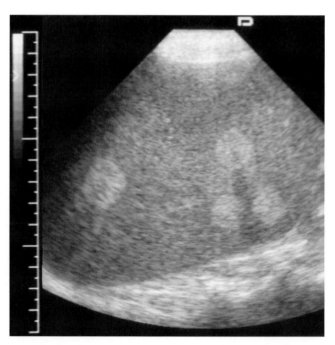

Fig. 17.143 Myelofibrosis. Multiple reflective splenic lesions in a patient with osteomyelofibrosis. This type of lesion is seen in extramedullary haematopoiesis.

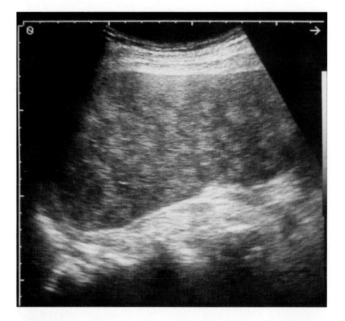

Fig. 17.144 Chronic myeloid leukaemia. Splenomegaly with multiple small-nodular, reflective splenic lesions in a patient with chronic myeloid leukaemia.

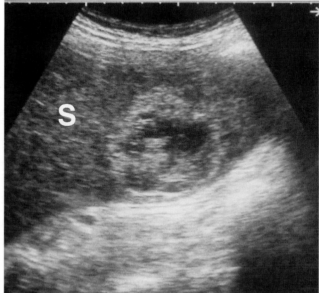

Fig. 17.145 Chronic myeloid leukaemia. A centrally liquefied, rounded, reflective lesion in a patient with chronic myeloid leukaemia; the mass remained constant for over a year. It is most likely the residue of a haemorrhage or an infarction. S – spleen.

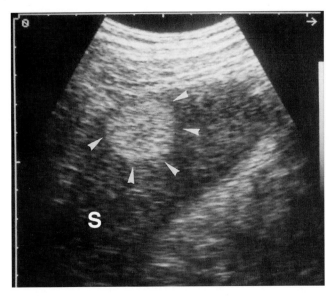

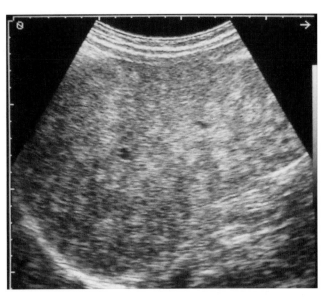

Fig. 17.146 Niemann-Pick disease. A reflective splenic lesion (arrowheads); a splenectomy established a storage disorder (Niemann-Pick disease, adult form). S – spleen.

Fig. 17.147 Gaucher's disease. Marked splenomegaly with multiple small-nodular, reflective splenic lesions in Gaucher's disease.

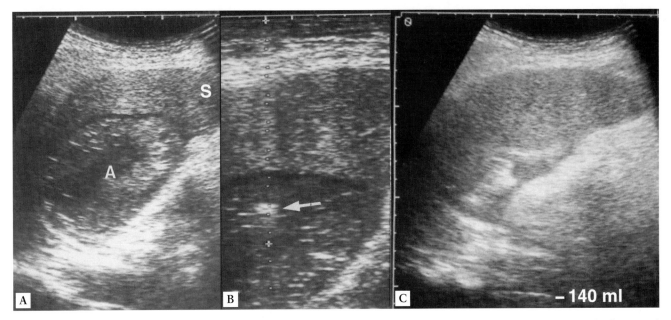

Fig. 17.148 Splenic abscess. A: An abscess (A) of the splenic hilum with faint reflections due to gas-forming bacteria; **B:** the arrow marks the point of the needle during aspiration drainage (middle). **C:** 140 ml of pus were evacuated. S – spleen.

Interventional sonography

Compared to other parenchymal organs, diagnostic and therapeutic puncture of the spleen is seldom used for various reasons.[32]

1 Splenic foci are rare.

2 If splenectomy is required, this provides histological diagnosis.

3 The risk of bleeding because of the spleen's vascularity has led to a general reluctance to carry out splenic puncture. There are no safety data from large series of splenic punctures.

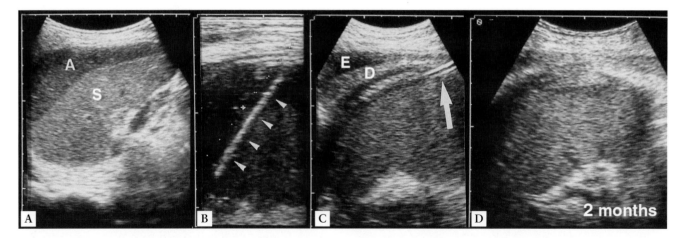

Fig. 17.149 Splenic abscess A: A subcapsular splenic abscess (A) due to alcoholic pancreatitis heals compleely after percutaneous catheter drainage. **B:** arrowheads mark the puncture needle; **C:** the large arrow points to the drainage catheter. **D:** Almost homogenous parenchyma was seen after 2 months. S – spleen, D – diaphragm; E – pleural effusion.

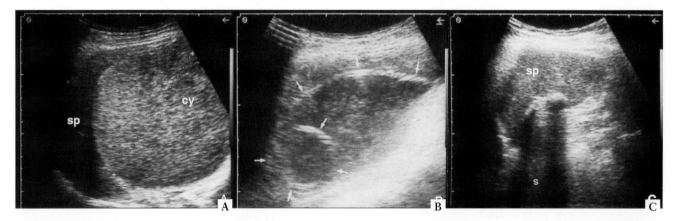

Fig. 17.150 Splenic cyst. A: Large, reflective splenic cyst (CY) with displacement of normal splenic parenchyma. **B:** Catheter drainage, note the intracystic echoes due to the catheter (arrows). **C:** Eventually the wall calcified. S – spleen.

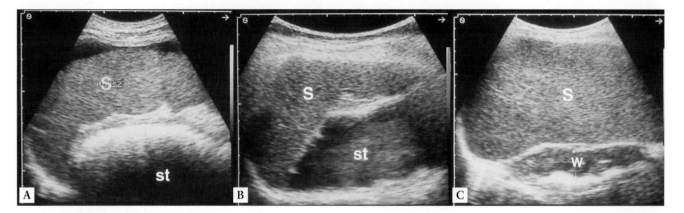

Fig. 17.151 Gastric lymphoma. A: Gas-filled stomach (st) with normal wall. **B:** Fluid-filled stomach (st). **C:** Pathological thickening of the gastric wall (W) in histologically confirmed lymphoma involvement of the stomach. S – spleen.

4 Access to the spleen is often difficult because of its position in the subphrenic space.

For these reasons, sonographic follow-up investigation is often used to confirm diagnoses. Despite this, interventional procedures (ultrasound-guided fine needle aspiration biopsy, ultrasound-guided catheter drainage using the Seldlinger technique) have established themselves, particularly for unexplained fluid masses[33,73,75,78,83] (Fig. 17.148). Repeated aspiration or catheter drainage, is the method of choice for macro-abscesses of the spleen and has a success rate of up to 90%.[78] Complications of catheter drainage, reported in 10–15% of cases, include empyema, fistulae, sepsis and haemorrhage (Figs 17.149 and 17.150).[135]

Perisplenic masses

Because of its close proximity to the pancreas, left kidney, adrenal gland, colon, stomach (Fig. 17.151) and the left hemidiaphragm, masses arising from these organs must be differentiated from splenic pathology. In particular, malignant tumous may infiltrate the spleen directly.

The differential diagnosis of echo-free splenic lesions includes renal cysts, hydronephrosis (Fig. 17.152), pancreatic pseudocysts (Fig. 17.153), splenic varices (Fig. 17.154), loculated ascites, necrosis and abscesses (Fig. 17.155) complicating acute pancreatitis,[136] as well as aneurysms of the splenic artery.

Poorly reflective lesions of the hilum may be caused by lymphoma, accessory spleens, splenic vein thrombosis and tumours of the pancreatic tail (Fig. 17.156) or adrenal gland (Fig. 17.157). The position and displacement of the spleen during respiration may be helpful in determining the origin of the perisplenic mass.

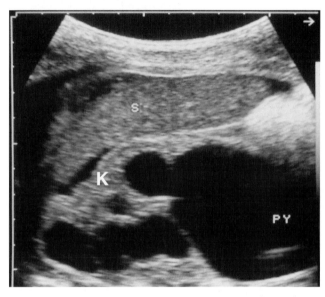

Fig. 17.152 Hydronephrosis. Cystic lesions apparently in the splenic hilum in hydronephrosis (PY). K – renal parenchyma. S – spleen.

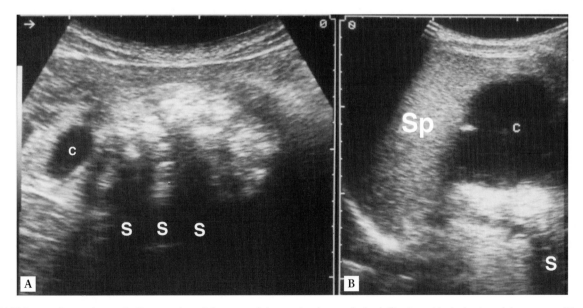

Fig. 17.153 Pancreatic pseudocyst. A: Cross-section of the upper abdomen showing marked calcification with shadowing of the pancreas (S) and a small pseudocyst (C) in the head region in a patient with chronic alcoholic pancreatitis. **B:** Larger pancreatic pseudocyst (C) in the region of the splenic hilum. Sp – spleen

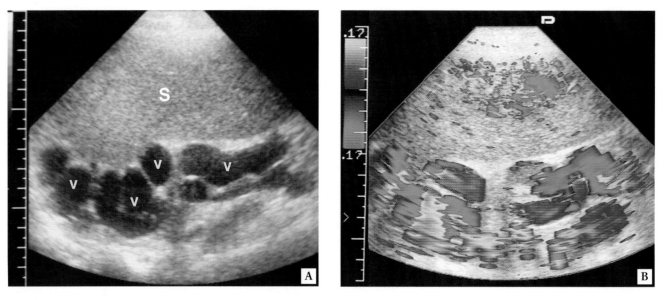

Fig. 17.154 Varices. A: Multiple, echo-free varices (V) of the splenic hilum in cirrhosis of the liver. **B:** Colour Doppler sonography confirmed the diagnosis. S – spleen.

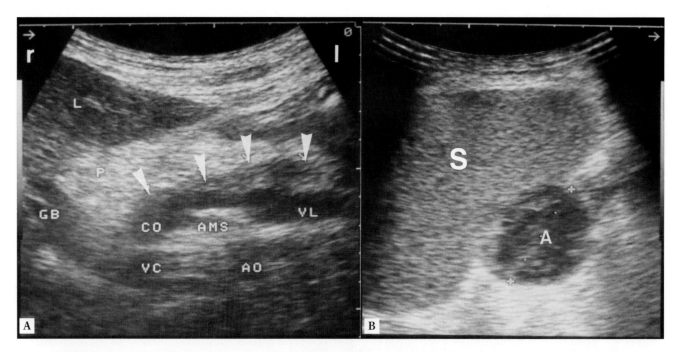

Fig. 17.155 Pancreatitis. A: A cross-section of the upper abdomen showing focal, poorly reflective, acute inflammation (arrowheads) of an otherwise reflective pancreas (P) in conjunction with chronic, recurrent alcoholic pancreatitis. **B:** A poorly reflective abscess (A) of the splenic hilum confirmed by aspiration drainage. L – liver, GB –gallbladder, CO – confluence, AMS – superior mesenteric artery, VL – splenic vein, VC – vena cava, AO – aorta.

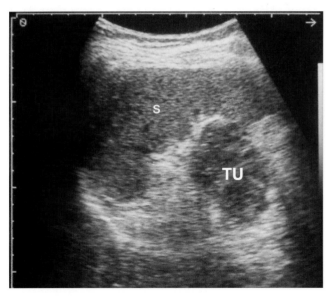

Fig. 17.156 Pancreatic carcinoma. Carcinoma of the pancreatic tail (TU) extending to the splenic hilum. S – spleen.

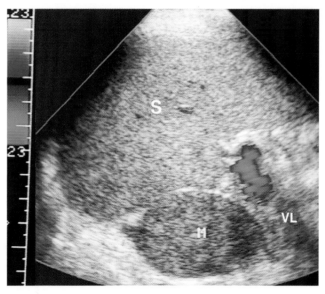

Fig. 17.157 Adrenal metastasis. Colour Doppler of an adrenal metastasis (M) in non-small-cell lung cancer showing its relationship to the splenic vein (VL).

REFERENCES

1 Dodds W J, Taylor A J, Erickson S J, Stewart E T, Lawson T L. Radiologic imaging of splenic anomalies. AJR 1990; 155: 805–810

2 Masamune A, Okano T, Satake K, Toyota T. Ultrasonic diagnosis of torsion of the wandering spleen. JCU 1994; 22: 126–128

3 Lamesch P, Lamesch A. Anomalies of the position of the spleen in the child: case report and review of the literature from 1896–1990. Langenbecks Arch Chir 1993; 378: 171–177

4 Koga T. Correlation between sectional area of the spleen by ultrasonic tomography and actual volume of the removed spleen. JCU 1979; 7: 119–120

5 Ishibashi H, Higuchi N, Shimamura R, Hirata Y, Kudo J, Niho Y. Sonographic assessment and grading of spleen size. JCU 1991; 19: 21–25

6 Kortsik C, Frank K, Schmidt H. Sonographische Milzgrößenbestimmung. In: Judmeier G, Frommhold H, Kratchowill A, eds. Ultraschalldiagnostik. Thieme Verlag, 1985

7 Weitzel D, Dinkel E, Dittrich M, Peters H. Pädiatrische Ultraschalldiagnostik. Berlin: Springer, 1984

8 Piekarski J, Federle M, Moss A, London S. Computer tomography of the spleen. Radiology 1980; 135: 683–689

9 Subramanyam B R, Balthazar E J, Horii S C. Sonography of the accessory spleen. AJR 1984; 143: 47–49

10 Bertolotto M, Gioulis E, Ricci C, Turoldo A, Convertino C. Ultrasound and Doppler features of accessory spleens and splenic grafts. Br J Radiol 1998; 71: 595–600

11 Glazer M, Sagar V V. Accessory splenic tissue, detection with Tc-99m labeled WBC in a post-splenectomy patient. Clin Nucl Med 1995; 20: 283

12 Schaffeldt J, Zimny M, Sabri O, Büll U. Die peritonealsplenose im antigranulozyten-AK-szintigramm. Fortschr Röntgenstr 1998; 168(1): 112–114

13 Wilson L S, Robinson D E, Griffiths K A. Evaluation of ultrasonic attentuation in diffuse diseases of spleen and liver. Ultrason Imaging 1987; 9: 236–247

14 Sommer G, Hoppe R, Fellingham L, Carroll B, Solomon H, Yousem S. Spleen structure in Hodgkin disease: ultrasonic characterization. Radiology 1984; 153: 219–222

15 Taylor K, Milan J. Differential diagnosis of chronic splenomegaly by gray scale ultrasonography. Clinical observations and digital A-scan analysis. Br J Radiol 1976; 49: 519–525

16 Manoharan A, Chen C F, Wilson L S, Griffiths K A, Robinson D E. Ultrasonic characterization of splenic tissue in myelofibrosis. Further evidence for reversal of fibrosis with chemotherapy. Eur J Haematol 1988; 40: 149–154

17 Bolondi L, Zironi G, Gaiani S, LiBassi S, Bemzi G, Barbara L. Caliber of splenic and hepatic arteries and spleen size in cirrhosis of different etiology. Liver 1991; 11: 198–205

18 Shah S H A, Hayes P C, Allan P L, Nicoll J, Finlayson N. Measurement of spleen size and its relation to hypertension and portal hemodynamics in portal hypertension due to hepatic cirrhosis. Am J Gastroenterol 1996; 91: 2580–2583

19 Mohr M, Gödderz W, Große A, Gerken G, Meyer zum Büschenfeld K H. Duplexsonographische untersuchungen zur pathogenese der lienalen hämodynamik bei leberzirrhose. Dtsch Med Wochenschr 1996; 121: 52–56

20 Bolognesi M, Sacerdoti D, Merkel C et al. Splenic Doppler impedance indices: influence of different portal hemodynamic conditions. Hepatology 1996; 23: 1035–1040

21 Schwerk W B. Portal vein thrombosis: real time sonographic demonstration and follow-up. Gastrointest Radiol 1986; 11: 312–318

22 Messinezy M, Chapman R, Dudley J M, Nunan T O, Pearson T C. Use of splenic volume estimation to distinguish primary thrombocythaemia from reactive thrombocytosis. Eur J Haematol 1988; 40: 339–342

23 Hehlmann R, Heimpel H, Hasford J et al. Randomized comparison of busulfan and hydroxyurea in chronic myelogenous leukemia: prolongation of survival by hydroxyurea. Blood 1993; 82: 398–407

24 Sokal J E, Cox E B, Baccarini M et al. Prognostic discrimination in 'good-risk' chronic granulocytic leukemia. Blood 1984; 63: 789–799

25 Pralle H. Treatment of hairy cell leukemia in the nineties. Onkologie 1995; 18: 219

26 Rai K R. A critical analysis of staging in CLL. In: Gale R P, Rai K R, eds. Chronic lymphocytic leukemia – recent progress and future directions. New Series 1987; 59: 253

27 Askergren J, Björkholm M, Holm G, Johanson B, Sundblad R. On the size and tumor involvement of the spleen in Hodgkin's disease. Acta Med Scand 1991; 209: 217–220

28 Falk S. Maligne lymphome in der milz. Stuttgart: Gustav Fischer Verlag, 1991

29 Stutte M J. Die Milz. In: Remmele W, ed. Pathologie. Berlin: Springer, 1984: 490

30 Hiller E, Gehartz H H, Löffler M et al. Ergebnisse und therapeutische konsequenzen der staging-laparotomie beim morbus Hodgkin. Onkologie 1991; 14: 171

31 Görg C, Schwerk W B, Görg K. Splenic lesions: sonographic patterns, follow-up, differential diagnosis. Eur J Radiol 1991; 13: 59

32 Börner N. Fokale milzveränderungen. In: Rettenmaier G, Seitz K M, eds. Sonographische differentialdiagnose. Weinheim: VCH Verlagsgesellschaft, 1990: 359

33 Solbiati L, Bossi M, Belotti E, Ravetto C, Montali G. Focal lesions in the spleen: sonographic patterns and guided biopsy. AJR 1983; 140: 59–65

34 Bostik W L. Primary splenic neoplasmas. Am J Pathol 1945; 21: 1143

35 Westhof M. Angiosarkom der milz. Dtsch Med Wochenscher 1992; 117: 1971

36 Nahman B, Cunningham J. Sonography of splenic angiosarcoma. JCU 1985; 13: 354–356

37 Wafula J M. Ultrasound and CT demonstration of primary angiosarcoma of the spleen. Br J Radiol 1985; 58: 903–905

38 Das Gubta T, Coombes B, Brasfeld R D. Primary malignant neoplasms of the spleen. Surg Gynecol Obstet 1969; 120: 947

39 Kehoe T, Straus D J. Primary lymphoma of the spleen. Clinical features and outcome after splenectomy. Cancer 1988; 62: 1433–1438

40 Weide R, Görg C, Pflüger K H et al. Concomitant primary low grade non-Hodgkin's lymphoma of the spleen and breast cancer. Leuk Lymph 1992; 7: 337–339

41 Berge T. Splenic metastasis – frequencies and patterns. Acta Pathol Microbiol Scand 1974; 82: 499–506

42 Carrington B M, Thomas N B, Johnson R J. Intrasplenic metastases from carcinoma of the ovary. Clin Radiol 1990; 41: 418–420

43 Görg C, Schwerk W B. Sonographic findings of splenic metastases. Bildgebung 1991; 58: 26–28

44 Mittelstaed C, Partain L. Ultrasonographic classification of splenic abnormalities gray scale patterns. Radiology 1980; 134: 697

45 Schwerk W B, Schmitz-Moormann P. Ultrasonically guided fine-needle biopsies in neoplastic liver disease: cytohistologic diagnosis and echopattern of lesions. Cancer 1981; 48: 1469–1477

46 Tsai C J. Ultrasound features of disseminated adenomucinosis. Br J Radiol 1998; 71: 564–566

47 Schwerk W B. Lebersonographie. In: Braun B, Günther R, Schwerk W B, eds. Ultraschalldiagnostik-lehrbuch und atlas. Landsberg: Ecomed Verlag, 1987: 75

48 Görg C, Schwerk W B, Görg K, Havemann K. Sonographic patterns of the affected spleen in malignant lymphoma. JCU 1990; 18: 569

49 Wernecke K, Peter P E, Krüger K G. Ultrasonographic pattern of focal hepatic and splenic lesions in Hodgkin's and non-Hodgkin's lymphoma. Br J Radiol 1987; 60: 655–660

50 Görg C, Weide R, Schwerk W B. Malignant splenic lymphoma: sonographic patterns, diagnosis, and follow-up. Clin Radiol 1997; 52: 535–540

51 Görg C, Schwerk W B, Neumann K, Görg K, Havemann K. Lymphommorphologie im ultraschall bei CLL. Ultraschall Klin Prax 1989; 4: 141

52 Ramani M, Reinhold C, Semelka R C et al. Splenic hemangiomas and haematomas: MR imaging characteristics of 28 lesions. Radiology 1997; 202: 166–172

53 Pines B, Rabinovitch J. Haemangioma of the spleen. Arch Pathol 1942; 33: 487

54 Husni E A. The clinical course of splenic hemangioma. Arch Surg 1961; 83: 681

55 Ros P R, Moser R P, Dachman A H, Murari P J, Olmsted W W. Hemangioma of the spleen. Radiologic-pathologic correlation in ten cases. Radiology 1987; 162: 73–77

56 Duddy M J, Calder C J. Cystic haemangioma of the spleen: findings on ultrasound and computed tomography. Br J Radiol 1989; 62: 180–182

57 Pinto P O, Advigo P, Garcia H et al. Splenic hamartoma: a case report. Eur J Radiol 1995; 5: 93

58 Iozzo R V, Haas J E, Chard R L. Symptomatic splenic hamartoma: a report of two cases and review of the literature. Pediatrics 1980; 66: 261–265

59 Meckler U, Wermke W. Sonographische differentialdiagnostik. Deutscher Ärzte-Verlag Köln, 1997

60 Brinkley A A, Lee J K T. Cystic hamartoma of the spleen: CT and sonographic findings. JCU 180; 9: 136–138

61 Rao B K, An Buchon J, Liebermann L B, Polcyn R E. Cystic lymphangiomatosis of the spleen: a radiologic–pathologic correlation. Radiology 1981; 41: 781–782

62 Wadsworth D T, Newman B, Abramson S J, Carpenter B L M, Lorenzo R L. Splenic lymphangiomatosis in children. Radiology 1997; 202: 173–176

63 Tsurni N, Ishida M, Morikawa P, Ishii N, Hoshino T, Masamune O. Splenic lymphangioma: report of two cases. JCU 1991; 19: 244–249

64 Sirinek K R, Evans W E. Non parasitic cysts. Am J Surg 1973; 126: 8–13

65 Walz M K, Metz K A, Eigler F W. Splenic cysts. Their morphology, diagnosis and therapy (German). Dtsch Med Wochenschr 1991; 116: 1377–1383

66 Bonakdarpour A. Echinococcus disease: report of 112 cases from Iran and review of 611 cases from the United States. AJR 1967; 99: 660–667

67 Franquet T, Montes M, Lecumberri F J, Esparza J, Bescos J M. Hydatid disease of the spleen. AJR 1990; 154: 525–528

68 Bürrig W L, Lucia S P. Non parasitic, non cancerous cystic tumors of the spleen. Am J Surg Pathol 1988; 12: 275–281

69 Dachman A H, Ros P R, Murari P J, Olmsted W W, Lichtenstein J E. Nonparasitic splenic cysts: a report of 52 cases with radiologic-pathologic correlation. AJR 1986; 147: 537–542

70 Weber J, Schmüdderich W, Harloff M, Kohler B, Riemann J F. Pankreasinduzierte Pseudozysten der milz: eine seltene komplikation. Ultraschall Med 1990; 11: 123–126

71 Lupien C, Sauerbrei E E. Healing in the traumatized spleen: sonographic investigation. Radiology 1984; 151: 181–185

72 Görg C, Schwerk W B. Splenic infarction: sonographic patterns, diagnosis, follow-up and complications. Radiology 1990; 194: 807

73 Görg C, Schwerk W B. Sonographic investigation in the diagnosis of intrasplenic fluid collections. Bildgebung 1991; 58: 76–82

74 Pachter M L, Hofstetter S R, Elkowitz A, Harris L, Liang H G. Traumatic cysts of the spleen: the role of cystectomy and splenic preservation: experience with seven consecutive patients. J Trauma 1993; 35: 430–436

75 Quinn S, van Sonnenberg E, Casola G et al. Interventional radiology in the spleen. Radiology 1986; 161: 289–291

76 Jequier S, Guttman F, Lafortune M. Non-surgical treatment of a congenital splenic cyst. Pediatr Radiol 1987; 17: 248–249

77 Akhan O, Baykan Z, Oguzkurt L, Sayek I. Özmen N. Percutaneous treatment of a congenital splenic cyst with alcohol: a new therapeutic approach. Eur Radiol 1997; 7: 1067–1070

78 Rogler G, Völk M, Strotzer M et al. Chronisches, pseudozystisch umgebautes milzhämatom als ursache linksseitiger thoraxschmerzen: erfolgreiche therapie mit alkoholinstillation. Dtsch Med Wochenschr 1998; 123: 792–797

79 Kiviniemi H, Ristkari S, Rämö J. Chemical peritonitis as caused by a rupture of a splenic cyst. Acta Chir Scand 1984; 150: 343–344

80 Elit L, Aylward B. Splenic cyst carcinoma presenting in pregnancy. Am J Hematol 1989; 32: 57–60

81 Chun C, Raff M, Contreras L et al. Splenic abcess. Medicine 1980; 59: 50–65

82 Simson J. Solitary abscess of the spleen. Br J Surg 1980; 67: 106–110

83 Schwerk W B, Görg C, Görg K, Restrepo I. Ultrasound-guided percutaneous drainage of pyogenic splenic abscesses. JCU 1994; 22: 161–166

84 Murray J G, Patel M D, Lee S, Sandhu J S, Feldstein V A. Microabscesses of the liver and spleen in AIDS: detection with 5 MHz sonography. Radiology 1995; 197: 723–727

85 Thaler M, Pastakia B, Shawker T H, O'Leary T, Pizzo P A. Hepatic candidiasis in cancer patients: the evolving picture of the syndrome. Ann Intern Med 1988; 108: 88–100

86 Görg C, Weide R, Schwerk W B, Köppler H, Havemann K. Ultrasound evaluation of hepatic and splenic microabscesses in the immunocompromised patient: sonographic patterns, differential diagnosis, and follow up. JCU 1994; 22: 525–529

87 Pastakia B, Shawker T H, Thaler M, O'Leary T, Pizzo P A. Hepatosplenic candidiasis: wheels within wheels. Radiology 1988; 166: 417–421

88 Görg C, Weide R, Schwerk W B, Eckstein E. Autosplenektomiesyndrom bei hämolytischer anämie. Ultraschall Klin Prax 1994; a: 149

89 Banani S A. Partial dearterialization of the spleen in thalassemia major. J Pediatr Surg 1998; 33: 449–453

90 Maresca G, Mirk P, De Gaetano A M, Babaro B, Colagrande C. Sonographic patterns in splenic infarct. JCU 1986; 14: 23–28

91 Weingarten M J, Fakhry J, McCarthy J, Freeman S J, Bisker J S. Sonography after splenic embolisation: the wedge-shaped acute infarct. AJR 1984; 141: 957–959

92 Görg C, Schwerk W B. Color Doppler imaging of focal splenic masses. Eur J Radiol 1994; 18: 214

93 Walker T M, Sergeant G R. Focal reflective lesions in the spleen in sickle cell disease. Clin Radiol 1993; 47: 114–116

94 Wetton C W N, Tran T L. Case report: splenic infarct in sickle cell disease. Clin Radiol 1995; 50: 573–574

95 Schwerk W B. Milzsonographie. In: Braun B, Günther R, Schwerk W B, eds. Ultraschalldiagnostik-lehrbuch und atlas. Landsberg: Ecomed Verlag, 1987: III.1.4

96 Black J J, Sinow R M, Wilson S E, Williams R A. Subcapsular hematoma as a predictor of delayed splenic rupture. Am Surg 1992; 58: 732–735

97 Seufert R M. Surgery of the spleen. Revised English edition. New York: Thieme, 1986

98 Scatamacchia S A, Raptopoulos V, Fuik M P, Silva W E. Splenic trauma in adults: impact of CT grading on management. Radiology 1989; 171: 725–729

99 Federle M P, Courcoulas A P, Powell M, Ferris J V, Peitzmann A B. Blunt splenic imaging in adults: clinical and CT criteria for management, with emphasis on active extravasation. Gastrointest Imag 1998; 206: 137–142

100 Thomas E A, Dubbins P A. Diagnosing splenic trauma (editorial). Clin Radiol 1991; 43: 297–300

101 Schwerk W B, Braun B. Ultraschalltomographie und gezielte Peritonealpunktion bei verzögerter traumatischer milzblutung. Fortschr Röntgenstr 1981; 134: 296–300

102 McKenney K L, Nunez D B, McKenney M G, Asher J, Zelnick K, Shipshak D. Sonography as the primary screening technique for blunt abdominal trauma: experience with 899 patients. AJR 1998; 170: 979–985

103 Goletti O, Ghiselli G, Lippolis P V. The role of ultrasonography in blunt abdominal trauma: results in 250 consecutive cases. J Trauma 1994; 36: 178–181

104 Nerlich M L, Hoffmann H. Ultrasonography in the diagnosis of abdominal trauma. In: Maull K I, ed. Advances in trauma and clinical care. Chicago: Mosby Year Book, 1991; 6: 415

105 Görg C, Schwerk W B. Splenic injury: sonographic investigation. Bildgebung 1991; 58: 199–204

106 Umlas S L, Cronan J J. Splenic trauma: can CT-grading systems enable prediction of successful non surgical treatment? Radiology 1991; 178: 481–487

107 Welk E, Stein U, Bindewald H, Glogowski P. Spontane milzruptur bei chronischer pankreatitis. Dtsch Med Wochenschr 1991; 1(6): 460–462

108 Hauenstein K H, Wimmer B, Billmann P, Nöldge G, Zavisic D. Die rolle der sonographie beim stumpfen bauchtrauma. Radiologe 1982; 22: 106–111

109 Sigel B, Coelko J C U, Spigos D G et al. Ultrasonography of blood during stasis and coagulation. Invest Radiol 1981; 16: 71–76

110 Van Sonnenberg E, Simeone J F, Mueller P R, Wittenberg J, Hall D A, Ferrucci J T. Sonographic appearance of hematoma in liver, spleen, and kidney: a clinical, pathologic and animal study. Radiology 1983; 147: 507–510

111 Crivello M S, Peterson I M, Austin R M. Left lobe of the liver mimicking perisplenic collections. JCU 1986; 14: 697–701

112 Wüstner M, Kühneit A, Brüggemann A. Das traumatische intralienale pseudoaneurysma (TILP) – eine häufige sonderform der gedeckten milzruptur. Ultraschall 1996; 17: 13.04

113 Benjamin C, Engrow L, Perry J. Delayed rupture or delayed diagnosis of rupture of the spleen. Surg Gynecol Obstet 1976; 142: 171–172

114 Johnson M A, Cooperberg P L, Boisvert J, Stoller J L, Winrob H. Spontaneous splenic rupture in infections mononucleosis: sonographic diagnosis and follow-up. AJR 1981; 136: 111–114

115 Falk S, Protz H, Köbrich U, Stutte H J. Spontane milzruptur bei akuter malaria tropica. Dtsch Med Wochenschr 1992; 117: 854

116 Shimono T, Yamaoka T, Nishimure K, Naya M, Hojo M, Yamamoto E. Peliosis of the spleen: splenic rupture with intraperitoneal hemorrhage. Abdom Imaging 1998; 23: 201–202

117 Crate I D, Payne M J. Is the diagnosis of spontaneous rupture of a normal spleen valid? J R Army Med Corps 1991; 137: 50–51

118 Börner N, Blank W, Bönhof J et al. Echoreiche milzprozesse: häufigkeit und differentialdiagnose. Ultraschall Med 1990; 11: 112–118

119 Moody A R, King D M. Splenic calcification following treatment of Hodgkin's disease. B J Radiol 1991; 64: 55–56

120 Halgrimson C G, Rustad D G, Zeligman E. Calcified hemangioma of the spleen. J Am Med Assoc 1984; 252: 2959–2960

121 Keane M A R, Finlayson C, Joseph A E A. A histological basis for the 'sonographic snowstorm' in opportunistic infection of the liver and spleen. Clin Radiol 1995; 50: 220–222

122 Kennan N M, Evans C. Case report: hepatic and splenic calcification due to amyloid. Clin Radiol 1991; 44: 60–61

123 Kedar R P, Merchant S A, Malde H H, Patel V H. Multiple reflective channels in the spleen: a sonographic sign of portal hypertension. Abdom Imaging 1994; 19: 453–458

124 Logan H, Meire H. Calcified splenic and portal vein thrombosis: an unusual cause of multiple high amplitude echoes in the spleen. Br J Radiol 1991; 64: 366–367

125 Porcel-Martin A, Rendon-Uncetas P, Bascunana-Quirell A et al. Focal splenic lesions in patients with AIDS: sonographic findings. Abdom Imaging 1998; 23: 196–200

126 Kessler A, Mitchel D G, Israel H L, Goldberg B B: Hepatic and splenic sarcoidosis: ultrasound and MR imaging. Abdom Imaging 1993; 18: 159–163

127 Kapoor R, Jain A K, Chatulvedi U, Saha M M. Case report: ultrasound detection of tuberculomas of the spleen. Clin Radiol 1991; 43: 128–129

128 Bradley M J, Metreweli C. Ultrasound appearance of extramedullary haematopoiesis in the liver and spleen. Br J Radiol 1990; 63: 816–818

129 Sinilnoto T M J, Hyvärinen S A, Päiväusalo M J, Alavaikko M J, Suramo I J I. Abdominal ultrasonography in myelofibrosis. Acta Radiol 1992; 33: 343–346

130 Gupta R, Woodham C H. Unusual ultrasound appearance of the spleen – a case of heridatary spherocytosis. Br J Radiol 1986; 59: 284–285

131 Görg C, Barth P, Weide R, Schwerk W B. Spontaneous splenic rupture in acute myeloid leukemia: sonographic follow-up study. Bildgebung 1994; 61: 37–39

132 Omarini L P A, Frank-Burkhardt S E, Seemayer T A, Mentha G, Terner F. Niemann-Pick disease type C: nodular splenomegaly. Abom Imaging 1995; 20: 157

133 Stevens P G, Kumari-Subaiya S S, Kahn L B. Splenic involvement in Gaucher's disease: sonographic findings. JCU 1987; 15: 397–400

134 Cerri G G, Alovis V A F, Magalhaes A. Hepatosplenic schistosomiasis mansoni: ultrasound manifestations. Radiology 1984; 153: 777–780

135 Neff C, Müeller P, Ferrucci J. Serious complications following transgression of the pleural space in drainage procedures. Radiology 1984; 152: 335–341

136 Laukisch P G. The spleen in inflammatory pancreatic disease. Gastroenterology 1990; 98: 509–516

The peritoneum and retroperitoneum

David O Cosgrove and Paul A Dubbins

PERITONEUM

Anatomy

The abdominal cavity is lined by a thin peritoneal membrane which lies deep to the transversalis fascia on the anterior abdominal wall and anterior to the retroperitoneal fascia on the posterior wall. The elongation, convolutions, rotations and glandular outpouchings from the embryological gastrointestinal tract result in the many loops of bowel and digestive glands that project into the abdominal cavity. All are covered by the peritoneal membrane, which they have evaginated. Where the evagination is most marked, bowel is suspended from the posterior abdominal wall by a mesentery. Where there is less evagination organs are directly attached to the abdominal wall by peritoneum, an example being the bare area of the liver. Some gastrointestinal structures remain retroperitoneal, such as the pancreas and the ascending and descending colon (see below). Knowledge of the anatomy of the peritoneal cavity, its mesenteries and ligaments is important for the proper understanding of the development and spread of pathology within the peritoneal cavity.[1]

The peritoneal cavity is a potential space and the peritoneum a thin membrane which can only be demonstrated on ultrasound in the presence of ascites, which allows the identification of many of the mesenteric and ligamentary layers and of the potential spaces.[2] The peritoneal reflections and mesenteric attachments determine the routes of spread of intraperitoneal fluid and serve as boundaries for its compartments (Fig. 18.1). The transverse mesocolon, the mesentery of the transverse colon, divides the abdominal cavity into supra- and inframesocolic compartments. The root of the small bowel mesentery further divides the lower compartment into two unequal inframesocolic spaces.[2] Although the transverse mesocolon may occasionally be demonstrated on ultrasound, neither it nor the root of the small bowel mesentery is usually seen, even in the presence of ascites, largely because of their situation posterior to multiple bowel loops, which usually contain some gas.

The supra- and inframesocolic spaces communicate via the paracolic gutters on the posterior abdominal wall, bounded medially by the ascending and descending colons, respectively. The right paracolic gutter is continuous with the right subhepatic space and its posterior extension, the hepatorenal fossa (Morrison's pouch) and, further superiorly, the right subphrenic space (Figs 18.2 and 18.3). The posterior aspect of a portion of the right lobe of the liver is in direct relationship with the diaphragm without intervening peritoneum (the bare area). If fluid is displayed posterior to the liver in this region it must be located within the pleural space; this sign may therefore help to differentiate

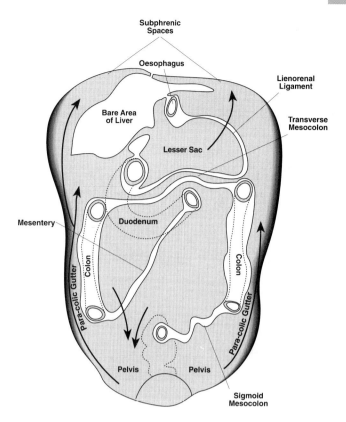

Fig. 18.1 The peritoneal cavity. The pathways along which infections tend to track are indicated in this diagram of the peritoneum. The commonest origins for infections are the pelvis and from the lower bowel and appendix.

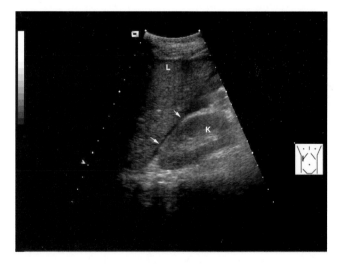

Fig. 18.2 Ascites. Fluid has collected in Morrison's pouch (arrows). K – kidney; L – liver.

pleural from peritoneal fluid (Fig. 18.4).[3] The falciform ligament separates the right and left subphrenic and subhepatic spaces. It appears as a thin strip between two fluid-containing areas. On the left the phrenocolic ligament fixes

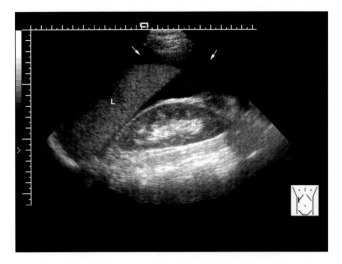

Fig. 18.3 Gross ascites. Fluid is demonstrated in Morrison's pouch and widely in the peritoneum (arrows). K – kidney; L – liver.

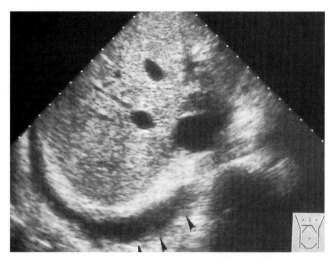

Fig. 18.4 Pleural fluid. Extension of pleural fluid (arrowheads) posterior and medial to the bare area of the liver, displacing the crus (C) of the diaphragm to the right and the inferior vena cava anteriorly.

the splenic flexure of the colon to the left hemidiaphragm, thereby partially obstructing communication between the left paracolic gutter and the left perisplenic space. This ligament may be identified above the upper pole of the spleen as a thick linear strip (Fig. 18.5).

The lesser omentum represents the mesentery of the stomach and, with the gastrocolic, splenogastric and splenopancreatic ligaments, delineates the lesser sac. Of these, only the lesser omentum is regularly visualised (in the presence of ascites), but its free edge is identified by the position of the portal vein and the common bile duct (Fig. 18.6). The separation of fluid layers between the lesser sac and the rest of the peritoneal cavity has been named the 'butterfly wings' sign by Weill[4] (Fig. 18.7). However, the compartmentalis-

ation of the lesser sac is so effective that pathologies arising elsewhere in the peritoneal cavity rarely involve it, and vice versa, with the exception of simple ascites which fills every part of the peritoneal cavity.

In the lower abdomen both inframesocolic spaces communicate with the pelvis, but the right is directly continuous with the pelvic cavity. In general, therefore, intraperitoneal spread occurs more commonly from pathology on the right than on the left side of the pelvis. The peritoneum is reflected over the dome of the bladder, the anterior and posterior surface of the uterus and the superior portion of the rectum (Fig. 18.8A). The peritoneal reflection over the fallopian tubes, the broad ligament, may be demonstrated in the presence of ascites (Fig. 18.8B). In men

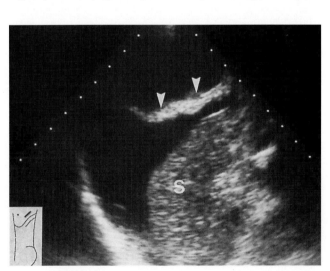

Fig. 18.5 The phrenolienal ligament is seen as a thick, highly reflective band (arrowheads). S – spleen.

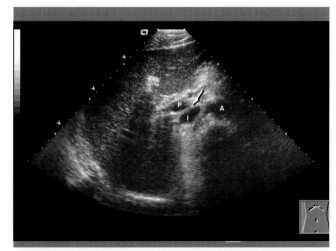

Fig. 18.6 The free edge of the lesser sac. The opening to the lesser sac (arrow) lies between the portal vein and the inferior vena cava. P – portal vein; I – inferior vena cava; A – aorta.

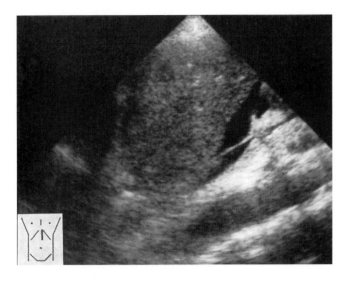

Fig. 18.7 **Fluid in the lesser sac** separated from fluid elsewhere in the peritoneum by the lesser omentum. This appearance has been described as 'butterfly wings'.

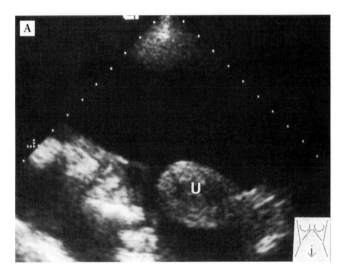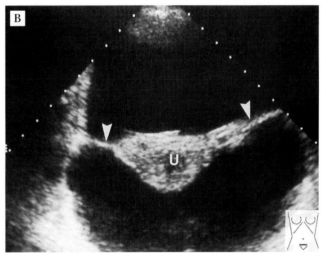

Fig. 18.8 **Pelvic ascites. A:** In longitudinal section the ascites surrounds the fundus of the uterus (U). **B:** In transverse section the broad ligaments (arrowheads) are clearly shown.

there is a single potential space for fluid collection, the rectovesical pouch, whereas in women there are two, the uterovesical pouch and the pouch of Douglas between the uterus and the rectum.

These anatomical features determine the route of spread of abdominal fluid, infections and tumours. Spread from the pelvis along the right paracolic gutter to the perihepatic spaces is the most common route, but anatomical variations, incompleteness of ligamentous obstacles and the presence of postoperative or postinfective adhesions may alter the pattern of spread.

Scanning technique

Ultrasound examination of the peritoneal cavity requires a meticulous and flexible approach.[5,6] Pathology affecting

the peritoneal cavity may be inflammatory or neoplastic, but the examination is aimed primarily at the detection of intra-abdominal fluid. If fluid collections are to be localised accurately, the anatomical basis of the spread within the abdomen needs to be fully understood, ultrasonic windows need to be appreciated, and the limitations of the ultrasound technique must be accepted.[7,8] Free fluid within the abdomen can be readily detected: it collects in the most dependent portion, and in the supine position this is Morrison's pouch (Fig. 18.9) or the pouch of Douglas or rectovesical pouch (Fig. 18.10). The detection of loculated fluid, particularly intra-abdominal abscesses, however, requires an approach designed to examine the likely sites of collection. Thus the right subphrenic and perihepatic spaces should be examined with the patient in the supine and left posterior oblique positions using the liver as an

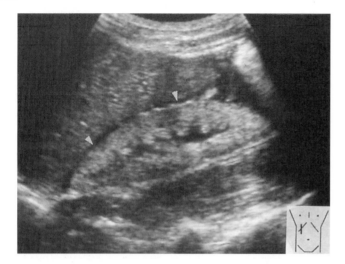

Fig. 18.9 Fluid in Morrison's pouch. A small amount of free fluid is present in Morrison's pouch (arrowheads) in this patient with renal failure secondary to glomerulonephritis. Note the highly reflective kidney.

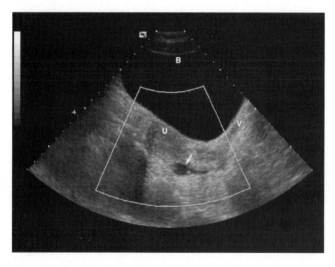

Fig. 18.10 Fluid in the pouch of Douglas. A trace of free fluid (arrow) lies behind the body and cervix of the uterus. Its sharp inferior limit indicates that it is peritoneal fluid rather than a collection which would have rounded margins. It contains a small amount of debris. B – bladder, U – uterus, V – vagina.

acoustic window, including scanning intercostally to obtain access to the right hemidiaphragm. A similar approach is used for the left upper quadrant and perisplenic regions, with the patient in the right posterior oblique and supine positions. The paracolic gutters are examined by placing the transducer on the flanks, and the pelvis can be imaged either using a filled urinary bladder as an acoustic window or trans-vaginally. Fluid collections loculated in the mid-abdomen are the most difficult to demonstrate with ultrasound as they are easily confused with bowel loops.

Ascites

Ultrasound is an extremely sensitive technique for the detection of free fluid within the peritoneum: although as little as 10 ml of fluid has been shown to be detectable in the pouch of Douglas and Morrison's pouch in experimental studies,[6,9] it is probable that several hundred millilitres must be present for routine clinical detection. Typically ascitic fluid is echo free, moves within the peritoneal cavity with change in patient position or compression by the transducer, and allows gas-containing bowel loops to float within the fluid (Fig. 18.11). The fluid tends to collect in the more dependent positions. Rotating the patient to a right decubitus position facilitates the demonstration of small amounts of fluid in Morrison's pouch. However, if only a very small quantity of ascites is present it may spread across the surface of a large organ, produc-

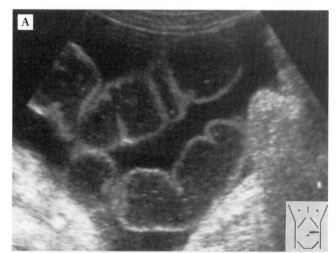

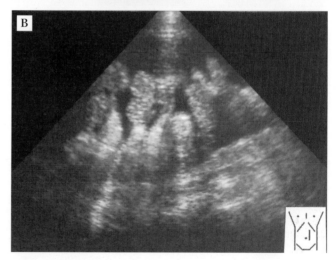

Fig. 18.11 Bowel loops in ascites. A: Scan of the mid-abdomen in a patient with ascites, showing multiple dilated loops of floating bowel. **B:** Scan in the mid-abdomen showing loops of bowel in ascites. The mesenteric attachments are well seen in this case.

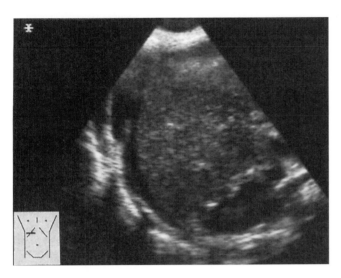

Fig. 18.12 Subtle ascites. A thin layer of ascitic fluid is shown over the surface of the liver.

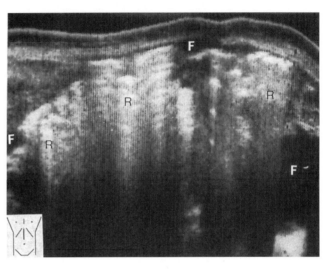

Fig. 18.14 Central abdominal bowel loops in ascites. The retroperitoneal structures are obscured by multiple loops of gas-containing bowel that float to the anterior abdominal wall and produce distal reverberation artefacts (R). Loculated ascitic fluid is noted (F).

ing a thin film over the lower or lateral border of the liver (Fig. 18.12). Careful scanning is required to elicit the subtle signs of small amounts of fluid.

The presence of ascites can improve the demonstration of many intra-abdominal structures (such as the peritoneal reflections and ligaments), though other features may be less well seen.[2] Whereas the female pelvic organs may be clearly outlined by ascitic fluid (Figs 18.8 and 18.13), the para-aortic regions and other retroperitoneal structures may become obscured by gas-containing bowel that floats towards the midline (Fig. 18.14). In some cases scanning through the flanks or changing the patient's position improves visualisation of retroperitoneal structures, but in many cases the patient must be re-examined after para-

centesis for an adequate study. Furthermore, ascites alters the appearances of some intra-abdominal organs on ultrasound. The right kidney may appear to be abnormally reflective as a result of increased through-transmission of ultrasound through non-attenuating fluid (Fig. 18.15): care must be taken not to confuse this artefactual appearance with a true increase in reflectivity caused by diffuse parenchymal renal disease.[10] Tense ascites pushes bowel to the middle of the abdomen, giving a classic appearance that helps the differentiation between ascites and a large cystic tumour (Figs 18.14 and 18.15).

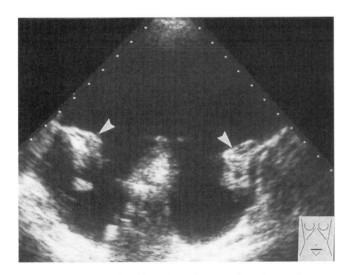

Fig. 18.13 Ovaries outlined by ascites. The normal ovaries are shown situated on the lateral pelvic walls (arrowheads), outlined by ascitic fluid.

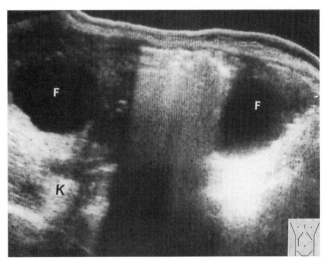

Fig. 18.15 Loculated ascites. Scan through the right abdomen showing partially loculated ascitic fluid (F). The loculated fluid in the right upper quadrant produces acoustic enhancement, obscuring the margins of the right kidney (K).

Occasionally it is difficult to differentiate between pleural and peritoneal fluid, especially when it is loculated. Features implying intrathoracic fluid are lateral displacement of the right crus of the diaphragm, anterior displacement of the inferior vena cava, and fluid immediately superior to the bare area of the liver (Fig. 18.4).[3] If the layers of the diaphragmatic muscle can be demonstrated, the level of the fluid can be ascertained.

Thickening of the gallbladder wall is a leading feature of acute cholecystitis (see Ch. 15), but thickening also occurs in a number of other conditions, including ascites.[11] The cause here is still a matter of debate: it may result from hypoalbuminaemia[12] or represent an artefact arising from the layer of ascites adjacent to the gallbladder, although a study in patients on peritoneal dialysis *in situ* did not substantiate this.[13] In patients with malignant ascites the gallbladder wall is only thickened when the serum albumin is decreased (Fig. 18.16).[14]

In uncomplicated ascites the fluid is freely mobile within the peritoneal cavity, allowing gas-containing bowel loops to float to the anterior abdominal wall. In complicated ascites (either infected or malignant) the fluid may become loculated and the bowel tethered to the abdominal wall (Fig. 18.17), with a thickened mesentery (Figs 18.18 and 18.19) and diminished or abolished peristalsis.[15] Thickening of the mesentery may follow malignant infiltration of the mesenteric root, and peritoneal seedlings can sometimes be demonstrated (Figs 18.17 and 18.18), though usually they are too small to be resolved by ultrasound, even when high-resolution transducers are used.

Uncomplicated ascitic fluid is echo free and produces increased through-transmission of sound. In malignant or infected ascites the fluid frequently contains blood or

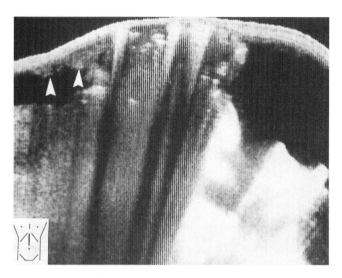

Fig. 18.17 **Malignant ascites.** There is loculated ascitic fluid and some tethering of bowel to the anterior abdominal wall; other gas-containing loops do not float freely. Peritoneal deposits are present (arrowheads).

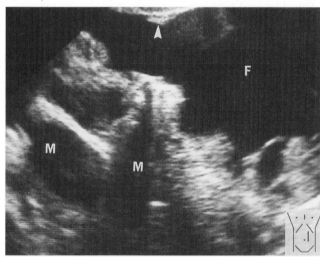

Fig. 18.18 **Malignant ascites.** Ascitic fluid is demonstrated (F) but the bowel loops are matted against the posterior abdominal wall by the thickened mesentery (M). There is a small peritoneal deposit (arrowhead).

pus, which produces mobile echoes (Fig. 18.20).[15] Septa within the fluid are typically seen in infection, especially tuberculosis (Fig. 18.21), but also occur in malignancy (Fig. 18.22). In the extreme form, pseudomyxomatous peritonitis, the entire cavity is filled with innumerable cystic spaces ranging from a few millimetres to several centimetres in diameter (Fig. 18.23).[16,17]

Occasionally it is possible to demonstrate the primary cause of the ascites, such as an ovarian carcinoma or metastatic disease within the liver (Fig. 18.24), thus allowing a confident diagnosis of the cause and nature of the

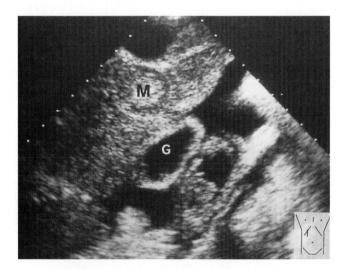

Fig. 18.16 **Thickened gallbladder wall in ascites.** There is free fluid in the right upper quadrant in this scan. There is a metastasis in the liver (M) and thickening of the wall of the gallbladder (G).

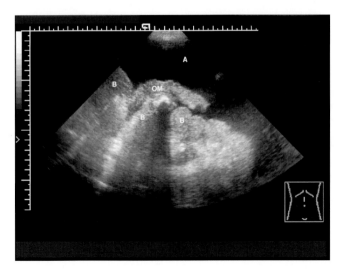

Fig. 18.19 Thickened omentum. The thickened omentum is surrounded by ascites in this patient with peritoneal tumour spread. The bowel loops are attached posteriorly. A – ascites, B – bowel loops, OM – omentum.

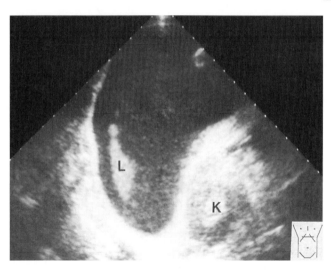

Fig. 18.20 Haemorrhagic malignant ascites. The inferior margin of the right lobe of the liver (L) and the right kidney (K) are seen. However, there is extensive intraperitoneal fluid which contains multiple low-level echoes. These appearances are characteristic of haemorrhagic ascites consistent with malignancy.

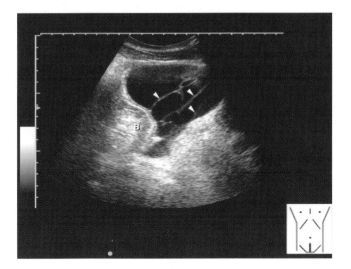

Fig. 18.21 Tuberculous peritonitis. Marked stranding is present within the ascites (arrowheads). Bowel loops have become attached to the posterior abdominal wall. B – bowel.

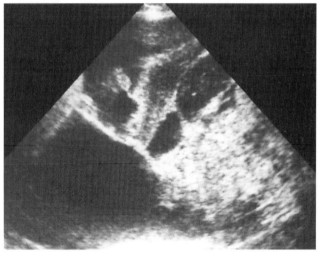

Fig. 18.22 Septa in malignant ascites.

ascitic fluid. The assessment of ancillary findings often allows differentiation of benign from malignant or complicated ascites. However, there are certain caveats. In the presence of severe hypoalbuminaemia, gallbladder wall thickening may be seen in both malignant and benign ascites. Gallbladder wall thickening and ascites are also frequently combined in severe acute hepatitis. Similarly, there may be difficulty with diagnosis when transudative ascites is associated with pre-existing bowel adhesions.

Paracentesis

Traditionally paracentesis has been performed via the insertion of a trocar and cannula in the left lower quadrant. However, the clinical diagnosis of ascites is unreliable, and although in gross ascites fluid is almost invariably present in the left lower quadrant, this may not be the safest site for drainage, as frequently bowel loops interpose between the anterior abdominal wall and the

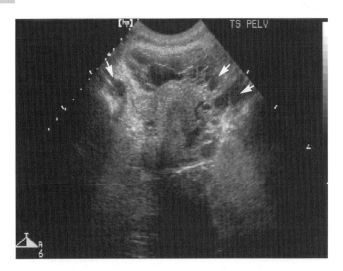

Fig. 18.23 Pseudomyxoma peritonei. Multiple septations and loculations (arrows) are seen within the intraperitoneal fluid in this patient with an ovarian carcinoma. Strictly, the term pseudomyxoma peritonei applies to non-malignant aetiologies (mostly following a ruptured mucinous appendicitis), but it is often loosely applied to any multicystic peritoneal condition.

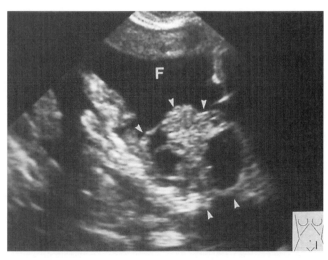

Fig. 18.24 Malignant ascites. Ascitic fluid (F) is noted in the pelvis in this patient with an empty bladder. A complex mass (arrowheads) replaces the left ovary

fluid collection in this location. Ultrasound-planned or -guided paracentesis is safer and more reliable: fluid can almost always be obtained.[18]

Intra-abdominal abscess

Despite advances in medical and surgical management there remains a significant morbidity and mortality from intra-abdominal abscess.[19,20] Symptoms and signs are often non-specific, and this is particularly true of postoperative abscesses.

Early diagnosis and effective treatment are important in the management of abscesses.[21–23] Ultrasound can play a role in both, but should not be considered in isolation. No single method of investigation is ideal. The sensitivity and specificity of CT, for example, is better than ultrasound in isolation. Isotope-labelled leukocyte studies are also sensitive in the detection of intra-abdominal abscess, but the specificity is low. Moreover, isotope imaging cannot be used as a guide for needle aspiration or catheter drainage, and this limits its role in management. The higher cost of CT, its more limited availability and the need to transport the patient to the CT unit are significant factors. Ultrasound is relatively cheap, almost universally available and mobile, making it suitable for the examination even of the very sick patient in the intensive care unit.

Examination of the patient with a suspected intra-abdominal abscess requires a careful approach.[7,8] The examination is often limited by poor access owing to abdominal wounds, dressings and drainage tubes. The examination should at first be directed towards any suspected abscess

site, suggested by symptoms, signs or plain radiological features, such as an elevated hemidiaphragm on a chest X-ray. If there are no such localising features a systematic examination of the various common sites for abscess collection must be made. The sub- and perihepatic regions are examined, using the liver as an acoustic window, with the patient in the supine and left posterior oblique positions (Figs 18.25

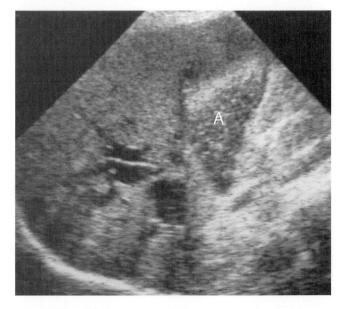

Fig. 18.25 Right subhepatic abscess. An abscess cavity (A) is shown in Morrison's pouch. This is predominantly echo free with distal enhancement, and contains a few low-level echoes.

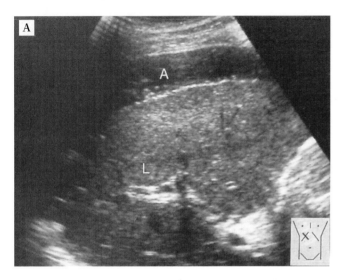
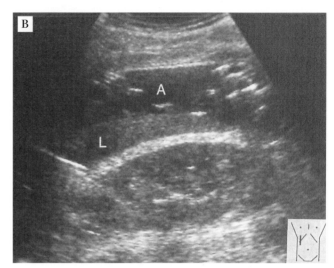

Fig. 18.26 Right subphrenic abscess. A: A fluid space with low level echoes (A) is interposed between the diaphragm and the liver (L). **B:** A longitudinal scan further laterally shows highly reflective echoes from gas within the fluid.

and 18.26). The left perisplenic region is examined using the spleen as a window in the supine and right posterior oblique positions. Care must be taken not to confuse a fluid-filled stomach or the left lobe of the liver with an abscess cavity.[7,24] The paracolic gutters are assessed with the patient supine; it is sometimes helpful to tilt the bed head-down in order to improve imaging of the upper abdominal organs. Pelvic scanning is best with a distended urinary bladder, which may have to be filled via a catheter if inadequate visualisation of the pelvis is achieved; trans-vaginal scanning does not require a filled bladder and gives higher-resolution images. Postoperative scanning is often severely hindered by traditional wound dressings: surgeons should be encouraged to use spray-on dressings to improve ultrasound access.

The operator must be conscious of the potential for auto- and cross-infection from open abdominal wounds throughout the examination.[25,26] Scrupulous cleaning and disinfection of the equipment (as well as of the operator's hands) before and after the examination is extremely important.

There is no unique appearance of an abscesses on ultrasound. The abscess cavity may appear echo free, thereby mimicking a cyst; it may have low-level echoes with an irregular margin (Fig. 18.27); or it may contain clumps of solid material within a predominantly fluid cavity. Occasionally, strong echoes within the fluid may suggest a solid mass (Fig. 18.25). Gas within the abscess can produce a confusing picture in which the abscess may be indistinguishable from adjacent bowel and thus rendered invisible to ultrasound investigation (Fig. 18.28).[27] Free intraperitoneal gas may be encountered in perforation of a viscus such as the duodenum, when it has been described as collecting preferentially in the region of the ligamentum teres.[28]

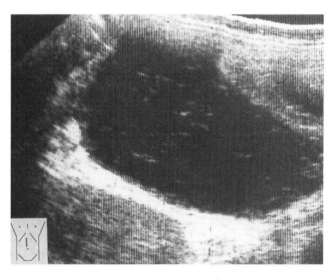

Fig. 18.27 Abdominal abscess. Large irregular fluid collection in the mid-abdomen communicating with the subcutaneous tissues and containing scattered low-level echoes.

Percutaneous aspiration and drainage

Because of the high morbidity of reoperation for intra-abdominal abscess[29] there has been increasing interest in percutaneous needle aspiration and catheter drainage (see Vol. 1, Ch. 7).[21,30–34] This provides the opportunity for bacteriological analysis of the aspirate to assist with the choice of antibiotics and to direct management, and this is particularly important as fungal abscesses respond poorly to percutaneous drainage.[35]

Whereas the fine needle used for aspiration can safely traverse bowel loops, the insertion of a catheter necessitates a clear bowel-free pathway. The type of procedure

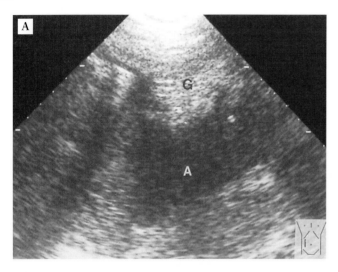 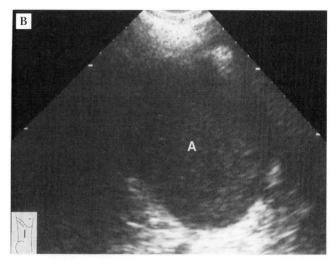

Fig. 18.28 Gas within an abdominal abscess. A: Much of the abscess cavity (A) in the mid-abdomen is obscured by superficially located gas (G). **B:** Scanning the abscess from a lateral approach the gas is avoided and the abscess cavity (A) can be identified.

chosen depends upon the size of the abscess and its position. Lesions smaller than 6 cm in diameter can usually be successfully aspirated with an 18 G needle under direct ultrasound control; in one series a success rate of greater than 95% was recorded. Larger abscesses, which are often more complex, require catheter insertion and yield poorer results, with success rates around 70% (which compares well with operative intervention and certainly shortens hospital stay). When a catheter must be inserted, planning the route for the guide needle generally requires CT to ensure that intervening gut is avoided. Fistulae require excision rather than drainage, and should be excluded by contrast studies.

Although ultrasound is valuable in the investigation and management of suspected intra-abdominal abscess, optimum management should follow a diagnostic algorithm. For patients too sick to be moved from intensive care, ultrasound is the only imaging technique available for investigation and aspiration or drainage of an abscess at the bedside, and can be life-saving. If there are clinical features or radiological signs pointing to a specific site for an abscess collection, ultrasound is the most cost-effective investigation. However, when the site of abscess is not clear (e.g. a fever of unknown origin), a radiolabelled leukocyte study or abdominal CT scan should be used.

Other fluid collections

Lymphoceles, haematomas and urinomas can all be demonstrated by ultrasound, but their sonographic appearances are variable, so that the nature of the collection cannot be determined by ultrasound alone.[3] The examination should be directed towards the site of the trauma, bearing in mind, as always, that fluids tends to collect in the most dependent portion of the peritoneum. *In vitro*, blood clots change with

time: initially echo free, they develop reflective regions with clot retraction. However, the variations in the rate of this process mean that the ultrasound appearances are not very reliable for estimating the age of the haematoma. Ultrasound is widely used to direct the tapping of peritoneal fluid in blunt abdominal trauma: if the fluid is bloodstained further investigation for ruptured viscera is required (usually either CT or laparoscopy/laparotomy), whereas a negative scan or aspiration of clear fluid supports conservative management.[36] However, in a proportion of cases rupture is not accompanied by peritoneal bleeding, and so follow-up ultrasound scans should be considered in 'negative' cases.[37]

Lymphoceles are frequently septated, but septa can also occur in haematomas and in abscesses (Fig. 18.29). Echogenic fluid within lymphoceles is suggestive of infection. As in abdominal abscesses, percutaneous aspiration is an important diagnostic technique and may be an alternative to surgical management.

Miscellaneous pathologies

Duplication cysts

Small bowel duplication cysts are rare but generally have the characteristic appearances of cysts. If they contain echogenic fluid they may be confused with other causes of intra-abdominal fluid collection. Bowel loops are displaced around the cyst and may partially or completely obscure it.

Mesenteric and peritoneal tumours

The difficulties of imaging peritoneal seedlings in intra-abdominal metastatic disease have already been described.

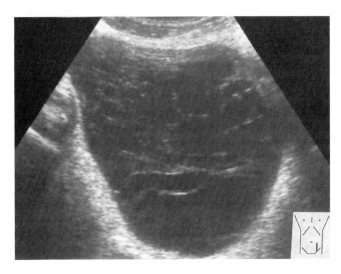

Fig. 18.29 Septated fluid collection in the left iliac fossa. This septated appearance is said to be characteristic of a lymphocele, but this was in fact a haematoma.

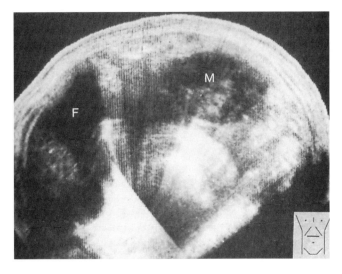

Fig. 18.30 Large mesenteric metastasis. A large mass is seen in the central abdomen (M) in a patient with ascites (F).

Occasionally large peritoneal deposits can be seen, particularly those in the mesentery (Fig. 18.30). They are usually solid, but may contain areas of necrosis with irregular cystic regions. Adjacent bowel loops are stretched around the mass in a similar fashion to duplication cysts.

Peritoneal metastases

Peritoneal spread of malignancies is not uncommon and is a particular feature of ovarian carcinoma (in which it receives its own staging classification) (Fig. 18.31). Intra-abdominal lymphoma is usually manifest as enlargement of the para-aortic and paracaval nodes, typically with a rounded shape and effacement of the vascular hilum.

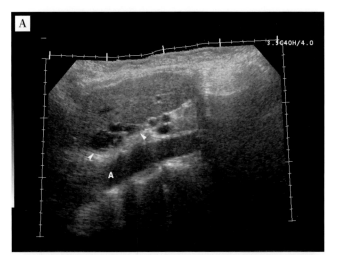

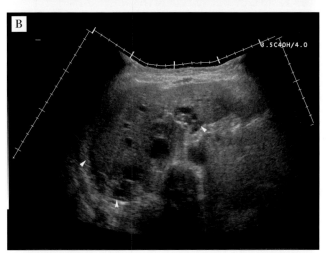

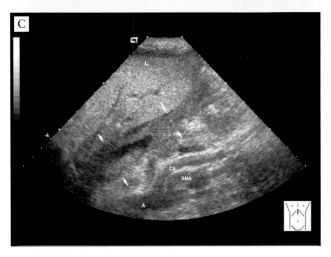

Fig. 18.31 Peritoneal tumour. A: Cystic masses (arrowheads) lie posterior to the liver in this patient with trans-coelomic spread of an ovarian cancer (extended field of view scan). **B:** Transverse scan in the same patient showing tumour (arrowheads) over the right lobe of the liver. **C:** In another patient, also with an ovarian carcinoma, the peritoneal spread is more solid in consistency (arrows). A – aorta, CA – coeliac axis, SMA – superior mesenteric artery.

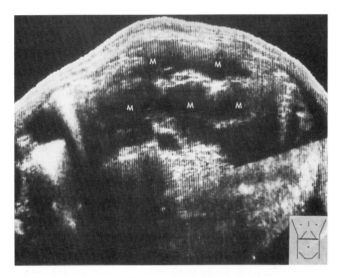

Fig. 18.32 The 'sandwich sign'. Multiple lymph node masses (M) envelop the mesenteric vessels (V) producing a sandwich effect.

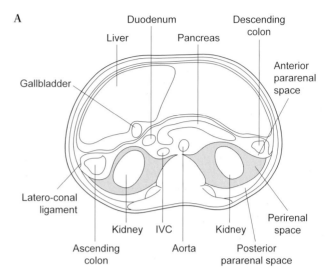

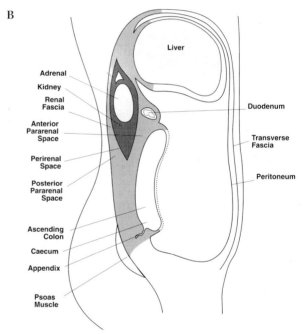

Fig. 18.33 The retroperitoneal spaces. Diagrammatic sections through the kidneys, A: transverse, B: parasagittal, to show the perirenal and pararenal spaces and the lateroconal ligaments. IVC – inferior vena cava. Reproduced with permission of Springer-Verlag from Meyer, MA. Dynamic radiology of the abdomen. Normal and pathologic anatomy, 3rd edn. New York: Springer-Verlag, 2000.

Assessment of the extent of nodal and extranodal disease is important in the staging of lymphoma: extension into the root of the mesentery is particularly important, as it represents a more advanced disease stage. These appearances have been described as the 'sandwich sign', with lymph node infiltration sandwiching the vessels of the mesentery (Fig. 18.32). Occasionally on ultrasound this sign can be mimicked by the presence of large amounts of fat in the mesentery, but generally fat tends to be more reflective than lymphomatous tissue.

RETROPERITONEUM

Anatomy

The retroperitoneum is that part of the abdomen which is bounded anteriorly by the posterior parietal peritoneum, posteriorly by the transversalis fascia and laterally by the lateroconal ligaments (Fig. 18.33). It is largest posteriorly but continues anteriorly as the properitoneal fat compartment, and extends from the pelvic brim inferiorly to the diaphragm superiorly. The retroperitoneum contains the adrenals, kidneys and ureters, the duodenal loop and the pancreas, the great vessels with their branches and associated lymph node chains, and the ascending and descending portions of the colon, including the caecum. It can be divided into three distinct compartments by the fascial planes it contains: these constrain the distribution of reteroperitoneal collections such as pseudocysts, haematomas and abscesses, and so an understanding of their arrangement has practical diagnostic value.

The anterior pararenal space lies between the posterior parietal peritoneum and the anterior renal fascia; the

lateroconal ligament lies laterally, blending with the parietal peritoneum anteriorly. The space is continuous across the midline and contains the pancreas, the duodenum, the ascending and descending colon, the caecum, and also the appendix when it lies in a retrocaecal position.

The perirenal space is confined by the anterior and posterior renal fasciae, which fuse laterally to form the lateroconal ligament. The precise site at which this blends with the renal fascia varies widely. The posterior renal fascia

(Gerota's fascia) is generally thicker than the anterior and has at least two layers, the anterior of which is continuous with the anterior renal fascia whereas the posterior layer continues into the lateroconal ligament. Superiorly the layers fuse above the adrenals and attach to the diaphragm. Inferiorly the renal fasciae extend into the pelvis, where they thin out so that the anterior and posterior pararenal spaces communicate in the iliac fossa. The fascial layers consist of dense connective tissue which blends with the connective tissue enveloping the aorta, the IVC and the roots of the superior mesenteric vessels. The perirenal space contains the kidneys, adrenals, fat and blood vessels.

The posterior pararenal space lies between the posterior renal and lateroconal ligaments anteriorly and the transversalis fascia posteriorly. Its medial border is formed by the psoas major and quadratus lumborum muscles. Laterally it communicates with the properitoneal fat compartment (flank stripe). It contains only fat.[38-41]

All the compartments of the retroperitoneal space contain varying amounts of adipose tissue, depending on body habitus, but the right anterior and both posterior pararenal spaces are usually thin compartments.

The diaphragmatic crura extend inferiorly as tendinous fibres that attach to the vertebrae and their transverse processes down as far as L3 on the right and L1 on the left. The right crus is more prominent and usually more lobular than the left. It is bounded by the IVC anterolaterally, and by the right adrenal gland and the right lobe of the liver posterolaterally. Its fibres diverge as they ascend: the lateral fibres insert on the central tendon of the diaphragm and the medial fibres ascend on the left side of the oesophageal hiatus, decussating with those of the left crus in front of the abdominal aorta. On parasagittal scans the right crus can be seen as a longitudinal echo-poor structure immediately posterior to the IVC or, to the left of the midline, anterior to the aorta. The intra-abdominal portion of the oesophagus begins at the cephalic end of the right crus. The left crus ascends along the anterior lumbar vertebral bodies and inserts into the central tendon of the diaphragm. It is closely related to the adrenal gland, the splenic vessels and the oesophagogastric junction. Occasionally the medial fibres of the left crus cross the aorta and run toward the IVC.

The right crus is more readily seen on ultrasound than the left, though both may be apparent on transverse scans.[42] The prevertebral spaces at the level of the crura contain the aorta, nerves, portions of the azygos venous system, lymph nodes and the cisterna chyli.

Scanning techniques and general appearances

Using transverse and longitudinal scans the superior reaches of the retroperitoneum are well seen because the liver and spleen can be used as acoustic windows. Little if any patient preparation is required for retroperitoneal ultrasound: fasting for 12 hours beforehand may reduce gas, but is not always necessary. Parenteral fluid or fluid enemas may occasionally be helpful, and the use of pharmaceutical gas-displacing liquids ('contrast agents') such as SonoRx (Bracco, Milan) improves visualisation.[43] Barium studies should be performed after rather than immediately before an ultrasound because barium is a strong reflector.

The diaphragmatic crura, pancreas, kidneys, duodenum, psoas muscles and prevertebral vessels are all detectable and, in the lower abdomen, the iliopsoas, quadratus lumborum and the prevertebral vessels can be visualised when scanning conditions are favourable. Oblique coronal views are a valuable addition to the standard views in visualising the retroperitoneum, particularly for the great vessels.[44-46] They are best performed from the right flank with the patient in a left posterior oblique position so that the right lobe of the liver and the right kidney move antero-inferiorly and act as acoustic windows. At the same time, fatty tissue and gas-filled bowel loops move anteriorly, facilitating acoustic access posterior to them. Similarly, scans can be performed from the left flank in the right posterior oblique position, but these are usually less successful than on the right, where a better window is provided by the liver.

Using oblique coronal views the proximal renal arteries can be demonstrated in up to 90% of patients, though success is lower in the presence of an aortic aneurysm (presumably because of the anatomical distortion it causes[44]) and the proximal portions of the common iliac arteries can be seen in 80% of patients. An anomalous (e.g. circumaortic) or duplicated vena cava can be displayed in sagittal or oblique coronal scans.

The general fat in the retroperitoneum is moderately reflective and this increases the contrast with the echo-poor lumina of vessels and ducts. Occasionally, however, the fat is relatively echo poor and its appearance as unexpectedly dark tissue, often with a striated structure from the fascial layers within it, can be confusing, creating the false impression of retroperitoneal pathology such as an infiltrating tumour. This is most often encountered in neonates (where it may be so echo poor as to suggest fluid) and in the obese (Fig. 18.34).

In easy-to-scan subjects normal retroperitoneal nodes are sometimes identified. These are bean-shaped, less than 1 cm in length, and their hilum can be demonstrated with a careful search as a reflective strip extending part-way into the echo-poor parenchyma.[47] On colour Doppler a vessel may be found in the hilum but there should be no vessels perforating the convexity of the node – this and a spherical shape suggest malignant involvement. Enlarged posterior abdominal lymph nodes can be detected with an accuracy, sensitivity and specificity of around 90% and

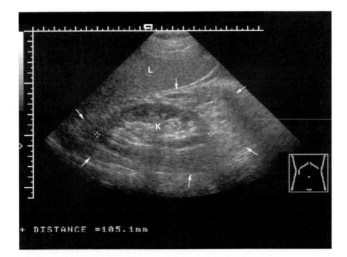

Fig. 18.34 Retroperitoneal fat. Retroperitoneal fat is usually moderately reflective but can be confusingly echo poor. In this obese patient the echo-poor fat around the right kidney (arrows) suggested an infiltrating malignancy: CT revealed low-density tissue in the retroperitoneum and around the gallbladder. K – kidney; L – liver.

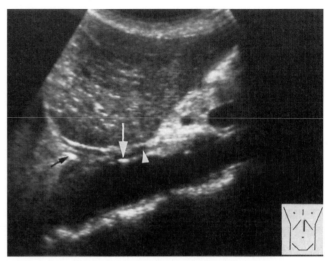

Fig. 18.36 The aorta and crus. The aorta is shown in longitudinal section as it enters the abdomen under the crus (arrowhead), with the lower thoracic oesophagus above it (black arrow). There is a small calcific plaque (white arrow) in the anterior wall of the aorta.

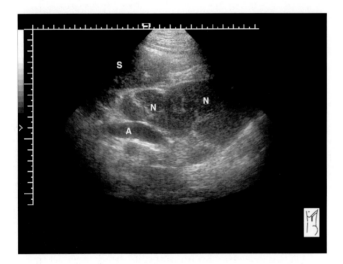

Fig. 18.35 Retroperitoneal lymphadenopathy. A large lobulated mass of confluent lymph nodes is seen in this left coronal section in a patient with abdominal Hodgkin's disease. A – aorta, N – nodes, S – spleen.

their oval or rounded shapes permit differentiation from the para-aortic vessels[40] (Fig. 18.35).

Aorta

The great vessels lie anterior to the spine in the retroperitoneum. The abdominal aorta enters the abdomen at approximately L1 level and descends to L4 (the level of the umbilicus), where it bifurcates into the common iliac arteries (Fig. 18.36). It is closely apposed to the anterior surface of the spine: any separation is suspicious, suggesting a space-occupying lesion such as a haematoma, lym-

phadenopathy or fibrosis. At the level of the crura the aortic lumen measures 2.5 cm in diameter, tapering to 1 cm at the bifurcation (Fig. 18.37). Apart from reverberant noise the lumen should be echo free, although phase-inversion harmonic techniques sometimes reveal flowing echoes from red cell rouleaux.

The coeliac axis, superior mesenteric artery and the origin of the renal arteries are all usually visualised on ultrasound (Fig. 18.38). The inferior mesenteric artery is harder to access, but is sometimes seen arising from the anterior surface of the aorta, several centimetres above its bifurcation. The common iliac arteries are often visible in decubitus views.

Congenital anomalies of the aorta are rare; in situs inversus all the abdominal contents are transposed so that the aorta lies on the right: apart from its position, the appearances are normal.

In atheroma the normally thin, smooth endothelial lining of the aorta thickens and becomes irregular, often with calcifications (Fig. 18.39). The aorta may also dilate slightly so that it loses its normal tapering configuration (Fig. 18.40). Such an ectatic aorta may present as a pulsatile epigastric 'mass' that suggests an aneurysm clinically; ultrasound makes the distinction clear. The ectatic aorta is often very tortuous (Fig. 18.41). Rarely atheroma causes stenosis of the aorta (Fig. 18.42).

Ultrasound has long been the diagnostic procedure of choice in evaluating abdominal aortic aneurysms.[48] It has found a role in screening in the elderly[49,50] and in differentiating aneurysms from other causes of a pulsatile mass, e.g. a hyperdynamic aorta in a thin person (Fig. 18.43) or a para-aortic mass. About a third of abdominal aortic aneurysms contain insufficient calcification to allow their

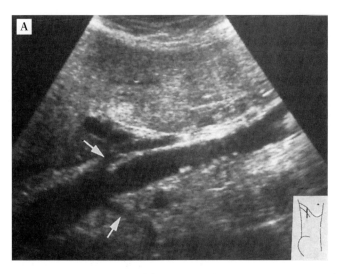

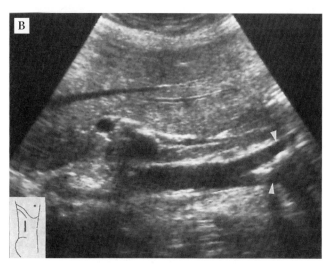

Fig. 18.37 Coronal sections of the aorta. A: The renal artery origins are shown (arrows). **B:** The bifurcation into the common iliac arteries (arrowheads).

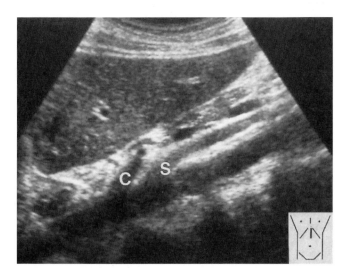

Fig. 18.38 Midline branches of the aorta. The coeliac axis (C) and the superior mesenteric artery (S) are seen in this sagittal section through the upper abdominal aorta.

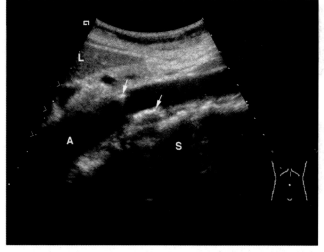

Fig. 18.39 Atheroma of the aorta. Intimal thickening is seen throughout this aorta, which is of normal calibre. In the most thickened plaques (arrows) the echoes are very intense, suggesting calcification. A – aorta, L – liver, S – spine.

measurement on a plain film, but ultrasound can be used to assess aneurysm size to within ±3 mm,[51] and has an advantage over angiography in that it demonstrates both the true lumen and the amount of mural thrombus (Fig. 18.44). An aneurysm with a true luminal diameter of 5 cm or more is at risk of rupture and half of those larger than 6 cm in diameter rupture within the first year. Both transverse and anteroposterior measurements should be taken, and the larger used for risk classification. It is important that the measurement be taken at right-angles to the aortic lumen and this is sometimes difficult to esti-mate, especially when the lumen is tortuous following elongation from atheroma. Ultrasound is useful for serial

measurements of the aneurysm: progressive expansion of more than 1 cm *per annum* is an indication for surgical intervention.[49,52] The relationship of the aneurysm and the renal arteries affects the surgical treatment as well as the associated morbidity and mortality, so that visualisation of the renal arteries is important. Although the origins of the renal arteries are usually seen in normal subjects, they are more difficult to visualise in the presence of an abdominal aortic aneurysm, so that aortography or dynamic CT may be required.[48] Extension of the aneurysm into the iliac arteries can usually be demonstrated on ultrasound.

Acute aortic rupture is a surgical emergency with a high mortality, so that imaging studies are not usually feasible.

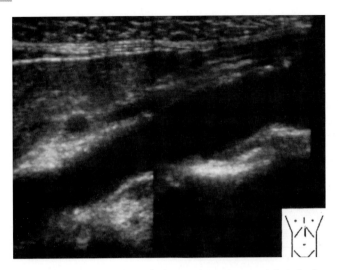

Fig. 18.40 Ectatic aorta. Instead of narrowing as it passes inferiorly, the ectatic aorta has the same calibre throughout its length or, as in this case, expands progressively. Such an aorta may be easily palpable and is readily confused within an aneurysm on clinical examination.

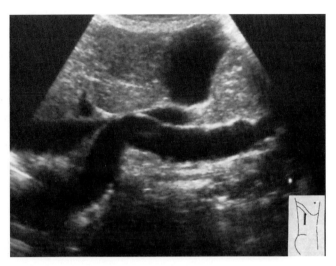

Fig. 18.41 Tortuous aorta. In this coronal section the extreme tortuosity that the aorta may achieve is well shown. Here the cava is compressed by the elongated tortuosity.

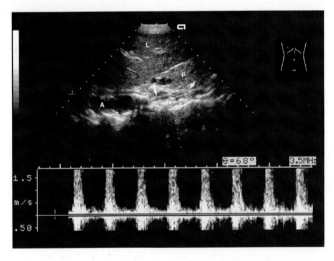

Fig. 18.42 Stenosis of the aorta. In this arteriopath the atheroma of the aorta has progressed to a tight stenosis (arrows). The spectral Doppler has aliased, so that the exact peak systolic velocity cannot be measured, but it is at least 1.5 m/s. This was an incidental finding: presumably the process developed sufficiently slowly that adequate collaterals had developed. A – aorta, L – liver, P – pancreas.

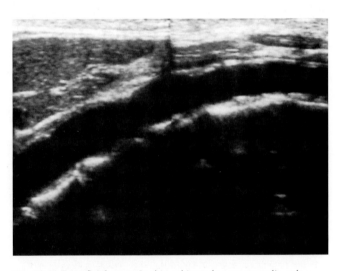

Fig. 18.43 Superficial aorta. In thin subjects the aorta may lie only a few centimetres deep because of the normal lumbar lordosis. This patient was referred to confirm an aortic aneurysm, but this is excluded by the normal tapering configuration.

However, in chronic aortic rupture a pulsating haematoma or a peri-aortic collection extending into the flanks may be demonstrated, though CT is more reliable than ultrasound for this problem.

Aortic dissection gives a characteristic ultrasound appearance, with a 'flapping' inner (media–intima) wall which has become separated from the outer (media–adventitia) wall, and the extent of the dissection within the abdomen can often be defined (Fig. 18.45).[53–57] Colour Doppler is particularly helpful in demonstrating the separate vascular channels, with their different flow velocities shown as distinct colour values, and microbubble contrast agents may assist in detecting the Doppler signals.[58] For the thoracic aorta, where dissections most often originate, transoesophageal ultrasound (TEE) has become established as the most useful technique.

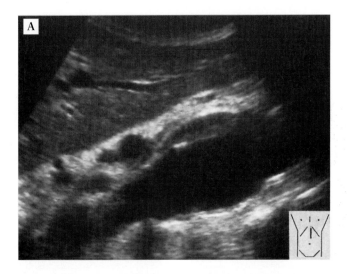

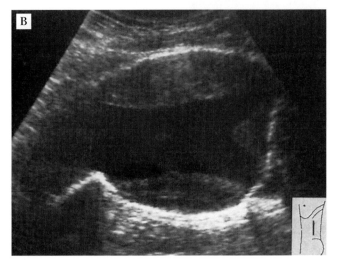

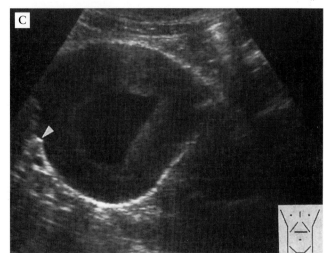

Fig. 18.44 Aortic aneurysm. A to C: All three components of an aneurysm, the wall, the lumen and the thrombus, are well shown on ultrasound. There is calcific atheroma (arrowhead) in the aortic wall in C.

In aortic occlusion the aorta typically remains anechoic but there is no pulsation.[59] Doppler studies are essential to confirm the occlusion.

Aortic grafts are identified by their sharply defined parallel reflective walls (Fig. 18.46). Abdominal aortic aneurysms are usually repaired by incising the aneurysm, implanting the graft, and then wrapping the aneurysm sac around the graft to stabilise it. Postoperative bleeding tends to track between the graft and the encircling aneurysm wall to produce a characteristic ultrasound 'lumen within a lumen' appearance,[60,61] which is better seen with intravascular ultrasound.[62] Usually, even recently implanted grafts are not associated with significant fluid collections. Any perigraft fluid, either proximal, distal or tracking along the length of the graft, is a serious and important finding that suggests an abscess, haematoma or lymphocele. Collections at the distal anastomoses can be aspirated under ultrasound control to exclude early infection. CT is more sensitive for graft abscesses because the characteristic gas pocket is readily detected. Small haematomas usually resorb within a few weeks of surgery. Persistent or enlarging collections suggest the formation of a false aneurysm or an abscess.[60] False aneurysms are a common complication of graft surgery. They occur at both anastomotic sites and are usually due to suture breakdown, but also occasionally to graft infection. Though less common at the proximal anastomotic site, these are more serious than those affecting the distal (femoral) anastomosis because they may erode into the overlying duodenum to produce an aorto-duodenal fistula, with massive gastrointestinal bleeding. In graft occlusion, as with aortic occlusion, the only grey scale ultrasound signs may be lack of pulsatility, and Doppler is required for a definitive diagnosis.[47,54]

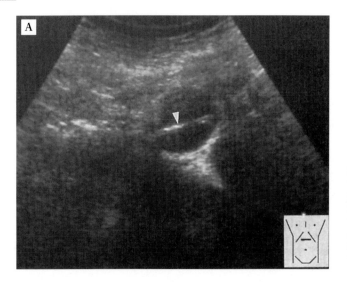

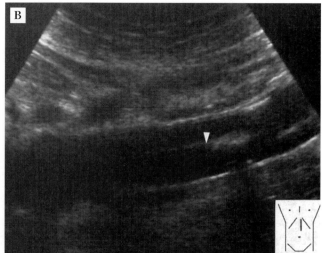

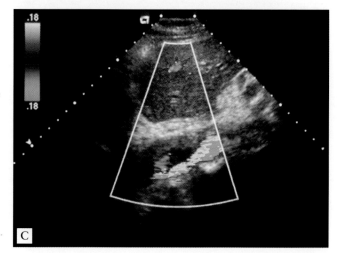

Fig. 18.45 Aortic dissection A: Longitudinal scan. **B:** Transverse scan. The intimal flap (arrowhead) is visualised as a fine mobile linear structure within the lumen; **C:** the differing flow patterns on either side of the flap can be demonstrated with colour Doppler (C).

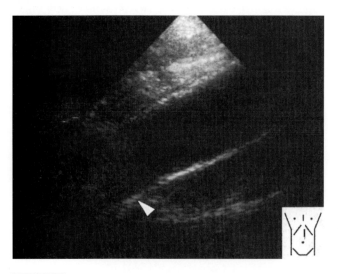

Fig. 18.46 Aortic graft. The graft's strong echoes and parallel walls are characteristic. In this case the texture of the weave of the Dacron (arrowhead) can be discerned in the graft wall.

Inferior vena cava

The inferior vena cava originates at the junction of the two common iliac veins to the right of L5 and continues cephalad on the right side of the spine, widening after receiving the renal veins (Fig. 18.47). It lies within a groove in the bare area of the liver and is occasionally enclosed by liver tissue. Just before penetrating the diaphragm at the level of T8–T9 it turns anteriorly towards the right atrium and receives the hepatic veins. Its walls are reflective and, apart from artefacts, its lumen should be echo free; however, with scanners using phase-inversion harmonics flowing echogenic streams may be detected, presumably arising from red cell rouleaux.

In the supine position the upper portion of the inferior vena cava is usually accessible, but it is often obscured distally by overlying bowel gas. The right coronal view often gives better visualisation of its entire length.

The calibre of the inferior vena cava varies with the cardiac and respiratory phases: it can normally appear thin and slit-like but typically opens in systole. A Valsalva manoeuvre can be used to increase the distension of a normal inferior vena cava so that it becomes more obvious on ultrasound. In congestive cardiac failure and cardiac tamponade the cava is distended and the respiratory variation damped, whereas in proximal caval obstruction both cardiac and respiratory calibre changes are lost.[63] If the lesion is above the hepatic veins these are also distended.[64]

Anomalies of the cava are common because of its complex embryological origins from several primitive segments. A left-sided cava has an incidence of 0.2% and occurs in various degrees of completeness, the commonest consisting of a left cava below renal level which drains into a large left renal vein that crosses over the aorta to a normal upper caval segment (Fig. 18.48).[65] The most obvious feature is often the attenuated infrarenal part of

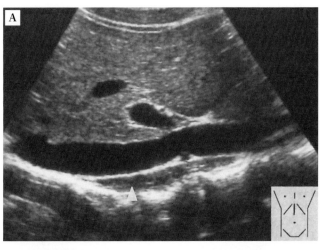

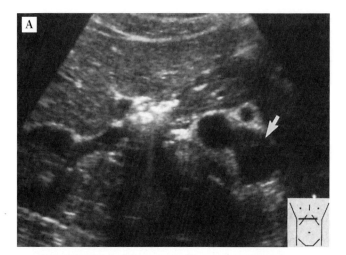

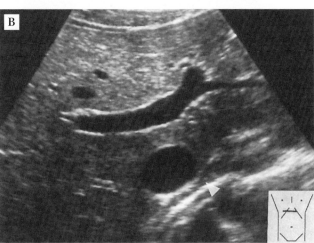

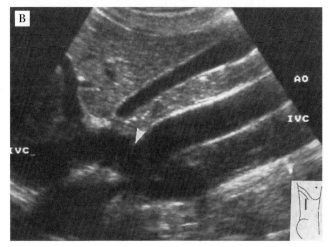

Fig. 18.47 Inferior vena cava. A: Longitudinal and **B:** transverse sections showing the normal cava in the distended state (held inspiration), closely applied to the posterior surface of the liver and lying over the right crus of diaphragm (arrowheads).

Fig. 18.48 Left-sided cava. A: Transverse and **B:** right coronal sections showing a left-sided cava (arrow) discharging into the left renal vein (arrowhead). AO – aorta, IVC – inferior vena cava.

the cava on the right, a finding that should prompt a search for the other features of the anomaly.

The inferior vena cava is invaded in approximately 10% of renal cell carcinomas. Reflective material may be visualised within its lumen and the connection with the tumour in the appropriate renal vein can be demonstrated (see Vol. 2, Ch. 23). However, the involvement is more clearly demonstrated with colour Doppler, which shows a flow void extending from the renal hilum sometimes as far as the right atrium. Colour Doppler also demonstrates whether the veins are occluded.

The inferior vena cava may be displaced anteriorly by posterior lesions, such as retrocaval lymphadenopathy and masses in the right kidney or adrenal gland. It is displaced posteriorly by anteriorly sited masses such as lymph nodes, masses in the pancreatic head, and caudate lobe enlargement from liver tumours or in the Budd–Chiari syndrome (see Chs 11 and 12, respectively). A large mass can severely compress or even obstruct the inferior vena cava, although flow often persists despite extreme distortion, a feature best demonstrated by colour Doppler.[64] Lack of distension on a Valsalva manoeuvre, with fixed dilatation below the apparent site of compression, is an indirect feature of occlusion.

Thrombus within the cava has the same general appearances as thrombus elsewhere, typically being seen as stationary reflective material within the lumen (Fig. 18.49).[66] However, fresh thrombus may be poorly reflective and hence difficult to distinguish from blood; colour Doppler is invaluable for revealing the position of the thrombus as well as demonstrating blood flowing through recanalisation channels. The distinction between blood and tumour thrombus can be difficult, but the demonstration of pulsatile arterial signals within the thrombus strongly suggests tumour neovascularisation.

Caval filters are strongly reflective and appear as a complex of linear echoes in the caval lumen (Fig. 18.50); ultrasound is useful to confirm the position of the 'umbrella' and the patency of the cava.

Retroperitoneal tumours

Most retroperitoneal tumours arise in the kidneys (see Vol. 2, Ch. 23) or adrenals (see Ch. 19). Of the remainder, primary retroperitoneal tumours other than lymphomas are uncommon.[64,67] Approximately 80% are malignant.[68,69] Most retroperitoneal tumours in the adult are mesenchymal in origin (Table 18.1), the three most common being liposarcoma, leiomyosarcoma and malignant fibrohistiocytoma.[70] Metastatic disease in the retroperitoneum is usually recurrence of a urological or gynaecological tumour.

Clinically, retroperitoneal tumours are insidious in onset with few early manifestations, so that they reach a large size by the time of diagnosis: in 80% of cases they are large enough to be palpable (Table 18.2). Abdominal pain is the commonest presentation, probably attributable to bowel and renal tract obstruction. Surgery offers the best hope of cure as there is limited response to radiotherapy or chemotherapy. However, most are invasive and cannot be resected completely, so the prognosis is poor.[71,72]

Although it is not always possible to confirm the retroperitoneal origin of the tumour with ultrasound, some characteristic features may be helpful in locating their origin. Anterior displacement of the pancreas, kidneys, great vessels, or the ascending or descending colon is highly suggestive of a retroperitoneal lesion (Fig. 18.51). Encasement of retroperitoneal structures such as the aorta, IVC, renal vessels, kidney and pancreas, or

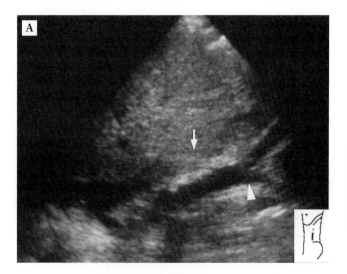

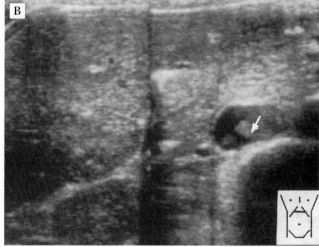

Fig. 18.49 Caval thrombus. A: Left coronal section at the pelvic brim. **B:** Transverse section in the epigastrium. The caval thrombus is seen as reflective material within the caval lumen (arrows). The aortic bifurcation (arrowhead in A) is seen.

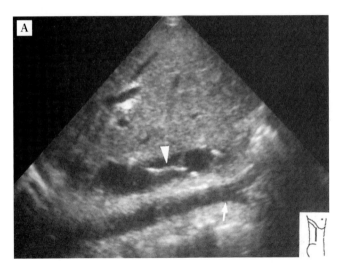

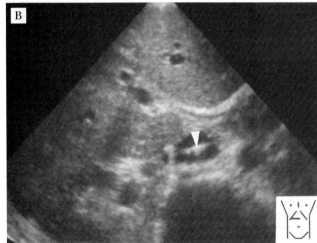

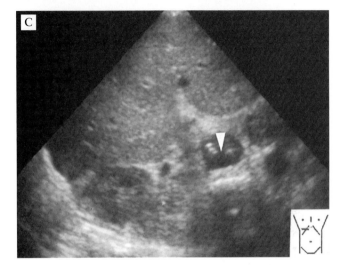

Fig. 18.50 Caval filter. A: Right coronal, **B** and **C:** low and high transverse sections showing the strong intracaval echoes (arrowheads) from a Greenberg filter. The aortic bifurcation is well seen (arrow in **A**).

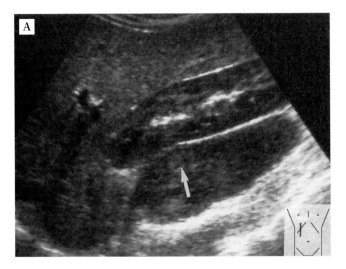

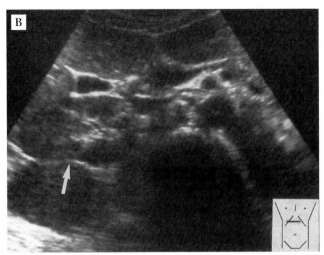

Fig. 18.51 Retroperitoneal sarcoma. A: Longitudinal right parasagittal and **B:** transverse sections of a retroperitoneal mass elevating the right kidney (arrow). The uniform echo texture is typical of a sarcoma.

Table 18.1 Classification of retroperitoneal tumours[67]

	Malignant	Benign
Mesenchymal		
	Liposarcoma	Lipoma
	Leiomyosarcoma	Leiomyoma
	Rhabdomyosarcoma	Rhabdomyoma
	Fibrosarcoma	Fibroma, fibromatosis
	Malignant fibrous histiocytoma	
Vascular		
	Haemangiopericytoma	
	Angiosarcoma	(Haemangioma)
	Lymphangiosarcoma	(Lymphangioma)
Neurogenic		
	Malignant schwannoma	Neurilemmoma
	Neurofibroma	
Tumours of sympathetic nerve origin		
	Neuroblastoma	
	Ganglioneuroblastoma	Ganglioneuroma
	Malignant paraganglionoma	Paraganglioneuroma
	Extra-adrenal phaeochromocytoma	
Germ cell tumours		
	Malignant teratoma	Benign teratoma
	Embryonal carcinoma	
	Seminoma*	

*Occasionally arises in the retroperitoneal space as a primary tumour. Very rare lesions are bracketed.

Table 18.2 Presenting features of retroperitoneal tumours[69]

Feature	Frequency (%)
Abdominal pain	88
Fatigue	44
Weight loss	32
Anorexia	24
Fever	20
Radiating nerve root pain	16
Back pain	12

compression of the iliopsoas or quadratus lumborum muscles are also typical features (Fig. 18.52).

The histology of the tumour cannot be determined from the ultrasound appearances, though in some cases there are features suggestive of a specific diagnosis. Many retroperitoneal tumours are large (particularly haemangiopericytomas), but functioning tumours (e.g. extra-adrenal phaeochromocytoma) and those associated with disease elsewhere (e.g. a Schwannoma in a patient with neurofibromatosis) may be small at diagnosis. Neurogenic tumours are generally paravertebral in position, whereas those of sympathetic nerve origin tend to lie in the para-aortic region. Extra-adrenal phaeochromocytomas or paraganglionomas often arise in the organs of Zuckerkandl, which are usually found below the renal hilum, or at the

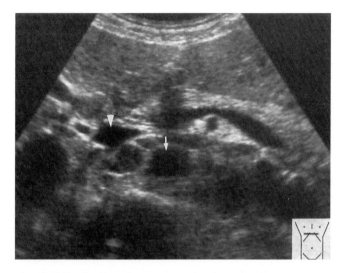

Fig. 18.52 Retroperitoneal tumour encasing the aorta. Numerous retroperitoneal masses are seen surrounding the aorta (arrow) and elevating the inferior vena cava (arrowhead).

origin of the inferior mesenteric artery. Teratomas often involve the sacrococcygeal area, whereas a malignant fibrohistiocytoma typically lies very close to the kidney (nephrectomy is needed in 50% of cases).[73] The patient's age may also provide a clue to the tumour type: rhabdomyosarcoma, neuroblastoma, ganglioneuroblastoma and teratomas tend to occur in children, whereas malignant fibrohistiocytoma is the commonest retroperitoneal soft tissue sarcoma of late adult life.

The ultrasound appearances are very variable, with strongly and poorly reflective or mixed tumours all occurring, both with and without anechoic zones from necrosis. Tumours with a uniform cell type and a paucity of connective tissue and fat have fewer internal echoes, so that they produce lesions that are echo-poor or nearly anechoic, as is typical of a malignant Schwannoma or fibrohistiocytoma. A highly reflective tumour suggests a liposarcoma, although this feature may be absent when the tumour is poorly differentiated.[74] The reflectivity of lipomas varies from highly intense to weak, depending on the content and distribution of fat and fibrous tissue (Fig. 18.53). Vascular tumours such as haemangiopericytomas are also reflective, presumably because of the abundant interfaces produced by the multiple vessel walls.[75]

A solid mass of mixed reflectivity with an echo-poor centre suggests a sarcoma, as these rapidly progressive tumours tend to outgrow their blood supply, causing central necrosis with haemorrhage. This is particularly true of leiomyosarcomas.

Teratomas have a characteristically heterogeneous mixed echo pattern with solid areas, calcification (50%) and cystic spaces (76%) (similar to ovarian teratomas). They occur in female infants under 6 months of age, with a second peak in incidence in young men. However, the

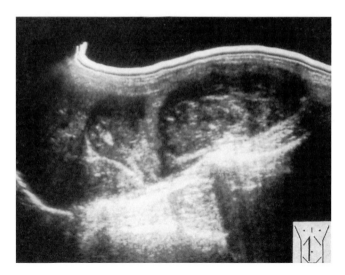

Fig. 18.53 Liposarcoma. The strong echoes that are typical of a liposarcoma are attributable to the admixture of fatty and watery soft tissue elements; for this reason, only well differentiated tumours (i.e. those that retain the ability to form fat) have this appearance.

latter are more likely to represent metastases from a testicular primary, and so the testes should also be scanned. Contrary to early reports, it is not possible to distinguish benign from malignant teratomas on the basis of whether they are predominantly cystic or solid.[76]

The benign or malignant nature of any retroperitoneal tumour cannot be reliably determined on ultrasound. A smooth, round, well demarcated cystic mass may be benign or malignant; however, an irregular lesion is more likely to be malignant, benign fibromatosis being an exception as it may be very irregular and show features of muscle invasion.

Retroperitoneal cysts

Primary retroperitoneal cysts are rare. They include simple inclusion cysts (teratomatous cysts) and cysts arising from embryonic gastrointestinal and genitourinary tract rests (e.g. Wolffian or Müllerian duct remnants). They may also be lymphatic, parasitic, traumatic or inflammatory, and are usually asymptomatic, being discovered incidentally

on routine physical examinations as a soft, non-tender abdominal mass, or detected on an abdominal X-ray because of calcification in their wall.

Retroperitoneal cysts meet the usual ultrasound criteria for simple cysts: they are smooth walled and echo free, with increased through-transmission of sound (Fig. 18.54).[3,77,78]

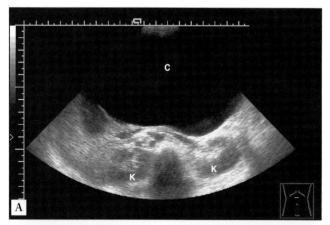

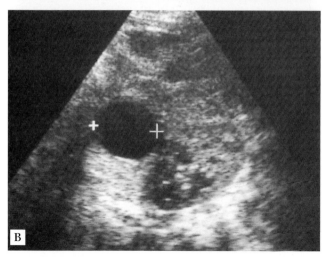

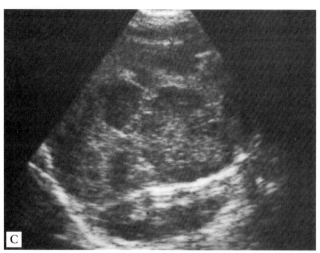

Fig. 18.54 Retroperitoneal cysts. A: A large cyst compressing the viscera posteriorly is seen in this transverse section through the epigastrium. The patient presented with abdominal swelling and a retroperitoneal cyst was removed at surgery. **B:** Transverse scan through a left intercostal space in a 4-month-old with a congenital retroperitoneal cyst. The distinction from a pancreatic cyst cannot be made on imaging, but at laparotomy the clear fluid that was aspirated had a very low amylase level. **C:** Scan through the liver showing multiple echo-poor lesions which were haemangioendotheliomas; the purpose of the laparotomy was to tie off the hepatic artery. The discovery of one developmental anomaly should prompt a careful search for others. C – cyst, K – kidney.

The absence of internal echoes helps distinguish them from abscesses, haematomas and complex cysts such as dermoids or hydatids, although a lymphangioma may consist of multiseptated cysts.[79] The history helps distinguish cysts from lymphoceles or urinomas, which are usually postoperative or follow an episode of ureteric obstruction.

The recommended treatment for retroperitoneal cysts is surgical removal, as they tend to recur after simple aspiration.

Retroperitoneal fluid collections

Retroperitoneal fluid collections tend to spread along the path of least resistance, namely between the fascial planes. Although occasionally more than one compartment is involved, or the fascia is destroyed by the disease process (e.g. in trauma), the fluid can generally be localised to a specific compartment, allowing its source to be deduced from anatomical considerations (see Fig. 18.33 and Table 18.3).[39]

Although ultrasound is reliable in detecting retroperitoneal collections it is often unhelpful in distinguishing between the types of collection, so that needle aspiration is an integral part of the examination. Subsequently ultrasound may be used to establish therapeutic drainage and to follow the progress of the lesion. Scans performed with the patient supine allow comparison between the two sides, but gas often obscures the views in this position and coronal decubitus and prone views (both transverse and longitudinal) may be more helpful.

Retroperitoneal abscesses are most commonly complications of surgery or extensions from renal, spinal or paraspinal infections (Fig. 18.55). Less often they follow septicaemia, trauma, or the perforation of an abdominal viscus such as the colon, appendix or duodenum. They often involve the psoas muscles (psoas abscess) and the perirenal spaces.[64] As elsewhere, abscesses typically have thick irregular walls, septa, layering of internal debris and, occasionally, contain diagnostic gas bubbles which may be observed floating upwards (Fig. 18.56). Large pockets of gas, although uncommon, may completely obscure views of the abscess so, where there is a clinical suspicion of a retroperitoneal abscess but a negative ultrasound, a CT scan should be performed. Gas may leak into the retroperitoneal space from a perforated viscus (typically the duodenum), where it obscures the right kidney.[80]

The psoas muscles are a relatively common site for abscess formation, tuberculosis being a common aetiology, but may also follow appendicitis, perirenal pathology and non-tuberculous bacterial spondylitis (Fig. 18.56). Clinically there is unilateral flank, hip or back pain, which is aggravated by hip extension. There may be a palpable and tender abdominal mass (particularly in children) or sometimes a lump in the anterior upper thigh. Typically there is fever, leukocytosis and a raised ESR. The radiograph may show bone destruction but this is a late and inconstant finding. Ultrasound reveals the psoas outline to be enlarged and rounded. The size and extent of the abscess can be assessed as well as its relationship to adjacent structures, particularly the kidneys and blood vessels. The muscle itself may be echo poor if the infection has spread diffusely, or may contain a localised fluid collection.

The right anterior pararenal space and the anterior perirenal fascia may become thickened and reflective as a result of extension of inflammation from retroperitoneal organs into the pararenal space. Although this is typical of acute pancreatitis, it has also been reported in association with acute cholecystitis and acute appendicitis.[64,81]

Retroperitoneal haematomas are not uncommon, especially in anticoagulated patients and those with bleeding diatheses, and in leaking abdominal aortic aneurysms (Fig. 18.57). Haematomas in the perirenal space most often follow renal trauma, whereas those in the posterior pararenal space or psoas muscle are more likely to occur spontaneously. There is a spectrum of ultrasound appearances: very fresh haematomas may be anechoic and thus difficult to differentiate from simple retroperitoneal fluid collections. A more chronic haematoma often develops complex multiseptate cystic spaces containing reflective material, which may layer and move with changes in the patient's position. Diffusely infiltrating haematomas may be very poorly defined in shape and size. A chronic haematoma may become so well organised that it cannot be distinguished from a solid mass; it may also calcify.

Table 18.3 Features of retroperitoneal collections

Compartment	Direction of movement	Renal displacement	Likely source
Perirenal	Dorsolateral to lower renal pole	Anteromedial and superior	Intrarenal infection Urine leak (hydronephrosis)
Posterior pararenal	Inferolaterally parallel to psoas	Anterior and superior	Retroperitoneal haemorrhage (bleeding diathesis, anticoagulant therapy)
Anterior pararenal	Bulges anteriorly into peritoneal cavity, displacing small bowel loops	Superior ± lateral (anterior or descending anterolaterally)	Exudates from lesions of colon, pancreas, duodenum, bile ducts, appendix or trauma. Haemorrhage from rupture of splenic or hepatic artery aneurysm

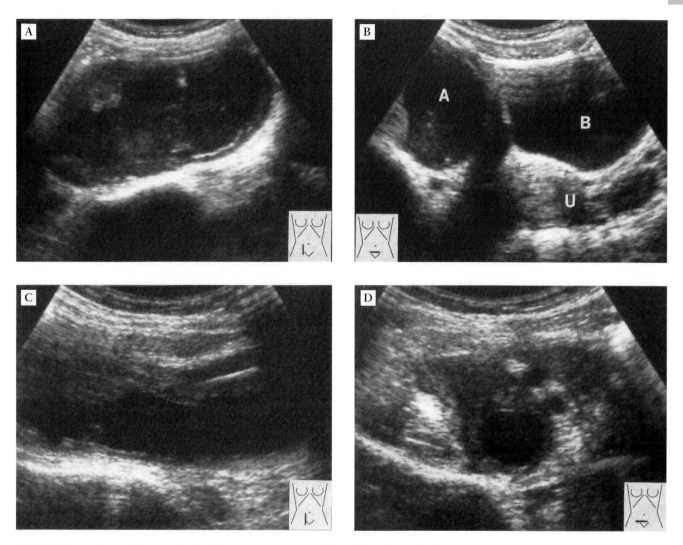

Fig. 18.55 Psoas abscess. A: Longitudinal and **B:** transverse section in the right iliac fossa. The abscess (A) is seen as a complex of fluid spaces, many with internal echoes, extending into the false pelvis. *Mycobacteria* were cultured and antituberculous drugs started. B – bladder, U – uterus. **C:** Longitudinal and **D:** transverse sections in similar positions 1 month later. The changes of organisation are seen with an increase in the solid elements.

The psoas muscle is a particular site for spontaneous retroperitoneal haemorrhage in haemophiliacs. Pain and stiffness in the flank, hip or groin are typical presenting symptoms, and flexion deformities of the hip may follow iliopsoas spasm. Large psoas haematomas may cause anorexia, constipation, fever, leukocytosis, dysuria and frequency (from pressure on the bladder), and may even mimic acute appendicitis or ureteric colic.[82] Femoral nerve entrapment can cause loss of sensation on the anterior surface of the thigh and, more seriously, paralysis of the quadriceps muscles. Early diagnosis of a psoas haematoma is particularly important in haemophiliacs as prompt treatment with factor VIII prevents femoral nerve damage. In addition to infection and haematoma, the differential diagnosis of psoas muscle enlargement includes invasion by retroperitoneal tumour and hemihypertrophy (occasionally also seen as a normal variant in young Caribbean males, when it is typically bilaterally symmetrical). It must also be differentiated from adjacent lymphadenopathy.

Urinomas and lymphoceles are mainly postoperative complications, although a urinoma may also result from urinary extravasation following ureteric obstruction (see Vol. 2, Ch. 24). Both appear as anechoic fluid spaces on ultrasound. Urinomas track along the perirenal space, following the line of the ureter, where they often produce a pattern of multiple layers representing the fluid separating the peri-ureteric tissues, whereas lymphoceles are more typically seen in the pelvis following renal transplantation (see Vol. 2, Ch. 26) or pelvic lymphadenectomy.

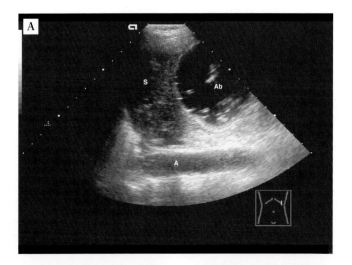

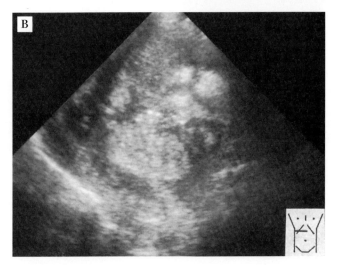
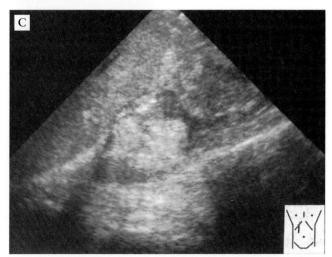

Fig. 18.56 Retroperitoneal abscess. A: A postoperative collection lying below the spleen in this left coronal section was considered suspicious for an abscess because of the intensely reflective mobile foci it contained. It was treated by guided drainage. In another case of an abscess that followed a nephrectomy, **(B)** transverse and **(C)** longitudinal sections in the right upper quadrant show a generally reflective mass that could be mistaken as a solid lesion. The intense echoes are due to multiple minute gas bubbles in the purulent fluid. A – aorta, Ab – abscess, S – spleen.

Retroperitoneal fibrosis

Retroperitoneal fibrosis is a proliferation of fibrous tissue generally confined to the central and paravertebral regions of the retroperitoneum in the perirenal space between the renal hila and the dome of the bladder.[83-86] It is typically thickest immediately anterior to the sacrum and lower lumbar spine. Rarely, extension into the mediastinum, porta hepatis and mesentery has been reported;[87] infiltration of the small bowel, uterus, vagina, bladder and rectum is also recognised.[88,89] The tissue is sharply delineated but not encapsulated. It tends to envelop rather than displace adjacent structures, such as the ureters, blood and lymphatic vessels and, rarely, bowel loops. Approximately 70% of cases are idiopathic,[83] whereas others are asso-

ciated with drugs (notably methysergide), inflammation, infection, trauma, retroperitoneal haemorrhage, and both primary and metastatic tumours. The rare association with Riedel's thyroiditis, sclerosing cholangitis and pseudotumour of the orbit suggests an immune basis in some cases. The incidence peaks in the fifth or sixth decade and it is commoner in males (2:1).

The insidious onset and progressive nature of the fibrosis make it difficult to diagnose. Presentation tends to be delayed until ureteric or vascular obstruction occurs. Symptoms are often vague and the clinical features are generally non-specific: patients present with abdominal or flank pain and tenderness, weight loss, anorexia, malaise, hypertension and renal failure. There may be scrotal or leg oedema from lymphatic obstruction. A palpable abdom-

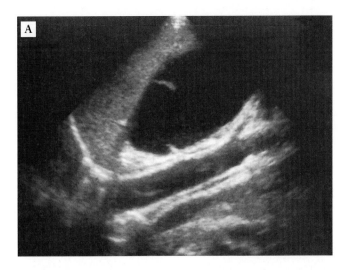

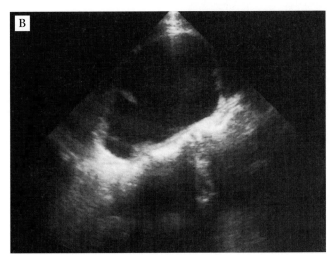
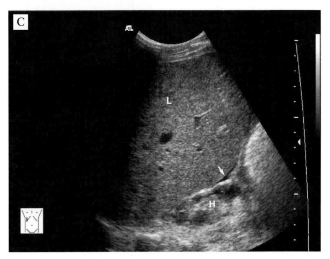

Fig. 18.57 Retroperitoneal haematoma. A and **B:** Left coronal sections showing two views of a well demarcated collection in the left para-aortic position. Note the low-level internal echoes and the septa. The bleed in this patient was from retroperitoneal metastases from a malignant melanoma. **C:** Right longitudinal section showing a post-adrenalectomy haematoma in the right adrenal bed. The relatively high level of echoes suggests organisation. Note also the trace of ascites (arrow). H – haematoma, L – liver.

inal or rectal mass is found in approximately 30%.[90] Laboratory investigations are also non-specific, with anaemia, a raised ESR and hypoalbuminaemia.

Ultrasound reveals a pre-aortic mass that is echo poor, presumably because of its homogeneous consistency, extending beyond the limits of the aorta (Fig. 18.58). It may be bulky, with an ill-defined irregular margin, or form a flat plaque with smooth margins. Adjacent solid organs such as the kidney may be displaced. Typically the plaque extends below the aortic bifurcation and across the pelvic brim.

The classic diagnostic triad of urographic findings in retroperitoneal fibrosis (upper tract dilatation with nar-

rowed and medially deviated ureters) is not entirely reliable: occasionally there is no hydronephrosis, and medial deviation of the ureters may be a normal variant,[83] so that further imaging is required when retroperitoneal fibrosis is suspected. CT is the investigation of choice to delineate the extent of the disease and to detect minimal or localised areas of fibrosis.[91] However, there is a role for ultrasound in follow-up, particularly in assessing the associated hydronephrosis. It may not always be possible to distinguish retroperitoneal fibrosis from other retroperitoneal masses such as lymphoma, sarcoma or haematoma. A needle biopsy, which can be performed under ultrasound guidance, is often needed.

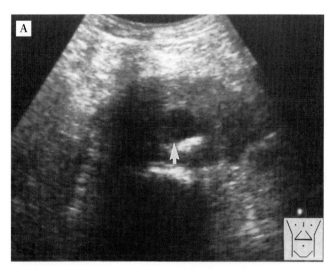
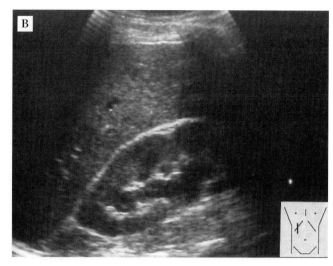

Fig. 18.58 Retroperitoneal fibrosis. A: Transverse section across the aorta (arrow) showing the echo-poor cuff of fibrous tissue which is thicker anteriorly. **B:** Right longitudinal section through the kidney showing the hydronephrosis.

REFERENCES

1 Meyer M A. Dynamic radiology of the abdomen. Normal and pathologic anatomy, 3 edn. New York: Springer Verlag, 2000

2 Weill F, Watrin J, Rohmer P et al. Ultrasound and CT of peritoneal recesses and ligaments: a pictorial essay. Ultrasound Med Biol 1986; 12: 977

3 Halvorsen R A, Thompson W M. Ascites or pleural effusion? CT and ultrasound differentiation. Crit Rev Diagn Imag 1986; 26: 201

4 Weill F, Perriguey G, Belloir A et al. Ultrasonic anatomical study of the lesser omental sac: a pictorial essay. Eur J Radiol 1983; 2: 143

5 Gerzof S G, Oates M E. Imaging techniques for infections in the surgical patient. Surg Infect 1968; 68: 147

6 Forsby J, Henriksson L. Detectability of intraperitoneal fluid by ultrasonography. Acta Radiol Diagn 1984; 25: 375

7 Dubbins P A, Kurtz A B. Intraabdominal fluid collections. In: Goldberg B B, ed. Abdominal ultrasonography 1984

8 Baker M E, Blinder R A, Rice R P. Diagnostic imaging of abdominal fluid collections and abscesses. Crit Rev Diagn Imag 1986; 25: 233

9 Paajanen H, Lahti P, Nordback I. Sensitivity of transabdominal ultrasonography in detection of intraperitoneal fluid in humans. Eur Radiol 1999; 9: 1423–1425

10 Fontaine S, Lafortune M, Breton G et al. Ascites as a cause of hyperechogenic kidneys. JCU 1985; 13: 633

11 Sanders R C. The significance of sonographic gallbladder wall thickening. JCU 1980; 8: 143

12 Fiske C E, Laing F C, Brown T W. Ultrasonographic evidence of gallbladder wall thickening in association with hypoalbuminemia. Radiology 1980; 135: 713

13 Kaftori J K, Pery M, Green J et al. Thickness of the gallbladder wall in patients with hypoalbuminemia: a sonographic study of patients on peritoneal dialysis. AJR 1987; 148: 1117

14 Tsujimoto T, Miyamoto T, Tada T. Differentiation of benign from malignant ascites by sonographic evaluation of gallbladder wall. Radiology 1985; 157: 503

15 Edell S L, Gefter W B. Ultrasonic differentiation of type of ascitic fluid. AJR 1979; 133: 111

16 Merrit C B, Williams S M. Ultrasound findings in a patient with pseudomyxoma peritonei. JCU 1978; 6: 417

17 Matsumi H, Kozuma S, Osuga Y et al. Ultrasound imaging of pseudomyxoma peritonei with numerous vesicles in ascitic fluid [letter]. Ultrasound Obstet Gynecol 1999; 13: 378–379

18 Bard C, Lafortune M, Breton G. Ascites: ultrasound guidance or blind paracentesis. Can Med Assoc J 1986; 135: 209

19 Lurie K, Plzak L, Deveney C W. Intraabdominal abscess in the 1980s. Surg Clin North Am 1988; 67: 621

20 Witzigmann H, Geissler F, Uhlmann D et al. Intra-abdominal abscess. Chirurgie 1998; 69: 813–820

21 Casola G, Vansonnenberg E. Diagnosis and percutaneous drainage of abdominal abscesses. Clin Gastroenterol 1985; 14: 469

22 Joseph A E. Imaging of abdominal abscesses. BMJ 1985; 291: 1447

23 Dobrin P B, Heer Gully P, Greenlee H B et al. Radiologic diagnosis of an intra-abdominal abscess. Arch Surg 1986; 121: 41

24 Crivello M S, Peterson I M, Austin R M. Left lobe of the liver mimicking perisplenic collection. JCU 1986; 14: 697

25 Ohara T, Itoh Y, Itoh K. Ultrasound instruments as possible vectors of staphylococcal infection. J Hosp Infect 1998; 40: 73–77

26 Tesch C, Froschle G. Sonography machines as a source of infection [letter; comment]. AJR 1997; 168: 567–568

27 Kressel H Y, Filly R A. Ultrasonographic appearance of gas-containing abscesses in the abdomen. AJR 1978; 130: 71

28 Patel S, Gopichandran T. Ultrasound evidence of gas in the fissure for the ligamentum teres: a sign of perforated duodenal ulcer. Br J Radiol 1999; 72: 901–902

29 Butler J A, Huang J, Wilson S E. Repeated laparotomy for postoperative intra-abdominal sepsis: an analysis of outcome predictors. Arch Surg 1987; 122: 702

30 Walters R, Herman C M, Neff R et al. Percutaneous drainage of abscesses in the postoperative abdomen that is difficult to explore. Am J Surg 1985; 149: 623

31 Brooke Jeffrey R, Wing V W, Laing F C. Real-time sonographic monitoring of percutaneoius abscess drainage. AJR 1985; 469

32 Worthen N J, Gunning J E. Percutaneous drainage of pelvic abscesses: management of the tubo-ovarian abscess. J Ultrasound Med 1986; 5: 551–556

33 Cadotte R N, Rankin R N. Percutaneous drainage and aspiration of fluid collections: emphasis on pancreatic collections and transplant patients. J Can Assoc Radiol 1988; 39: 121

34 Pruett T L, Rotstein O D, Crass J. Percutaneous aspiration and drainage for suspected abdominal infection. Surgery 1984; 96: 731

35 Jansen M, Truong S N, Sparenberg P et al. Ultrasound-controlled, percutaneous drainage: a safe and simple method for treatment of intra-abdominal abscesses. Langenbecks Arch Chir 1997; 114: 1205–1206

36 Rozycki G. Abdominal ultrasonography in trauma. Surg Clin North Am 1995; 75: 175–191

37 Shanmuganathan K, Mirvis S, Sherbourne C et al. Hemoperitoneum as the sole indicator of abdominal visceral injuries: a potential limitation of screening abdominal US for trauma. Radiology 1999; 212: 423–430

38 Belli A M, Joseph A E. The renal rind sign: a new ultrasound indication of inflammatory disease in the abdomen. Br J Radiol 1988; 61: 806–810

39 Meyers M A, Whalen J P, Peele K. Radiological features of extraperitoneal effusions. Radiology 1972; 104: 249–257

40 Raptopoulos V, Kleinman P K, Marks S, Snyder M, Silverman P M. Renal fascial pathway: posterior extension of pancreatic effusions within the anterior pararenal space. Radiology 1986; 158: 367–374

41 Raskin M. Combination of CT and ultrasound in the examination of the retroperitoneum and pelvis. Crit Rev Diag Imag 1980; 13: 173–228

42 Callen P W, Filly R A, Sarti D A, Sample W F. Ultrasonography of the diaphragmatic crura. Radiology 1979; 130: 721–724

43 Lev-Toaff A, Goldberg B. Gastrointestinal ultrasound contrast. In: Ultrasound contrast agents. London: Martin Dunitz, 1997

44 Pardes J G, Auh Y H, Kneeland J B. The oblique coronal view in sonography of the retroperitoneum. AJR 1985; 144: 1241–1247

45 Creagh-Barry M, Adam E J, Joseph A E. The value of oblique scans in the ultrasonic examination of the abdominal aorta. Clin Radiol 1986; 37: 239–241

46 Grunebaum M, Ziv N, Kornreich L. The sonographic evaluation of the great vessels' interspace in the pediatric retroperitoneum. Pediatr Radiol 1986; 16: 384–387

47 Dietrich C F, Zeuzem S, Caspary W F, Wehrmann T. Ultrasound lymph node imaging in the abdomen and retroperitoneum of healthy probands. Ultraschall Med 1998; 19: 265–269

48 LaRoy L L, Cormier P J, Matalon T A, Patel S K, Turner D A, Silver B. Imaging of abdominal aortic aneurysms. AJR 1989; 152: 785–792

49 Grimshaw G M, Thompson J M. Changes in diameter of the abdominal aorta with age: an epidemiological study. JCU 1997; 25: 7–13

50 Jaakkola P, Hippelainen M, Farin P, Rytkonen H, Kainulainen S, Partanen K. Interobserver variability in measuring the dimensions of the abdominal aorta: comparison of ultrasound and computed tomography. Eur J Vasc Endovasc Surg 1996; 12: 230–237

51 Leopold G R, Goldberger L E, Bernstein E F. Ultrasonic detection and evaluation of abdominal aortic aneurysms. Surgery 1980; 72: 939–945

52 Mittlestaed C A, Vascular Ultrasound, in 6. 1987. Abdominal ultrasound: Mittlestaed, CA. 441–580

53 King P S, Cooperberg P L, Madigan S M. The anechoic crescent in abdominal aortic aneurysms: not a sign of dissection. AJR 1986; 146: 345–458

54 Bondestam S, Hekali P, Landtman M. Sonographic diagnosis of dissection of the descending thoracic aorta. Ann Chir Gynaecol 1981; 70: 210–212

55 Schopp D, Wimmer B. Current diagnosis of dissecting aortic aneurysm. Radiology 1989: 237–244

56 Williams D M, Lee D Y, Hamilton B H et al. The dissected aorta: part III. Anatomy and radiologic diagnosis of branch-vessel compromise. Radiology 1997; 203: 37–44

57 Lee D Y, Williams D M, Abrams G D. The dissected aorta: part II. Differentiation of the true from the false lumen with intravascular US. Radiology 1997; 203: 32–36

58 Voci P. Opacification of the thoracic aorta after venous injection of sonicated albumin microbubbles. Implications for aortic dissection. Cardiologia 1997; 42: 299–304

59 Harter L P, Gross B H, Callen P W, Barth R A. Ultrasonic evaluation of abdominal aortic thrombus. J Ultrasound Med 1982; 1: 315–318

60 Gooding G A, Effeney D J, Goldstone J. The aortofemoral graft: detection and identification of healing complications by ultrasonography. Surgery 1981; 29: 94–101

61 Sato D T, Goff C D, Gregory R T et al. Endoleak after aortic stent graft repair: diagnosis by color duplex ultrasound scan versus computed tomography scan. J Vasc Surg 1998; 28: 657–663

62 White R A, Donayre C, Kopchok G, Walot I, Wilson E, de Virgilio C. Intravascular ultrasound: the ultimate tool for abdominal aortic aneurysm assessment and endovascular graft delivery. J Endovasc Surg 1997; 4: 45–55

63 Katzarski K S, Nisell J, Randmaa I, Danielsson A, Freyschuss U, Bergstrom J. A critical evaluation of ultrasound measurement of inferior vena cava diameter in assessing dry weight in normotensive and hypertensive hemodialysis patients [see comments]. Am J Kidney Dis 1997; 30: 459–465

64 Koenigsberg M et al. Sonographic evaluation of the retroperitoneum. Semin Ultrasound 1982; 3: 79–95

65 Applegate K, Goske M, Pierce G, Murphy D. Situs revisited: imaging of the heterotaxy syndrome. Radiographics 1999; 19: 837–852

66 Cavanna L, Civardi G, Vallisa D. Ultrasound image of massive inferior vena cava thrombosis causing asymptomatic subclinical disseminated intravascular coagulation. Haematologica 1998; 83: 1041–1042

67 Yeh H C. Adrenal gland and non-renal retroperitoneum. Urol Radiol 1987; 9: 127–140

68 Felix E L et al. Tumours of the retroperitoneum. Curr Probl Cancer 1981; 6: 3–47

69 Jacobsen S, Juul-Jorgensen P. Primary retroperitoneal tumours. Acta Chir Scand 1974; 140: 498–500

70 Davidson A J, Hartman D S. Imaging strategies for tumors of the kidney, adrenal gland, and retroperitoneum. Cancer 1987; 37: 151–164

71 Kryger-Baggesen N, Kjaergaard J, Sehested M. Nonchromaffin paraganglionoma of the retroperitoneum. J Urol 1985; 134: 536–537

72 Goldman S M, Davidson A J, Neal J. Retroperitoneal and pelvic haemangiopericytomas: clinical, radiologic and pathologic correlation. Radiology 1988; 168: 13–17

73 Goldman S M, Hartman D S, Weiss S W. The varied radiographic manifestations of retroperitoneal malignant fibrous histiocytoma revealed through 27 cases. J Urol 1986; 135: 33–38

74 Skaane P. The right iliac fossa features of a large retroperitoneal liposarcoma. Fortschr Rontgenstr 1986; 145: 351–353

75 Bertolotto M, Cittadini G Jr, Crespi G, Perrone C, Pastorino R. Hemangiopericytoma of the greater omentum: US and CT appearance. Eur Radiol 1996; 6: 454–456

76 Davidson A J, Hartman D S, Goldman S M. Mature teratoma of the retroperitoneum. Radiologic, pathologic and clinical correlation. Radiology 1990; 172: 421–425

77 Derchi L E. Rizzatto G, Banderali A, Sala P, Larghero G C, Solbiati L. Sonographic appearance of primary retroperitoneal cysts, J Ultrasound Med 1989; 8: 381–384

78 Kehagias D T, Karvounis E E, Fotopoulos A, Gouliamos A D. Retroperitoneal mucinous cystadenoma. Eur J Obstet Gynecol Reprod Biol 1999; 82: 213–215

79 Davidson A J, Hartman D S. Lymphangioma of the retroperitoneum: CT and sonographic characteristic. Radiology 1990; 175: 507–510

80 McWilliams R G, Blakeborough A, Johnson M I, Weston M. Case report: The 'veiled right kidney sign' – an ultrasound finding in retroperitoneal perforation of the duodenum. Br J Radiol 1996; 69: 1061–1063

81 Hoddick W, Jeffrey R B, Goldberg H I, Federle M P, Laing F C. CT and sonography of severe renal and perirenal infections. AJR 1983; 140: 517–520

82 Kumari S, Pillari G, Phillips G, Pochachaczevsky R. Fluid collections of the psoas in children. Semin Ultrasound 1982; 3: 139–155

83 Fagan C J, Amparo E G, Davis M. Retroperitoneal fibrosis. Semin Ultrasound 1982; 3: 123–138

84 Sanders R C, Duffy T, McLoughlin M G, Walsh P C. Sonography in the diagnosis of retroperitoneal fibrosis. J Urol 1977; 118: 944–946

85 Gilkeson G S, Allen N B. Retroperitoneal fibrosis. A true connective tissue disease. Rheum Dis Clin North Am 1996; 22: 23–38

86 Kottra J J, Dunnick N R. Retroperitoneal fibrosis. Radiol Clin North Am 1996; 34: 1259–1275

87 Arger P H, Stolz J L, Miller W T. Retroperitoneal fibrosis: an analysis of the clinical spectrum and roentgenographic signs. AJR 1973; 119: 812–821

88 Coleman P K. Radiologic/pathologic correlation conference. Case 15: abdominal mass in a 73 year old man. Appl Radiol 1980; 12: 121–126

89 Kittredge R D, Nash A D. The many facets of sclerosing fibrosis. AJR 1974; 122: 288

90 Fagan C J, Larrieu A J, Amparo E G. Retroperitoneal fibrosis: ultrasound and CT features. AJR 1979; 133: 239–243

91 Brooks A P. Computed tomography of idiopathic retroperitoneal fibrosis ('periaortitis'): variants, variations, patterns and pitfalls. Clin Radiol 1990; 4: 75–79

The adrenals

Keith C Dewbury

Introduction

Demonstration of the normal adrenal glands and small adrenal lesions remains a challenge for abdominal ultrasound. These small organs are high in location, deep within the ribcage and adjacent to the vertebrae. They are, therefore, easily obscured by the ribs, transverse processes and by stomach and bowel gas. A clear understanding of the anatomy and careful technique are essential to show them. Successful demonstration of the normal glands was reported by Sample in 1977[1] and by Yeh in 1980.[2] Both authors used static grey scale equipment and achieved high success rates of about 80% for the right adrenal gland and rather less for the left gland. These results were not universally achieved and computed tomography became preeminent for the routine examination of the adrenals.[3–6] The routine availability of real-time ultrasound equipment with its ease and flexibility of use, particularly for intercostal scanning, has rekindled interest in adrenal ultrasound imaging. The progressive technical improvements in transducers, and particularly beam focusing capabilities, have led to a further reappraisal of the situation. There can be no doubt that routine visualisation of the adrenal glands during abdominal ultrasound is now commonplace and worthwhile.[7]

The normal adrenal gland

The adrenal glands are a pair of rather small, flat organs lying anteromedial to the upper pole of the kidneys, extending partly over the kidneys.

Each gland consists of three parts: an anteromedial ridge from which two thin wings extend posteriorly. These are the lateral and medial wings which straddle the anteromedial aspect of the upper pole of the kidney. The general shape of the glands is illustrated diagrammatically in Figure 19.1.

The right adrenal gland is triangular or pyramidal in shape. The medial wing is largest superiorly and may be absent inferiorly; the opposite is true of the lateral wing. The anteromedial ridge of the gland is located immediately posterior to the inferior vena cava (IVC). It lies between

the crus of the diaphragm and the posteromedial margin of the right lobe of the liver.

The left adrenal gland is more crescentic in shape and more cranial than the right. The anteromedial ridge of the gland may be slightly convex in outline and the lateral and medial wings are shorter than on the right. The gland lies lateral or slightly posterior to the aorta and lateral to the left crus of the diaphragm. It is posterior to the lesser sac superiorly and posterior to the pancreas inferiorly. As on the right, the adrenal is anteromedial to the upper pole of the kidney. The bulk of the adrenal gland is composed of the adrenal cortex with a thin central medulla. The glands are 3–6 cm in overall length and 2–3 cm in width but only 2–6 mm in thickness.

Scanning technique and normal appearances

The position of the adrenals as described (Fig. 19.2A) dictates an intercostal approach using the acoustic window of the liver on the right and the spleen on the left. Figure 19.2B diagrammatically illustrates the preferred scanning approach with the patient lying supine. For the right side the transducer is placed in the ninth or tenth intercostal space in the mid or anterior axillary line. Scanning transversely the transducer is gently rotated to move the field of view from the renal hilum upwards to a few centimetres above the kidney, concentrating on the region behind the IVC and lateral to the right diaphragmatic crus. The adrenal area will be completely covered in such a sequence. In the upper transverse section on the right a vertical linear or curvilinear structure corresponding to the anteromedial ridge and medial wing is seen. In the middle section both wings are seen as an inverted 'V' or 'Y' (Fig. 19.3). Through the inferior portion of the gland only the lateral wing may be seen as a horizontal band. Coronal or longitudinal sections are obtained by rotating the transducer through 90°. The upper pole of the right kidney is located and the transducer angled medially. Both wings of the gland may be simultaneously displayed as a thin, long inverted 'V'- or 'Y'-shaped structure up to 6 cm in length (Fig. 19.4). A further small medial angulation is necessary to visualise the anteromedial ridge of the gland in this plane where it lies posterior to the IVC (Fig. 19.5).

The left adrenal gland is more difficult to image because of the smaller acoustic window available through the spleen. The transducer is placed on the eighth or ninth intercostal space in the posterior axillary line, avoiding stomach or bowel gas, to give a coronal scan. The upper pole of the kidney should first be located through the spleen. A small angulation of the transducer towards the anterior aspect of the kidney will demonstrate the left adrenal gland in the perirenal space between spleen, kidney and left diaphragmatic crus. This is best recognised

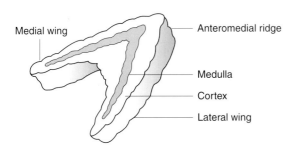

Fig. 19.1 Anatomy of the adrenals. Diagrammatic representation of the general shape and make-up of the adrenal gland.

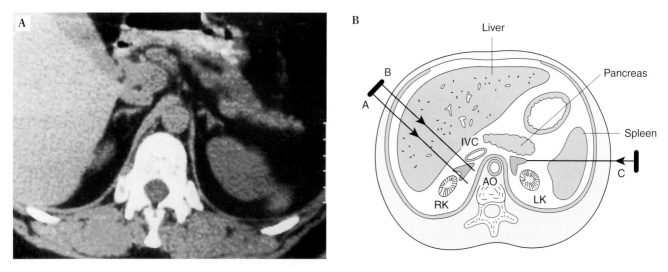

Fig. 19.2 Anatomy of the adrenals. A: CT scan showing the position of the normal adrenal glands. **B:** Diagrammatic section taken at the same level as the CT scan to show the ideal scanning approach to the two sides. Scan lines A and B will show the wings and anteromedial ridge of the right gland respectively. Scan line C through the spleen will show the left adrenal gland.

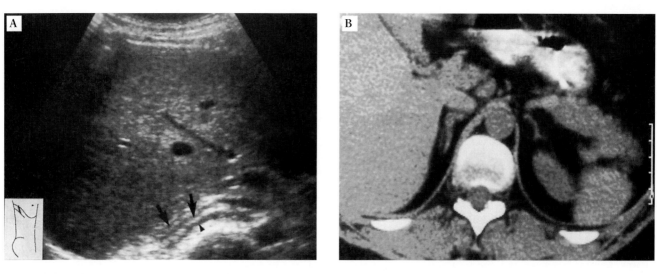

Fig. 19.3 Right adrenal – transverse sections. A: A slightly oblique transverse view through a right intercostal space showing both wings of the adrenal gland (arrows) lying parallel to the diaphragmatic crus (arrowhead). **B:** CT scan at the corresponding level.

when both wings are shown, displaying the characteristic 'V' shape (Fig. 19.6). A transverse section is obtained by rotating the transducer through 90°. Because of the relative difficulty in demonstrating the left adrenal gland, additional views in right lateral decubitus and erect positions may be helpful. With high resolution real-time scanning, the right adrenal gland is demonstrated in 92% of patients and the left gland in 71%.[7]

The adrenal cortex appears echo-poor on ultrasound. The medulla is regularly seen as a thin reflective structure in the centre of the cortex in up to 13% of adults (Fig. 19.7).[7] This is a particularly prominent feature in the neonatal or

fetal adrenal gland (Fig. 19.8). At birth the neonatal adrenal cortex is relatively thick and is composed of two layers: the thick fetal zone occupying 80% of the gland and the thin peripheral zone that becomes the adult cortex.[8] The fetal cortex synthesises most of the precursors for maternal oestrogens and is one of the main consumers of placental progesterone. It involutes after birth. The neonatal adrenal gland is readily visualised for several reasons:

1   The infant gland is proportionally larger. At birth it is one-third of the size of the kidney for which it can be mistaken if the kidney does not lie in its normal

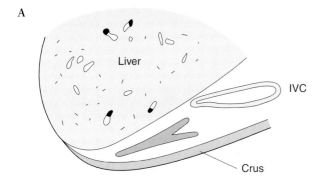

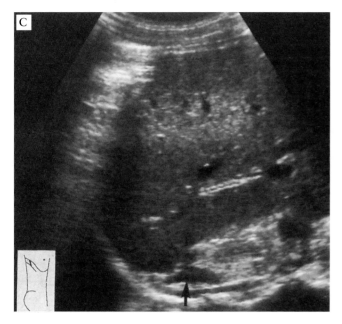

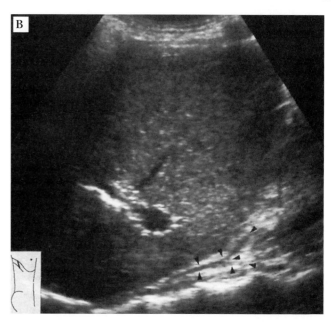

Fig. 19.4 Right adrenal – coronal sections. A: Diagrammatic representation of the shape and appearance of the right adrenal gland shown on a coronal section. **B:** Corresponding ultrasound section where both wings of the gland are displayed as a long inverted 'Y'-shaped structure lying above the diaphragmatic crus. **C:** A similar section in another patient shows the gland to be more 'V' shaped and with rather bulkier limbs.

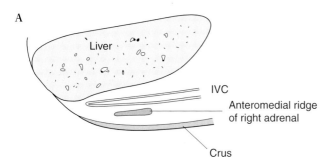

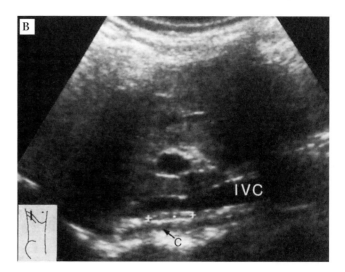

Fig. 19.5 Right adrenal – coronal sections. A: Diagrammatic representation of the position and appearance of the anteromedial ridge of the right adrenal gland lying sandwiched between the IVC and the diaphragmatic crus. **B:** Corresponding ultrasound section (c – crus). Small crosses mark the position of the anteromedial ridge.

A

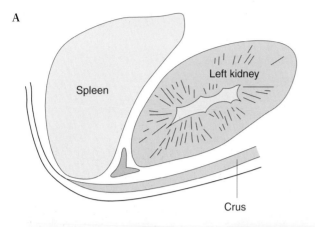

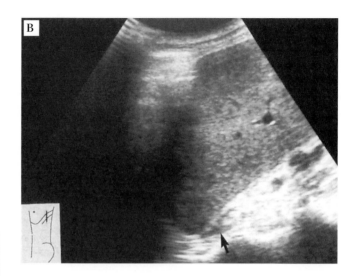

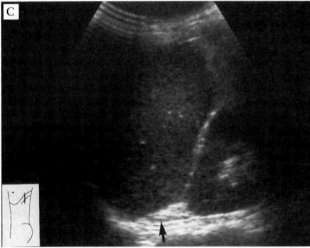

Fig. 19.6 Left adrenal – coronal section. A: Diagrammatic representation of a coronal view of the left adrenal gland. **B and C:** Corresponding ultrasound sections in different patients mirroring this appearance (arrows).

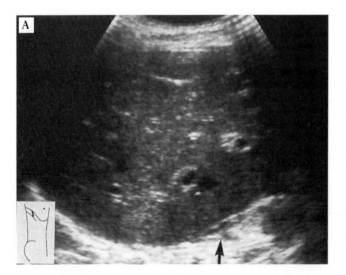

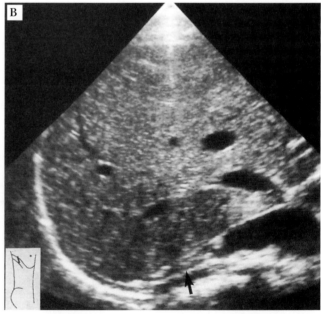

Fig. 19.7 Structure of the adrenal gland. A and B: Views of the right adrenal gland (arrow) in two adults clearly showing the distinction between cortex and medulla.

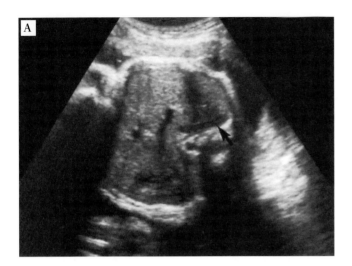

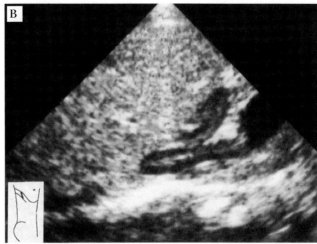

Fig. 19.8 Fetal and neonatal adrenal. A: Transverse scan through the fetal abdomen at 32 weeks of gestation. The right adrenal gland is well visualised (arrow) with clear distinction between cortex and medulla. **B:** Coronal view of the right adrenal gland in a neonate which shows the relatively large size of the gland at this age and the marked contrast between cortex which has a low reflectivity and the central medulla having a high reflectivity.

position. During the first week of life, the adrenal reduces in size.[8]

2   The small amount of perirenal fat in neonates allows for better resolution.

3   The small size of the subject means that higher frequency transducers are routinely used, further optimising overall resolution.[9]

The contours of the normal adrenal glands are straight or concave and convexity should be regarded with suspicion. It is important to examine the whole of each gland since small masses may affect only part of the gland leaving the remainder with a normal appearance.

Congenital anomalies

Agenesis

Unilateral adrenal agenesis is described[10] but is rare. The contralateral gland will characteristically show compensatory hypertrophy. Bilateral renal agenesis is not compatible with life but has also been described.

Hyperplasia (adrenogenital syndromes)

Congenital adrenal hyperplasia is an autosomal recessive disorder due to an inborn error of metabolism. A number of syndromes are described;[11] the most common are termed 'adrenogenital syndromes' and demonstrate clinical manifestations of virilisation. Ultrasound is useful in assessing adrenal size in this situation.

Discoid adrenal (renal agenesis)

The adrenal gland is normally present in patients with renal agenesis. The absence of the kidney may be associ-

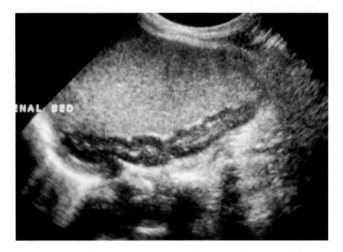

Fig. 19.9 Discoid left adrenal (left renal agenesis). A longitudinal scan in the left flank in a neonate. There is left renal agenesis. The flattened elongated left adrenal gland is well visualised through the spleen. Note the pronounced corticomedullary differentiation.

ated with the loss of the normal folding of the adrenal gland into a medial and lateral wing. The gland becomes flattened and elongated, producing a typical discoid shape. This may be particularly well seen in neonates when the gland is proportionally larger and the zonal architecture is still seen (Fig. 19.9).

Pathology

Adrenal cystic lesions

The most common adrenal cyst is an endothelial cyst, accounting for nearly half of all reported cases.[12] These are mostly lymphangiomatous in origin but some are

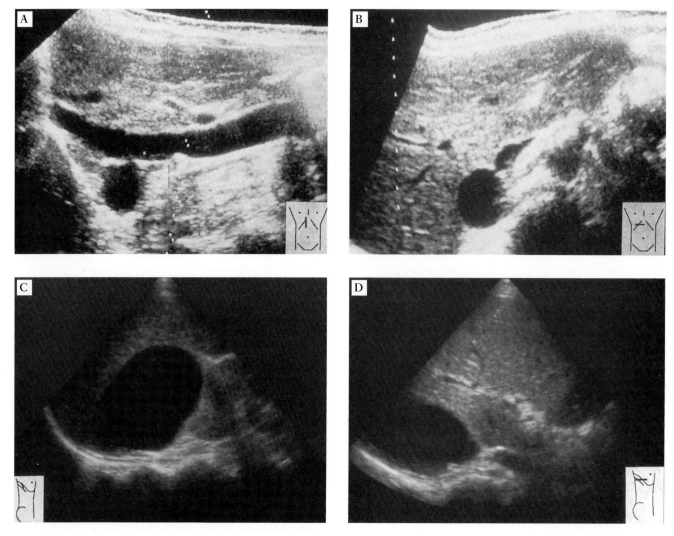

Fig. 19.10 Adrenal cysts. A: Longitudinal and **B:** transverse scans showing a 2.5 cm right adrenal cyst. **C** and **D:** Intercostal views of the right adrenal gland showing a larger adrenal cyst. Note the clear plane between the cyst and the upper pole of the kidney.

angiomatous. Some adrenal cysts are sequelae of haemorrhage or epithelial glandular cysts. Occasionally, the cyst wall may calcify. Adrenal cysts are rarely symptomatic, most being encountered as incidental findings (Fig. 19.10) which do not require active intervention.[13]

Adrenal haemorrhage

The large adrenal gland of the neonate undergoes a marked reduction in size following birth. The vessels in the primitive adrenal cortex become distended and are prone to haemorrhage. The exact cause of haemorrhage in neonates is unknown, but stress and birth trauma, anoxia and systemic disease are all implicated. Infants usually present within 2–7 days of birth (Fig. 19.11). Haemorrhage is more commonly seen on the right side although up to 10% are bilateral.[14–16]

In adults the hypertrophic adrenal gland caused by adrenocorticotrophic hormome (ACTH) therapy or severe stress may also be more prone to haemorrhage. Sepsis secondary to meningococcal infection and anticoagulant therapy may also predispose to haemorrhage. The resulting adrenal haematoma is usually echo-free, but may be more reflective due to fibrin strand formation as resolution occurs (Fig. 19.12). The haematoma may resolve, calcify or remain as a residual adrenal cyst.[14]

Adrenal tumours

It is most common for adrenal tumours to enlarge the adrenal gland focally, although diffuse enlargement may occur. A focal mass is usually oval or round and may vary in size from 0.5 to 20 cm. A small adrenal mass is easier to delineate than the normal adrenal gland because its

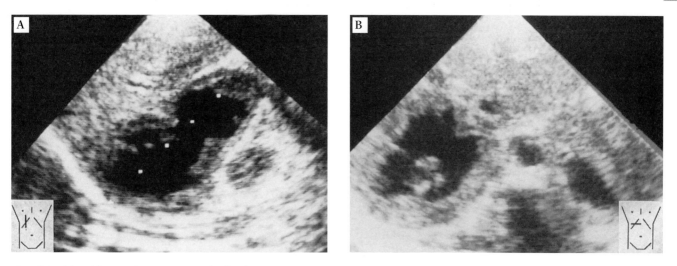

Fig. 19.11 Adrenal haemorrhage. A: Longitudinal and **B:** transverse scans in a neonate showing a large lobular right adrenal haemorrhage. This has a low reflectivity overall with a slightly irregular wall and a few centrally placed high-level echoes.

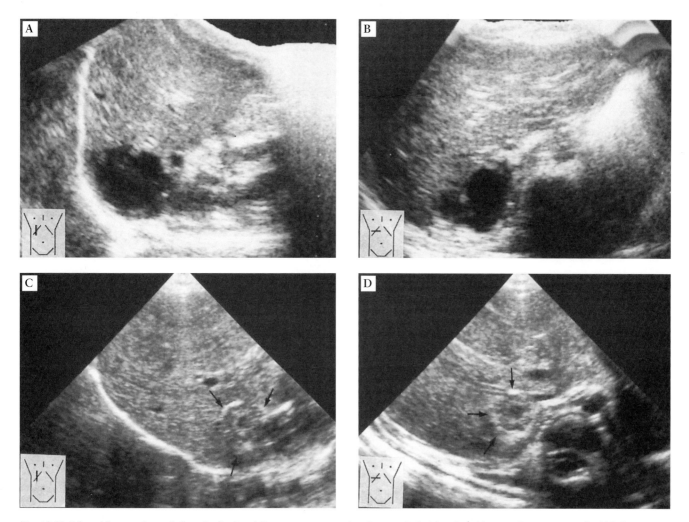

Fig. 19.12 Adrenal haemorrhage. A: Longitudinal and **B:** transverse scans showing a typical right adrenal haemorrhage in a 6-week-old baby. **C** and **D:** Longitudinal and transverse scans taken 2 months later showing almost complete resolution of the haemorrhage which is now replaced by an area of higher reflectivity with the suggestion of a peripheral calcific rim (arrows).

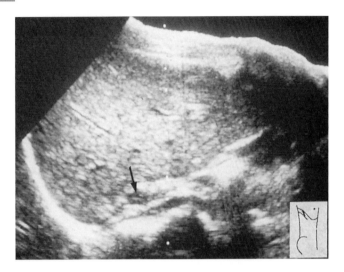

Fig. 19.13 Adenoma. An oblique scan showing a tiny echo-poor mass arising within one limb of the right adrenal gland. This measures <1 cm in diameter. It proved to be a small Conn's tumour.

diameter usually exceeds that of the adrenal. Its overall reflectivity is low, in contrast to the high reflectivity of the surrounding fat (Fig. 19.13). Ultrasound has been reported to have an overall accuracy of 95% in the evaluation of adrenal masses.[17] Even when a normal adrenal gland is not visualised, if the adrenal area is thoroughly scanned and no mass can be identified, tumour can be fairly confidently excluded.[18] To differentiate an adrenal from a renal mass, a separating interface must be demonstrated (Fig. 19.14). A right adrenal tumour typically compresses or displaces the IVC forwards (Fig. 19.15).[19] A large adrenal tumour usually displaces the upper pole of the kidney laterally or the whole kidney inferiorly.

Occasionally, the tumour may extend downwards anterior to the kidney without much displacement (Fig. 19.16). Larger masses may indent liver or kidney. While smaller tumours are usually fairly homogeneous, focal areas of necrosis or haemorrhage are more likely to occur in larger masses. This produces heterogeneity (Fig. 19.17).[19]

Cortical adenoma

These tumours are common incidental findings, being reported in up to 2% of adult autopsies. While most are non-steroid producing, they may be part of an endocrine neoplastic syndrome (MEN type 2). They are usually small, 1–2 cm in diameter (Fig. 19.18).[20]

Carcinoma

Adrenal carcinomas in children usually produce steroids and are associated with one of the hyperadrenal syndromes. In adults, adrenal carcinomas are only rarely endocrinologically active and are therefore large and commonly have invaded the adrenal vein and IVC by the time they present (Fig. 19.19). Nodal and blood-borne metastases are common.[20]

Myelolipoma

Adrenal myelolipoma is a rare cortical tumour composed of varying proportions of fat and bone marrow elements.[21] There is no malignant potential and the lesions are endocrinologically non-functioning. On ultrasound these rare tumours are characteristically highly reflective, which may confirm the fatty nature of the lesion (Fig. 19.20).[22,23]

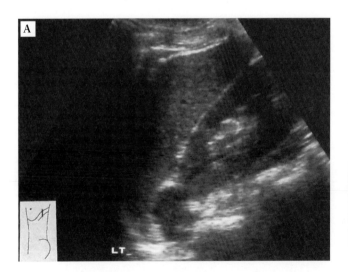
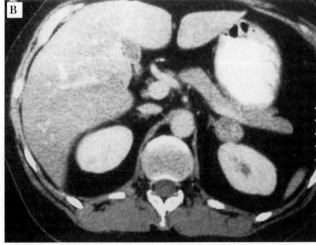

Fig. 19.14 Adrenal mass. A: Coronal ultrasound view of the left adrenal gland and kidney. There is a very well defined 2 cm mass in the left adrenal gland. Clear separation from the left kidney is shown. **B:** Corresponding CT scan.

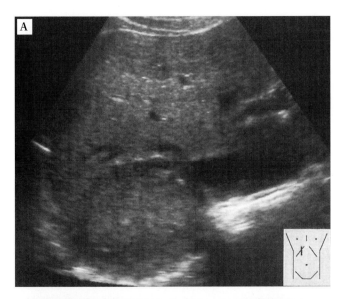

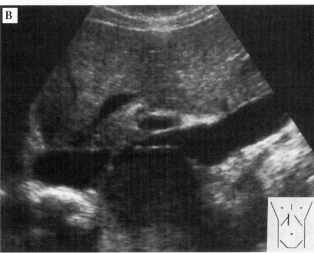

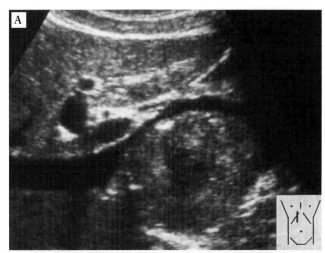

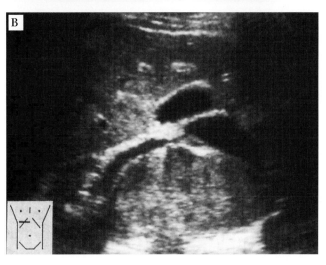

Fig. 19.16 Adrenal tumour. A: Longitudinal and **B:** transverse scans showing a relatively homogeneous right adrenal tumour which is causing anterior displacement and bowing of the IVC. The tumour has extended downwards anterior to the kidney producing very little renal displacement. In the transverse section the bowing of the renal vessels is well shown.

Fig. 19.15 Adrenal tumour. A: Longitudinal and **B:** oblique views showing a 5 cm mass in the right adrenal gland causing marked anterior bowing of the posterior wall of the IVC. The IVC has been compressed by the tumour.

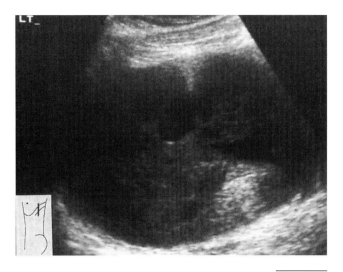

Fig. 19.17 Adrenal metastasis. Coronal view of a large left adrenal metastasis. The tumour mass is heterogeneous. This is a typical pattern, often seen as tumours increase in size.

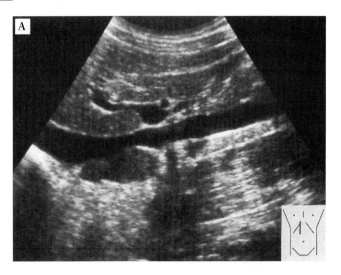
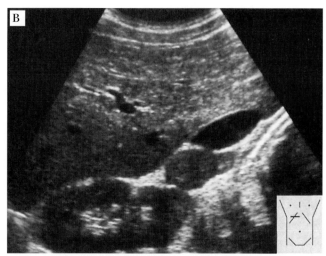

Fig. 19.18 Adrenal adenoma. A: Longitudinal and **B:** transverse scans showing two small, rounded masses in the right adrenal gland. The upper and more medial mass measures under 1 cm in diameter and the inferior and more laterally placed mass about 2 cm in diameter. Note the characteristic position behind the IVC which is slightly bowed by the small cortical adenoma.

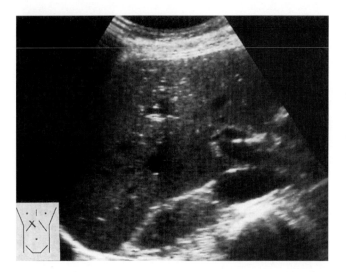
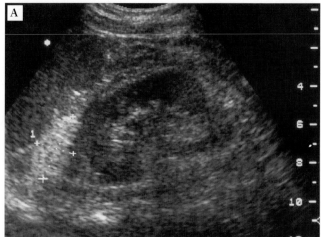
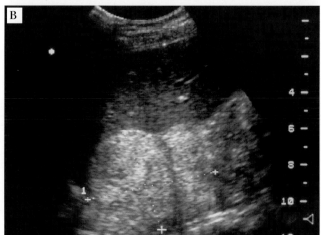

Fig. 19.19 Adrenal carcinoma. Oblique scan showing a moderate-sized right adrenal carcinoma. This has a relatively uniform reflectivity and its typical position tucked posterior to the IVC is clearly shown.

Fig. 19.20 Myelolipoma (bilateral). A: Longitudinal scan through the right kidney and adrenal showing a typical highly reflective adrenal mass. **B:** Longitudinal scan in the left flank in the same patient showing a 7.6 cm highly reflective adrenal mass typical of a fatty tumour.

Phaeochromocytoma

Phaeochromocytomas are uncommon tumours occurring in up to 1% of patients with hypertension. The majority arise within the chromaffin cells of the adrenal medulla but up to 10% arise in the autonomic nervous tissue, particularly in the organs of Zuckerkandl.[24,25] The majority of phaeochromocytomas are benign but 5–10% are malignant and up to 5% are multiple. Multiple lesions are frequently associated with various hereditary syndromes, e.g. Sipple's syndrome and von Hippel–Lindau syndrome. The clinical presentation is typically with paroxysmal hypertension. The diagnosis may be confirmed by biochemical assay for catecholamines in the urine.[25] Phaeochromocytomas may present when small (<2 cm in diameter; Fig. 19.21) or when larger. Typically, when small they are well-defined round or oval masses with a uniform reflectivity. Larger tumours frequently undergo necrosis or haemorrhage with loss of homogeneity (Fig. 19.22).

Neuroblastoma

The neuroblastoma is one of the most common tumours of childhood with 80% occurring in children under 5 years of age and one-third under 2 years of age. Under 1 year of age the tumour may spontaneously regress or differentiate into a ganglioneuroma.[25] The great majority of neuroblastomas arise in the adrenal medullary tissue, but the posterior mediastinum is the second most common site. The clinical presentation of neuroblastoma is related to its rapid growth and its secretions. There may be generalised debility with weight loss and fever. An abdominal mass may be palpable. Most tumours produce catecholamines.

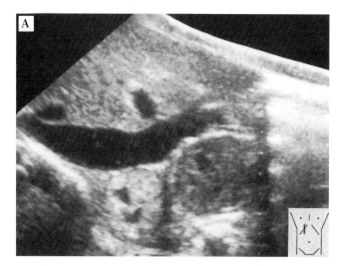

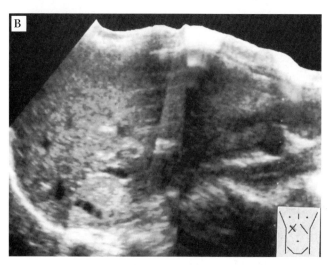

Fig. 19.22 Phaeochromocytoma. A: Longitudinal and B: oblique scans showing a 3 cm phaeochromocytoma of the right adrenal gland. Note the slightly high reflectivity of the main tumour mass with small central echo-poor necrotic areas. This is a typical pattern of phaeochromocytomas.

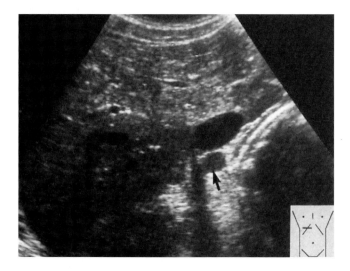

Fig. 19.21 Phaeochromocytoma. Transverse scan showing a tiny phaeochromocytoma only 1 cm in diameter lying posterior to the IVC and on the diaphragmatic crus.

Up to three-quarters of patients have metastases at the time of presentation.[25] Neuroblastoma is often well demonstrated by ultrasound and must be distinguished from the other common childhood abdominal tumour, the Wilms' tumour (see Vol. 2, Ch. 49). Neuroblastomas are typically heterogeneous with areas of high reflectivity which may represent calcification and areas of lower reflectivity (Figs 19.23 and 19.24). The margins of the tumour are ill-defined. Neuroblastoma will often cross the midline (Fig. 19.25).[26] It is important to delineate the relationship of the mass to the IVC and aorta before surgery is planned. Ultrasound is particularly valuable in the follow-up of those children who undergo chemotherapy to monitor the response of the tumour.

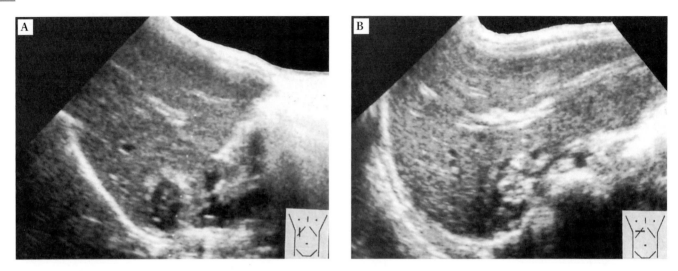

Fig. 19.23 Neuroblastoma. A: Longitudinal and **B:** transverse scans of a right neuroblastoma. This shows the typical appearances of marked heterogeneity and areas of high reflectivity within and on the periphery of the tumour, which lies above the right kidney as shown on the longitudinal scan.

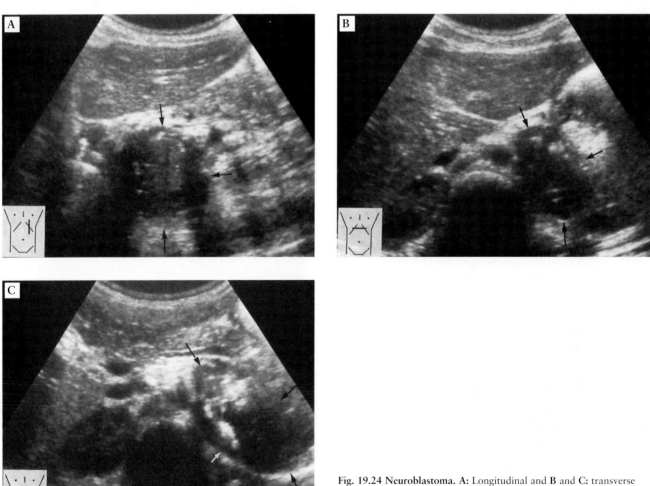

Fig. 19.24 Neuroblastoma. A: Longitudinal and **B** and **C:** transverse scans through the upper abdomen of a 3-year-old child showing a left neuroblastoma (arrows). Note the marked heterogeneity of the tumour with areas of very high reflectivity within the tumour mass.

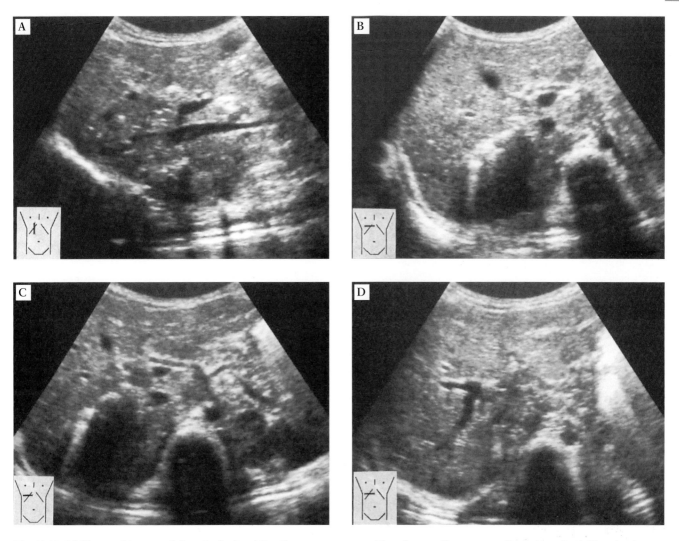

Fig. 19.25 Calcific neuroblastoma. A: Longitudinal and **B** to **D:** transverse scans with each succeeding scan at a slightly lower level. There is a large right neuroblastoma which contains calcification with distal acoustic shadowing. The tumour has infiltrated diffusely across the midline, around the coeliac axis and up towards the hilum of the liver. The tumour margins are extremely poorly defined. This pattern of extension of neuroblastoma around the IVC and aorta is typical and a more precise delineation may often be made with CT.

Adrenal metastases

The adrenal glands are the fourth most common site in the body for metastases after the lungs, liver and bones. Common primaries to metastasise to the adrenals include bronchial and breast carcinomas. The adrenals are also commonly involved with non-Hodgkin's lymphoma. Metastases are usually rounded or oval and poorly reflective.[27-29] Visualisation of both adrenal areas should be part of the routine assessment of any patient with primary malignancy (Fig. 19.26). Imaging alone will not differentiate between a metastasis and a benign adenoma and colour Doppler ultrasound is not helpful in this differentiation.[30,31]

Diffuse adrenal enlargement

Diffuse adrenal enlargement may occur in diffuse bilateral hyperplasia in conditions such as Cushing's syndrome. In most patients the enlargement will be slight and this is extremely difficult to detect with confidence using ultrasound. When the glands are significantly enlarged, demonstration of the medulla allows differentation of hyperplasia from a diffuse infiltrative process such as lymphoma, when the medulla cannot be identified (Fig. 19.27).[32,33]

Adrenal calcification

Adrenal calcification is not uncommonly noted as an incidental finding on plain abdominal X-rays or on standard

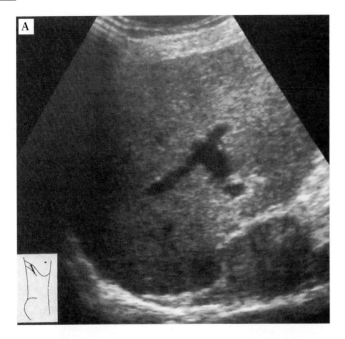

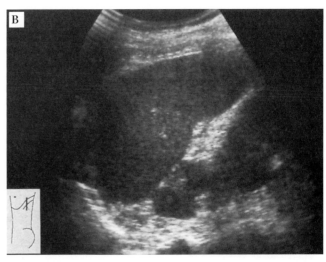

Fig. 19.26 Adrenal metastases. A: Coronal scan through the right and B: left adrenal glands. These sections are taken from a patient with a known bronchial carcinoma and the appearances are typical of metastases. No focal lesions were demonstrated in either liver or spleen.

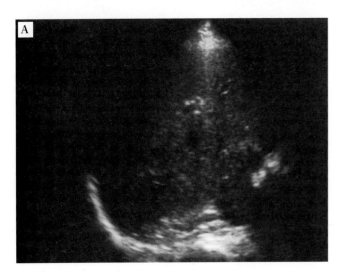

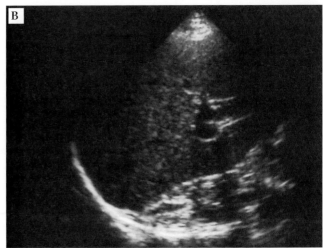

Fig. 19.27 Adrenal hyperplasia. A and B: Minor enlargement of the right adrenal gland affecting the echo-poor peripheral cortex resulting in exaggeration of the trilaminar appearance.

examination of the upper abdomen (Fig. 19.28). It is a recognised sequel of adrenal haemorrhage and, perhaps more commonly in the past, of adrenal tuberculous infection. A less commonly seen pattern of curvilinear calcification may be seen in the wall of an adrenal cyst.

REFERENCES

1 Sample W F. A new technique for the evaluation of the adrenal gland with grey scale ultrasonography. Radiology 1977; 124: 463–469

2 Yeh H C H. Sonography of the adrenal glands: normal glands and small masses. AJR 1980; 135: 1167–1177

3 Hattery R R, Sheedy P F 2nd, Stevens D H. Computed tomography of the adrenal glands. Semin Roentgenol 1981; 16: 290–300

4 El-Sherief M A, Hemmingson A. Computed tomography of the normal adrenal gland. Acta Radiol 1982; 23: 433–442

5 Wilms G, Baert A L, Marchal G. Computed tomography of the normal adrenal glands: correlative study with autopsy specimens. J Comput Assist Tomogr 1979; 3: 467–469

6 Abrams H L, Siegelman S S, Adams D F. Computed tomography versus ultrasound of the adrenal glands: a prospective study. Radiology 1982; 143: 121–128

7 Marchal G, Gelin J, Verbeken E, Baert A, Lauwerijns J. High resolution real time sonography of the adrenal glands: a routine examination? J Ultrasound Med 1986; 5: 65–68

8 Scott E M, Thomas A, McGarrigle H H, Lachelin G C. Serial adrenal ultrasonography in normal nenates. J Ultrasound Med [Am] 1990; 9: 279–283

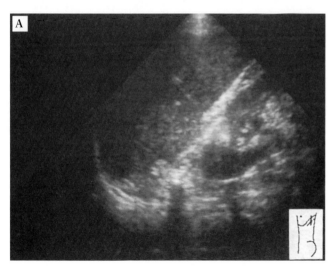

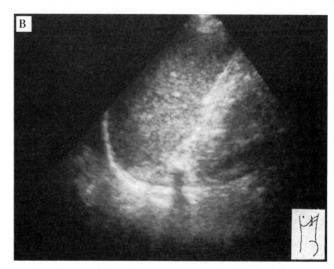

Fig. 19.28 Adrenal calcification. A and B: Coronal views of the left kidney showing a small area of calcification in the region of the left adrenal gland beyond which there is clear acoustic shadowing. A small amount of calcification was visible on the plain abdominal X-ray in this patient who was asymptomatic.

9 Oppenheimer D A, Carroll B A, Yousem S. Sonography of the normal neonatal adrenal glands. Radiology 1983; 146: 157–160

10 Mitty H A. Adrenal embryology, anatomy and imaging techniques. In: Pollack H M, ed. Clinical urography: an atlas and textbook of urologic imaging. Philadelphia: 1990; 2291–2305

11 White P C, New M I, Dupont B. Congenital adrenal hyperplasia. N Engl J Med 1987; 316: 1519–1524

12 Foster D G. Adrenal cysts: review of literature and report of case. Arch Surg 1986; 92: 131–143

13 Scheible W, Coel M, Siemers P T, Siegel H. Percutaneous aspiration of adrenal cysts. AJR 1977; 128: 1013–1016

14 Pery M, Kaftori J K, Bar-Maor J A. Sonography for diagnosis and follow up of adrenal haemorrhage. JCU 1981; 9: 397–401

15 Mittelstaedt C A, Volberg F M, Merten D F, Brill P W. The sonographic diagnosis of neonatal haemorrhage. Radiology 1979; 131: 453–457

16 Mineau D E, Koehler P R. Ultrasound diagnosis of neonatal adrenal haemorrhage. AJR 1979; 132: 443–444

17 Sample W F. Adrenal ultrasonography. Radiology 1978; 127: 461–466

18 Yeh H C. Ultrasonography of normal adrenal gland and small adrenal masses. AJR 135: 1980; 1167–1177

19 Yeh H C, Mitty H A, Rose J et al. Ultrasonography of adrenal masses: unusual manifestations. Radiology 1978; 127: 475–483

20 Robbins S L, Cotran R S. The endocrine system – adrenal cortex. In: Pathologic basis of disease. Philadelphia: Saunders, 1979: 1387

21 Behan M, Martin E C, Meucke E C, Kazam E. Myelolipoma of the adrenal: two cases with ultrasound and CT findings. AJR 1977; 129: 993–996

22 Vick C W, Zeman R K, Mannes E et al. Adrenal myelolipoma: CT and ultrasound findings. Urol Radiol 1984; 6: 7–13

23 Musante F, Derchi L E, Zappasodi F et al. Myelolipoma of the adrenal gland: sonographic and CT features. AJR 1988; 151: 961–964

24 Bowerman R A, Silver T M, Jaffee M H. Sonography of adrenal phaeochromocytoma. AJR 1981; 137: 1227–1237

25 Robbins S L, Cotran R S. The endocrine system – adrenal medulla. In: Pathologic basis of disease. Philadelphia: Saunders, 1979: 1402

26 White S J, Stuck K J, Blane C E, Silver T M. Sonography of neuroblastoma. AJR 1983; 141: 465–468

27 Cunningham J J. Ultrasonic findings in 'primary' lymphoma of the adrenal area. J Ultrasound Med 1983; 2: 467–469

28 Antoniou A, Spetseropoulos J, Vlahos L, Pontifex G. The sonographic appearance of adrenal involvement in non-Hodgkins lymphoma. J Ultrasound Med 1983; 2: 235–236

29 Forsythe J R, Gosink B B, Leopold G R. Ultrasound in the evaluation of adrenal metastases. JCU 1977; 5: 31–34

30 Dunnick N R, Korobkin M, Francis I. Adrenal radiology: distinguishing benign from malignant adrenal masses. AJR 1996; 167: 861–867

31 Ghiatas A A, Chopra S, Schnitker J B. Is sonographic flow imaging useful in the differential diagnosis of adrenal masses? Br J Radiol 1996; 69: 1005–1008

32 Paling M R, Williamson B R J. Adrenal involvement in non-Hodgkins lymphoma. AJR 1983; 141: 303–305

33 Yeh H C. Ultrasonography of the adrenals. Semin Roentgenol 1988; 23: 250–258

20

The lymph nodes

Keith C Dewbury

Introduction

The lymphatic system consists of a series of valved vessels with lymph nodes distributed along their course. Flow within the lymphatics is controlled by the valves; however, its direction can be changed by tumour or infection. There are thousands of lymph nodes within the body and they may enlarge in response to infection or when invaded by tumour, hence their great importance in disease assessment and staging. The marked improvement in resolution of ultrasound equipment in recent years has led to the demonstration of both normal and abnormal nodes both more easily and in exquisite detail, particularly in relatively accessible and superficial areas such as the neck and groin. Colour Doppler also allows assessment of blood flow to these lymph nodes.

Neck nodes

Normal appearances

The hundreds of normal lymph nodes in the neck are found in standard locations which include the submental region, the submandibular and parotid regions, the deep cervical chain anterior and medial to the internal jugular vein, the transverse cervical nodes over the upper clavicular margin and anterior cervical nodes around the midline structures of the neck. More posteriorly placed nodes are less frequently assessed by ultrasound.

Once searched for, normal neck nodes in any of the above locations will be readily demonstrated. Normal lymph nodes typically have a smooth margin, even mid-reflectivity with a reflective central hilus and are oval or elongated in shape. In the neck, normal lymph nodes usually are 7 mm or less in length (Fig. 20.1).

Malignant nodes

The size of the lymph node is an important indicator for abnormality but, while 7 mm is often taken as the upper limit, nodes of up to 3 cm are found in normal subjects, particularly children. Other factors must be taken into consideration including the number of nodes in a particular area, a cluster of several being more suspicious than an isolated node.[1]

The shape of the lymph node is a better indicator of malignancy than size. Malignant nodes are more rounded in shape; benign nodes are elongated. This has led to the use of the long:short access ratio with a ratio less than 2.0 being an indication of malignancy.[2,3] In the neck an exception to this rule is the submandibular and submental nodes which typically are normally rather rounder. Many normal lymph nodes demonstrate a central reflective hilus which has been shown to be due to the arrangement of lymphatics in the central area of the gland.[4] Demonstration depends on the orientation of the nodes to the transducer and it is not always a prominent feature in ultrasound of neck nodes. The reflectivity of normal nodes is homogeneous and of

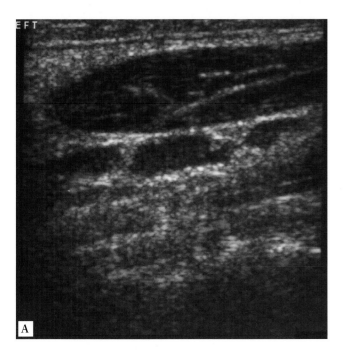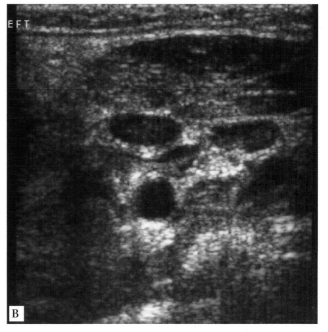

Fig. 20.1 Normal lymph nodes in the neck. A: Longitudinal scan and **B:** transverse scan showing a small node of 5–7 mm in diameter in the deep cervical chain.

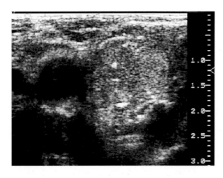
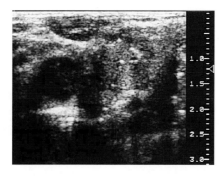
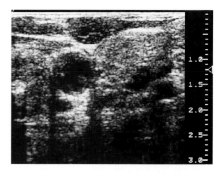

Fig. 20.2 Metastatic papillary carcinoma of the thyroid. Transverse scans at various levels on the left side of the neck above the thyroid gland showing enlarged, rounded lymph nodes lateral to the carotid artery. These nodes all contain small punctate foci of high reflectivity typical of the psammomatous calcification seen in papillary carcinoma of the thyroid.

mid-reflectivity. Lymphomatous infiltration of lymph nodes typically produces a reduction in reflectivity. This may be very marked and associated with increased through-transmission of sound.[5,6] In metastatic nodes the architecture is abnormal and heterogeneous and intranodal cystic necrosis may be seen.[7] Perhaps the most characteristic feature of a malignant lymph node in the neck is the presence of microcalcification in an enlarged and rounded node (Fig. 20.2).[7]

The improved sensitivity of colour Doppler is proving promising with regard to assessment of flow patterns in benign and malignant nodes. Benign (inflammatory) nodes show a central hilar or longitudinal vessel from which branching may be seen. Malignant nodes show displacement of vessels performing a focal absence of perfusion and peripheral vessels.[8]

The criteria for defining malignant nodes have become much more accurate in recent years. However, the great advantage of ultrasound is that if a doubtful or suspicious node is identified, guided fine needle aspiration can readily be performed to reach a definitive pathological diagnosis.

Groin and axilliary nodes

The general discussion in the preceding section applies in large part to the groin and axilliary nodes. The nodes in these regions tend to be slightly larger than in the neck. Since minor infections of the limbs is a common occurrence, inflammatory enlargement of these nodes may often be seen and may be chronic. Accumulation of fat at the hilus of the normal nodes in these regions is typical, producing a prominent reflective central hilus. This may sometimes be so prominent and large as to let the node 'merge in' with adjacent soft tissue fat and so not be easily recognised (Fig. 20.3).

In these regions the criteria for malignancy remain as discussed for lymph nodes in the neck. Enlargement, rounding and a heterogeneous reflectivity are typical metastatic features (Fig. 20.4).

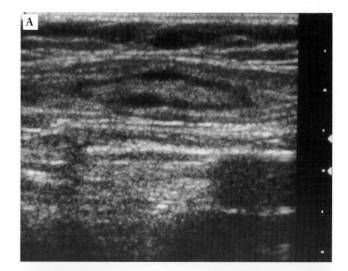
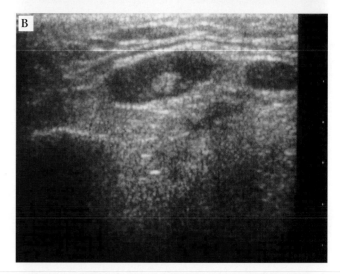

Fig. 20.3 Groin lymph nodes. A: A normal groin lymph node with a large reflective central hilus and a small peripheral poorly reflective margin. **B:** An inflammatory groin lymph node which is slightly enlarged but a central hilar area is still demonstrated.

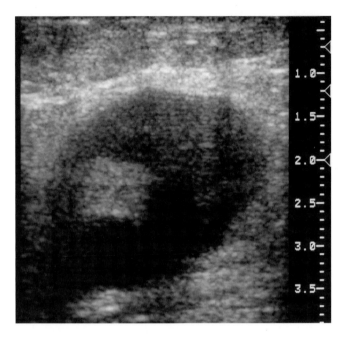

Fig. 20.4 Metastatic malignant melanoma. This groin node shows considerable enlargement and rounding. There is a heterogeneous pattern within it.

Abdominal nodes

Hepatoduodenal ligament nodes

Lymph nodes demonstrated in the hepatoduodenal ligament (HDL) were first described by Lyttkens *et al* in 1990.[9] Ninety patients with nodes demonstrated in the HDL were reviewed to define their association with disease and the majority were to be found in the benign group. In a more recent study in normal subjects, nodes in the HDL were documented in approximately 60% of subjects. Demonstration was more frequent in younger subjects, which has been attributed to the more homogeneous perinodal fat in the younger subjects and the larger size of these nodes.[10] Our own experience also suggests an increased node size and therefore visualisation in patients with inflammatory liver disease (Fig. 20.5).

Mesenteric lymph nodes

Massive central mesenteric nodal enlargement is a typical feature of many lymphomas and is detailed and illustrated in the next section. More recent studies have demonstrated mesenteric lymph nodes in a normal paediatric population.[11] The technique is of graded compression in the lower abdomen and pelvis, particularly on the right (see Vol. 2 Ch. 50). In the majority of children, mesenteric nodes were documented ranging in size from 10 to 20 mm (Fig. 20.6).

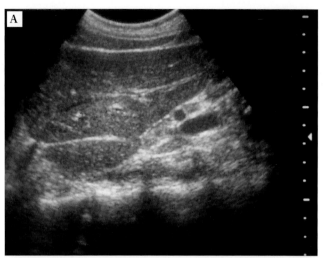

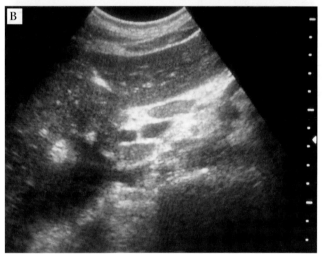

Fig. 20.5 Hepatoduodenal lymph nodes. A: Longitudinal scan. **B:** Transverse scan.

Para-aortic nodes

Lymphatic glands surround the major vessels such as the abdominal aorta and its branches, the inferior vena cava (IVC) and the splanchnic system. Para-aortic nodes may lie directly anterior to the spine while some of the splanchnic nodes lie in the gut mesentery and are difficult to image with ultrasound. The special drainage of the gonads should be borne in mind: as a consequence of their descent from the mid-abdomen, the first nodes from the testes lie at renal level. For the ovaries the arrangement is the same except that they also drain to the uterus along the uterine tubes.

Since normal para-aortic lymph nodes are rarely identified on ultrasound, to search for lymphadenopathy it is necessary to identify the associated vessels and trace their abdominal course looking for paravascular masses (Fig. 20.7).[12] Enlarged nodes may be found at the porta

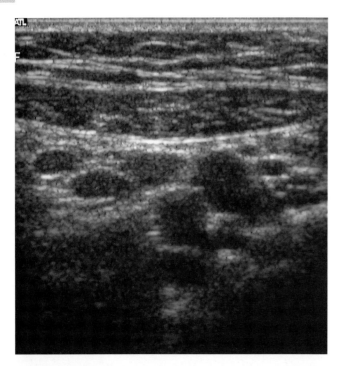

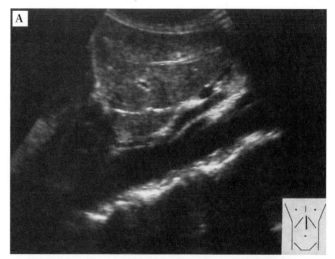

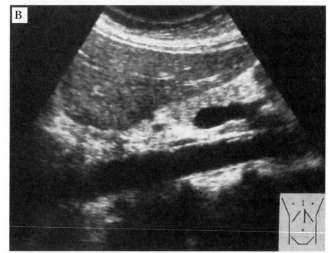

Fig. 20.6 Mesenteric lymph nodes in the right iliac fossa of a child. Graded compression scanning in the right iliac fossa of this child shows small lymph nodes of 6–10 mm in the right iliac fossa. These nodes may enlarge in mesenteric adenitis.

Fig. 20.7 Normal great vessels. A: Longitudinal scan showing the upper aorta and the origins of the coeliac axis, superior and inferior mesenteric arteries. Note the anomalous hepatic artery. **B:** Longitudinal scan of the abdominal aorta. **C:** Longitudinal scan through the IVC. Note the normal common bile duct and the prominent right diaphragmatic crus lying behind the IVC. With clear crural visualisation, retrocrural nodes may be easily detected. **D:** A coronal section taken from the right side showing a portion of the IVC proximal to the aorta. Note the origin of the renal arteries (arrows).

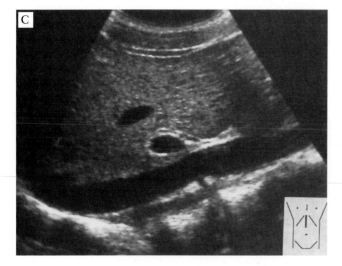

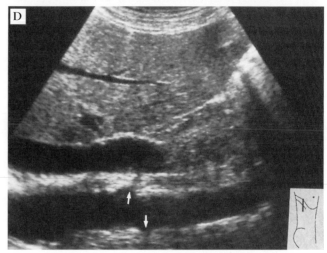

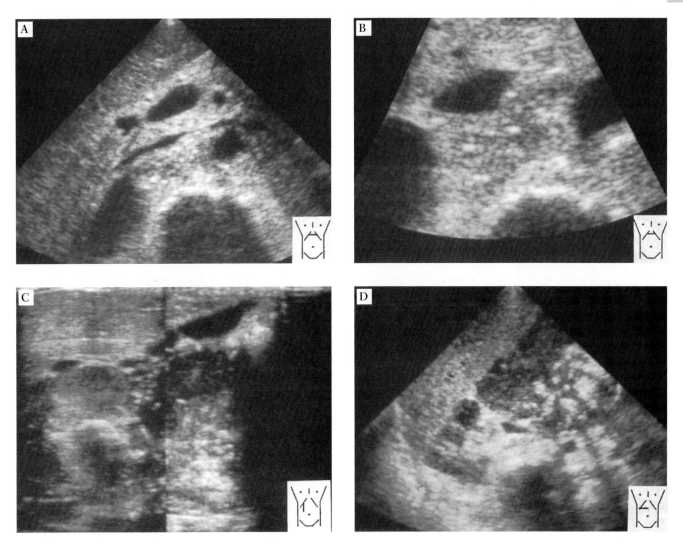

Fig. 20.8 Calcific nodes. A: Reflective masses surround the aorta and IVC; these were calcific nodes in a patient with carcinoma of the prostate following successful endocrine therapy. **B:** Magnification of A. **C** and **D:** Calcific mass in neuroblastoma (longitudinal and transverse sections); these are either retroperitoneal nodes or infiltration from the primary tumour – the distinction is impossible and not clinically important.

hepatis, renal hila, splenic hilum and in the mesentery as well as around the coeliac axis and along the pancreas.

Enlarged nodes typically have low and uniform reflectivity on ultrasound; indeed they may be almost anechoic, especially when very large. This is presumed to be because of their relatively homogeneous structure so that there are few interfaces to produce echoes. When there is calcification or, rarely, lipid deposition (e.g. Whipple's disease[13]) they may have the same reflectivity as fat or even be more strongly reflective (Fig. 20.8). Abnormal nodes as small as 1.5 cm may be visualised with ultrasound, particularly if they distort the normal anatomy, for example, in the retrocrural or retrocaval spaces (Fig. 20.9). Apart from the intense echoes due to calcification and lipids, there is no correlation between the ultrasound appearances of the lymph nodes and the histology, unlike in neck nodes.

Lymphadenopathy in lymphoma, metastatic disease or in inflammatory reactions such as retroperitoneal fibrosis, are all difficult to distinguish from each other. The most florid nodal involvement is characteristically seen in non-Hodgkin's lymphoma (Fig. 20.10).[14]

Lymphomatous involvement of para-aortic nodes occurs in approximately 25% of patients with Hodgkin's disease and in 40% with non-Hodgkin's lymphoma.[15] Effective therapeutic management in these patients requires accurate histological classification and reliable definition of the anatomical regions involved in the disease process.[15–17] Classically lymphangiography was used, but CT scanning and MRI have now become the gold standard for the abdomen and pelvis. Ultrasound, however, has been shown to detect retroperitoneal nodal lymphoma with an 80–90% accuracy.[18] It is also capable of demonstrating

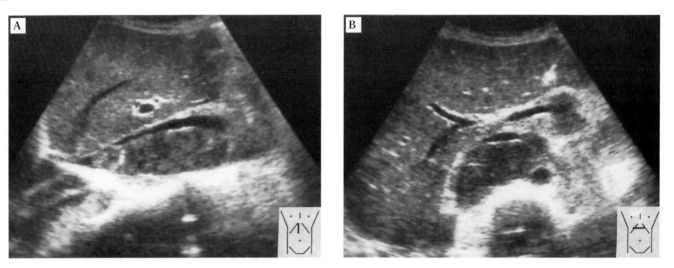

Fig. 20.9 **Enlarged retrocaval nodes. A:** A longitudinal scan showing a retrocrural and retrocaval nodal mass. There is anterior bowing of the IVC. **B:** A transverse scan showing the same nodal mass. There is some extension anteriorly across the front of the aorta.

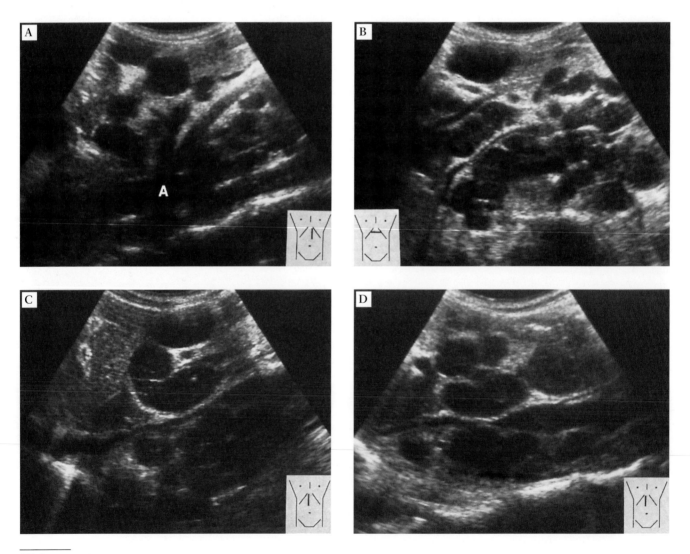

lymphadenopathy in the coeliac, perisplenic, mesenteric and perihepatic areas with an accuracy similar to that of CT, although the reliability is not as good due to intervening gas. The ease and cost effectiveness of ultrasound suggest a continuing role in the assessment of nodal disease and its follow-up in selected cases.

A variety of patterns of nodal enlargement may be seen in the retroperitoneum:

1 discrete enlargement of individually identifiable nodes occurs when a small number of individual nodes is enlarged, retaining the overall morphology (Fig. 20.11),
2 a homogeneous confluent mass extending anteriorly from the prevertebral space, enveloping and often elevating the great vessels (Fig. 20.12). The normal outline of the aorta may be lost; this is sometimes misleadingly called the 'silhouette sign' (Fig. 20.13),

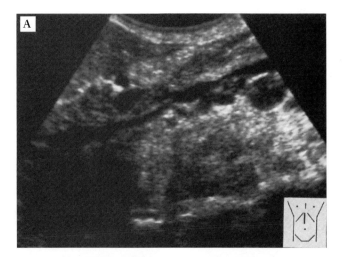

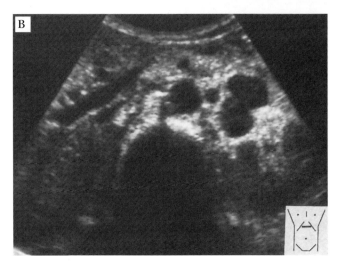

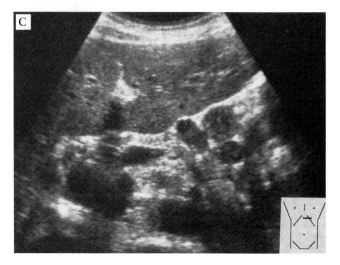

Fig. 20.11 Discrete nodal enlargement. A: Longitudinal and **B** and **C:** transverse scans. These sections all show discrete nodal enlargement of a relatively small number of individual nodes that can be separately identified. The pattern in each case is similar with a uniform low reflectivity.

Fig. 20.10 Non-Hodgkin's lymphoma. A: A longitudinal section through the abdominal aorta. Note the origins of the coeliac axis and superior mesenteric artery which is elevated by enlarged nodes posterior to it. There is a sheet of nodes lying behind the aorta (A) and large nodal masses are seen above the coeliac axis. **B:** A transverse section taken at about the level of the coeliac axis showing lobular nodal enlargement extending around the para-aortic area and laterally towards the flanks. There is anterior extension up towards the liver. **C:** A longitudinal scan through the IVC showing nodes in the region of the porta hepatis. There is also a large mass of nodes behind the IVC causing elevation and compression. **D:** A similar longitudinal section showing greater detail of the retrocaval nodal mass.

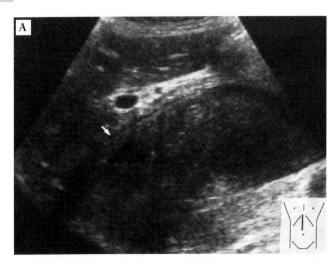

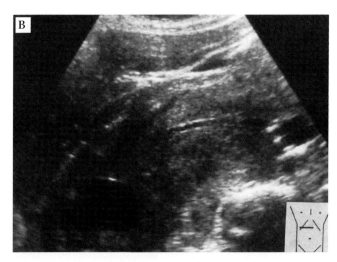

Fig. 20.12 Confluent nodal mass. A: Longitudinal and **B:** transverse scans showing a huge amorphous nodal mass extending from the right kidney to cross the midline and elevate and envelop the IVC (arrow). No single discrete node can be identified, in contrast to Figure 20.11.

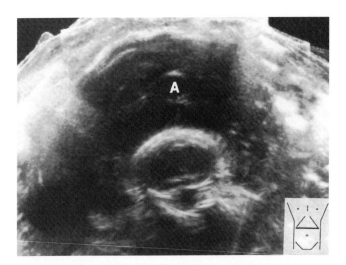

Fig. 20.13 Lost aortic outline. A compounded transverse section through the mid-abdomen showing partial loss of the outline of the normal aorta (A) and IVC which are elevated and enveloped by a lobular echo-poor nodal mass. This is misleadingly known as the 'silhouette sign'.

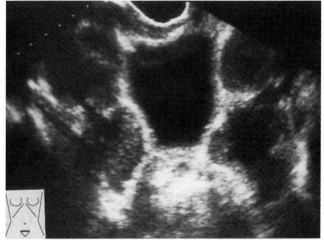

Fig. 20.14 Pelvic lymphadenopathy. A transverse scan through the pelvis showing the filled bladder which is elevated and distorted by large echo-poor lobular nodal enlargement on the pelvic side walls.

3 compression or displacement of adjacent organs by a nodal mass. Extensive pelvic nodal enlargement characteristically distorts and elevates the bladder (Fig. 20.14) or other contiguous structures, especially those that are less well supported, such as the ureters and veins (both portal and systemic),

4 very rarely, vascular invasion from malignant lymphadenopathy may occur (Fig. 20.15).

Associated nodal enlargement at other sites in the abdomen is commonly seen in lymphoma. Mesenteric lymphomatous involvement characteristically produces a lobulated, confluent, anechoic mass surrounding a central, more reflective region. This appearance is the result of the nodal mass infiltrating the mesenteric layers and encasing the mesenteric vessels to produce the so-called 'sandwich sign' (Fig. 20.16).[19] Mesenteric nodal involvement is rare in Hodgkin's disease but occurs commonly in non-Hodgkin's lymphoma (Fig. 20.17). Generally, mesenteric lymphadenopathy is associated with retroperitoneal or para-aortic adenopathy which should be evaluated systematically.

Peripancreatic, perihepatic and coeliac axis nodes, as well as nodes at the splenic and renal hilum, manifest a spectrum of appearances similar to retroperitoneal lymphadenopathy. Portal nodes may cause biliary obstruction

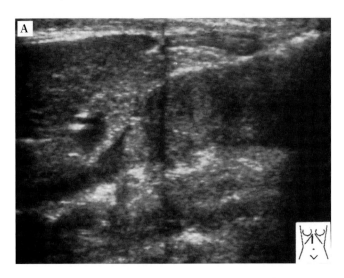
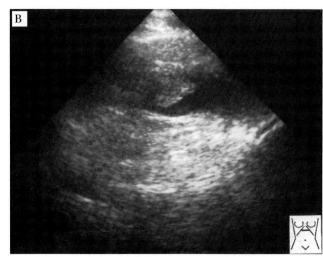

Fig. 20.15 **Nodal invasion of the IVC. A:** Longitudinal and **B:** transverse sections. Solid tissue in the upper cava is due to tumour extension from retroperitoneal lymphadenopathy in this patient with carcinoma of the ovary. This is an uncommon occurrence.

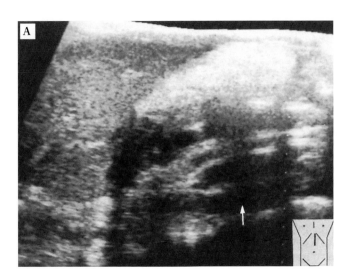
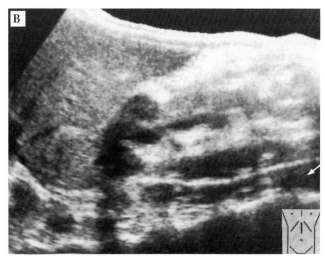

Fig. 20.16 **Mesenteric lymphadenopathy. A** and **B:** Longitudinal scans showing confluent echo-poor nodal masses extending into the mesentery. Both the mesenteric artery and vein can be identified producing a relatively reflective central core which is sometimes described as the 'sandwich sign'. Prespinal nodes (arrow) are also identified.

and are characteristic of hepatic lymphomatous involvement (Fig. 20.18). Nodes that are demonstrated by ultrasound may be accessible to percutaneous biopsy. The enlarged node in the porta (the 'cholecystitis node') is typically observed in patients with viral hepatitis; though not clinically significant, its demonstration is helpful in differential diagnosis.

Differential diagnosis

Generally the appearances of lymphadenopathy are distinctive, an isolated echo-poor nodule or the multi-lobulated appearance of multiple enlarged nodes being diagnostic. However, occasionally masses in the same spaces produce confusing appearances. For example, small neurofibromata may be identical (Fig. 20.19). Retroperitoneal fibrosis also produces an echo-poor mass related to the aorta; the differentiation from nodal enlargement may be impossible but the lack of lobulation and the typical thickening of retroperitoneal fibrosis below the sacral promontory are suggestive (Figs 20.20 and 20.21). An abdominal aortic aneurysm may also be confusing, the echo-poor thrombus easily being mistaken for para-aortic lymphadenopathy. The internal echo

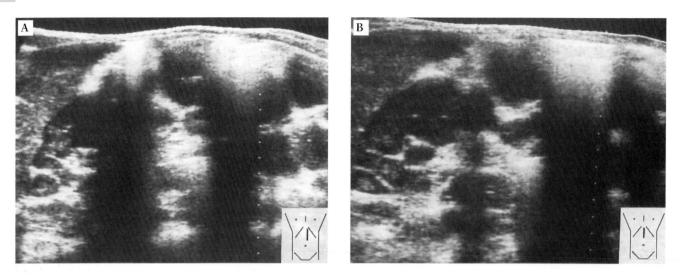

Fig. 20.17 Mesenteric lymphadenopathy. A and **B:** Longitudinal scans showing large discrete nodal enlargement involving the mesentery in a patient with non-Hodgkin's lymphoma.

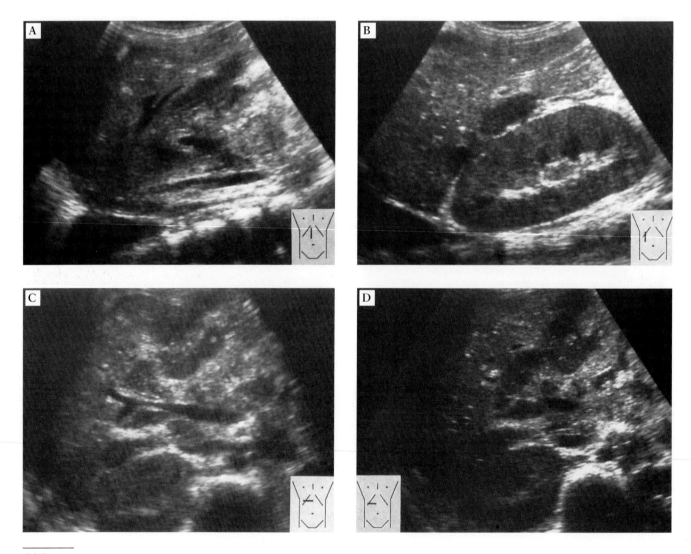

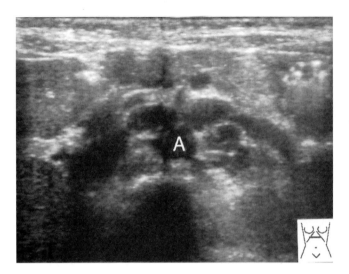

Fig. 20.19 Neurofibroma. Echo-poor retroperitoneal masses with a pattern indistinguishable from lymphadenopathy were seen in this patient with Von Recklinghausen's disease. A – aorta.

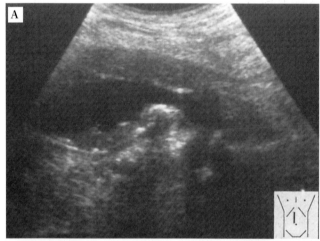

Fig. 20.20 Retroperitoneal fibrosis. A: Longitudinal and **B:** transverse scans. An echo-poor mass surrounding the lower abdominal aorta is typical of retroperitoneal fibrosis (the aorta was atheromatous). **C:** Associated hydronephrosis is shown.

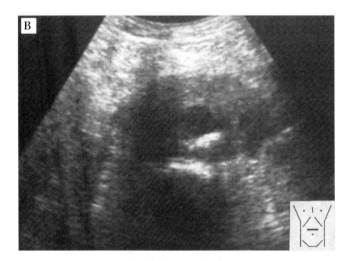

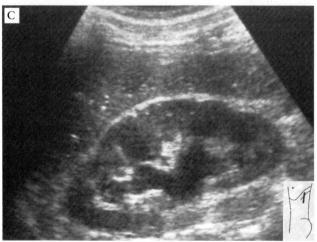

Fig. 20.18 Widespread lymphoma. A: A longitudinal scan through the IVC. **B:** A longitudinal scan through the right kidney. **C:** A transverse scan through the right branch of the portal vein. **D:** A similar, slightly lower transverse section. Widespread abnormalities are demonstrated on these scans with diffuse lymphomatous involvement of the kidney, deposits in the liver and more discrete nodal enlargement particularly around the porta hepatis and in the para-aortic region. A right pleural effusion is also demonstrated in images A and B.

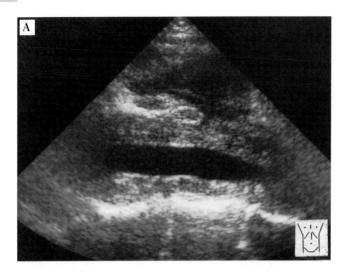
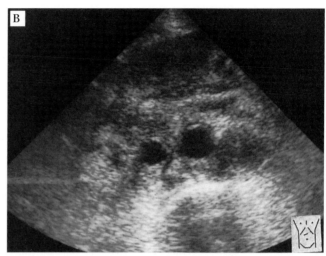

Fig. 20.21 Peri-aortic lymphadenopathy. A: Longitudinal and **B:** transverse sections showing a cuff of tissue surrounding both great vessels. Biopsy showed lymphoma. Note the unusual lack of compression of the vessels. Compare this appearance with that shown in Figure 20.20.

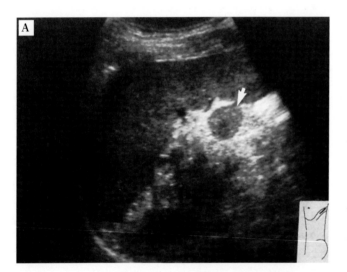
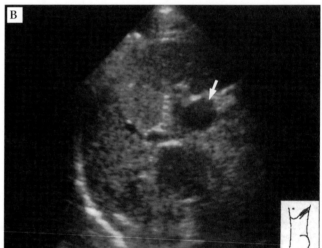

Fig. 20.22 Splenunculus. A: A rounded mass (arrow) near the hilum with an echo pattern identical to the spleen is typical of a splenunculus. **B:** An echo-poor mass (arrow) in a similar position, but due to lymphadenopathy.

texture of the solid region may be distinctive if the whorled pattern of the thrombus in an aneurysm can be demonstrated, but otherwise the pattern in a transverse section showing the conformity of the 'mass' to the circular shape of the aorta by comparison with the lateral extension of lymphadenopathy can be helpful.

Masses in organs adjacent to the expected position of nodes can also be very confusing. An example is the way an adrenal mass, especially on the right, simulates high retrocaval lymphadenopathy. The differential diagnosis may be impossible unless the adrenal gland itself can be demonstrated. Similarly, lymphadenopathy in or close to the pancreas can be difficult to distinguish from a pancre-

atic mass. The uniform echo-poor texture of enlarged nodes can be helpful, while demonstration of multiple masses is very suggestive of lymphadenopathy since multicentric pancreatic masses are rare. A splenunculus (accessory spleen) can be very confusing; usually these are solitary and have exactly the same reflectivity and texture as the spleen itself but lymphadenopathy is difficult to exclude (Fig. 20.22).

Nodes often compress adjacent ducts such as the bile and pancreatic ducts and the ureter. Where anatomically appropriate, features of these should be searched for both because of their diagnostic importance and because they may be important in management.

REFERENCES

1 Van den Brekel M, Castlijns J A, Stel H V et al. Occult metastatic neck disease: detection with US and US guided fine needle aspiration cytology. Radiology 1991; 180: 457–461

2 Solbiati L. Rizatto G, Belloti E et al. High-resolution sonography of cervical lymph nodes in head and neck cancers: criteria for differentiation of reactive versus malignant nodes. Radiology 1988; 169 (P): 113 (abstr)

3 Van den Brekel M, Castelijns J A, Stel H et al. Cervical lymph node metastasis: assessment of radiologic criteria. Radiology 1990; 177: 379–384

4 Rubaltelli L, Proto E, Salmaso R, Bortoletto P, Candiani F, Pierpaolo C. Sonography of abnormal lymph nodes in vitro: correlation of sonographic and histological findings. AJR 1990; 155: 1247–1244

5 Bruneton J N, Norman F. Cervical lymph nodes. In: Bruneton J N, ed. Ultrasonography of the neck. Berlin: Springer Verlag, 1987: 81–92

6 Ahuja A, Ying M, Yang W T, Evans R M, King W, Metreweli C. The use of sonography in differentiating cervical lymphomatous lymph nodes from cervical metastatic lymph nodes. Clin Radiol 1996; 51: 186–190

7 Ahuja A, Chow L, Mok C O, King W, Metreweli C. Metastatic cervical lymph nodes in papillary carcinoma of the thyroid; ultrasound and histological correlation. Clin Radiol 1995; 50: 391–395

8 Tschammler A, Ott G, Schant T, Seelbach-Goebel B, Schwager K, Hahn D. Lymphadenopathy: differentiation of benign from malignant disease – colour Doppler US assessment of intranodal angioarchitecture. Radiology 1998; 208: 117–123

9 Lyttkens K, Forsberg L, Hederstrom E. Ultrasound examination of lymph nodes in the hepatoduodenal ligament. J Radiol 1990; 63(745): 26–30

10 Metreweli C, Ward S C. Ultrasound demonstration of lymph nodes in the hepatoduodenal ligament ('daisy chain nodes') in normal subjects. Clin Radiol 1995; 50(2): 99–101

11 Healy M V, Graham P M. Assessment of abdominal lymph nodes in a normal paediatric population: an ultrasound study. Australas Radiol 1993; 37(2): 171–172

12 Ritchie W G N. The sonographic demonstration of abdominal visceral lymph node enlargement. AJR 1982; 138: 517–521

13 Davis S J, Patel A. Distinctive echogenic lymphadenopathy in Whipple's disease. Clin Radiol 1990; 42: 60–62

14 Kaude J V, Joyce P H. Evaluation of abdominal lymphoma by ultrasound. Gastrointest Radiol 1980; 5: 249–254

15 Carroll B A. Ultrasound in lymphoma. In: Raymond H W, Zwiebel W J, eds. Seminars in ultrasound, vol. 3. New York: Grune & Stratton, 1982: 114

16 Carroll B A, Ta H N. The ultrasound appearance of extranodal abdominal lymphoma. Radiology 1980; 136: 419–425

17 Carroll B A. Lymphoma. In: Goldberg B B, ed. Clinics in diagnostic ultrasound: ultrasound in cancer. New York: Churchill Livingstone, 1981: 52

18 Beyer D, Peter P E. Real time ultrasonography: an efficient screening method for abdominal and pelvic lymphadenopathy. Lymphology 1980; 13: 142–149

19 Mueller P R, Ferrucci J T Jr, Harbin W P et al. Appearances of lymphomatous involvement of the mesentery by ultrasonography and body computed tomography: the 'sandwich sign'. Radiology 1980; 134: 467–473

Index